Advances in the Medicinal Chemistry of Neglected Tropical Disease and Related Infectious Diseases

Edited by

Igor Jose dos Santos Nascimento
Programa de Pós-Graduação em Ciências Farmacêuticas
Departamento de Farmácia
Universidade Estadual da Paraíba
Campina Grande-PB, Brasil

&

Ricardo Olimpio de Moura
Programa de Pós-Graduação em Ciências Farmacêuticas
Departamento de Farmácia
Universidade Estadual da Paraíba
Campina Grande-PB, Brasil

Advances in the Medicinal Chemistry of Neglected Tropical Disease and Related Infectious Diseases

Editors: Igor Jose dos Santos Nascimento and Ricardo Olimpio de Moura

ISBN (Online): 978-981-5324-78-5

ISBN (Print): 978-981-5324-79-2

ISBN (Paperback): 978-981-5324-80-8

need for a court order if at any point you breach any terms of this License Agreement. In no event will any delay or failure by Bentham Science Publishers in enforcing your compliance with this License Agreement constitute a waiver of any of its rights.

3. You acknowledge that you have read this License Agreement, and agree to be bound by its terms and conditions. To the extent that any other terms and conditions presented on any website of Bentham Science Publishers conflict with, or are inconsistent with, the terms and conditions set out in this License Agreement, you acknowledge that the terms and conditions set out in this License Agreement shall prevail.

Bentham Science Publishers Pte. Ltd.
No. 9 Raffles Place
Office No. 26-01
Singapore 048619
Singapore
Email: subscriptions@benthamscience.net

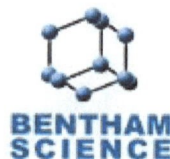

**BENTHAM
SCIENCE**

CONTENTS

Karla Joane da Silva Menezes, Arthur Gabriel Corrêa de Farias, Marianny de Souza, Éric de Oliveira Rios, Igor José dos Santos Nascimento and *Ricardo* **Olimpio de Moura**

Salma Darwish, Mohamed Teleb, Sherry N. Nasralla, Sherine N. Khattab and *Adnan A. Bekhit*

FOREWORD

Infectious diseases caused by neglected tropical pathogens continue to present significant global health challenges, especially in regions with limited economic and healthcare resources. The chemical structures of therapeutic agents targeting these diseases often rely heavily on heteroatom-rich scaffolds, notably structures that contain nitrogen, which provide a foundation for improved pharmacokinetic and pharmacodynamic properties.

This volume presents a comprehensive account of the critical advancements in medicinal chemistry aimed at addressing Neglected Tropical Diseases (NTDs) and related infections, emphasizing the significance of innovative strategies in drug design, scaffold-hopping methodologies, and target-based approaches utilizing both natural and synthetic compounds. Particular emphasis is placed on the incorporation of heteroatoms to improve solubility, lipophilicity, and hydrogen bonding capacity, as well as to optimize the ADME/Tox profiles of prospective drug candidates. Moreover, the distinctive biological functions of several chemical scaffolds offer molecular mimicry of natural metabolites, thereby facilitating the identification of agents with broad-spectrum bioactivity and enhanced therapeutic indices.

In addition to reviewing the core structures and biological targets, this work explores diverse synthetic methodologies employed to expand the drug-like chemical space. It highlights the significance of Structure-Activity Relationship (SAR) studies in optimizing lead compounds for efficacy and selectivity. Through the integration of classical medicinal chemistry with emerging approaches, including computational modeling and high-throughput screening, new avenues are being unveiled for addressing diseases that have historically been neglected due to limited commercial interest.

KEY FEATURES

1. Comprehensive insights into innovative compounds for NTDs and related infectious diseases.

2. Integration of natural products, synthetic compounds, and drug repurposing approaches.

3. Insights into target-based drug design and mechanistic pathways.

4. Application of advanced computational, experimental, and screening techniques.

5. Multidisciplinary strategies to address drug resistance and improve therapeutic outcomes.

It is our firm belief that this volume will stand as a valuable reference and an enduring source of inspiration for medicinal chemists, pharmacologists, and global health researchers committed to overcoming the burden of neglected diseases through advances in molecular innovation.

Fátima Nogueira
Instituto de Higiene e Medicina Tropical (IHMT)
Universidade NOVA de Lisboa
Lisbon, Portugal

PREFACE

Neglected tropical diseases are a conjunct of infectious diseases that affect several countries around the world, mainly those with tropical and subtropical conditions, affecting the population living in poverty and without basic sanitation, causing severe damage to the health of the population and economy of the countries. They are considered "*neglected*" due to the low investment of pharmaceutical companies in P&D for new drugs against these diseases. Thus, despite alarming statistics, there are few drugs to treat these conditions, with scientific research institutions being the main ones for developing new agents against these conditions [1 - 4].

In view of this, the book "*Advances in the Medicinal Chemistry of Neglected Tropical Disease and Related Infectious Diseases*" appears, highlighting the main developments in recent years against this disease, mainly in innovative compounds and molecular targets that can be explored in subsequent drug design studies.

This first edition is organized into ten chapters, namely:

Chapter 1 "*Medicinal Chemistry of Neglected Tropical Diseases (NTDs): From Targets to Drugs,*" briefly introduces these diseases and some actual drug targets explored in the drug design process. The authors provide great material focusing on epidemiological, clinical manifestations, and current treatments. In addition, the structure, functions, and the most promising inhibitors of the *N*-myristoyltransferase, nitroreductases, topoisomerases, pyrimidine synthesis pathway, and mitochondrial alterations are shown and provide its importance in the drug design and development process. Finally, this chapter can guide research worldwide to discover a promising drug against several NTDs.

Chapter 2 "*Advancements in Antileishmanial Drug Discovery: Targeting Druggable Pathways and Overcoming Treatment Challenges*" explores the latest developments in synthetic, semi-synthetic, and natural compounds identified in *in silico*, *in vitro*, and *in vivo* assays against leishmaniasis and a brief introduction about some new targets used in the design process. In addition, the authors provide information about the primary chemical scaffolds explored against leishmaniasis, such as flavonoids and chalcones, naphthoquinones and iridoids, saponins, quinolines, lignans, terpenes and terpenoids, and others synthetic nucleus. Finally, the drug target of each scaffold is proposed, and this information can be used in the drug design of further compounds.

Chapter 3 "*Chagas Diseases: State Of the Art and New Perspectives*," provides new information about Chagas diseases, including the physiopathology and the drugs used in the clinical treatment. In addition, the authors provide new insights into the drug design and discovery process, highlighting the main explored drug targets, the chemical scaffolds used, and novel promising drugs in clinical practice.

Chapter 4 "*Novel Agents against Human African Trypanosomiasis: Updates on Medicinal Chemistry and Target Identification,*" highlights the clinical manifestations and current treatments against *Trypanosoma brucei*, an etiological agent of the sleeping sickness, or human African trypanosomiasis. Furthermore, the most prominent drug targets are shown, such as protein tyrosine kinases (PTKs), mitogen-activated protein kinases (MAPKs), heat shock proteins (HSPs), kinetoplastid proteasome, Tb Cathepsin L (TbCatL), Tb UDP-Glucose 4'-Epimerase (TbGalE), and others that provide new insights in drug design to researchers worldwide.

Chapter 5 "*Schistosomiasis: State Of the Art and New Perspectives*" similar to the previous chapters, provides information about the life cycle of the schistosome and other parameters such as clinical manifestations and the current drug treatment. In addition, some repurposed drugs are explored as having promising potential against this disease, and the main research focuses on new drug targets, highlighting HDAC and Sirtuin inhibitors, histone methylation, protein kinases, protease, CYP450, transporters inhibitors, and others that can be a promising intervention in the drug design of antischistosomal drugs.

Chapter 6 "*Progress In Medicinal Chemistry For Neglected Tropical Diseases: A Focus On DENV Drug Discovery (2014 - 2023),*" explores the potential of classical drug targets of dengue virus and highlights the main features to design anti-dengue drugs. Similar to the chapters above, the functions of some non-structural targets, such as protease, RdRp, methyltransferase, and structural targets, such as E protein and others, were characterized. Thus, this chapter provides critical information for designing innovative anti-dengue compounds.

Chapter 7, "*Malaria: State Of the Art and New Perspectives*," discusses the actual drug treatment and its difficulties due to the parasite's resistance and the urgency to discover new drugs to overcome this. For this, it is necessary to explore new targets, as shown in the manuscript, such as channels/transporters, aquaporin channel, Plasmodial surface anion channel, hexose transporter, choline transporter, apicoplast, cyclin-dependent protein kinases (CDKs), nucleic acid metabolism, mitochondrial system, redox system, shikimate pathway, isoprenoid biosynthesis, parasite proteases, membrane biosynthesis, and pfTBP–pfTFIIB interface. Finally, the authors highlight the main chemical scaffolds explored that can provide an innovative drug against this disease.

Chapter 8 "*On The Trail of Zika Virus: Understanding its Druggable Targets,*" explores the structural and non-structural proteins used in the drug design against the Zika virus. Thus, the authors provide critical information about the structure, functions, and main inhibitors of the NS1, NS2A, NS2B, NS3, NS2B/NS3, NS4B, NS5, envelop (E) protein, prM, capsid (C) protein, and some alternatives pathways that can be promising to discover an innovative anti-Zika drug.

Chapter 9 "*Mycobacterium tuberculosis: Recent Advances in Drug Discovery and Targets – A SAR-Based Approach,*" explores the epidemiology and insights into drug design and development against tuberculosis. Thus, the authors highlight the importance of identifying new targets to provide an innovative drug and overcome the parasite's resistance to the actual clinical drugs of this disease. For this, targets such as DNA gyrase, shikimate pathway, adenosine kinases, and others are shown, highlighting their structure and functions. In addition, the authors provide exceptional work on the structure-activity relationship (SAR) to provide critical information on the structural features of the most actual discovered inhibitors.

Chapter 10 "*Drug discovery in Fasciola hepatica: Few Steps in the Last Ten Years,*" highlights the urgency to discover new flukicide drugs and explores the drug design and discovery against Fasciola hepatica. For this, the authors provide excellent material about the explored drug targets, such as cathepsin Ls, triosephosphate isomerase, thioredoxin glutathione reductase, and other biological structures of the fasciola that do not have an experimental inhibitor, as well as the inhibitors identified in phenotypic drug screenings, and the function of the drug repurposing to discover drugs against fasciola. This chapter can provide new horizons for the readers and critical information to use in drug design against these diseases.

We hope our book will serve as a guide for researchers worldwide and help discover drugs against these diseases, ending these threatening agents.

Igor Jose dos Santos Nascimento
Programa de Pós-Graduação em Ciências Farmacêuticas
Departamento de Farmácia
Universidade Estadual da Paraíba
Campina Grande-PB, Brasil

&

Ricardo Olimpio de Moura
Programa de Pós-Graduação em Ciências Farmacêuticas
Departamento de Farmácia, Universidade Estadual da Paraíba
Campina Grande-PB, Brasil

REFERENCES

[1]   Nascimento IJ, dos S, Cavalcanti M, de AT, de Moura RO. Exploring nmyristoyltransferase as a promising drug target against parasitic neglected tropical diseases. Eur J Med Chem 2023; 258: 115550.

[2]   De Souza M, Medeiros DC, de Moura RO, dos Santos Nascimento IJ. Pharmacokinetic limitations to overcome and enable K777 as a potential drug against chagas disease. Curr Pharm Des 2023; 29: 2359-60.

[3]   Dos Santos Nascimento IJ, de Moura RO. Targeting cysteine and serine proteases to discover new drugs against neglected tropical diseases. Curr Med Chem 2024; 31: 2133-4.

[4]   Dos Santos Nascimento IJ, de Aquino TM, da Silva-Júnior EF. Cruzain and rhodesain inhibitors: Last decade of advances in seeking for new compounds against american and african trypanosomiases. Curr Top Med Chem 2021; 21: 1871-99.

List of Contributors

Arthur Gabriel Corrêa de Farias
Drug Development and Synthesis Laboratory, Department of Pharmacy, State University of Paraíba, Campina Grande 58429-500, Brazil

Adnan A. Bekhit
Department of Pharmaceutical Chemistry, Faculty of Pharmacy, Alexandria University, Alexandria 21521, Egypt
Pharmacy Program, Allied Health Department, College of Health and Sport Sciences, University of Bahrain, Sakhir 32038, Kingdom of Bahrain

Akankcha Gupta
Integrated Drug Discovery Research Laboratory, Department of Pharmaceutical Sciences, Dr. Harisingh Gour University (A Central University), Sagar (MP), India

Aviral Kaushik
Department of Life Sciences, Parul Institute of Applied Sciences and Biophysics & Structural Biology Laboratory, Research & Development Cell, Parul University, Vadodara, Gujarat, India

Claudiu T. Supuran
Neurofarba Department, Pharmaceutical and Nutraceutical Section, University of Florence, Firenze FI, Sesto Fiorentino, Italy

C. Ratna Prabha
Department of Biochemistry, Maharaja Sayajirao University of Baroda, Vadodara, Gujarat, India

Dickson Mambwe
Department of Chemistry, School of Natural Sciences, University of Zambia, Lusaka, Zambia

Evelyn Funjika
Department of Chemistry, School of Natural Sciences, University of Zambia, Lusaka, Zambia

Éric de Oliveira Rios
Pharmacy Departament, Cesmac University Center, Maceió, Brazil

Edeildo Ferreira da Silva-Júnior
Research Group on Biological and Molecular Chemistry, Institute of Chemistry and Biotechnology, Federal University of Alagoas, Lourival Melo Mota Avenue, 57072-970, Maceió, Brazil

Fabrizio Carta
Neurofarba Department, Pharmaceutical and Nutraceutical Section, University of Florence, Firenze FI, Sesto Fiorentino, Italy

Gioele Renzi
Neurofarba Department, Pharmaceutical and Nutraceutical Section, University of Florence, Firenze FI, Sesto Fiorentino, Italy

Godfrey Mayoka
Department of Pharmacology and Pharmacognosy, School of Pharmacy, Jomo Kenyatta University of Agriculture and Technology, Nairobi, Kenya

Gourav Rakshit
Department of Pharmaceutical Sciences & Technology, Birla Institute of Technology, Mesra, Ranchi, JH, India

Igor José dos Santos Nascimento
Pharmacy Department, State University of Paraíba, Campina Grande, Brazil
Drug Development and Synthesis Laboratory, Department of Pharmacy, State University of Paraíba, Campina Grande 58429-500, Brazil
Pharmacy Departament, Cesmac University Center, Maceió, Brazil

Ileana Corvo
Laboratorio de I+D de Moléculas Bioactivas, Departamento de Ciencias Biológicas, Centro Universitario Regional Litoral Norte, Universidad de la República, Paysandú, Uruguay

Karla Joane da Silva Menezes	Pharmacy Department, State University of Paraíba, Campina Grande, Brazil Drug Development and Synthesis Laboratory, Department of Pharmacy, State University of Paraíba, Campina Grande 58429-500, Brazil
Krupanshi Bharadava	Department of Life Sciences, Parul Institute of Applied Sciences and Biophysics & Structural Biology Laboratory, Research & Development Cell, Parul University, Vadodara, Gujarat, India
Leandro Rocha Silva	Research Group on Biological and Molecular Chemistry, Institute of Chemistry and Biotechnology, Federal University of Alagoas, Lourival Melo Mota Avenue, 57072-970, Maceió, Brazil
Marianny de Souza	Pharmacy Department, Cesmac University Center, Maceió, Brazil
Mohamed Teleb	Department of Pharmaceutical Chemistry, Faculty of Pharmacy, Alexandria University, Alexandria 21521, Egypt
Mohd Usman Mohd Siddique	Department of Pharmacy, SVKM's Institute of Pharmacy, Dhule, MH, India
Mitali Mishra	Integrated Drug Discovery Research Laboratory, Department of Pharmaceutical Sciences, Dr. Harisingh Gour University (A Central University), Sagar (MP), India
Mauricio Cabrera	Laboratorio de I+D de Moléculas Bioactivas, Departamento de Ciencias Biológicas, Centro Universitario Regional Litoral Norte, Universidad de la República, Paysandú, Uruguay
Nigam Vyas	Department of Microbiology, Parul Institute of Applied Sciences, Parul University, Vadodara, Gujarat, India Department of Life Sciences, Parul Institute of Applied Sciences and Biophysics & Structural Biology Laboratory, Research & Development Cell, Parul University, Vadodara, Gujarat, India
Peter Mubanga Cheuka	Department of Chemistry, School of Natural Sciences, University of Zambia, Lusaka, Zambia
Priyanshu Nema	Integrated Drug Discovery Research Laboratory, Department of Pharmaceutical Sciences, Dr. Harisingh Gour University (A Central University), Sagar (MP), India
Ricardo Olimpio de Moura	Pharmacy Department, State University of Paraíba, Campina Grande, Brazil Drug Development and Synthesis Laboratory, Department of Pharmacy, State University of Paraíba, Campina Grande 58429-500, Brazil
Rajendra Prasad Chatterjee	National Institute of Cholera and Enteric Diseases, Indian Council of Medical Research, Kolkata, WB, India
Radhey Shyam Kaushal	Department of Life Sciences, Parul Institute of Applied Sciences and Biophysics & Structural Biology Laboratory, Research & Development Cell, Parul University, Vadodara, Gujarat, India
Salma Darwish	Department of Pharmaceutical Chemistry, Faculty of Pharmacy, Alexandria University, Alexandria 21521, Egypt
Sherry N. Nasralla	Pharmacy Program, Allied Health Department, College of Health and Sport Sciences, University of Bahrain, Sakhir 32038, Kingdom of Bahrain
Sherine N. Khattab	Chemistry Department, Faculty of Science, Alexandria University, Alexandria 21321, Egypt

Silvia Selleri Neurofarba Department, Pharmaceutical and Nutraceutical Section, University of Florence, Firenze FI, Sesto Fiorentino, Italy

Sheikh Murtuja Department of Pharmaceutical Technology, School of Health and Medical Science, Adamas University, Kolkata, WB, India

Shilpa Chatterjee Department of Pharmaceutical Technology, School of Health and Medical Science, Adamas University, Kolkata, WB, India

Samyak Bajaj Integrated Drug Discovery Research Laboratory, Department of Pharmaceutical Sciences, Dr. Harisingh Gour University (A Central University), Sagar (MP), India

Sushil Kumar Kashaw Integrated Drug Discovery Research Laboratory, Department of Pharmaceutical Sciences, Dr. Harisingh Gour University (A Central University), Sagar (MP), India

Tarun Kumar Upadhyay Department of Life Sciences, Parul Institute of Applied Sciences and Immuno-biochemistry Laboratory, Research & Development Cell, Parul University, Vadodara, Gujarat, India

Medicinal Chemistry of Neglected Tropical Diseases (NTDs): From Targets to Drugs

Karla Joane da Silva Menezes[1,2,†], Arthur Gabriel Corrêa de Farias[2,†], Marianny de Souza[3], Éric de Oliveira Rios[3], Igor José dos Santos Nascimento[1,2,3,*] and Ricardo Olimpio de Moura[1,2]

[1] *Pharmacy Department, State University of Paraíba, Campina Grande, Brazil*

[2] *Drug Development and Synthesis Laboratory, Department of Pharmacy, State University of Paraíba, Campina Grande 58429-500, Brazil*

[3] *Pharmacy Departament, Cesmac University Center, Maceió, Brazil*

Abstract: Neglected Tropical Diseases (NTDs) are a group of infectious diseases that affect thousands of people all over the world. These diseases mainly affect the population that lives in poverty and lack sanitation, prevalent mainly in tropical and subtropical countries. In this sense, they are called "neglected" due to the low investment in P&D in pharmaceutical companies' discovery and development of new agents. Thus, developing new drugs against these diseases is one of the two biggest challenges for academic researchers around the world, and increasingly, there is a need for advances in medicinal chemistry methods and the identification of molecular targets for the design of innovative drugs that can put an end to these threats. Finally, here we will present methods used in medicinal chemistry in recent years in the design of drugs against these agents, with a focus on the development of new compounds against *N*-myristoyltransferase, nitroreductases, topoisomerases, pyrimidine synthesis pathway, and mitochondrial alterations constantly explored against various NTDs. We hope this chapter serves as a guide for researchers worldwide searching for innovative drugs that can finally help these people and improve the health of the world's population.

Keywords: CADD, Chagas diseases, Chikungunya, Dengue, Drug design, Drug discovery, Fasciola, leprosy, Leishmaniasis, Malaria, NTDs, Schistosomiasis, Sleeping sickness, Tuberculosis, Zika.

* **Corresponding author Igor José dos Santos Nascimento:** Pharmacy Department, State University of Paraíba, Campina Grande, Brazil; Tel: (+55)8299933-5457; E-mails: igor.nascimento@cesmac.edu.br; igorjsn@hotmail.com
† These authors contributed equally to this work

INTRODUCTION

Neglected Tropical Diseases (NTDs) are a group of 20 infectious diseases prevalent worldwide, recognized by the World Health Organization (WHO) [1]. These diseases are intrinsically linked to the socioeconomic situation and environment of the patient's residence, affecting the poor population and those without basic sanitation [2]. NTDs pose a significant threat to public health in tropical, subtropical, and rural regions due to the conducive environment for the etiological agent of these diseases [3]. Poverty, particularly the lack of proper sanitation and limited access to medical care and follow-up, is another contributing factor to the high incidence of these diseases [4]. In general, NTDs can contribute to the perpetuation of poverty in a region. This is because the symptoms of NTDs can impede an individual's productivity and professional development, significantly impacting the regional economy [2, 5].

NTDs affect approximately 1.7 billion people worldwide, with Africa being the continent most vulnerable to these diseases, accounting for 40% of the population affected by NTDs globally [6]. This is primarily due to environmental conditions conducive to developing these diseases and inadequate sanitation. However, urbanization has led to a significant increase in NTDs in urban and peri-urban regions over the years, which has generated greater attention and caution towards these diseases [7]. Another risk factor in the spread of NTDs is the environmental impact caused by deforestation, fires, and climate change due to global warming. Many of these diseases go through complex transmission cycles between humans and animals, which can be induced to leave or expand their habitats due to these global stigmas [3, 8].

Due to these factors, public health organizations are developing new intervention strategies to control, eliminate, or eradicate these diseases [9]. These approaches offer a holistic and multisectoral approach to treating and preventing NTDs [10 - 12]. Strategies to control NTDs include preventive chemotherapy and transmission control (PCT), innovative and intensified disease management (IDM), vector ecology and management (VEM), veterinary public health measures, and the provision of safe water, sanitation, and hygiene (WASH) [13]. Other strategies, such as conditional cash transfer programs and social marketing interventions, can also reduce the incidence of NTDs. These programs aim to improve access to medical care and raise awareness among the population [13, 14].

However, the development of new drugs to mitigate NTDs remains the most promising strategy for controlling and eliminating these diseases despite the diverse intervention strategies employed [15]. Addressing the challenges of developing these drugs is crucial to achieving this objective. Among the challenges associated with NTD treatment are the lengthy duration of therapy, which can exceed two months, the high incidence of adverse effects that require treatment during and after drug use, and various contraindications that can directly affect patient adherence to NTD treatment [16]. In addition to clinical factors, the discovery of new drugs faces a long, complex, and costly journey through several rigorous stages. Together, these factors indicate the key challenges that must be addressed in developing new drugs for NTDs [17].

In the face of numerous challenges, medicinal chemistry seeks new techniques and methods for developing drugs for NTDs [18]. These include implementing machine learning, applying pharmacogenomics in the development process, and the Target-Based Drug Design (TBDD) approach [19]. The increased availability of data from high-throughput screening (HTS) has made machine learning an essential tool in discovering new drugs, enabling models to be trained to predict the biological activities of compounds before laboratory work [20]. Pharmacogenomics has been applied at various stages in developing new drugs and analyzing the interactions between compounds and DNA through *in vitro* and *in silico* assays [21]. The Target-Based Drug Design (TBDD) approach involves testing selected drugs against biological targets of parasites. This approach is a critical stage in the discovery and development of new drugs, as using inappropriate targets is a leading cause of failure in the final stages of the new drug discovery process [1]. Therefore, validating a promising biological target is crucial in discovering new drugs [22].

Designing and discovering new drugs against NTDs is a challenge and is necessary to improve new approaches to obtain success in a short time and with less financial investment. From this perspective, this chapter will approach the main advances in medicinal chemistry to discover new drugs against NTDs, focusing on new drug targets such as *N*-myristoyltransferase, nitroreductases, topoisomerases, pyrimidine synthesis pathway, and mitochondrial alterations. We hope our findings help researchers worldwide search for an innovative drug to stop these threatening agents and improve the world population's health.

NEGLECTED TROPICAL DISEASES: A CONSTANT THREAT

In 2005, the WHO distributed a list of neglected tropical diseases. The list included a diverse group of tropical infections, predominantly chronic and parasitic, that disproportionately affect people living in poverty. The list consists of leishmaniasis - cutaneous (CL), mucocutaneous (MCL), and visceral (VL), trypanosomiasis (Chagas disease and sleeping sickness), which are caused by the infectious agents *Leishmania* spp. and *Trypanosomacruzi* or *Trypanosoma brucei*, and other parasitics, viral and bacterial diseases [23]. Thus, the following topics will approach a brief explanation of epidemiology, consequences, treatment, and drug design against these diseases.

Epidemiology

NTDs affect over one billion people around the world with several social and economic impacts. The epidemiology of NTDs is complex and often related to environmental conditions. Although they are caused by different agents (bacteria, viruses, helminths, and protozoa), NTDs include common characteristics related to their social, political, and economic impacts. All these factors make their public health control challenging [24, 25]. Furthermore, the COVID-19 pandemic has exacerbated the impact of NTDs, bringing numerous social, economic, epidemiological, and health challenges [26].

Although these diseases are currently concentrated in Africa, Asia, and Latin America, they can also be found in developed countries in Europe, North America, Southeast Asia, and Australasia due to local poverty, immigration, and other factors. Therefore, NTDs comprise a broad group of diseases with the highest prevalence in tropical and subtropical regions, specifically in underdeveloped or developing countries, since female vector flies use the decomposing organic materials and moist places for oviposition [25, 27].

Given that these diseases are neglected, there are considerable uncertainties regarding global burden estimates. Due to climate change and globalization, the incidence of parasitic and protozoa diseases, for example, is increasing, especially in Europe. *Cystic echinococcosis*, endemic in Mediterranean and Eastern countries, and *Alveolar echinococcosis*, restricted to the northern hemisphere in temperate climate zones, can be considered emerging public health problems in Europe [28].

In 2019, over 128,000 irregular arrivals of migrants to Europe were recorded, coming mainly from African and Asian countries *via* Mediterranean migration routes. An observational, prospective study of infectious disease prevalence showed that the two NTDs targeted by European and national screening guidelines, Strongyloidiasis and Schistosomiasis, are highly prevalent among African refugee asylum seekers in Rome and the Lazio region, Italy [29].

Human African trypanosomiasis (HAT), leishmaniasis, and Chagas disease (CD) are three neglected tropical diseases for which current treatments are inadequate and even cause toxic side effects, leading to thousands of deaths in the poorest countries [30]. Leishmaniasis and trypanosomiasis are endemic neglected diseases in South America and Africa and are considered a significant public health problem, mainly in poor communities [25]. Millions of people are living in areas where these diseases are endemic and urgently need new drugs to stop these agents [17, 31].

Leishmaniasis is caused by different species of the genus *Leishmania* that can produce very severe infections, being fatal if untreated [32]. The parasite *T. brucei*, the causing agent of HAT, invades the Central Nervous System (CNS) and is relatively spread throughout Africa. At the same time, *T. cruzi* is the parasite responsible for CD in Latin American countries [33]. With 6 to 7 million infections worldwide, most cases of CD are found in rural areas of Latin America, with others found in the United States of America, Canada, Europe, and Africa [26].

As a critical NTD, a zoonosis, a vector-borne infection and considered a global public health problem, occurring in around 98 countries with 1.3 million cases per year and 350 million people at risk of infection, leishmaniasis is a challenging burden to control in developing countries [34]. More than 90% of the total number of leishmaniasis patients worldwide are reported in six countries: Brazil, Ethiopia, India, Somalia, South Sudan, and Sudan. In recent years, Nicaragua has experienced alarmingly high numbers of patients and high incidence rates [35].

Consequences on the Health System

NTDs are a diverse group of diseases caused by various etiological agents. Some diseases are easily accessible through pattern recognition or clinical assessment of physical symptoms, but identification in early stages and asymptomatic diseases is often difficult. NTDs result in substantial disability, stigma, and loss of livelihood, in addition to the deaths caused. Given that these diseases are neglected, there are considerable uncertainties regarding global burden estimates. They are related to significant costs in terms of health and care, but they also negatively impact the economic activities of the poorest people [36].

The clinical manifestations of leishmaniasis are divided into cutaneous (CL), mucocutaneous (MCL), and visceral (VL). Although parasites alter their morphology depending on the environmental conditions, promastigote and amastigote are the primary forms during the life cycle of *Leishmania* spp [25]. CL and ML generally involve uncovered areas of the body, such as the face and extremities, generating social stigma and psychological repercussions even after healing. At the same time, LV presents a high lethality and mainly affects internal organs, such as the liver and spleen, making it the second most dangerous parasitic tropical disease after malaria [35, 37].

CD, in turn, can clinically progress acutely or chronically. The acute phase is marked by intense parasitemia, which can be asymptomatic or oligosymptomatic, with nonspecific systemic symptoms, such as fever, anorexia, and tachycardia, among other characteristic signs. On the other hand, the progression to chronicity leads to multisystem manifestations that mainly affect the digestive and cardiovascular systems, causing cardiomyopathy, megaesophagus, and megacolon [38, 39].

Pharmacological Intervention and Prevention

The complex biology of many of these parasites and their need for vectors for development and transmission makes traditional industrial-scale drug discovery programs challenging [30]. In addition, the widespread distribution of drugs, free of charge, to people in need of treatment also does not guarantee that these people will be treated due to the lack of information about the treatment [40]. In addition, the drugs available to treat these diseases do not reflect the clinical need. Therefore, a comprehensive approach must be used, combining mass administration of drugs with access to treatment on demand, as well as a more significant commitment on the part of endemic countries to enable equitable access, efficient use of existing drugs, and effort for the discovery of new targets and development of new drugs [30, 40].

The search for new drugs against NTDs focuses on discovering drugs mainly against the organisms derivative from kinetoplastids, helminths, and Plasmodium. In this way, some strategies are more relevant and most used, such as high-throughput screening (HTS) by *in vitro* assay targeting the microorganism of interest; HTS targeting the microorganism enzymes through enzymatic assays screening; and *in silico* works for inhibitor-structure optimizations, and target-based and phenotypic approaches [30, 41].

In addition to the actual strategies, natural products remain an excellent source of compounds against these diseases [42, 43]. For example, seven medicinal plants from the flora of Uganda were tested as traditional ethnomedicinal and ethnoveterinary therapies or in zoo pharmacognosy to evaluate *in vitro* antiplasmodial, antitrypanosomal, and antileishmania activities, presenting promising candidates for additional cell-based and systems pharmacology studies [44].

On the other hand, nifurtimox and benznidazole are effective and are used in current antiChagas therapies. However, they are highly toxic and ineffective in eradicating parasites in the final stages of diseases. Thus, new drug targets must be explored in searching for new drugs. For example, cruzain, the main cysteine protease of *T. cruzi*, is an attractive drug target and has been explored in several to be essential for intracellular parasite survival and infectivity [30].

DNA topoisomerases play vital roles in the survival of many protozoan parasites that cause fatal diseases. The structures of topoisomerases in protozoan parasites are different from those in humans. Therefore, they act as an essential target for developing effective drugs for parasitic diseases. Several studies have already revealed the therapeutic potential of these drugs targeting parasitic topoisomerases, including Leishmania, Trypanosoma, Plasmodium, Giardia, Entamoeba, Babesia, Theileria, Crithidia, Cryptosporidium, Toxoplasma, *etc* [51].

Currently, used antileishmanial drugs include pentavalent antimonials, first-line therapy due to affordable price and high cure rate, pentamidine, amphotericin B, and miltefosine, which are known to target different metabolic pathways. Mitochondria emerge as a potential target for developing therapies for this infection, given their unique properties and proteins that differ from those of mammalian hosts [52].

Leishmania parasite has several molecules to protect it from oxidative damage and the hydrolytic activity within the phagolysosome, including lipophosphoglycans (LPG), which modulate the immune response by modifying the levels of produced cytokines, LPG glycosylinositol phospholipids, proteophosphoglycans, acid phosphatases, zinc-dependent metalloprotease GP63, and cysteine proteases [25].

Cysteine proteases have caught the attention of researchers and are being proposed as promising targets for drug discovery [25]. These enzymes, members of the papain-like peptidase family, are essential for different cellular processes such as nutrition, reproduction, host cell invasion, and evading the host's immune system. They are validated drug targets for developing safe and effective pharmacological agents for trypanosomiasis diseases, as they are expressed throughout the life cycle of these parasites. Several genetic and chemical validation studies confirmed the essentiality of these enzymes in the different phases of the life cycle of *T. cruzi* and *T. brucei* [53].

Histone deacetylase enzymes (HDACs) are validated drug targets for treating cancer and other diseases. They have also become relevant for NTDs in developing new potential antiparasitic treatments in recent years. However, knowledge about HDACs in cestodes is very scarce [54].

Benznidazole and nifurtimox are prodrugs activated by the reduction of the nitro group, catalyzed by the *T. cruzi* type I nitroreductase enzyme (TcNTR). In the literature, the enzyme already has a validated role in reducing the metabolism of these prodrugs available against Chagas diseases. However, the exact physiological role of NTRs in bacteria or trypanosomatids is still unknown [55]. This drug target will be discussed in detail in the next section.

Treating gastrointestinal CD is also challenging, with limited options once symptoms become apparent. Recently, researchers used an innovative metabolomics approach to define mechanisms of disease tolerance and identify therapeutic targets against Chagas diseases [39, 56]. Despite concerted efforts to develop effective and safe medicines, treat patients, and eliminate vectors, correct and rapid diagnosis is the first necessary step to accelerate treatment [27]. Ongoing research in biosensors applied to neglected tropical diseases presents promising and exciting results [27].

SOME EXPLORED DRUG TARGETS AND PATHWAYS

N-myristoyltransferase (NMT)

Myristoylation is a lipidation process that attaches the myristate, a 14-carbon saturated fatty acid chain, to proteins, allowing them to target membranes and become fully available inside or outside cells. Then, these proteins can interact with others, acting as sensors and participating in signal transduction [57]. In this way, the universally conserved enzyme *N*-myristoyltransferase (NMT), classified as an *N*-acetyltransferase, is required to catalyze this co and post-translational protein modification, which is essential for its function, stability, and membrane partitioning [1, 58, 59]. This enzyme is crucial for the survival of several protozoa parasites, including *Plasmodium* spp [60 - 63], *Leishmania* spp [64, 65], *Trypanosoma brucei* [64, 66], *Trypanosoma cruzi* [67, 68], *Giardia lamblia* [69, 70], *Entamoeba histolytica* [70], and *Toxoplasma gondii* [71], as well as some nematodes, such as *Caenorhabditis elegans* and *Brugia malayi* [72].

The *N*-myristoyltransferase is an exclusive eukaryote enzyme that evolved between the archaeal and the eukaryotic common ancestors. Lower eukaryotes possess only one isoform, whereas some mammals, such as humans and mice, present two, NMT1 and NMT2 [59]. The myristoylation process occurs through the recognition of myristoyl-CoA by the apo-enzyme, followed by a conformational modification of NMT, in which the substrate binding pocket is exposed, allowing the interaction with a protein. Then, its *N*-terminal glycine is attached to myristate. Both products are released from the enzyme, the *N*-myristoylated protein, and the free CoA, using a bi-bi mechanism (Fig. 1). For this, the saturated carbon chain is placed inside a deep and hydrophobic pocket. In contrast, the thioester from myristoyl-CoA is located inside the "oxyanion hole" of the enzyme to activate the carbonyl for the following nucleophilic attack of the amine moiety from glycine of the peptide substrate. Concurrently, the glycine is deprotonated by the *C*-terminal residue of NMT, turning the ammonium into an amine group, essential for initiating this nucleophilic addition-elimination reaction. Ultimately, after the release of the products, the substrate binding pocket becomes hidden again, restoring the initial conformation of NMT [59, 73].

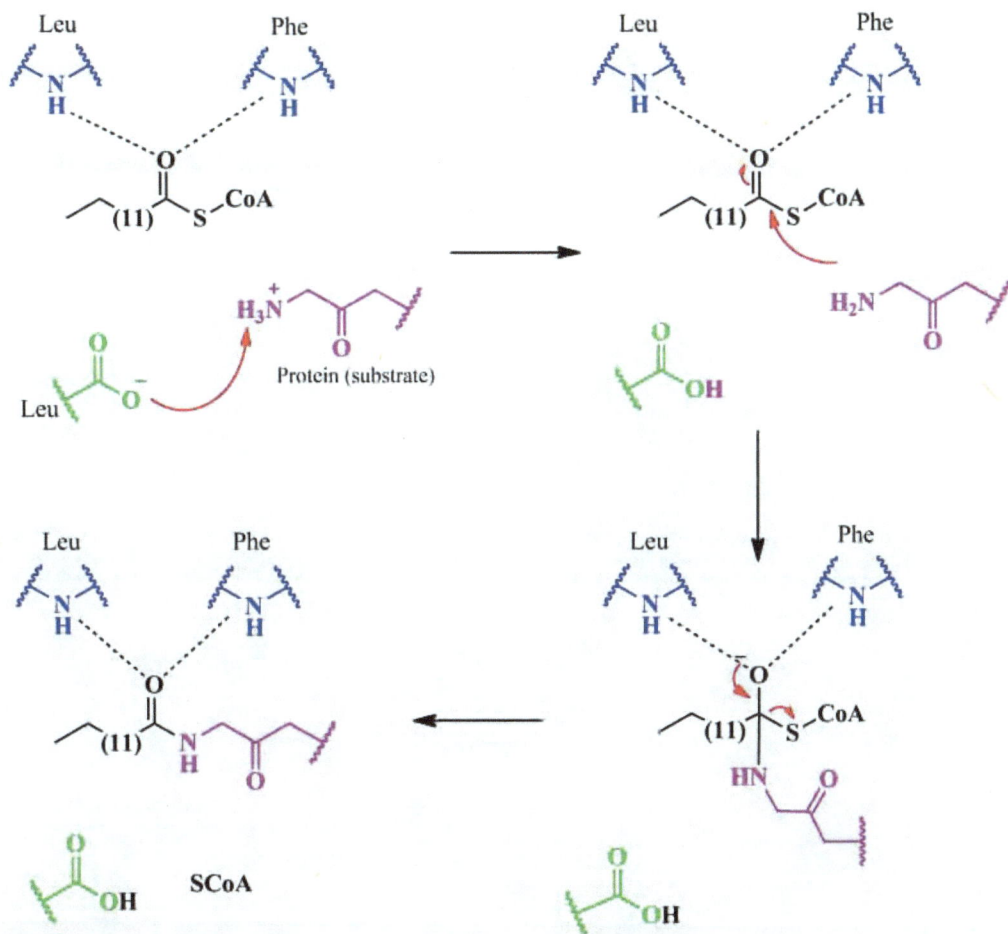

Fig. (1). The structure and catalytic mechanism of action of *N*-myristoyltransferase.

For an appropriate design of new NMT inhibitors, it is fundamental to understand the catalytic mechanism of the enzyme, as well as the substrate binding mode, since selective compounds against NMT have been developed toward the peptide active site through the analysis of the different residues and its positions [65]. Selective antiparasitic molecules can be designed due to the differences through which protein substrates bind to the active site of human and parasite NMT (Fig. 2). In the human NMT, Phe[247] and Leu[248] residues stabilize the thioester group of myristoyl-CoA inside the oxyanion pocket, and Thr[282] and Gln[496] enable deprotonation of the *N*-terminal Gly. It was possible through crystallographic analysis to determine that C-terminal Leu[410] is responsible for deprotonate glycine as Asn[161] and Thr[197] stabilize the rising amino group, making it readily available to attack the MysCoA carbonyl group in *P. vivax* NMT. Thus, the catalytic mechanism depends on Leu[410], and its interaction with it enhances the selectivity of the inhibitor. Similarly, Phe[162] and Leu[163] are crucial for stabilizing the tetrahedral oxyanion intermediate that undergoes further elimination to release CoA and the *N*-myristoylated protein. Furthermore, key residues such as His[213], Ser[319], and Asn[365] in P*v*NMT play a crucial role in interacting with selective inhibitors. H-bond with His[213] and Asn[365] is possible if the ligand could interact with Tyr[211] and Tyr[334] in the active site and thus assume the ideal position for interaction [1].

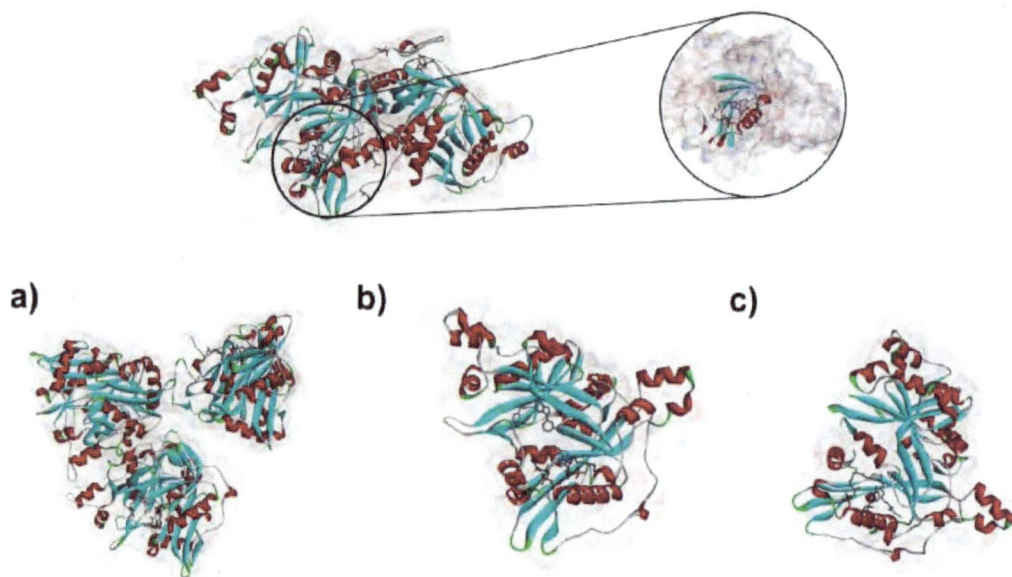

Fig. (2). Comparison between human NMT (PDB id: 4C2Y) and *a)P. vivax* NMT (PDB id: 5V0W); *b)L. major* NMT (PDB id: 4CGN); and *c)L. donovani* NMT (PDB id: 5WUU).

A set of eleven carbonyl thiourea derivatives was synthesized and biologically evaluated against *L. major* promastigotes by Mohammadi-Ghalehbin *et al.* (2023) [74]. Since NMT is an essential target for developing novel antileishmanial agents, the authors assessed the interactions between their molecules and the L*m*NMT through docking and molecular dynamics simulations. The derivatives were obtained from different substitution patterns on the carbonyl thiourea scaffold. The compound **(1)** Fig. **(3)** presented higher antileishmanial activity, although it was lower than the positive control amphotericin B ($IC_{50} = 0{,}19 \pm 0{,}01$

µg/mL). Ultimately, the molecular docking results revealed that thiazole derivatives, such as compound (2) Fig. (3), show the lowest Gibbs free energy (ΔG), similar to that of the co-crystallized ligand of the protein. In addition, compound (3) Fig. (3) exhibited the lowest ΔG, and molecular docking revealed predominantly apolar interactions with the protein. It was pointed out that π-stacking interactions emerged between the thiazole ring and Phe[90] of the LmNMT. In contrast, the *p*-bromophenyl group occupied a hydrophobic pocket in the enzyme with the bromine atom, enabling the interaction with Gly[205].

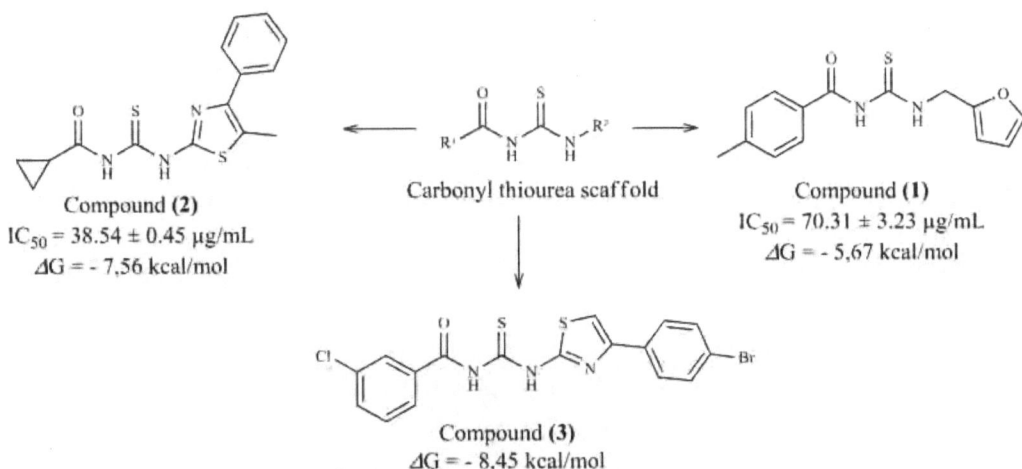

Compound (2)
IC_{50} = 38.54 ± 0.45 µg/mL
ΔG = - 7,56 kcal/mol

Carbonyl thiourea scaffold

Compound (1)
IC_{50} = 70.31 ± 3.23 µg/mL
ΔG = - 5,67 kcal/mol

Compound (3)
ΔG = - 8,45 kcal/mol

Fig. (3). Chemical structures of thiourea derivatives (1), (2), and (3) with potential against LmNMT.

One of the problems in developing new NMT inhibitors is to achieve selectivity over human NMT. Exploring this perspective, Rodríguez-Hernández *et al.* (2023) [75] applied a molecular hybridization in two previously characterized P*v*NMT inhibitors and assessed its *in vitro* activity against *P. vivax* hypnozoites. In this way, different substituents were attached to a biaryl scaffold to improve potency and selectivity (Fig. 4). The head region of the core (R^1) was intended to interact with *C*-terminal Leu[410] using head groups such as piperazine and dimethylaminoethanol capable of ionically interacting with this residue. Meanwhile, the groups R^2 were placed to interact with the critical residue Ser[319] in the active site. Among those containing piperazine, compounds (4) and (5) Fig. (4) presented the best selectivity indexes (259.2 and 269.8, respectively). Both share a structural feature in common: a 1,3,5-trimethylaminopyrazole group, which can interact with Ser[319] through H-bond, as demonstrated in the molecular docking.

Bell and coworkers (2020) [76] developed a structure-activity relationship (SAR) study to improve the selectivity of a series of thienopyrimidine inhibitors of

Leishmania NMT. The authors chose as scaffold the compound IMP-083 (Fig. **5**), an analog of a previously characterized hit compound against L*d*NMT. It was possible to assess the effect on activity and selectivity upon different variations in the nucleus and substituents of the thienopyrimidine scaffold. The exchange of the thienopyrimidine nucleus by a quinazoline in compound **(6)** (Fig. **5**) or pyridopyrimidine nucleus did not affect the potency and selectivity profile. At the same time, activity was lost by exchange with purine and pyrimidine in compounds **(7)** and **(8)**, respectively (Fig. **5**). It was suggested that this was due to the reduced lipophilicity of these two last nuclei. When the C2 substituent was exchanged by a tetrahydropyran in compound **(9)** (Fig. **5**) or a hydroxypropyl group in compound **(10)** (Fig. **5**), activity against L*d*NMT was lost due to the loss of an essential basic center. Furthermore, decreased activity is followed by extending this basic moiety due to steric factors in compound **(11)** < compound **(12)** < compound **(13)** (Fig. **5**). The authors also reported that enhancing flexibility by substituting this moiety for an acyclic amine side-chain in compounds **(14)**, **(15)**, and **(16)** (Fig. **5**) had no effect on activity against L*d*NMT but slightly decreased activity against L*m*NMT compared to compound **(13)**.

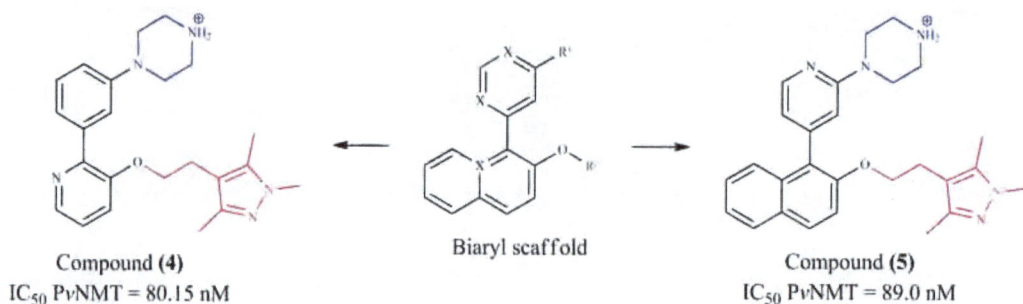

Compound (4)
IC_{50} P*v*NMT = 80.15 nM

Biaryl scaffold

Compound (5)
IC_{50} P*v*NMT = 89.0 nM

Fig. (4). Structure of promising biaryl hybrids to target *P. vivax* *N*-miristoyltransferase (P*v*NMT).

To identify novel *L. major* NMT inhibitors, Khalil *et al*. (2019) [77] performed a multistage virtual screening, and selected compounds were subject to docking and molecular dynamics simulations. The study identified twelve hit molecules, and their chemical features and binding modes were analyzed to see their interactions with the L*m*NMT. Most compounds reportedly interacted with Tyr[217] through H-bond or π-stacking interaction and with some hydrophobic and aromatic residues such as Phe[88], Phe[90], and Phe[232]. Molecular dynamics simulations showed that Van der Waals contributed significantly to the stability of ligand-protein complexes, and the compounds **(17)**, **(18)**, and **(19)** Fig. **(6)** presented great binding free energies and can explored in further works of drug design against this drug target.

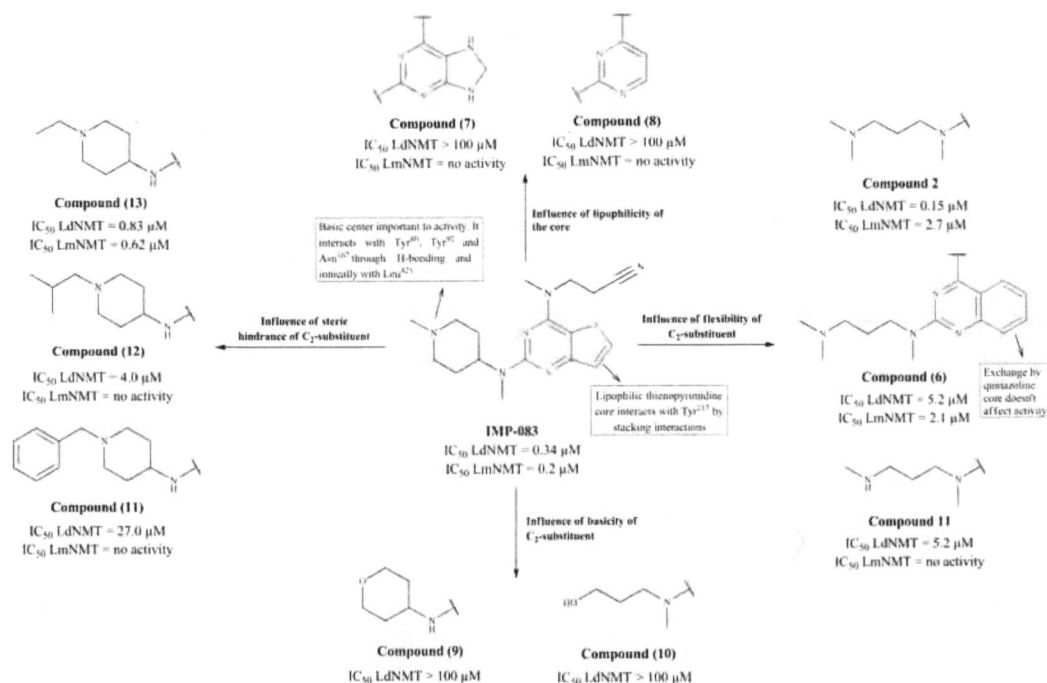

Fig. (5). Development strategy of selective thienopyrimidine *Leishmania* NMT inhibitors by Bell and colleagues (2020).

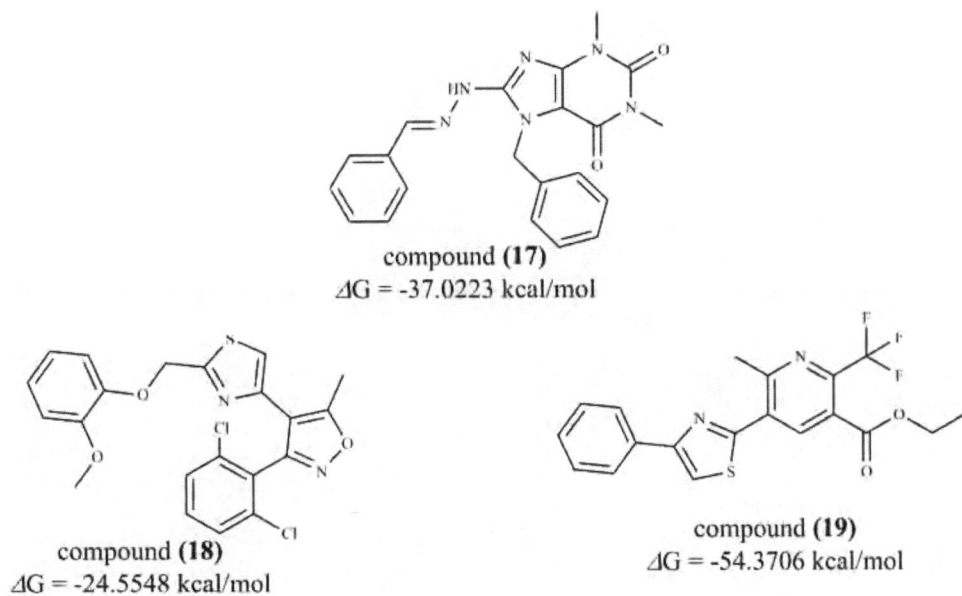

compound **(17)**
ΔG = -37.0223 kcal/mol

compound **(18)**
ΔG = -24.5548 kcal/mol

compound **(19)**
ΔG = -54.3706 kcal/mol

Fig. (6). Chemical structure of the most promising compounds against L*m*NMT identified by Khalil *et al.* (2019).

Utilizing molecular docking and molecular dynamics simulation, Orabi *et al.* (2023) [78] identified potential L*m*NMT inhibitors from *Withania somnifera* L., a plant reported with antileishmanial activity. The authors searched for previously reported phytoconstituents of the medicinal plant, and these compounds were evaluated against L*m*NMT. According to binding affinity and deviation calculation with the reference ligand, three compounds **(21)**, **(22)**, and **(23)** (Fig. 7) were chosen as the most active. The highest affinity was attributed to 4,16-dihydroxy-5,6-epoxyphysagulin D **(21)** (dock score = -24,0 kcal/mol). In addition, due to the hydroxy groups, this compound interacted with the target mainly through H-bond and hydrophobic interactions due to the steroid scaffold. Since *W. somnifera* extract demonstrated antileishmanial activity *in vitro* and *in silico* techniques revealed an excellent interaction with L*m*NTR, these compounds are suggested to be potential antileishmanial for further evaluation and optimization.

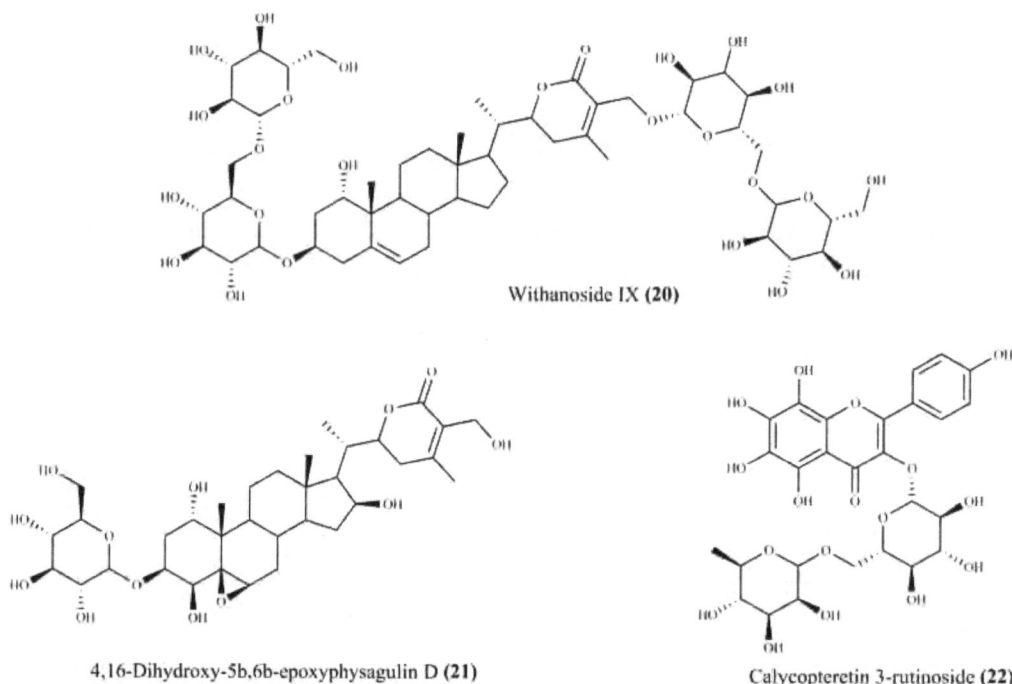

Withanoside IX **(20)**

4,16-Dihydroxy-5b,6b-epoxyphysagulin D **(21)**

Calycopteretin 3-rutinoside **(22)**

Fig. (7). Chemical structure of the most active compounds isolated from *Withania somnifera* L. by Orabi and coworkers (2023).

Finally, the NMT is a critical target that can be explored in the drug design against NTDs, and several scaffolds can be used against it. In addition, discovering a drug against this target can be innovative because there is still no approved drug against this target, providing a new therapeutic option against this disease.

Nitroreductases

Nitroreductases (NTR) are enzymes found in bacteria, fungi, and some species of lower eukaryotes, such as *Trypanosoma* sp. and *Leishmania* sp. Comparative studies with bacterial NTR suggest that *Trypanosoma cruzi* NTR (TcNTR) is an enzyme containing 312 residues divided into 3 domains, one of which is the catalytic domain [55]. Furthermore, it includes an Arg^{90} essential for flavin-based cofactor binding, with the same function as Arg^{96} in *Leishmania major* NTR. Based on its substrate specificity, cellular localization, and sequence, these enzymes must play an essential role in controlling the balance of $NADH/NAD^+$ concentration within the mitochondria. For both *L. major* and *L. donovani*, NTR function substantially replicates these parasites' amastigote and promastigote forms. In contrast, the TcNTR function is only essential to the replicating forms in the mammalian host [79].

There are two types of nitroreductases based on the mechanism of the nitro group reduction reaction and the required cofactors. Type I NTR is known as oxygen-insensitive because it acts through a mechanism that does not require an oxygen molecule, only reduced nicotinamide adenine dinucleotide phosphate (NADPH) and flavin mononucleotide (FMN) as cofactor, which binds to the enzyme through a non-covalent interaction. The electrons gained from reducing equivalents (NADH or NADPH) are used to reduce FMN to $FMNH_2$, reducing a nitroaromatic or quinone-based substrate (the already mentioned bi-bi mechanism). On the other hand, type II NTR requires oxygen to reduce the substrate through a one-electron transfer from FAD, or FMN, generating a nitro radical product. The oxygen can now react with the radical, becoming a superoxide anion and regenerating the nitro group [55, 79]. Many nitro-based prodrugs (Ex. nifurtimox, benznidazole, fexinidazole) must be activated by type I NTR to produce highly reactive species such as nitroso or hydroxylamine-based compounds that exert their cytotoxic activity against bacteria and parasites [55, 79 - 81].

In this context, a series of 4-nitroimidazole derivatives of benznidazole was assessed by Mello and coworkers (2020) [82] for *in vitro* trypanocidal activity against *T. cruzi* trypomastigotes and amastigotes. These derivatives were designed by ring and group bioisosterism strategies, and the 4-nitroimidazole moiety of benznidazole **(23)** (Fig. **8**) was kept unchanged. In contrast, the amide group was replaced by its bioisostere 1,2,3-triazole ring. Furthermore, different substituents were attached to the triazole ring, and their contributions to the trypanocidal activity were evaluated. The derivative with a cyclopropyl substituent, compound **(24)** (Fig. **8**), in the triazole ring, was reported as 1.6 times more active than benznidazole against the trypomastigotes of the Y strain of *T. cruzi*. Next, molecular dynamics simulations revealed the interactions between this compound and TcNTR. The nitro group made a H-bond with His[503] and FMN cofactor. One of the nitrogen atoms of the triazole ring made an H bond with Tyr[545] along with π-π interactions with the aromatic amino acid Trp[235] and the FMN isalloxazine system. Furthermore, the compound presented the ideal fit to the ligand cavity of the enzyme, highlighting the importance of considering hydrophobic and steric parameters of substituents throughout the design of new drug candidates.

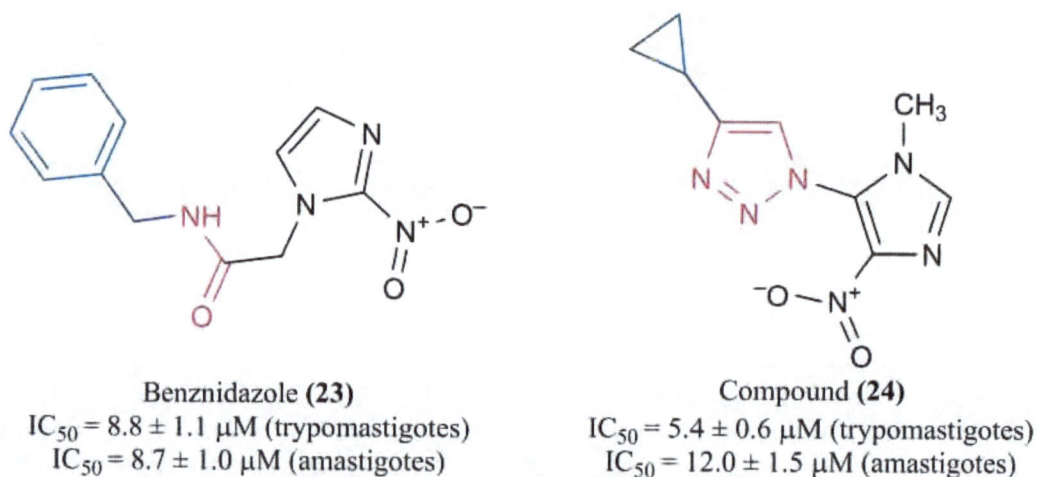

Benznidazole (23)
$IC_{50} = 8.8 \pm 1.1$ µM (trypomastigotes)
$IC_{50} = 8.7 \pm 1.0$ µM (amastigotes)

Compound (24)
$IC_{50} = 5.4 \pm 0.6$ µM (trypomastigotes)
$IC_{50} = 12.0 \pm 1.5$ µM (amastigotes)

Fig. (8). Chemical structure of benznidazole and a 4-nitroimidazole derivative synthesized by Mello and colleagues (2020).

A study was performed to explore the activity against *T. cruzi* and *T. brucei* and the role of NTR in the bioactivation of *N*-acylhydrazones derivatives carrying a nitrofuran group and a metallocene moiety. Four new compounds were synthesized from an *N*-acyl hydrazone scaffold by adding a ferrocenyl or cyrhetrenyl hydrazide to a 2-formyl- or 2-acetyl-5-nitrofuran (Fig. 9). Those with Rhenium complex in compound (25), (26) (Fig. 9) had shown better activity than those with a ferrocenyl group in compound (27), and (28) (Fig. 9) against *T. cruzi* epimastigotes and *T. brucei* trypomastigotes. Furthermore, the methylated compounds in (28) and (26) (Fig. 9) were more active than their analogs (27) and (25), respectively, compared to standard compound nifurtimox (29) (Fig. 9). To assess the participation of NTR in the trypanocidal activity of these derivatives, the authors performed an essay in which the susceptibility of a type I NTR-overexpressed *T. brucei* recombinant form was measured. The susceptibility of the NTR-overexpressed trypanosomes was more significant than the control group for compounds (28) and (26), indicating that these were substrates for the enzyme [83].

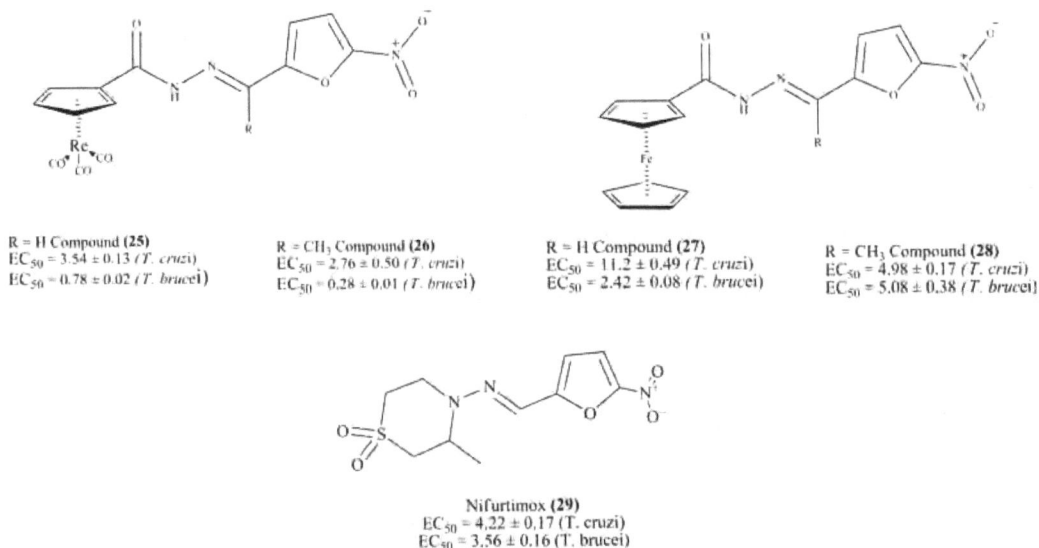

R = H Compound **(25)**
EC_{50} = 3.54 ± 0.13 *(T. cruzi)*
EC_{50} = 0.78 ± 0.02 *(T. brucei)*

R = CH₃ Compound **(26)**
EC_{50} = 2.76 ± 0.50 *(T. cruzi)*
EC_{50} = 0.28 ± 0.01 *(T. brucei)*

R = H Compound **(27)**
EC_{50} = 11.2 ± 0.49 *(T. cruzi)*
EC_{50} = 2.42 ± 0.08 *(T. brucei)*

R = CH₃ Compound **(28)**
EC_{50} = 4.98 ± 0.17 *(T. cruzi)*
EC_{50} = 5.08 ± 0.38 *(T. brucei)*

Nifurtimox **(29)**
EC_{50} = 4.22 ± 0.17 (T. cruzi)
EC_{50} = 3.56 ± 0.16 (T. brucei)

Fig. (9). Chemical structure of the four metallocene derivatives synthesized by Toro and coworkers (2021) to target Trypanosome NTR.

Topoisomerases and DNA

Eukaryotic parasites such as *Leishmania* sp. and trypanosomes have two types of DNA, the nuclear DNA and the mitochondrial DNA, which is contained within the kinetoplast, a specific region of the mitochondria. This DNA is made up of larger and smaller circles. Closely spaced AT sequences at the minicircles are responsible for their curved structure. Pentamidine is a bisbenzamidine drug that is currently available to treat parasitic diseases such as leishmaniasis and trypanosomiasis. However, it presents severe side effects related to its toxic metabolites. In addition, along with berenil and other diamidines, pentamidine is suggested to interact with AT-rich sequences of the minor groove of DNA because of their structural features, such as H-bond donating groups and slight flexibility of a linking chain. Phenylamidine moieties of pentamidine can interact with H-bond acceptors such as adenine (A) and thymine (T) and stack within the minor groove. At the same time, positively charged amidine groups counterbalance the negatively charged phosphate groups of DNA [84]. Understanding these characteristics makes it possible to design effective and more selective molecules to target specific regions of parasite genetic material [21, 85].

During replication and other processes, topological tension can arise in the DNA structure, and if not released, this tension can drastically affect the normal cell's functioning. Topoisomerases are responsible for maintaining the suitable DNA topology and are classified as type I and II based on their structure features and catalytic mechanism. To release the twisting tension and solve the supercoiled DNA, type I topoisomerase catalyzes the scission of a single strand of DNA, passes the other strand through the gap, and splices the ends back together (Fig. **10A**). On the other hand, type II topoisomerase uses ATP molecules to break a double-stranded DNA, passes another segment though the break and reconnects the ends of the first DNA (Fig. **10B**). Kinetoplastid parasites have three types of topoisomerases: IA, IB e II. Topoisomerase IB of *L. donovani* and *T. cruzi* was the first kinetoplastid topoisomerase to be elucidated and was found to be an ATP-independent heterodimeric enzyme and sensitive to the anticancer drug camptothecin. There are two subunits that form this parasite topoisomerase, but the sequence that codifies the catalytic tyrosine residue is conserved at the small subunit gene. This tyrosine molecule plays a pivotal role in the mechanism of DNA strand cleavage [86]. Type I and type II topoisomerases are found and recognized in other parasites such as *Plasmodium*, *Toxoplasma*, *Cryptosporidium*, *Giardia*, *etc*. The DNA metabolism of these parasites is dependent on the action of these enzymes, and inhibition of the mitochondrial type II topoisomerase is reported to lead to the disruption of the minicircles structure due to the loss of the kinetoplastid DNA (kDNA) [51].

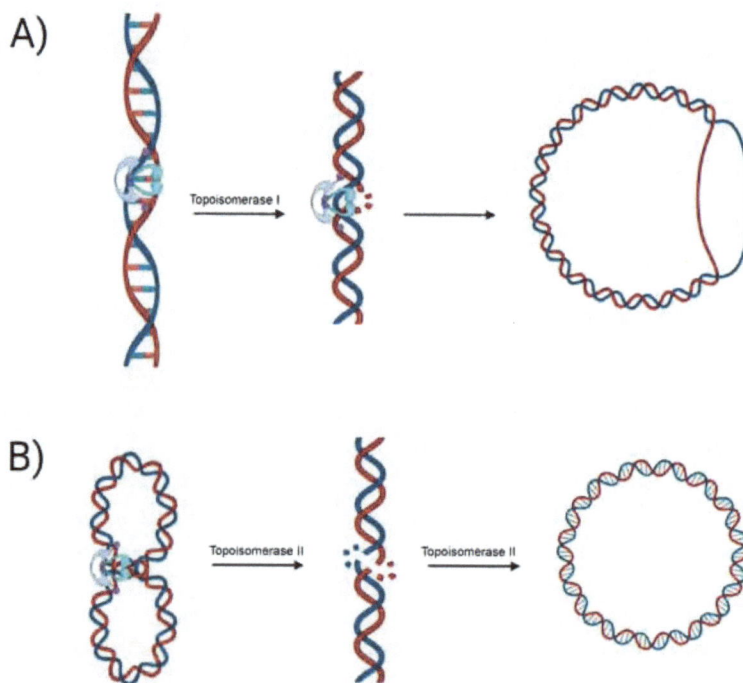

Fig. (10). Catalytic mechanism of *A)* DNA topoisomerase I; *B)* DNA topoisomerase II.

One of the most promising ways of developing selective parasitic topoisomerase inhibitors is based on the structure analysis of the enzyme. Although parasite and human topoisomerase I share a remarkable structural similarity, parasitic topoisomerases such as *L. donovani, T. cruzi,* and *T. brucei* Topoisomerase IB possess this unique aforementioned bi-subunit structure. The essential amino acid residues of the active site are located in both subunits; thus, these subunits must be attached to take place in the catalytic mechanism. Therefore, molecules capable of blocking the interaction between the subunits can be promising selective parasitic topoisomerase inhibitors [87].

Holarrhena pubescens is a medicinal plant widely used in Asia to treat parasitic infections, and it was demonstrated that its extract possesses anthelmintic and antimalarial properties [88]. In view of this, Goel and coworkers (2022) [89] investigated the antileishmanial activity of the steroidal alkaloids isolated from the bark of *H. pubescens*. Holanamine (**30**) Fig. (**11**) demonstrated a cytotoxic effect on AG83 and BHU-575 (multidrug-resistant) strains of *L. donovani* promastigotes, with growth inhibition of 97% and 91%, respectively. Through a plasmid relaxation assay, holanamine (**30**) has been shown to inhibit LdTopIB in a concentration-dependent manner, achieving 98% inhibition of catalytic activity at 10 µM. Holanamine (**30**) inhibited the DNA-LdTopIB complex in a non-competitive manner, as revealed by a time course relaxation assay when both enzyme and substrate were assessed simultaneously. Under preincubation conditions, this alkaloid could also interact with the free topoisomerase. Fortunately, holanamine (**30**) did not inhibit human topoisomerase I up to 250 µM. Molecular docking revealed that holanamine (**30**) interacted with both the hinge region and the *N*-terminal of the large subunit of LdTopIB with a binding affinity similar to that of camptothecin (-8.3 and -8.4 kcal/mol, respectively).

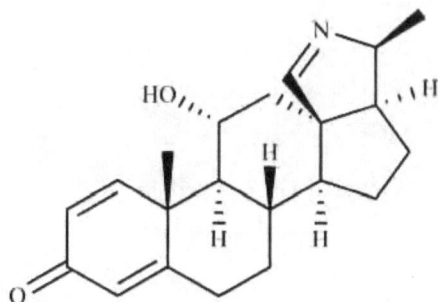

Holanamine (30)

Fig. (11). Chemical structure of the steroidal alkaloid Holanamine (**30**).

Drug instability and resistant strains are significant problems in developing new topoisomerase I inhibitors. In this way, Reguera and coworkers (2019) [90] investigated the antileishmanial activity of aromathecins, which are hybrids of indenoisoquinolines and camptothecins. The authors assessed the *in vitro* activity of two series of aromathecins (Fig. **12**) against promastigotes and amastigotes forms of *L. infantum*. Next, different nitrogenated substituents were attached to the planar ring system to improve solubility and enhance the stability of the enzyme-DNA-inhibitor complex. Series 2 compounds carry an ethylenedioxy bridge to enhance Top IB inhibitory activity. Compounds **(31)**, **(32)**, **(33)**, **(34)**, and **(35)** Fig. **(12)** presented moderate inhibition activity of *L. infantum* Top IB, and the relaxation activity assay results suggested that they act as inhibitors rather than topoisomerase poisons. Also, the ethylenedioxy bridge in series 2 did not improve Top IB inhibitory activity as desired. Finally, the resistant strain was susceptible to all the aromathecins designed, suggesting that these compounds can overcome the drug-protein efflux-mediated resistance.

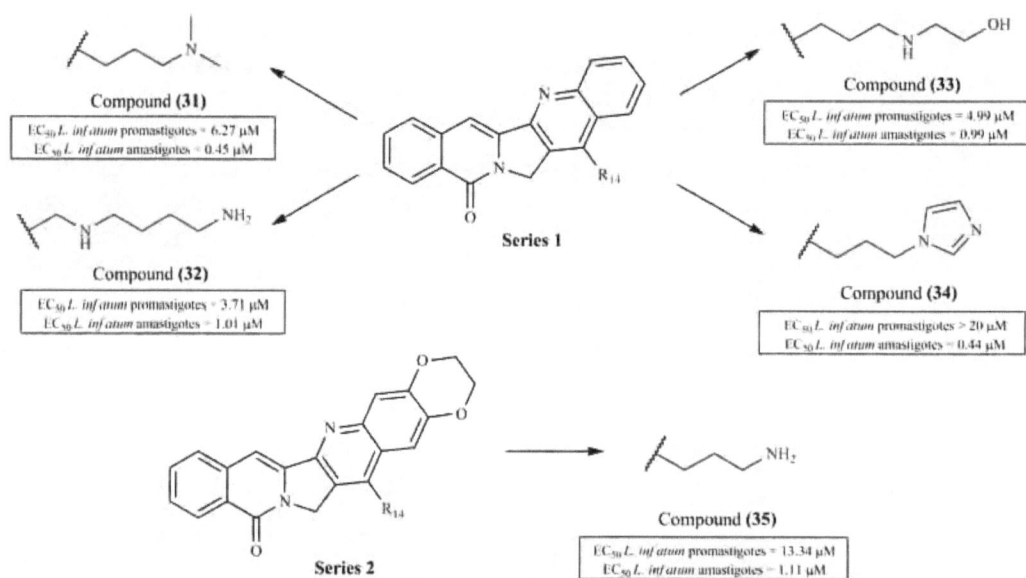

Compound (31)

EC$_{50}$ *L. infantum* promastigotes = 6.27 µM
EC$_{50}$ *L. infantum* amastigotes = 0.45 µM

Compound (32)

EC$_{50}$ *L. infantum* promastigotes = 3.71 µM
EC$_{50}$ *L. infantum* amastigotes = 1.01 µM

Compound (33)

EC$_{50}$ *L. infantum* promastigotes = 4.99 µM
EC$_{50}$ *L. infantum* amastigotes = 0.99 µM

Compound (34)

EC$_{50}$ *L. infantum* promastigotes > 20 µM
EC$_{50}$ *L. infantum* amastigotes = 0.44 µM

Series 1

Series 2

Compound (35)

EC$_{50}$ *L. infantum* promastigotes = 13.34 µM
EC$_{50}$ *L. infantum* amastigotes = 1.11 µM

Fig. (12). Chemical structures and antileishmanial activity of aromathecins assessed by Reguera and colleagues (2019).

In another work, Gutiérrez-Corbo *et al*. (2019) [91] assessed the antileishmanial activity of indenoisoquinoline derivatives varying the N-6 substituent. Almost all compounds were active against *L. infantum* promastigotes and amastigotes. Compound **(36)** (Fig. **13**) was the most active of the N-6 aminoalkyl derivatives against intracellular amastigotes and had an excellent selective index (SI) of 24.4 based on cytotoxicity (CC$_{50}$) over murine splenocytes. Comparing compounds

(36), (37), (38), and (39) (Fig. 13), increasing the length of the N-6 substituent decreases the activity against the amastigote form. The N-6 imidazole and morpholine derivatives were less active against promastigotes but maintained activity against *L. infantum* amastigotes. On the other hand, compounds (40), (41), and (42) (Fig. 13) were the most active and selective of these groups with SI = 33, 29 and 29.3, respectively. All the compounds inhibited the relaxation of DNA at tested concentrations. Furthermore, compounds (41) and (42) (Fig. 13) were the most potent at generating precipitable DNA-TopIB cleavage complexes.

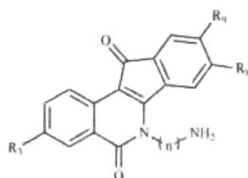

Compound	n	R_3	R_8	R_9	EC_{50} (mM)	
					Promastigotes	Amastigotes
(36)	2				0.94	0.04
(37)	3	H	H	H	0.34	0.12
(38)	4				0.43	0.73
(39)	5				2.40	2.29

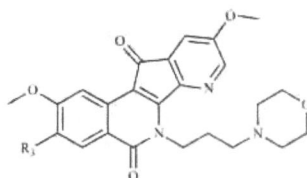

Compound	R_1	EC_{50} (nM)	
		Promastigotes	Amastigotes
(41)	H	2.92	0.27
(42)	-OCH₃	0.53	0.13

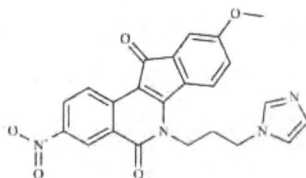

Compound (40)

EC_{50} (mM)	
Promastigotes	Amastigotes
> 10	0.01

Fig. (13). Rational design and antileishmanial activity of indenoisoquinoline derivatives.

Pérez-Pertejo and coworkers (2019) [92] evaluated the activity of quinone/hydroquinone derivatives against free-living promastigotes and intracellular amastigotes of *L. infantum*. These derivatives were planned by attaching different substituents to nine different quinone/hydroquinone scaffolds (Fig. 14), of which four are derived from monoterpenoid myrcene and five from the diterpenoid myrceocommunic acid. Thus, six of the twenty-three monoterpenoid derivatives, compounds (43), (44), (45), (46), (47), and (48) Fig. (14), showed growth inhibitory activity of intracellular amastigotes with an $EC_{50} < 10$ μM. Most of the diterpenoid derivatives demonstrated to be active against *L. infantum*, but they exhibited greater cytotoxicity to host hepatocytes. Despite the low antileishmanial activity of the naphthoquinone derivatives, they presented the

best inhibitory activity of TopIB. Molecular docking analysis with DNA-TopI-
-CPT as a template revealed that the compounds intercalate with DNA,
showingπ-stacking interactions with the predominant ones. As they can also
interact with the enzyme by H-bond and other interactions, results suggest that
these compounds act as topoisomerase poisons.

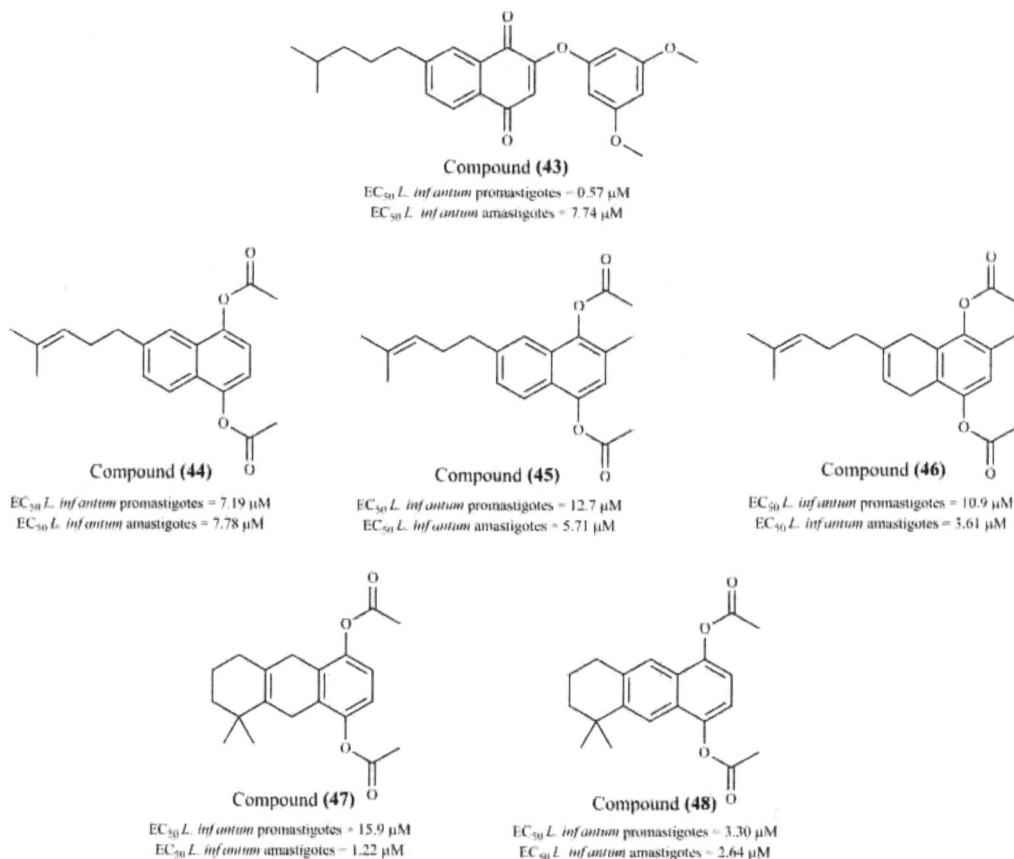

Compound **(43)**

EC$_{50}$ *L. infantum* promastigotes = 0.57 µM
EC$_{50}$ *L. infantum* amastigotes = 7.74 µM

Compound **(44)**

EC$_{50}$ *L. infantum* promastigotes = 7.19 µM
EC$_{50}$ *L. infantum* amastigotes = 7.78 µM

Compound **(45)**

EC$_{50}$ *L. infantum* promastigotes = 12.7 µM
EC$_{50}$ *L. infantum* amastigotes = 5.71 µM

Compound **(46)**

EC$_{50}$ *L. infantum* promastigotes = 10.9 µM
EC$_{40}$ *L. infantum* amastigotes = 3.61 µM

Compound **(47)**

EC$_{50}$ *L. infantum* promastigotes = 15.9 µM
EC$_{50}$ *L. infantum* amastigotes = 1.22 µM

Compound **(48)**

EC$_{50}$ *L. infantum* promastigotes = 3.30 µM
EC$_{50}$ *L. infantum* amastigotes = 2.64 µM

Fig. (14). Quinone derivatives designed by Pérez-Pertejo and coworkers (2019) to target *L. infantum* TopIB.

A set of hybrids of different tetrahydroquinolines and quinolines derivatives
carrying phosphorus-containing substituents were assessed for antileishmanial
activity by Tejería and coworkers (2019) [93]. Most of the compounds presented
antileishmanial activity against intracellular amastigotes of *L. infantum*.
Compounds **(49)**, **(50)**, and **(51)** (Fig. **15**) had good activity maintaining a good
selective index (SI > 50) since they presented low cytotoxicity on uninfected
macrophages. A higher selective index was shown for compound **(50)**, which
showed the best activity against intracellular amastigotes. Results from the

supercoiled plasmid relaxation assay showed that 1,2,3,4-tetrahydroquinollynilphospines were the most active inhibitors of LTopIB with emphasis on compound **(52)** (IC_{50} 23.64 μM) (Fig. **15**), which was also more selective over human TopIB (IC_{50} 84.56 μM).

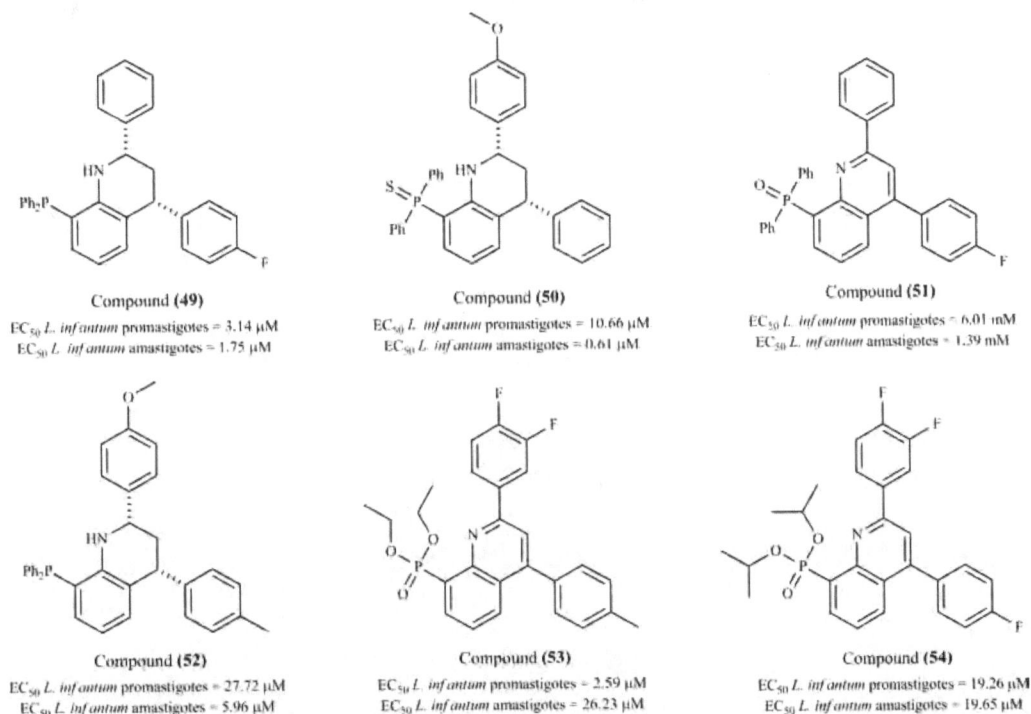

Compound **(49)**
EC_{50} *L. infantum* promastigotes = 3.14 μM
EC_{50} *L. infantum* amastigotes = 1.75 μM

Compound **(50)**
EC_{50} *L. infantum* promastigotes = 10.66 μM
EC_{50} *L. infantum* amastigotes = 0.61 μM

Compound **(51)**
EC_{50} *L. infantum* promastigotes = 6.01 mM
EC_{50} *L. infantum* amastigotes = 1.39 mM

Compound **(52)**
EC_{50} *L. infantum* promastigotes = 27.72 μM
EC_{50} *L. infantum* amastigotes = 5.96 μM

Compound **(53)**
EC_{50} *L. infantum* promastigotes = 2.59 μM
EC_{50} *L. infantum* amastigotes = 26.23 μM

Compound **(54)**
EC_{50} *L. infantum* promastigotes = 19.26 μM
EC_{50} *L. infantum* amastigotes = 19.65 μM

Fig. (15). Chemical structure of the tetrahydroquinolines with antileishmanial potential identified by Tejería and coworkers (2019) and Selas and colleagues (2021).

Using a CPT-hTopIB-DNA ternary complex as a template, the authors performed molecular docking to assess the binding modes of the compounds. Compound **(52)** had an excellent binding affinity energy of -8.699 kcal/mol with its C4-substituent directed to the minor groove of DNA and interacting with base pairs through π-stacking interactions. The C2-methoxyphenyl group interacted with Glu[356] and made π-stacking interactions with the DNA. Furthermore, its diphenylphosphine group was oriented towards the major groove and interacted with some hydrophobic amino acids such as Ile[424], Ile[427], Ala[351], and Leu[429]. On the other hand, in another work, Selas and colleagues (2021) [94] showed the compounds **(53)** and **(54)** Fig. **(15)** presented a higher percentage of inhibition of LTopIB (77.02% and 73.27%, respectively).

Several existing compounds, such as antitumor drugs, are being repurposed for leishmaniasis treatment. In this way, Fernandez-Rubio *et al.* (2023) [95] evaluated the antileishmanial activity of previously reported selenium derivatives. The compounds were first submitted for an analysis of their druggability and cytotoxicity. The most promising and less toxic compounds were assessed for their *in vitro* activity against promastigotes and intracellular amastigotes of *L. major* and *L. amazonensis*. NISC-6 **(55)** (Fig. **16**) was the parasites' most active compound against amastigotes and promastigotes. Furthermore, the authors tested the inhibitory activity of this compound on *L. major* Top II through the precipitation of induced cleavable complexes after adding potassium chloride (KCl) solution. NISC-6 **(55)** significantly enhanced the formation of cleavable complexes. Finally, the increased number of cells in the G_1 phase supported the cell cycle arrest effect of NISC-6 **(55)**.

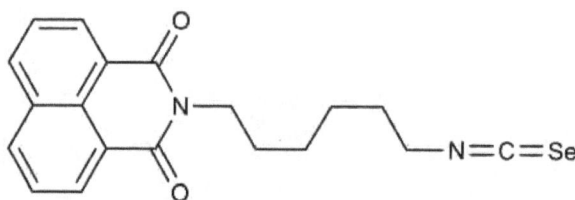

NISC-6 **(55)**

IC_{50} *L. major* promastigotes = 0.03 μM

IC_{50} *L. amazonensis* promastigotes = 0.2 μM

Fig. (16). The Chemical structure of NISC-6 is a selenium derivative with potential antileishmanial activity.

Alkyl and aryl derivatives of p-coumaric acid, a hydroxycinnamic acid, were assessed for their *in vitro* activity against *L. braziliensis* amastigotes and *P. falciparum* by Lopes and coworkers (2020) [96]. Compounds **(56-61)** (Fig. **17**) were the most active against *L. braziliensis*, but none of the compounds presented significant activity against *P. falciparum*. Activity decreased with increased branching, as seen with compounds **(59, 60)** and **(62, 63)**. Being the most active of the set, the researchers submitted compound **(60)** to a molecular docking analysis to see its potential targets in the parasite. Results suggested *Leishmania* topoisomerase II as one of the possible targets of the molecule, and the best compound interacted with the Top II with a −6.15 kcal/mol binding energy. The hexyl group of compound **(60)** fit in the bottom of the binding cavity of the enzyme, while the phenyl group interacted with the entrance residues.

An investigation of the antileishmanial activity of spiroacridine compounds with potential antitumor and topoisomerase inhibitory action was performed by

Almeida and colleagues (2021) [97]. In this way, AMTAC 11 **(64)** (Fig. **18A**) was the most active compound against *L. infantum* promastigotes (EC_{50} = 0.974 µg/mL), possibly due to the electron-donor effect of the *p*-dimethylamino group attached to the phenyl ring. Its planarity and polar character make acridine a promising scaffold for molecules capable of intercalating the DNA. Therefore, molecular docking was performed using LdTopI-DNA as a template, revealing the potential of AMTAC 11 **(64)** in inhibiting the enzyme, and this is one of the possible mechanisms that explain its antileishmanial activity. Among the compounds, AMTAC 11 **(64)** had the highest fitness score of 62.99. Docking also revealed essential interactions, such as H-bonds between the compound and Lys[211] and Arg[190]. Furthermore, low cytotoxicity was observed in PBMC cells treated with different concentrations of AMTAC 11 **(64)** (EC_{50} > 100 µg/mL; SI > 102.67).

Compound	R	EC_{50} (µM)	
		L. braziliensis amastigotes	*P. falciparum*
(56)	-CH₃	8.28	
(57)	-CH₂CH₃	4.91	
(58)	-CH₂CH₂CH₃	6.3	~ 60
(59)	-CH₂CH₂CH(CH₃)₂	6.02	
(60)	-CH₂(CH₂)₄CH₃	4.14	
(61)	-CH₂(CH₂)₁₀CH₃	16.34	

Compound	R	EC_{50} (µM)	
		L. braziliensis amastigotes	*P. falciparum*
(62)	-CH₃	5.69	> 80
(63)	-CH(CH₃)₂	11.21	

Fig. (17). Chemical structures of the alkyl and aryl derivatives of *p*-coumaric acid designed by Lopes and colleagues (2020).

Some HIV-1 protease inhibitors demonstrate antileishmanial and antimalarial activity. Therefore, Roy and coworkers (2021) [98] assessed the inhibitory activity of Amprenavir **(65)** (Fig. **18B**) on *L. donovani* topoisomerase I. Firstly, it was tested for its antileishmanial effect *in vitro* using *L. donovani* AG83 strain promastigotes. Amprenavir **(65)** exhibited 95% growth inhibition of amastigotes at 20 µM after 24h of incubation. The same concentration was acceptable in the cytotoxicity assay, maintaining more than 80% of THP-1 macrophage viability. Furthermore, Amprenavir **(65)** at 20 µM inhibited by 90% the catalytic activity of LdTopI in the simultaneous plasmid DNA relaxation assay as well as stabilized 95% cleavable complex of DNA-LdTopIB, suggesting it acts as a topoisomerase poison. Molecular docking analysis revealed several non-covalent interactions between Amprenavir **(65)** and the active site residues of LdTopI. Its sulphonamide group interacted with Tyr[222] and Lys[353] by H-bond, whereas aminophenyl, oxolan, and phenyl moieties established connections mainly through hydrophobic interactions.

Erigeron multiradiatus (Asteraceae) is a medicinal plant used in traditional medicine to treat several conditions due to its antimicrobial, antidiabetic, and anti-inflammatory properties. The essential oil of *E. multiradiatus* is a source of several bioactive compounds, such as Matricaria ester and other oxygenated terpenoids. The antileishmanial activity of trans-2-cis-8-matriarca ester **(66)** (Fig. **18C**) was assessed by Pandey and colleagues (2019) [99] as well as the mode of action through *in silico* screening of the phytoconstituents of the essential oil. The matriarca ester inhibited the growth of *L. donovani* promastigotes and amastigotes with IC_{50} of 55.09 and 61.2 μM, respectively. The compound reduced 50% of the peritoneal hamster macrophages at a much higher concentration (CC_{50} 609 μM). Therefore, a reasonable selective index > 10. Molecular docking analysis revealed that this compound could target the *L. donovani* DNA Topoisomerase II with a binding energy score of -3.741 kcal/mol and can be explored in further works.

Through high throughput screening (HTS), selective inhibitors of LdTopIB were selected, and their antileishmanial activity was assessed by Lee *et al.* (2021) [87]. Since LdTopIB is a bi-subunit enzyme, the motif containing the residues responsible for uniting both subunits was identified and used as a template in the DNA relaxation assay. Thus, the compounds LRT-TP-85 **(67)** and LRT-TP-94 **(68)** (Fig. **18D**) exhibited good inhibition of DNA relaxation with no inhibition of human TopIB at the concentrations tested. LRT-TP-85 **(67)** and LRT-TP–94 **(68)** inhibited LdTopIB with IC_{50} values of 1.3 and 2.9 μM, respectively. Both compounds are pyridine rings carrying a 4-(3-(piperidin-1-ylmethyl)phenyl) substituent. Molecular docking analysis revealed the presence of an electrostatic interaction between the protonated nitrogen atom of the piperidine ring of both compounds and the hydroxyl group of Ser[415] residue in the LdTopIB. Moreover, an H-bond interaction between the pyrazole ring and Asp[419] and a cation-π interaction between pyridine and Arg[274] was observed. Finally, both compounds were active against *L. donovani* promastigotes, exhibiting activity comparable to the current antileishmanial drug miltefosine.

Pyrimidine Synthesis Pathway

Pyrimidine biosynthesis is essential in every living organism, as it provides precursors of RNA and DNA nucleotide, glycoprotein synthesis, and membrane lipids, which are conducted by *de novo* and rescue pathways. *De novo* pathway involves six sequential enzymatic reactions, in which driidoorotate dehydrogenase (DHODH) is involved in the fourth step and is the only redox reaction in the cascade. This flavoenzyme catalyzes the oxidation of (S)-dihydroorotate to orotate in a cycle comprising two half-reactions. The first half-reaction is similar in humans and *Trypanosoma cruzi*. In the second half-reaction, the products differ (succinate in the parasite and ubiquinol in humans). Among all the fundamental mechanisms, nucleotide biosynthesis is distinct in most trypanosomatids, species of *Leishmania* and *Trypanosoma*, because they are unable to synthesize purines *de novo*, except for *T. cruzi*, which has both pathways and can be explored in further works of most selective drugs [100, 101].

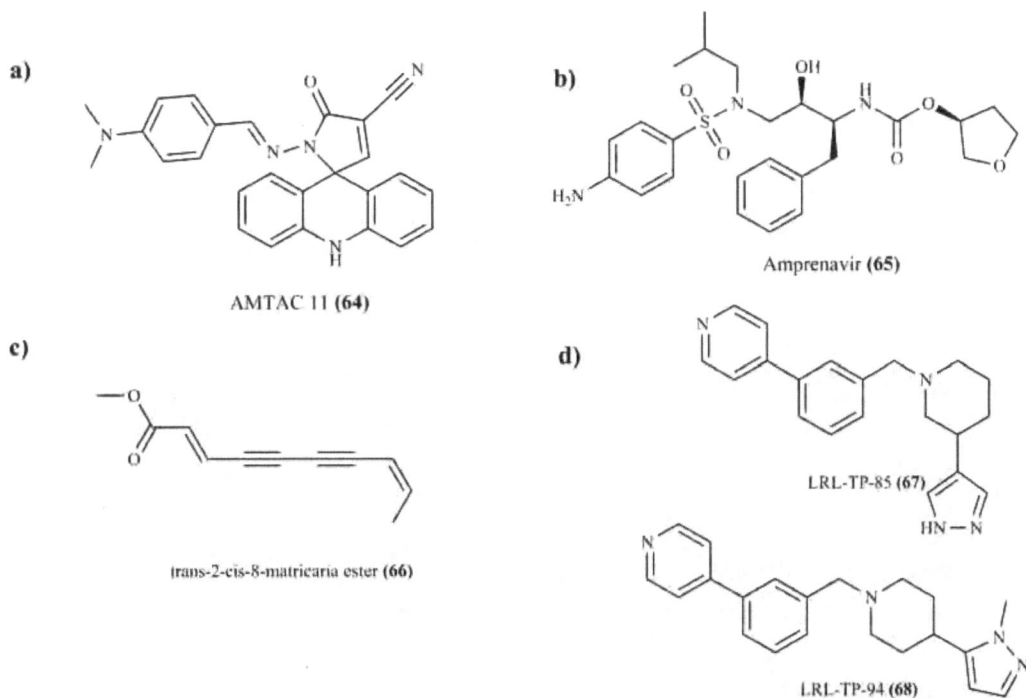

Fig. (18). Chemical structure of *A)* AMTAC 11 (**64**) investigated by Almeida and coworkers (2021); *B)* Amprenavir (**65**); *C)* trans-2-cis-matricaria ester (**66**) isolated by Pandey and colleagues (2019) from *E. multiradiatus*; and *D)* LRT-TP-85 (**67**) and LRT-TP-94 (**68**) from a screening developed by Lee and coworkers (2021).

DHODH is subdivided into classes 1 (cytosolic) and 2 (membrane-bound) according to sequence similarity, location, and substrate preference. Class 1 DHODH can be found in several living beings, such as *Trypanosoma cruzi*, *Lactococcus lactis*, *Leishmania major*, *Leishmania donovani*, *Leishmania braziliensis*, *Trypanosoma brucei* and *Streptococcus mutans*. In contrast, class 2 DHODH is found in other parasites, such as *Plasmodium falciparum*, and in humans. Metabolic pathways are attractive targets for drug development due to the selective inhibition of DHODH, which is essential for the *de novo* biosynthesis of pyrimidine and the cellular redox balance of the protozoan, directly affecting its survival, and can be considered an attractive therapeutic target against leishmaniasis and trypanosomiasis [100, 102]. Fig. (**19**) shows the DHODH pathway.

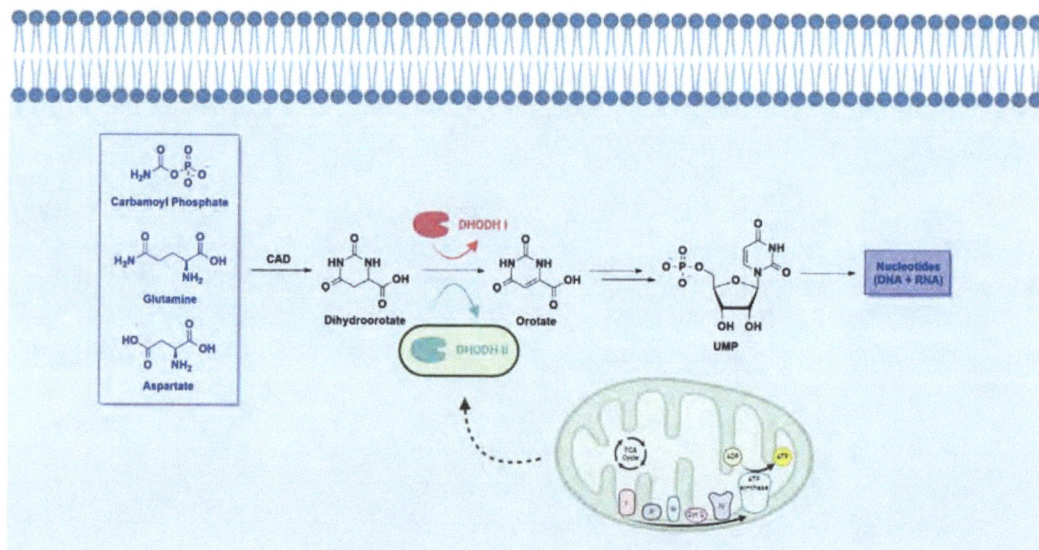

Fig. (19). DHODH pathway as the primary target related to the Pyrimidine.

Some works have allowed the co-crystallography of DHODH from *Leishmania* with its substrates [103, 104], enabling the observation of the active site in which orotate and fumarate bind (Lm-DHODH-ORO, PDB id: 3GZ3) and (Lm-DHODH fum, PDB id: 3TQ0). However, there are few studies involving *Leishmania* DOHDH, which is a limitation in finding drugs that act through this pathway.

The general structure of DHODH from *Trypanosoma cruzi* is very similar to that of other class 1A DHODHs. Several amino acid residues, including Lys[43], Asn[67], and Asn[194], form H-bonds with ORO and are essential for substrate binding. Pharmacophore characteristics were performed using the fragment molecular orbital (FMO) method, and the interaction energy between TcDHODH, ORO, and oxonate (a competitive inhibitor of DHODH) was analyzed. From the crystallographic coordinates, FMO analysis confirmed that all H-bonds between ORO and Lys[43], Asn[67], and Asn[194] are essential and significantly contribute to ligand binding. These results suggest that *Tc*DHODH inhibitors should preferably contain an aromatic moiety functionalized with H-bond donors or acceptors, which is necessary to form additional hydrogen bonds and hydrophobic interactions. Furthermore, an interaction between Lys^{214} and an H-bond accepting functional group was predicted. Thus, it was found that interactions with the aforementioned amino acid residues are fundamental in anti-Chagas drugs [100, 105].

Inaoka and collaborators [106] observed the active site of *T.cruzi* DHODH is small, and its loop is highly flexible (residues from Leu^{128} to Asp^{142}), which makes it challenging to discover potent inhibitors. Cheleski *et al.* (2010) [65] performed additional topological studies to identify novel regions capable of interacting with ligands beyond the active site, thereby expanding the scope for designing selective ligands. The author's analysis identified four new regions capable of accommodating ligands, which affect the catalytic capacity of the enzyme. Despite the few molecular modeling studies carried out against *Tc*DHODH, the reported inhibitors' primary binding mode was in the substrate's active site [101]. All compounds studied for this target must present interactions with catalytic residues of the enzyme, such as Gly^{70}, Lys^{43}, Asp^{53}, Asn^{47}, and Asn^{194}.

DHDOH from *Plasmodium falciparum*, although class 2, is also an exciting target, as it has a vital function in the *de novo* synthesis of pyrimidine. The *Pf*DHODH crystal structures of PfDHODH are different from the structures of DHODH in humans, and the binding sites of the inhibitors are different. *Pf*DHODH has a hydrophobic *N*-terminal extension that is quite a sequence variable and a conserved α/β barrel structure consisting of eight β-sheets wrapped by eight α-helices. Due to the packaging, there is a tunnel-shaped pouch. The enzyme's active site is inside the barrel, containing a flavin mononucleotide (FMN)-binding site. Enzyme inhibitors may bind to the enzyme barrel, blocking access to the substrate or the tunnel-like pocket near the *N*-terminal extension and blocking the passage of electrons from FMN and CoQ. Three areas constitute the tunnel binding site: a hydrophilic pocket containing His^{185} and Arg^{265} residues; a hydrophobic pocket containing the fundamental aromatic residues Phe^{188} and Phe^{227}, involved in inhibitor binding; and a small hydrophobic channel that leads to the FMN and is lined by Val^{532}, Ile^{272}, and Ile^{263} [107, 108].

Pippione and colleagues (2019) [109] synthesized a series with a 3-hydroxypyrazol-4-carboxylic acid modulation, a scaffold previously explored for *Pf*DHODH inhibition. The authors initially carried out a recombinant *Pf*DHODH assay to evaluate the inhibitory activity of the compounds. They found that the presence of the 3-hydroxy and 4-carboxy functions in the pyrazole ring is essential for the activity since compounds with this characteristic presented reduced IC_{50} values, such as compound **(69)** Fig. **(20)**, which presented the closest value to the DSM1 reference inhibitor (IC_{50}= 2.8 and 0.065 μM, respectively).

works [18, 45]. Given the urgent need for new antichagasic therapeutics, several strategies, such as computer-aided drug design, have proven critical in identifying and characterizing cruzain inhibitors as promising potential as antichagasic compounds [46].

Other diseases are related to liver flukes, for example, and although they cause a significant global burden of disease, therapeutic options are limited, and vaccines are not expected to be available soon due to the complex immunological context and low economic incentive [47]. Although millions of people are infected with Helminths, there are limited tools to control infections caused by these parasitic worms [30]. Of the 1,556 new chemical entities marketed between 1975 and 2004, only four drugs (albendazole, oxamniquine, praziquantel, and ivermectin) were developed to treat helminthiasis [48].

Considering that there are still no vaccine available for these diseases, preventive actions and pharmacological interventions are the current approaches for their treatment. However, the drugs available to treat these diseases have several limitations, such as low efficacy, high toxicity, adverse reactions, prolonged administration regimens, and also drug resistance, driving the constant search for new targets and therapeutic options [25].

Research in Drug Design and Development Focuses on New Targets

The lack of investment in research and development for the treatment and prevention of NTDs contributes to the greater invisibility of these diseases. Less than 0.5% of drugs and vaccines in the discovery phase and clinical trials proceed to market launch and target NTDs [24]. Therefore, initiatives all around the world have been pivotal in the fight against NTDs [49].

Advances in the knowledge of parasite biology have revealed essential enzymes involved in the replication, survival, and pathogenicity of *Leishmania* and *Trypanosoma* species and can be explored to discover new drugs [25]. Currently, only two drugs are marketed for treating Chagas diseases in the acute phase. Two of the most promising targets against this disease are trypanothione reductase (TR) and iron-containing superoxide dismutase (Fe-SOD), which protect the parasite against oxidative damage by reactive oxygen species [50].

One of the targets used is the enzyme 3′,5′-cyclic nucleotide phosphodiesterase (PDE) type B1 from the *T. brucei* parasite (TbrPDEB1). Another target for *T. brucei* is methionyl-tRNA synthetase (MetRS), which has already been validated in a mouse model. Other examples of target-based assays are sterol 14-α-demethylase inhibitors, which are active against Chagas diseases, and *Leishmania* casein kinase 1.2 (LmCK1.2), an exoprotein kinase that has recently been shown

The compounds were also evaluated for hDHODH inhibitory activity to verify selectivity between species, and all showed $IC_{50} > 200$ µM, demonstrating high selectivity for *Pf*DHODH. With an emphasis on compound **(69)**, which presented the highest hDHODH/*Pf*DHODH activity ratio (ratio >71). The authors also determined the crystal structure of *Pf*DHODH with compound 7e, with a resolution of 1.98 Å (PDB id: 6I4B), and it was found that the replacement of residues Ala[59] and Pro[364] in hDHODH with bulkier residues: Phe[188] and Met[536], found in *Pf*DHODH, makes the pocket inaccessible in hDHODH. Compound 7e occupies this pocket formed by Phe[171], Leu[172], Leu[187], Phe[188] and Met[536]. These interactions are essential for selectivity since the biggest differences in the hDHODH and *Pf*DHODH enzymes are found in this region [109].

Using molecular hybridization, Silveira *et al.* (2021) [110] designed and synthesized different series of *Pf*DHODH inhibitors, of which triazolopyrimidine derivatives were considered the most potent. The [1, 2, 4]triazolo [1,5-α]pyrimidine structure is a privileged scaffold against DHODH enzymes. Therefore, the hDHODH and *Pf*DHODH inhibitory activities of the triazolopyrimidine derivatives were evaluated. The evaluation of the enzymatic inhibitory activity was carried out in two stages. The first involved evaluating each compound's inhibitory activity against hDHODH and *Pf*DHODH enzymes at a single concentration (50 µM). The compounds that inhibited the enzymatic activity with ≥ 80% inhibition were evaluated in a second step. In this stage, IC_{50} values against *Pf*DHODH were determined.

The IC_{50} values of the [1, 2, 4]triazolo [1,5-α]pyrimidine derivatives spanned from 0.08 to 1.3 µM, of which compound **(70)** Fig. **(20)** presented an IC_{50} of 0.08 µM, being 8.75-fold more potent than prototype without replacement (Ic50= 0.70 µM), whose enzymatic assay was carried out in another work [111]. The compounds did not show significant inhibition against the hDHODH enzyme (0-30% at 50 µM), indicating selectivity for *Pf*DHODH. The results found by the authors suggest that this is the mechanism of action of this new [1, 2, 4]triazolo [1,5-α]pyrimidine derivatives.

Mitochondrial Alterations

Parasite mitochondria are essential targets for antiparasitic drugs because of the occurrence of glycolysis in these organelles. Drugs that act on this pathway can interfere with metabolism, altering the enzymatic function or mitochondrial membrane potential, resulting in a lack of energy [112]. Trypanosomatids have only one mitochondrion along their body, and a region known as the kinetoplast contains 30% of their DNA material (k-DNA). Mitochondria are essential in regulating diverse physiological processes such as bioenergetics, ATP generation, control of redox metabolism, calcium homeostasis, growth, differentiation, and biosynthesis pathways [113 - 115].

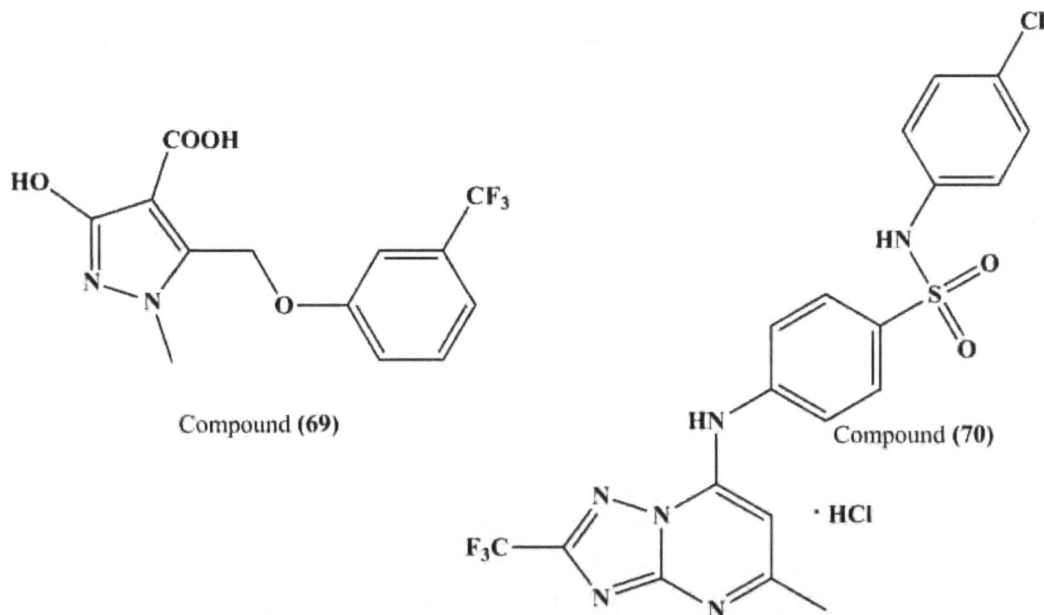

Fig. (20). Chemical structure of compounds **(69)** and **(70)** as promising inhibitors of parasitic DHODH.

Dysfunctions in this organelle can lead to leakage in the electron transport chain (ETC) and accelerate the generation of reactive oxygen species (ROS), such as superoxide anions, hydrogen peroxide, and hydroxyl radicals. Interruption in mitochondrial functioning can quickly result in a decline in the parasite's bioenergetic metabolism, reducing ATP synthesis and cell death [115]. Thus, drugs that alter the mitochondrial functions of trypanosomatids, such as *Leishmania* and *Trypanosoma*, are of great pharmaceutical interest (Fig. **21**).

In the study carried out by Glanzmann *et al.* (2021), hybridization between two rings whose derivatives already had activity was favorable. The authors synthesized a hybrid of 4-aminoquinoline and 1,2,3-triazole and tested it against *Leishmania amazonensis*, in which the compound presented IC_{50} values lower than non-hybrid precursors, in addition, to be promising in the membrane potential analysis assay, indicating an attractive strategy to develop new antileishmanial drugs [115]. Similarly, Santana-Filho *et al.* (2023) designed indole scaffolds merged with selenium functional groups in the C-3 position of the indole ring based on structures already related in the literature with antileishmanial activity [116].

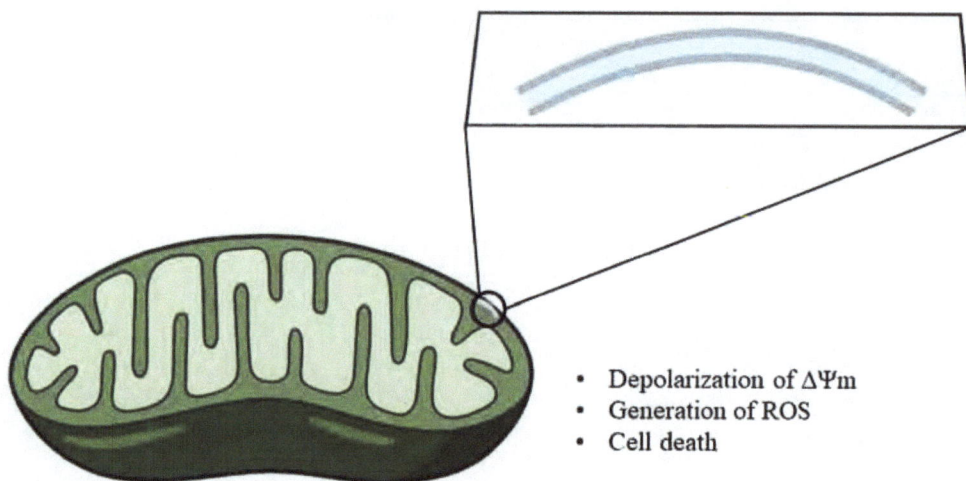

Mitochondrion of *Trypanosoma* spp. and *Leishmania* spp.

Fig. (21). Mitochondrial alterations explored to discover new drugs against trypanosomatids.

Some authors suggest that nitro substituent (-NO$_2$) compounds confer effective antiparasitic potential against *Leishmania*. The nitro group in these compounds is called parasitophorous, which is critical for the antiparasitic action [117 - 120]. Several antiparasitic drugs, such as metronidazole, tinidazole, benznidazole, and nifurtimox, present the process of enzymatic bioreduction of the nitro group as a possible mechanism of action, resulting in the formation of free radicals with more evident toxicity for bacterial and parasitic cells [121, 122].

Regarding the molecules evaluated against *Leishmania* species, some are more prominent, and Glanzmann and colleagues (2021) [115] synthesized and evaluated a set of quinoline derivatives compounds: 1,2,3-triazole derivatives and quinoline-triazole hybrids in the promastigote and amastigote stage of *Leishmania amazonensis*, in which analog **(71)** (Fig. **22**) stood out in all assays. Derivative **(71)** showed the best antileishmanial effect, with IC$_{50}$ values of 5.7 µM (against promastigotes) and 1.1 µM (against amastigotes), being better than the reference drug miltefosine (IC$_{50}$ of 22.0 µM and 4.2 µM, respectively). Furthermore, compound **(71)** showed moderate cytotoxicity in murine peritoneal macrophages, with a CC$_{50}$ of 18.2 µM and a selectivity index (SI) of at least 16 times more potency against the amastigote forms of *L. amazonensis* than against the host cell. Thus, its mechanism of action was investigated based on the analysis of the depolarization of the mitochondrial membrane potential ($\Delta\Psi$m) of *L. amazonensis* and the induction of oxidative stress.

Analysis of mitochondrial membrane potential ($\Delta\Psi$m) by flow cytometry, using the fluorescent marker JC-1, demonstrated that compound **(71)** provided a decrease in $\Delta\Psi$m, indicated by the increase in green fluorescence, which corresponded to 5.2% and 46.2% of parasites after treatment with 5 and 10 μM of compound **(71)**, respectively. In addition, the relative value of $\Delta\Psi$m was quantified using the ratio of red and green fluorescence, in which the JC-1 ratio was 42.09 in the untreated control and decreased to 18.1 and 1.21 in the groups treated with 5 and 10 μM of compound **(71)**, respectively. This result was supported by the fluorimetric result using the Mitotracker red, in which the compound showed a significant reduction of $\Delta\Psi$m of 23.9% (5 μM) and 37.6% (10 μM). In contrast, in promastigotes incubated with FCCP, a known respiratory chain inhibitor (5 μM), there was a 55.6% reduction in $\Delta\Psi$m. Thus, compound **(71)** affected the mitochondrial function of *L. amazonensis* through the marked decrease in its hydrogen membrane potential, which also induced a significant increase in the generation of ROS [115].

Gouveia *et al.* (2022) [120] synthesized and evaluated thiazolidine derivatives in different stages of *Leishmania infantum*. The authors carried out cytotoxicity tests on the promastigote forms of *Leishmania in vitro* to obtain compounds that showed leishmanicidal activity and observed that the results were concentration-dependent. These values were evaluated according to the scale described by Upegui *et al.* (2014) [123], in which compounds with an $IC_{50} < 20$ μM were considered active, compounds that exhibited an IC_{50} between 20 and 50 μM were moderately active, and compounds that presented an $IC_{50} > 50$ μM were considered inactive.

It was found that the most promising compound against antipromastigote activity was compound **(72)** (Fig. **22**) ($IC_{50}= 0.42 \pm 0.15$). Therefore, a kinetic study was carried out on the variation of its concentration (0.105, 0.21, 0.42, 0.84, and 1.68 μM) with time (0, 24, 48, and 72 h) to obtain the best condition for the inhibition of promastigote forms. The authors observed that in the first 24 hours of treatment, there was a significant leishmanicidal action in 48 hours of treatment, concentrations of 1.68, 0.84, and 0.42 μM promoted 70% inhibition. In the period of 72 h, inhibition of around 95% was observed for the three concentrations, showing that in 72 h, there is no significant difference between the highest concentrations (1.68, 0.84, and 0.42 μM).

Considering the antipromastigote potential of the compound **(72)**, it was selected to carry out microscopy experiments, including Transmission Electron Microscopy (TEM), to investigate the possible intracellular targets of the compound and its action on the parasite's cell membrane. The effects of this compound were evaluated using its IC_{50} and double the $IC_{50}= 0.42$ and 0.84 μM, respectively. TEM analysis showed that, in the untreated group, the promastigote forms of *L. infantum* had standard shape and morphology and well-preserved organelles and cytoplasm, containing a central cytoplasmic nucleus, a single mitochondrion containing a kinetoplast and flagellar pocket. The control group with cells treated with Amphotericin B, a standard drug for treating leishmaniasis, showed mitochondrial swelling and the presence of electron-dense and electrotransparent regions. Cells treated with 0.42 μM of compound (72) showed intense vacuolization, while treatment with 0.84 μM caused intense mitochondrial swelling and cellular disorganization with nucleus migration towards the periphery. The compound was responsible for causing several structural changes in the promastigote forms of *L. infantum*, like other studies on different species of *Leishmania*, indicating its effectiveness in the action of these parasites.

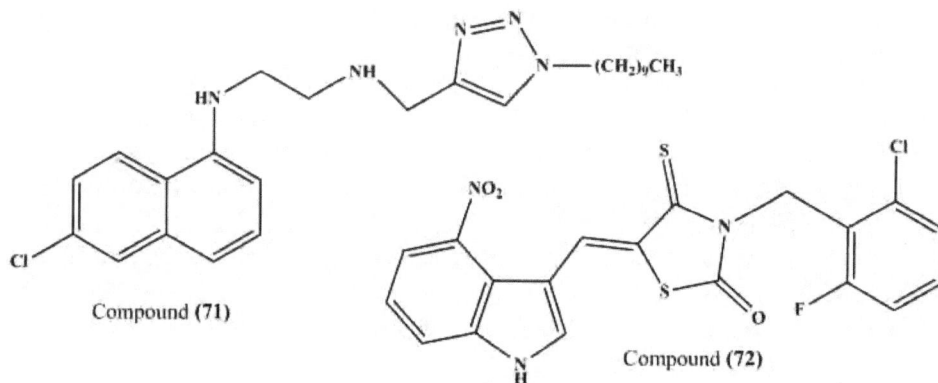

Fig. (22). Chemical structure of the compounds (71) and (72) related to the mitochondrial alterations as the antiparasitic mechanism.

Cytotoxicity assays of compound (72) on amastigotes were performed using Amphotericin B as a control. The results were concentration-dependent, and IC_{50} values were also classified according to the scale described by Upegui *et al.* (2014) [123]. Once again, compound (72) presented an IC_{50} of 0.65 ± 0.01, being classified as active. In addition, the compound's selectivity index (SI) and the specificity index (IPS) for the promastigote and amastigote forms were also determined. SPI values > 2.0 indicate that the compound was more active for the amastigote forms. Values < 0.4 suggest that the compound was more effective for the promastigote forms, and values between 0.4 and 2.0 indicate activity for both stages. Among the active compounds evaluated for anti amastigote activity, compound (72) presented a selectivity index close to the standard drug amphotericin B (13.11 and 13.48, respectively). Furthermore, according to the scale proposed by Don and Ioset (2014) [124], this compound was considered active for both parasite forms, obtaining an SPI of 0.65.

Over the years, several promising drug targets have been explored against NTDs, and the drugs that interfere with mitochondrial alterations and pyrimidine synthesis pathways provide new horizons in the drug discovery process. In addition, the targeting of nitroreductases shows the importance of its metabolic pathway in the drug design and discovery process.

CONCLUSION

Neglected tropical diseases (NTDs) remain a serious public health problem, and more investment is needed to contain these agents. Despite preventive measures and vector control, these diseases continue to increase worldwide, and efforts to discover new drugs are necessary to protect the population. Therefore, new targets are constantly explored to be validated and as potential in the development of drugs against NTDs. Among them, those presented in this chapter stand out, such as *N*-myristoyltransferase, nitroreductases, topoisomerases, pyrimidine synthesis pathway, and mitochondrial alterations, explored for different parasites and can offer great opportunities in the identification and development of drugs. Interestingly, the parasitic NMT stands out here, exploited against leishmania, Chagas, and malaria. Inhibitors such as thienopyrimidine, thiazoles, and metal complexes have shown their importance, and their scaffolds can be explored in future developments. We hope that our chapter can inspire researchers around the world and serve as a guide in discovering an innovative and affordable drug that can stop these threatening agents.

ACKNOWLEDGMENTS

The authors thank the Coordenação de Aperfeiçoamento de Pessoal de Nível Superior (CAPES), the National Council for Scientific and Technological Development (CNPq), and Fundação de Apoio à Pesquisa do Estado da Paraíba the National (FAPESQ) for their support to the Brazilian Postgraduate Programs.

REFERENCES

[1]   Nascimento IJ dos S. Cavalcanti M de AT, de Moura RO. Exploring N-myristoyl transferase as a promising drug target against parasitic neglected tropical diseases. Eur J Med Chem 2023; 258: 115550.
[http://dx.doi.org/10.1016/j.ejmech.2023.115550] [PMID: 37336067]

[2]   Hotez PJ, Aksoy S, Brindley PJ, Kamhawi S. World neglected tropical diseases day. PLoS Negl Trop Dis 2020; 14(1): e0007999.
[http://dx.doi.org/10.1371/journal.pntd.0007999] [PMID: 31995572]

[3]   Tidman R, Abela-Ridder B, de Castañeda RR. The impact of climate change on neglected tropical diseases: a systematic review. Trans R Soc Trop Med Hyg 2021; 115(2): 147-68.
[http://dx.doi.org/10.1093/trstmh/traa192] [PMID: 33508094]

[4]   Engels D, Zhou XN. Neglected tropical diseases: an effective global response to local poverty-related disease priorities. Infect Dis Poverty 2020; 9(1): 10.

[http://dx.doi.org/10.1186/s40249-020-0630-9] [PMID: 31987053]

[5]   Rinaldo D, Perez-Saez J, Vounatsou P, Utzinger J, Arcand JL. The economic impact of schistosomiasis. Infect Dis Poverty 2021; 10(1): 134.
[http://dx.doi.org/10.1186/s40249-021-00919-z] [PMID: 34895355]

[6]   Semahegn A, Manyazewal T, Getachew E, *et al.* Burden of neglected tropical diseases and access to medicine and diagnostics in Ethiopia: a scoping review. Syst Rev 2023; 12(1): 140.
[http://dx.doi.org/10.1186/s13643-023-02302-5] [PMID: 37580784]

[7]   Klohe K, Koudou BG, Fenwick A, *et al.* A systematic literature review of schistosomiasis in urban and peri-urban settings. PLoS Negl Trop Dis 2021; 15(2): e0008995.
[http://dx.doi.org/10.1371/journal.pntd.0008995] [PMID: 33630833]

[8]   Magalhães AR, Codeço CT, Svenning JC, Escobar LE, Van de Vuurst P, Gonçalves-Souza T. Neglected tropical diseases risk correlates with poverty and early ecosystem destruction. Infect Dis Poverty 2023; 12(1): 32.
[http://dx.doi.org/10.1186/s40249-023-01084-1] [PMID: 37038199]

[9]   De Souza M, Medeiros DC, de Moura RO, dos Santos Nascimento IJ. Pharmacokinetic Limitations to Overcome and Enable K777 as a Potential Drug against Chagas Disease. Curr Pharm Des 2023; 29(30): 2359-60.
[http://dx.doi.org/10.2174/0113816128267517231010061552] [PMID: 37828665]

[10]   Banda GT, Deribe K, Davey G. How can we better integrate the prevention, treatment, control and elimination of neglected tropical diseases with other health interventions? A systematic review. BMJ Glob Health 2021; 6(10): e006968.
[http://dx.doi.org/10.1136/bmjgh-2021-006968] [PMID: 34663634]

[11]   Bodimeade C, Marks M, Mabey D. Neglected tropical diseases: elimination and eradication. Clin Med (Lond) 2019; 19(2): 157-60.
[http://dx.doi.org/10.7861/clinmedicine.19-2-157] [PMID: 30872302]

[12]   Peterson JK, Bakuza J, Standley CJ. One health and neglected tropical diseases—multisectoral solutions to endemic challenges. Trop Med Infect Dis 2020; 6(1): 4.
[http://dx.doi.org/10.3390/tropicalmed6010004] [PMID: 33383621]

[13]   Aya Pastrana N, Lazo-Porras M, Miranda JJ, Beran D, Suggs LS. Social marketing interventions for the prevention and control of neglected tropical diseases: A systematic review. PLoS Negl Trop Dis 2020; 14(6): e0008360.
[http://dx.doi.org/10.1371/journal.pntd.0008360]

[14]   Ahmed A, Aune D, Vineis P, Pescarini JM, Millett C, Hone T. The effect of conditional cash transfers on the control of neglected tropical disease: a systematic review. Lancet Glob Health 2022; 10(5): e640-8.
[http://dx.doi.org/10.1016/S2214-109X(22)00065-1] [PMID: 35427521]

[15]   José dos Santos Nascimento I, Mendonça de Aquino T, Fernando da Silva Santos-Júnior P, Xavier de Araújo-Júnior J, Ferreira da Silva-Júnior E. Molecular modeling applied to design of cysteine protease inhibitors – a powerful tool for the identification of hit compounds against neglected tropical diseases. Front. Comput. Chem 2020; pp. 63-110.
[http://dx.doi.org/10.2174/9789811457791120050004]

[16]   Porta EOJ, Kalesh K, Steel PG. Navigating drug repurposing for Chagas disease: advances, challenges, and opportunities. Front Pharmacol 2023; 14: 1233253.
[http://dx.doi.org/10.3389/fphar.2023.1233253] [PMID: 37576826]

[17]   dos Santos Nascimento IJ, de Aquino TM, da Silva-Júnior EF. Cruzain and rhodesain inhibitors: last decade of advances in seeking for new compounds against american and african trypanosomiases. Curr Top Med Chem 2021; 21(21): 1871-99.
[http://dx.doi.org/10.2174/18734294MTE10MTEoz] [PMID: 33797369]

[18]   dos Santos Nascimento IJ, Santana Gomes JN, de Oliveira Viana J. de Medeiros e Silva YMS, Barbosa EG, de Moura RO. The power of molecular dynamics simulations and their applications to discover cysteine protease inhibitors. Mini Rev Med Chem 2023; 23.
[http://dx.doi.org/10.2174/1389557523666230901152257] [PMID: 37680157]

[19]   Nascimento IJS, de Aquino TM, da Silva-Júnior EF. The new era of drug discovery: The power of computer-aided drug design (CADD). Lett Drug Des Discov 2022; 19(11): 951-5.
[http://dx.doi.org/10.2174/1570180819666220405225817]

[20]   Breslin W, Pham D. Machine learning and drug discovery for neglected tropical diseases. BMC Bioinformatics 2023; 24(1): 165.
[http://dx.doi.org/10.1186/s12859-022-05076-0] [PMID: 37095460]

[21]   Albino SL, da Silva Moura WC, Reis MML, *et al.* ACW-02 an acridine triazolidine derivative presents antileishmanial activity mediated by dna interaction and immunomodulation. Pharmaceuticals (Basel) 2023; 16(2): 204.
[http://dx.doi.org/10.3390/ph16020204] [PMID: 37259353]

[22]   dos Santos Nascimento IJ, da Silva Rodrigues ÉE, da Silva MF, de Araújo-Júnior JX, de Moura RO. Advances in computational methods to discover new NS2B-NS3 inhibitors useful against dengue and zika viruses. Curr Top Med Chem 2022; 22(29): 2435-62.
[http://dx.doi.org/10.2174/1568026623666221122121330] [PMID: 36415099]

[23]   Narayanasamy S, Dat VQ, Thanh NT, *et al.* A global call for talaromycosis to be recognised as a neglected tropical disease. Lancet Glob Health 2021; 9(11): e1618-22.
[http://dx.doi.org/10.1016/S2214-109X(21)00350-8] [PMID: 34678201]

[24]   da Conceição JR, Lopes CPG, Ferreira EI, Epiphanio S, Giarolla J. Neglected tropical diseases and systemic racism especially in Brazil: from socio-economic aspects to the development of new drugs. Acta Trop 2022; 235: 106654.
[http://dx.doi.org/10.1016/j.actatropica.2022.106654] [PMID: 35988823]

[25]   Judice WAS, Ferraz LS, Lopes RM, *et al.* Cysteine proteases as potential targets for anti-trypanosomatid drug discovery. Bioorg Med Chem 2021; 46: 116365.
[http://dx.doi.org/10.1016/j.bmc.2021.116365] [PMID: 34419821]

[26]   Pradhan AU, Uwishema O, Wellington J, *et al.* Challenges of addressing neglected tropical diseases amidst the COVID-19 pandemic in Africa: A case of Chagas Disease. Ann Med Surg (Lond) 2022; 81: 104414.
[http://dx.doi.org/10.1016/j.amsu.2022.104414] [PMID: 36035600]

[27]   Cordeiro TAR, de Resende MAC, Moraes SCS, Franco DL, Pereira AC, Ferreira LF. Electrochemical biosensors for neglected tropical diseases: A review. Talanta 2021; 234: 122617.
[http://dx.doi.org/10.1016/j.talanta.2021.122617] [PMID: 34364426]

[28]   Peters L, Burkert S, Grüner B. Parasites of the liver – epidemiology, diagnosis and clinical management in the European context. J Hepatol 2021; 75(1): 202-18.
[http://dx.doi.org/10.1016/j.jhep.2021.02.015] [PMID: 33636243]

[29]   Marrone R, Mazzi C, Ouattara H, *et al.* Screening for neglected tropical diseases and other infections in african refugees and asylum seekers in rome and lazio region, Italy. Travel Med Infect Dis 2023; 56: 102649.
[http://dx.doi.org/10.1016/j.tmaid.2023.102649] [PMID: 37820947]

[30]   Lage OM, Ramos MC, Calisto R, Almeida E, Vasconcelos V, Vicente F. Current screening methodologies in drug discovery for selected human diseases. Mar Drugs 2018; 16(8): 279.
[http://dx.doi.org/10.3390/md16080279] [PMID: 30110923]

[31]   Nascimento IJ dos S, Santos MB. Marinho WPDJ, Moura RO de. Insights to design new drugs against human african trypanosomiasis targeting rhodesain using covalent docking, molecular dynamics simulations, and MM-PBSA calculations. Curr Comput Aided Drug Des 2024; 20.

[http://dx.doi.org/10.2174/0115734099274797231205055827]

[32]   Barrett MP, Croft SL. Management of trypanosomiasis and leishmaniasis. Br Med Bull 2012; 104(1): 175-96.
[http://dx.doi.org/10.1093/bmb/lds031] [PMID: 23137768]

[33]   Rassi A Jr, Rassi A, Marin-Neto JA. Chagas disease. Lancet 2010; 375(9723): 1388-402.
[http://dx.doi.org/10.1016/S0140-6736(10)60061-X] [PMID: 20399979]

[34]   Kamhawi S. The yin and yang of leishmaniasis control. PLoS Negl Trop Dis 2017; 11(4): e0005529.
[http://dx.doi.org/10.1371/journal.pntd.0005529] [PMID: 28426716]

[35]   Hernández-Bojorge SE, Blass-Alfaro GG, Rickloff MA, Gómez-Guerrero MJ, Izurieta R. Epidemiology of cutaneous and mucocutaneous leishmaniasis in Nicaragua. Parasite Epidemiol Control 2020; 11: e00192.
[http://dx.doi.org/10.1016/j.parepi.2020.e00192] [PMID: 33313430]

[36]   Ehrenberg N, Ehrenberg JP, Fontes G, *et al.* Neglected tropical diseases as a barometer for progress in health systems in times of COVID-19. BMJ Glob Health 2021; 6(4): e004709.
[http://dx.doi.org/10.1136/bmjgh-2020-004709] [PMID: 33849898]

[37]   Savoia D. Recent updates and perspectives on leishmaniasis. J Infect Dev Ctries 2015; 9(6): 588-96.
[http://dx.doi.org/10.3855/jidc.6833] [PMID: 26142667]

[38]   Tameirão CMB, Miranda LJ, Gomes MEF, D'Assumpção MGE, Junior MHG. A doença de chagas e a cardiopatia chagásica crônica: uma revisão de literatura / Chagas disease and chronic chagas heart disease: literature review. Brazilian Journal of Development 2021; 7(12): 112598-615.
[http://dx.doi.org/10.34117/bjdv7n12-172]

[39]   Hossain E, Khanam S, Dean DA, *et al.* Mapping of host-parasite-microbiome interactions reveals metabolic determinants of tropism and tolerance in Chagas disease. Sci Adv 2020; 6(30): eaaz2015.
[http://dx.doi.org/10.1126/sciadv.aaz2015] [PMID: 32766448]

[40]   Chami GF, Bundy DAP. More medicines alone cannot ensure the treatment of neglected tropical diseases. Lancet Infect Dis 2019; 19(9): e330-6.
[http://dx.doi.org/10.1016/S1473-3099(19)30160-4] [PMID: 31160190]

[41]   Bajorath J. Selected concepts and investigations in compound classification, molecular descriptor analysis, and virtual screening. J Chem Inf Comput Sci 2001; 41(2): 233-45.
[http://dx.doi.org/10.1021/ci0001482] [PMID: 11277704]

[42]   Santos-Júnior PFS, Nascimento IJS, Neto GJS, *et al.* Design of antimalarial compounds on quinoline scaffold: From plant to drug. 2023; pp. 189-237.
[http://dx.doi.org/10.2174/9789815123678123030010]

[43]   da Silva-Júnior EF, dos Santos Nascimento IJ. TNF-α inhibitors from natural compounds: An overview, CADD approaches, and their exploration for Anti-inflammatory agents. Comb Chem High Throughput Screen 2022; 25(14): 2317-40.
[http://dx.doi.org/10.2174/1386207324666210715165943] [PMID: 34269666]

[44]   Obbo CJD, Kariuki ST, Gathirwa JW, Olaho-Mukani W, Cheplogoi PK, Mwangi EM. *in vitro* antiplasmodial, antitrypanosomal and antileishmanial activities of selected medicinal plants from Ugandan flora: Refocusing into multi-component potentials. J Ethnopharmacol 2019; 229: 127-36.
[http://dx.doi.org/10.1016/j.jep.2018.09.029] [PMID: 30273736]

[45]   Silva LR, Guimarães AS, do Nascimento J, *et al.* Computer-aided design of 1,4-naphthoquinone-based inhibitors targeting cruzain and rhodesain cysteine proteases. Bioorg Med Chem 2021; 41: 116213.
[http://dx.doi.org/10.1016/j.bmc.2021.116213] [PMID: 33992862]

[46]   Durrant JD, Keränen H, Wilson BA, McCammon JA. Computational identification of uncharacterized cruzain binding sites. PLoS Negl Trop Dis 2010; 4(5): e676.
[http://dx.doi.org/10.1371/journal.pntd.0000676] [PMID: 20485483]

[47] dos Santos Nascimento IJ, Albino SL, da Silva Menezes KJ, *et al.* Targeting SmCB1: Perspectives and insights to design antischistosomal drugs. Curr Med Chem 2024; 31(16): 2264-84.
[http://dx.doi.org/10.2174/0109298673255826231011114249] [PMID: 37921174]

[48] Hotez PJ, Bottazzi ME, Kaye PM, Lee BY, Puchner KP. Neglected tropical disease vaccines: hookworm, leishmaniasis, and schistosomiasis. Vaccine 2023; 41(Suppl 2) (Suppl. 2): S176-9.
[http://dx.doi.org/10.1016/j.vaccine.2023.04.025] [PMID: 38407985]

[49] dos Santos Nascimento IJ, de Moura RO. Targeting cysteine and serine proteases to discover new drugs against neglected tropical diseases. Curr Med Chem 2024; 31(16): 2133-4.
[http://dx.doi.org/10.2174/0929867331162402141435111] [PMID: 38785275]

[50] Beltran-Hortelano I, Perez-Silanes S, Galiano S. Trypanothione reductase and superoxide dismutase as current drug targets for trypanosoma cruzi: An overview of compounds with activity against chagas disease. Curr Med Chem 2017; 24(11): 1066-138.
[http://dx.doi.org/10.2174/0929867323666161227094049] [PMID: 28025938]

[51] Lamba S, Roy A. DNA topoisomerases in the unicellular protozoan parasites: Unwinding the mystery. Biochem Pharmacol 2022; 203: 115158.
[http://dx.doi.org/10.1016/j.bcp.2022.115158] [PMID: 35780829]

[52] J B, M BM, Chanda K. An overview on the therapeutics of neglected infectious diseases—leishmaniasis and chagas diseases. Front Chem 2021; 9: 622286.
[http://dx.doi.org/10.3389/fchem.2021.622286]

[53] Ferreira LG, Andricopulo AD. Targeting cysteine proteases in trypanosomatid disease drug discovery. Pharmacol Ther 2017; 180: 49-61.
[http://dx.doi.org/10.1016/j.pharmthera.2017.06.004] [PMID: 28579388]

[54] Vaca HR, Celentano AM, Toscanini MA, *et al.* The potential for histone deacetylase (HDAC) inhibitors as cestocidal drugs. PLoS Negl Trop Dis 2021; 15(3): e0009226.
[http://dx.doi.org/10.1371/journal.pntd.0009226] [PMID: 33657105]

[55] Cirqueira ML, Bortot LO, Bolean M, *et al.* Trypanosoma cruzi nitroreductase: Structural features and interaction with biological membranes. Int J Biol Macromol 2022; 221: 891-9.
[http://dx.doi.org/10.1016/j.ijbiomac.2022.09.073] [PMID: 36100001]

[56] Poveda C, Bottazzi ME, Jones KM. Mining the metabolome for new and innovative chagas disease treatments. Trends Pharmacol Sci 2021; 42(1): 1-3.
[http://dx.doi.org/10.1016/j.tips.2020.11.007] [PMID: 33248705]

[57] Giglione C, Meinnel T. Mapping the myristoylome through a complete understanding of protein myristoylation biochemistry. Prog Lipid Res 2022; 85: 101139.
[http://dx.doi.org/10.1016/j.plipres.2021.101139] [PMID: 34793862]

[58] Dian C, Pérez-Dorado I, Rivière F, *et al.* High-resolution snapshots of human N-myristoyltransferase in action illuminate a mechanism promoting N-terminal Lys and Gly myristoylation. Nat Commun 2020; 11(1): 1132.
[http://dx.doi.org/10.1038/s41467-020-14847-3] [PMID: 32111831]

[59] Wang B, Dai T, Sun W, *et al.* Protein N-myristoylation: functions and mechanisms in control of innate immunity. Cell Mol Immunol 2021; 18(4): 878-88.
[http://dx.doi.org/10.1038/s41423-021-00663-2] [PMID: 33731917]

[60] Gunaratne RS, Sajid M, Ling IT, Tripathi R, Pachebat JA, Holder AA. Characterization of N-myristoyltransferase from Plasmodium falciparum. Biochem J 2000; 348(2): 459-63.
[http://dx.doi.org/10.1042/bj3480459] [PMID: 10816442]

[61] Wright MH, Clough B, Rackham MD, *et al.* Validation of N-myristoyltransferase as an antimalarial drug target using an integrated chemical biology approach. Nat Chem 2014; 6(2): 112-21.
[http://dx.doi.org/10.1038/nchem.1830] [PMID: 24451586]

[62]   Schlott AC, Knuepfer E, Green JL, *et al.* Inhibition of protein N-myristoylation blocks Plasmodium falciparum intraerythrocytic development, egress and invasion. PLoS Biol 2021; 19(10): e3001408.
[http://dx.doi.org/10.1371/journal.pbio.3001408] [PMID: 34695132]

[63]   Pino P, Sebastian S, Kim EA, *et al.* A tetracycline-repressible transactivator system to study essential genes in malaria parasites. Cell Host Microbe 2012; 12(6): 824-34.
[http://dx.doi.org/10.1016/j.chom.2012.10.016] [PMID: 23245327]

[64]   Price HP, Menon MR, Panethymitaki C, Goulding D, McKean PG, Smith DF. Myristoyl-CoA:protein N-myristoyltransferase, an essential enzyme and potential drug target in kinetoplastid parasites. J Biol Chem 2003; 278(9): 7206-14.
[http://dx.doi.org/10.1074/jbc.M211391200] [PMID: 12488459]

[65]   Brannigan JA, Smith BA, Yu Z, *et al.* N-myristoyltransferase from Leishmania donovani: structural and functional characterisation of a potential drug target for visceral leishmaniasis. J Mol Biol 2010; 396(4): 985-99.
[http://dx.doi.org/10.1016/j.jmb.2009.12.032] [PMID: 20036251]

[66]   Price HP, Güther MLS, Ferguson MAJ, Smith DF. Myristoyl-CoA:protein N-myristoyltransferase depletion in trypanosomes causes avirulence and endocytic defects. Mol Biochem Parasitol 2010; 169(1): 55-8.
[http://dx.doi.org/10.1016/j.molbiopara.2009.09.006] [PMID: 19782106]

[67]   Roberts AJ, Torrie LS, Wyllie S, Fairlamb AH. Biochemical and genetic characterization of *Trypanosoma cruzi N* -myristoyltransferase. Biochem J 2014; 459(2): 323-32.
[http://dx.doi.org/10.1042/BJ20131033] [PMID: 24444291]

[68]   Herrera LJ, Brand S, Santos A, *et al.* Validation of N-myristoyltransferase as potential chemotherapeutic target in mammal-dwelling stages of trypanosoma cruzi. PLoS Negl Trop Dis 2016; 10(4): e0004540.
[http://dx.doi.org/10.1371/journal.pntd.0004540] [PMID: 27128971]

[69]   šarić-et-al-2009-dual-acylation-accounts-for-the-localization-of-α19-giardin-in-the-v-ntral-flagellum-pair-of-giardia.pdf n.d.

[70]   Maurer-Stroh S, Eisenhaber B, Eisenhaber F. N-terminal N -myristoylation of proteins: refinement of the sequence motif and its taxon-specific differences 1 1Edited by J. Thornton. J Mol Biol 2002; 317(4): 523-40.
[http://dx.doi.org/10.1006/jmbi.2002.5425] [PMID: 11955007]

[71]   Alonso AM, Turowski VR, Ruiz DM, *et al.* Exploring protein myristoylation in Toxoplasma gondii. Exp Parasitol 2019; 203: 8-18.
[http://dx.doi.org/10.1016/j.exppara.2019.05.007] [PMID: 31150653]

[72]   Galvin BD, Li Z, Villemaine E, *et al.* A target repurposing approach identifies N-myristoyltransferase as a new candidate drug target in filarial nematodes. PLoS Negl Trop Dis 2014; 8(9): e3145.
[http://dx.doi.org/10.1371/journal.pntd.0003145] [PMID: 25188325]

[73]   Tate EW, Bell AS, Rackham MD, Wright MH. *N*- Myristoyltransferase as a potential drug target in malaria and leishmaniasis. Parasitology 2014; 141(1): 37-49.
[http://dx.doi.org/10.1017/S0031182013000450] [PMID: 23611109]

[74]   Mohammadi-Ghalehbin B, Shiran JA, Gholizadeh N, Razzaghi-Asl N. Synthesis, antileishmanial activity and molecular modeling of new 1-aryl/alkyl-3-benzoyl/cyclopropanoyl thiourea derivatives. Mol Divers 2023; 27(4): 1531-45.
[http://dx.doi.org/10.1007/s11030-022-10508-3] [PMID: 36001225]

[75]   Rodríguez-Hernández D, Vijayan K, Zigweid R, *et al.* Identification of potent and selective N-myristoyltransferase inhibitors of Plasmodium vivax liver stage hypnozoites and schizonts. Nat Commun 2023; 14(1): 5408.
[http://dx.doi.org/10.1038/s41467-023-41119-7] [PMID: 37669940]

[76]   Bell AS, Yu Z, Hutton JA, *et al.* Novel thienopyrimidine inhibitors of *Leishmania N* - Myristoyltransferase with on-target activity in intracellular amastigotes. J Med Chem 2020; 63(14): 7740-65.
[http://dx.doi.org/10.1021/acs.jmedchem.0c00570] [PMID: 32575985]

[77]   Khalil R, Ashraf S, Khalid A, Ul-Haq Z. Exploring novel *N* -myristoyltransferase inhibitors: A molecular dynamics simulation approach. ACS Omega 2019; 4(9): 13658-70.
[http://dx.doi.org/10.1021/acsomega.9b00843] [PMID: 31497683]

[78]   Orabi MAA, Alshahrani MM, Sayed AM, Abouelela ME, Shaaban KA, Abdel-Sattar ES. Identification of Potential *Leishmania* N-Myristoyltransferase Inhibitors from *Withania somnifera* (L.) Dunal: A Molecular Docking and Molecular Dynamics Investigation. Metabolites 2023; 13(1): 93.
[http://dx.doi.org/10.3390/metabo13010093] [PMID: 36677018]

[79]   Voak AA, Gobalakrishnapillai V, Seifert K, *et al.* An essential type I nitroreductase from Leishmania major can be used to activate leishmanicidal prodrugs. J Biol Chem 2013; 288(40): 28466-76.
[http://dx.doi.org/10.1074/jbc.M113.494781] [PMID: 23946481]

[80]   Papadopoulou MV, Bloomer WD, Rosenzweig HS, *et al.* Discovery of potent nitrotriazole-based antitrypanosomal agents: *in vitro* and *in vivo* evaluation. Bioorg Med Chem 2015; 23(19): 6467-76.
[http://dx.doi.org/10.1016/j.bmc.2015.08.014] [PMID: 26344593]

[81]   Fersing C, Boudot C, Pedron J, *et al.* 8-Aryl-6-chloro-3-nitro-2-(phenylsulfonylmethyl)imid-zo[1,2-a]pyridines as potent antitrypanosomatid molecules bioactivated by type 1 nitroreductases. Eur J Med Chem 2018; 157: 115-26.
[http://dx.doi.org/10.1016/j.ejmech.2018.07.064] [PMID: 30092366]

[82]   do Vale Chaves e Mello F, Castro Salomão Quaresma BM, Resende Pitombeira MC, *et al.* Novel nitroimidazole derivatives evaluated for their trypanocidal, cytotoxic, and genotoxic activities. Eur J Med Chem 2020; 186: 111887.
[http://dx.doi.org/10.1016/j.ejmech.2019.111887] [PMID: 31787363]

[83]   Toro PM, Peralta F, Oyarzo J, *et al.* Evaluation of trypanocidal properties of ferrocenyl and cyrhetrenyl N-acylhydrazones with pendant 5-nitrofuryl group. J Inorg Biochem 2021; 219: 111428.
[http://dx.doi.org/10.1016/j.jinorgbio.2021.111428] [PMID: 33774450]

[84]   Wilson WD, Tanious FA, Mathis A, Tevis D, Hall JE, Boykin DW. Antiparasitic compounds that target DNA. Biochimie 2008; 90(7): 999-1014.
[http://dx.doi.org/10.1016/j.biochi.2008.02.017] [PMID: 18343228]

[85]   Santos MB, de Azevedo Teotônio Cavalcanti M, de Medeiros e Silva YMS, dos Santos Nascimento IJ, de Moura RO. Overview of the new bioactive heterocycles as targeting topoisomerase inhibitors useful against colon cancer. Anticancer Agents Med Chem 2024; 24(4): 236-62.
[http://dx.doi.org/10.2174/0118715206269722231121173311] [PMID: 38038012]

[86]   Saha S, Chowdhury SR, Majumder HK. Dna topoisomerases of kinetoplastid parasites: Brief overview and recent perspectives. Curr Issues Mol Biol 2019; 31: 45-62.
[http://dx.doi.org/10.21775/cimb.031.045] [PMID: 31165719]

[87]   Lee H, Baek KH, Phan TN, *et al.* Discovery of Leishmania donovani topoisomerase IB selective inhibitors by targeting protein-protein interactions between the large and small subunits. Biochem Biophys Res Commun 2021; 569: 193-8.
[http://dx.doi.org/10.1016/j.bbrc.2021.07.019] [PMID: 34256188]

[88]   Zahara K, Panda SK, Swain SS, Luyten W. Metabolic diversity and therapeutic potential of holarrhena pubescens: An important ethnomedicinal plant. Biomolecules 2020; 10(9): 1341.
[http://dx.doi.org/10.3390/biom10091341] [PMID: 32962166]

[89]   Goel N, Gupta VK, Garg A, *et al.* Holanamine, a Steroidal Alkaloid from the Bark of *Holarrhena pubescens* Wall. ex G. Don Inhibits the Growth of *Leishmania donovani* by Targeting DNA Topoisomerase 1B. ACS Infect Dis 2023; 9(1): 162-77.

[http://dx.doi.org/10.1021/acsinfecdis.2c00562] [PMID: 36417798]

[90]   Reguera RM, Álvarez-Velilla R, Domínguez-Asenjo B, *et al*. Antiparasitic effect of synthetic aromathecins on Leishmania infantum. BMC Vet Res 2019; 15(1): 405.
[http://dx.doi.org/10.1186/s12917-019-2153-9] [PMID: 31706354]

[91]   Gutiérrez-Corbo C, Álvarez-Velilla R, Reguera RM, *et al*. Topoisomerase IB poisons induce histone H2A phosphorylation as a response to DNA damage in Leishmania infantum. Int J Parasitol Drugs Drug Resist 2019; 11: 39-48.
[http://dx.doi.org/10.1016/j.ijpddr.2019.09.005] [PMID: 31563118]

[92]   Pérez-Pertejo Y, Escudero-Martínez JM, Reguera RM, *et al*. Antileishmanial activity of terpenylquinones on Leishmania infantum and their effects on *Leishmania topoisomerase* IB. Int J Parasitol Drugs Drug Resist 2019; 11: 70-9.
[http://dx.doi.org/10.1016/j.ijpddr.2019.10.004] [PMID: 31678841]

[93]   Tejería A, Pérez-Pertejo Y, Reguera RM, *et al*. Antileishmanial activity of new hybrid tetrahydroquinoline and quinoline derivatives with phosphorus substituents. Eur J Med Chem 2019; 162: 18-31.
[http://dx.doi.org/10.1016/j.ejmech.2018.10.065] [PMID: 30408746]

[94]   Selas A, Fuertes M, Melcón-Fernández E, *et al*. Hybrid quinolinyl phosphonates as heterocyclic carboxylate isosteres: Synthesis and biological evaluation against topoisomerase 1b (top1b). Pharmaceuticals (Basel) 2021; 14(8): 784.
[http://dx.doi.org/10.3390/ph14080784] [PMID: 34451880]

[95]   Fernández-Rubio C, Larrea E, Peña Guerrero J, *et al*. Leishmanicidal activity of isoselenocyanate derivatives. Antimicrob Agents Chemother 2019; 63(2): e00904-18.
[http://dx.doi.org/10.1128/AAC.00904-18] [PMID: 30478164]

[96]   Lopes SP, Yepes LM, Pérez-Castillo Y, Robledo SM, de Sousa DP. Alkyl and aryl derivatives based on p-coumaric acid modification and inhibitory action against leishmania braziliensis and plasmodium falciparum. Molecules 2020; 25(14): 3178.
[http://dx.doi.org/10.3390/molecules25143178] [PMID: 32664596]

[97]   Almeida FS, Sousa GLS, Rocha JC, *et al*. in vitro anti-Leishmania activity and molecular docking of spiro-acridine compounds as potential multitarget agents against Leishmania infantum. Bioorg Med Chem Lett 2021; 49: 128289.
[http://dx.doi.org/10.1016/j.bmcl.2021.128289] [PMID: 34311084]

[98]   Roy A, Behera S, Mazire PH, *et al*. The HIV − 1 protease inhibitor Amprenavir targets Leishmania donovani topoisomerase I and induces oxidative stress-mediated programmed cell death. Parasitol Int 2021; 82: 102287.
[http://dx.doi.org/10.1016/j.parint.2021.102287] [PMID: 33515743]

[99]   Chandra Pandey S, Dhami DS, Jha A, Chandra Shah G, Kumar A, Samant M. Identification of *trans* - 2- *cis* -8-Matricaria-ester from the Essential Oil of *Erigeron multiradiatus* and Evaluation of Its Antileishmanial Potential by *in vitro* and in Silico Approaches. ACS Omega 2019; 4(11): 14640-9.
[http://dx.doi.org/10.1021/acsomega.9b02130] [PMID: 31528820]

[100]   Boschi D, Pippione AC, Sainas S, Lolli ML. Dihydroorotate dehydrogenase inhibitors in anti-infective drug research. Eur J Med Chem 2019; 183: 111681.
[http://dx.doi.org/10.1016/j.ejmech.2019.111681] [PMID: 31557612]

[101]   Beltran-Hortelano I, Alcolea V, Font M, Pérez-Silanes S. Examination of multiple Trypanosoma cruzi targets in a new drug discovery approach for Chagas disease. Bioorg Med Chem 2022; 58: 116577.
[http://dx.doi.org/10.1016/j.bmc.2021.116577] [PMID: 35189560]

[102]   Annoura T, Nara T, Makiuchi T, Hashimoto T, Aoki T. The origin of dihydroorotate dehydrogenase genes of kinetoplastids, with special reference to their biological significance and adaptation to anaerobic, parasitic conditions. J Mol Evol 2005; 60(1): 113-27.
[http://dx.doi.org/10.1007/s00239-004-0078-8] [PMID: 15696374]

[103] Cordeiro AT, Feliciano PR, Pinheiro MP, Nonato MC. Crystal structure of dihydroorotate dehydrogenase from Leishmania major. Biochimie 2012; 94(8): 1739-48.
[http://dx.doi.org/10.1016/j.biochi.2012.04.003] [PMID: 22542640]

[104] Reis RAG, Lorenzato E Jr, Silva VC, Nonato MC. Recombinant production, crystallization and crystal structure determination of dihydroorotate dehydrogenase from *Leishmania (Viannia) braziliensis*. Acta Crystallogr F Struct Biol Commun 2015; 71(5): 547-52.
[http://dx.doi.org/10.1107/S2053230X15000886] [PMID: 25945707]

[105] Yoshino R, Yasuo N, Inaoka DK, *et al.* Pharmacophore modeling for anti-Chagas drug design using the fragment molecular orbital method. PLoS One 2015; 10(5): e0125829.
[http://dx.doi.org/10.1371/journal.pone.0125829] [PMID: 25961853]

[106] Inaoka DK, Iida M, Tabuchi T, *et al.* The open form inducer approach for structure-based drug design. PLoS One 2016; 11(11): e0167078.
[http://dx.doi.org/10.1371/journal.pone.0167078] [PMID: 27893848]

[107] Hurt DE, Widom J, Clardy J. Structure of *Plasmodium falciparum* dihydroorotate dehydrogenase with a bound inhibitor. Acta Crystallogr D Biol Crystallogr 2006; 62(3): 312-23.
[http://dx.doi.org/10.1107/S0907444905042642] [PMID: 16510978]

[108] Sharma M, Pandey V, Poli G, Tuccinardi T, Lolli ML, Vyas VK. A comprehensive review of synthetic strategies and SAR studies for the discovery of PfDHODH inhibitors as antimalarial agents. Part 1: triazolopyrimidine, isoxazolopyrimidine and pyrrole-based (DSM) compounds. Bioorg Chem 2024; 146: 107249.
[http://dx.doi.org/10.1016/j.bioorg.2024.107249] [PMID: 38493638]

[109] Pippione AC, Sainas S, Goyal P, *et al.* Hydroxyazole scaffold-based Plasmodium falciparum dihydroorotate dehydrogenase inhibitors: Synthesis, biological evaluation and X-ray structural studies. Eur J Med Chem 2019; 163: 266-80.
[http://dx.doi.org/10.1016/j.ejmech.2018.11.044] [PMID: 30529545]

[110] Silveira FF, de Souza JO, Hoelz LVB, *et al.* Comparative study between the anti-P. falciparum activity of triazolopyrimidine, pyrazolopyrimidine and quinoline derivatives and the identification of new PfDHODH inhibitors. Eur J Med Chem 2021; 209: 112941.
[http://dx.doi.org/10.1016/j.ejmech.2020.112941] [PMID: 33158577]

[111] Boechat N, Pinheiro LCS, Silva TS, *et al.* New trifluoromethyl triazolopyrimidines as anti-Plasmodium falciparum agents. Molecules 2012; 17(7): 8285-302.
[http://dx.doi.org/10.3390/molecules17078285] [PMID: 22781441]

[112] Martín-Montes Á, Aguilera-Venegas B, Mª Morales-Martín R, *et al.* in vitro assessment of 3-alkox--5-nitroindazole-derived ethylamines and related compounds as potential antileishmanial drugs. Bioorg Chem 2019; 92: 103274.
[http://dx.doi.org/10.1016/j.bioorg.2019.103274] [PMID: 31539744]

[113] da Silva PR, de Oliveira JF, da Silva AL, *et al.* Novel indol-3-yl-thiosemicarbazone derivatives: Obtaining, evaluation of *in vitro* leishmanicidal activity and ultrastructural studies. Chem Biol Interact 2020; 315: 108899.
[http://dx.doi.org/10.1016/j.cbi.2019.108899] [PMID: 31738906]

[114] Amaral M, de Sousa FS, Silva TAC, *et al.* A semi-synthetic neolignan derivative from dihydrodieugenol B selectively affects the bioenergetic system of Leishmania infantum and inhibits cell division. Sci Rep 2019; 9(1): 6114.
[http://dx.doi.org/10.1038/s41598-019-42273-z] [PMID: 30992481]

[115] Glanzmann N, Antinarelli LMR, da Costa Nunes IK, *et al.* Synthesis and biological activity of novel 4-aminoquinoline/1,2,3-triazole hybrids against Leishmania amazonensis. Biomed Pharmacother 2021; 141: 111857.
[http://dx.doi.org/10.1016/j.biopha.2021.111857] [PMID: 34323702]

[116] Santana Filho PC, Brasil da Silva M, Malaquias da Silva BN, *et al.* Seleno-indoles trigger reactive oxygen species and mitochondrial dysfunction in Leishmania amazonensis. Tetrahedron 2023; 135: 133329.
[http://dx.doi.org/10.1016/j.tet.2023.133329]

[117] Barrientos-Salcedo C, Espinoza B, Soriano-Correa C. Computational study of substituent effects on the physicochemical properties and chemical reactivity of selected antiparasitic 5-nitrofurans. J Mol Struct 2018; 1173: 92-9.
[http://dx.doi.org/10.1016/j.molstruc.2018.06.089]

[118] Da Silva AS, Paim FC, Santos RCV, *et al.* Nitric oxide level, protein oxidation and antioxidant enzymes in rats infected by Trypanosoma evansi. Exp Parasitol 2012; 132(2): 166-70.
[http://dx.doi.org/10.1016/j.exppara.2012.06.010] [PMID: 22771866]

[119] Genestra M, Guedes-Silva D, Souza WJS, *et al.* Nitric oxide synthase (NOS) characterization in Leishmania amazonensis axenic amastigotes. Arch Med Res 2006; 37(3): 328-33.
[http://dx.doi.org/10.1016/j.arcmed.2005.07.011] [PMID: 16513480]

[120] Gouveia ALA, Santos FAB, Alves LC, *et al.* Thiazolidine derivatives: *in vitro* toxicity assessment against promastigote and amastigote forms of Leishmania infantum and ultrastructural study. Exp Parasitol 2022; 236-237: 108253.
[http://dx.doi.org/10.1016/j.exppara.2022.108253] [PMID: 35381223]

[121] de Mello MVP, Abrahim-Vieira BA, Domingos TFS, *et al.* A comprehensive review of chalcone derivatives as antileishmanial agents. Eur J Med Chem 2018; 150: 920-9.
[http://dx.doi.org/10.1016/j.ejmech.2018.03.047] [PMID: 29602038]

[122] Pacheco JS, Costa DS, Cunha-Júnior EF, *et al.* Monocyclic nitro-heteroaryl nitrones with dual mechanism of activation: Synthesis and antileishmanial activity. ACS Med Chem Lett 2021; 12(9): 1405-12.
[http://dx.doi.org/10.1021/acsmedchemlett.1c00193] [PMID: 34531949]

[123] Upegui Y, Gil J, Quiñones W, *et al.* Preparation of rotenone derivatives and *in vitro* analysis of their antimalarial, antileishmanial and selective cytotoxic activities. Molecules 2014; 19(11): 18911-22.
[http://dx.doi.org/10.3390/molecules191118911] [PMID: 25412039]

[124] Don R, Ioset JR. Screening strategies to identify new chemical diversity for drug development to treat kinetoplastid infections. Parasitology 2014; 141(1): 140-6.
[http://dx.doi.org/10.1017/S003118201300142X] [PMID: 23985066]

CHAPTER 2

Advancements in Antileishmanial Drug Discovery: Targeting Druggable Pathways and Overcoming Treatment Challenges

Salma Darwish[1], **Mohamed Teleb**[1], **Sherry N. Nasralla**[2], **Sherine N. Khattab**[3] and **Adnan A. Bekhit**[1,2,*]

[1] *Department of Pharmaceutical Chemistry, Faculty of Pharmacy, Alexandria University, Alexandria 21521, Egypt*

[2] *Pharmacy Program, Allied Health Department, College of Health and Sport Sciences, University of Bahrain, Sakhir 32038, Kingdom of Bahrain*

[3] *Chemistry Department, Faculty of Science, Alexandria University, Alexandria 21321, Egypt*

Abstract: Over the last decades, neglected tropical diseases (NTDs), especially leishmaniasis, have been the focus of several drug discovery programs. The identification of the pathogen druggable targets and the ability to map the differences between parasites and human enzymes have contributed to the increased interest in the development of new lead compounds. Despite this progress, there remain substantial gaps with respect to developing efficient medications that can be the foundation for surmounting the acquired resistance and overcoming treatment failure. With this background in mind, this chapter will discuss the validated drug targets with a special focus on the reported structural determinants of activity of novel antileishmanial agents. The aim is to introduce an updated overview of the medicinal chemistry aspects of leishmaniasis to the scientific community.

Keywords: Current treatment, Leishmaniasis, Natural antiparasitic agents, Neglected tropical diseases, Semisynthetic antileishmanial agents, Synthetic drugs.

INTRODUCTION

Leishmaniasis is a neglected tropical disease (NTD) endemic in Asia, Africa, the Americas, and the Mediterranean region [1]. The causative agent of the disease is an intracellular parasite related to the order *Kinetoplastidae*, the family

* **Corresponding author Adnan A. Bekhit:** Department of Pharmaceutical Chemistry, Faculty of Pharmacy, Alexandria University, Alexandria 21521, Egypt and Pharmacy Program, Allied Health Department, College of Health and Sport Sciences, University of Bahrain, Sakhir 32038, Kingdom of Bahrain; E-mail: adnbekhit@pharmacy.alexu.edu.eg

Igor Jose dos Santos Nascimento & Ricardo Olimpio de Moura (Eds.)

Trypanosomatidae, and the genus *Leishmania* [2, 3]. On the other hand, the vector responsible for the transmission of the parasite to humans through its bite is the infected female sandfly, mainly of the *Phlebotomus* and *Lutzomyia* genera, belonging to the subfamily *Phlebotominae* [1]. Based on the development site of the parasite in the gut of the sandfly, the mammalian *Leishmania* species are divided into two subgenera: *Leishmania*, which includes the species that develop only in the midgut and foregut, and *Viannia*, which develop in the *Phlebotomus* hindgut before migrating to the midgut and foregut [1, 4]. According to the WHO (12 January 2023), an estimated 700,000 to 1 million new cases occur annually, although only a small fraction of those infected by parasites eventually develop the disease [5]. The disease can be categorized into four clinical forms: Visceral leishmaniasis (VL), Cutaneous leishmaniasis (CL), Mucocutaneous leishmaniasis (MCL), and post kala-azar dermal leishmaniasis (PKDL), caused by over 20 *Leishmania* species. However, the clinical manifestations and their severity depend on the *Leishmania* species involved and the triggered immune response of the host. Generally, while cutaneous leishmaniasis is the most common, visceral leishmaniasis is the most severe form that can be fatal if left untreated [6].

LIFE CYCLE

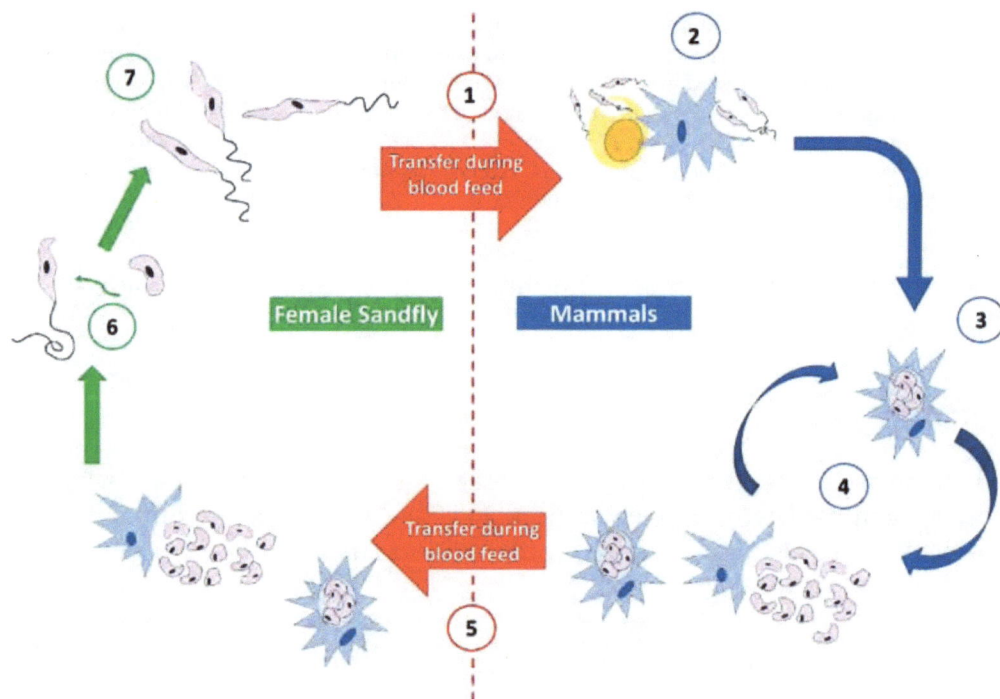

Fig. (1). Life cycle of Leishmania.

According to the Fig. (**1**), the life cycle of *Leishmania* follows the following steps: 1) Infected female sandfly, the insect vector, bites a healthy host and takes a blood meal, thereby injecting the infective stage (*i.e.*, motile promastigotes) through their proboscis. 2) At the puncture wound, the promastigotes are phagocytosed by macrophages and other types of mononuclear phagocytic cells. 3) Promastigotes transform into non-motile amastigotes, which multiply by simple division inside the phagolysosome. 4) The amastigotes are released because of the host immune response-mediated cytolytic environment and proceed to infect other mononuclear phagocytic cells, where they survive as intracellular parasites. 5) Sandfly takes a blood meal from an infected person, thereby ingesting infected cells. 6) In the gut (in the foregut, midgut, and hindgut for leishmanial organisms in the *Viannia* subgenus; in the midgut and foregut for organisms in the *Leishmania* subgenus), the amastigotes transform into flagellated promastigotes. These survive extracellularly and multiply by binary fission. 7) After multiplication, the virulent promastigotes migrate to the proboscis, ready to infect a healthy host during the next blood meal. The presence of an anticoagulant in the saliva of the vector prevents the blood from coagulating at the bite site, thereby allowing a successful transmission of the parasite [1, 2, 6, 7].

FORMS OF THE DISEASE

Leishmaniasis is a vector-borne disease with various clinical manifestations that depend on the virulence characteristics of the parasite and the effectiveness of the host's immune response. Four main clinical forms can be identified: A) cutaneous leishmaniasis (CL), B) mucocutaneous leishmaniasis (MCL), C) visceral or kala-azar (VL), and D) Post-kala-azar dermal leishmaniasis (PKDL) [6].

Cutaneous Leishmaniasis (Localized Cutaneous Leishmaniasis)

This form of the disease occurs in the body areas exposed to insects' bites; in decreasing order of frequency, the ears, nose, upper lip, cheeks, legs, hands and forearms, and ankles are affected. After exposure, the incubation period can range from 1 to 4 weeks. However, it can last up to several years [1]. Generally, skin lesions that develop in cutaneous leishmaniasis can persist for months, but in some cases, they can last for years before they spontaneously heal, leaving flat, hypopigmented scars [6, 8].

Mucocutaneous Leishmaniasis (MCL)

MCL is a rare and severe variant of CL that can take place years after the initial cutaneous manifestations have resolved. It can result in facial deformities due to mucosal lesions, which lead to partial or complete destruction of mucosal linings of the nose, throat, and mouth. This form of disease is caused by the spread of the parasites (amastigotes) from the skin to the naso-oropharyngeal mucosa through the hematogenous or lymphatic system. The symptoms of MCL can be associated with the hyperallergic immune response targeting host tissues.

Generally, MCL is harder to diagnose and treat than cutaneous leishmaniasis [6, 9]. Although the mortality associated with mucosal leishmaniasis is low, the morbidity connected to the resulting disfigurement can be significant [8].

Visceral or Kala-azar (VL)

Visceral leishmaniasis is a form of the disease that includes a wide range of symptoms of different degrees of severity. Because the infection affects visceral organs like the spleen, liver, and bone marrow, it can be fatal either from the disease or indirectly from complications. Generally, the incubation period ranges from weeks to months; however, in some cases, the disease can be asymptomatic during the initial phase and can be diagnosed years later when the patients become immunocompromised. Clinical symptoms of the disease encompass fever, weight loss, anemia, hyper-gammaglobulinemia, and hepatosplenomegaly, mainly as a result of increased parasite burden in these visceral organs [6, 8, 9].

Post kala-azar Dermal Leishmaniasis (PKDL)

Post kala-azar dermal leishmaniasis (PKDL) is a complication of the skin that occurs months or even years after visceral leishmaniasis has resolved. In this case, patients develop cutaneous papules and nodular rashes, usually found on the face around the mouth and gradually spreading to other parts of the body [6, 10].

CURRENT TREATMENT

As indicated previously, the severity of the disease is related to the infecting *Leishmania* species and the triggered host-immune response. In the current antileishmanial therapy, the visceral disease that may result in PKDL is treated systemically, while cutaneous leishmaniasis, which may further progress into MCL, is treated either systemically or locally.

In the current antileishmanial therapy regimen, the following drugs are used:

Pentavalent Antimonials

Sodium stibogluconate **1** and meglumine antimoniate **2** (Fig. **2**) have been recommended for decades as first-line treatment for both major forms of the disease (VL and CL). They are still used as drugs of choice in endemic areas where resistance has not developed. However, the occurrence of resistance in some areas limits their use [11, 12]. Pentavalent antimonials are administered daily, parenterally, for 20-30 days. The recommended dose is 20 mg per kg body weight [13].

Till now, the exact mechanism of action of antimonials is being investigated, and two main models have been proposed. Some studies suggest that these drugs act as prodrugs that are activated by reduction to active trivalent form [14, 15]. On the other side, there are studies that suggest that the pentavalent form possesses intrinsic antileishmanial activity [16].

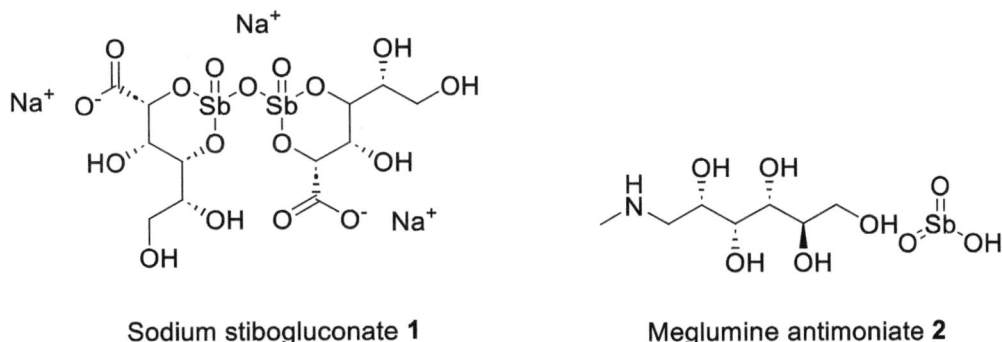

Sodium stibogluconate **1**   Meglumine antimoniate **2**

Fig. (2). Structures of sodium stibogluconate 1 and meglumine antimoniate 2.

Because of the long parenteral administration, in addition to several side effects, the use of the pentavalent antimonials decreased. The reported side effects include pancreatitis during treatment, pancytopenia, reversible peripheral neuropathy, elevations in serum aminotransferases, pain at the site of injection, stiff joints, gastrointestinal problems, and hepatic and renal insufficiency (nephrotoxicity). Moreover, sudden death due to cardiotoxicity may take place. Also, accumulation of the drug in the liver and spleen can result from the long duration of treatment [13, 17 - 22].

Amphotericin B

Another first-line drug, especially used in areas where resistance to antimonials antileishmanial treatment is common, is amphotericin B **3** (Fig. **3**). Originally, this drug was a macrolide polyene antifungal antibiotic, and its use in antileishmanial therapy was a result of drug repurposing [23, 24]. Amphotericin B is used effectively in the treatment of VL [25, 26], PKDL [27], CL, and MCL [28].

It has been reported that the host-parasite interaction is specific. Studies show that the binding and internalization of the *Leishmania* parasite into the macrophages require the membrane cholesterol. Therefore, any cholesterol depletion results in a decrease in the number of the intracellular amastigote load of the parasite [29 -

31]. Moreover, amphotericin B, as an anti-fungal, possesses the ability to bind ergosterol, which is a major component of the cell wall of the leishmanial cell membrane. Interfering with ergosterol results in the formation of aqueous pores permeable to monovalent cations, anions, and small metabolites, leading to the death of the *Leishmania* promastigotes [23, 32]. These results indicate that the effect of amphotericin B treatment can be a result of its interaction with both the ergosterol of the leishmanial cell membrane and with the cholesterol of the cell membrane of the host macrophage.

Amphotericin B desoxycholate (Fungizone®) [33] and various liposomal formulations (such as AmBisome®) [34 - 36] are the intravenous preparations of amphotericin B currently used. Liposomal formulations of the drug were developed to improve its bioavailability and pharmacokinetic properties, thereby reducing side effects, including infusion-related adverse effects such as nephrotoxicity, fever, bone pain, hypotension, and anorexia, and increasing its efficacy [35 - 37].

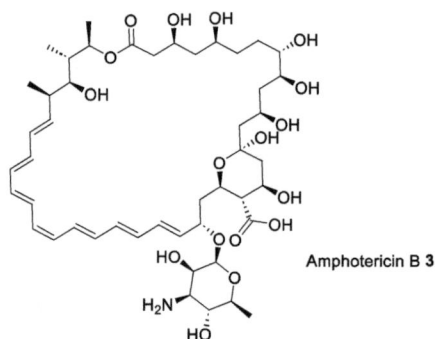

Fig. (3). Structure of amphotericin B 3.

Miltefosine

Originally, miltefosine **4** (Fig. **4**) was developed as an anticancer agent used in topical treatment of skin metastases of breast cancer [38]. Drug repurposing to find new treatments for leishmaniasis led to the use of miltefosine as the first oral drug to be administered for the treatment of visceral and cutaneous leishmaniasis [39, 40]. Although not all the involved pharmacological targets were identified, the mode of action of miltefosine is associated with the induction of apoptosis-like cell death in both human cancer cells and *Leishmania* parasites. However, the drug was found to possess the ability to disturb lipid-dependent cell signaling pathways and to affect the host's immune responses to the parasites [41, 42]. On the other hand, the most beneficial characteristic of miltefosine is its pharmacokinetics, which allows its high bioavailability after oral administration, decreasing the need for hospitalization [42, 43].

Concerning its side effects, the use of miltefosine has been associated with severe gastrointestinal disturbances, hepatotoxicity, and renal toxicity. In addition, it was reported to cause teratogenicity; therefore, its use during pregnancy is prohibited [42]. Till now, resistance has been reported only in laboratory strains. Recently, relapse after 6 to 12 months after successful treatment using miltefosine has been reported [44]. Studies show that there is potential in using miltefosine in combination therapy with amphotericin B and paromomycin, especially in the treatment of antimonial-resistant VL patients [45].

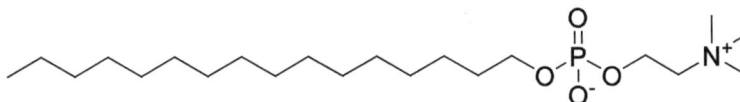

Miltefosine **4**

Fig. (4). Structure of miltefosine 4.

Paromomycin

Paromomycin **5** (Fig. **5**) is a broad-spectrum aminoglycoside antibiotic originally developed for the treatment of intestinal protozoans; however, its use was extended to include the treatment of several parasitic infections, including amoebiasis, cryptosporidiosis, and giardiasis. It is effective against both visceral and cutaneous leishmaniasis [46, 47]. Especially in combination with miltefosine, it was found to be effective against human visceral leishmaniasis [48]. Although its activity is known to involve inhibition of protein synthesis, its exact mechanism of action still requires further elucidation [47]. It requires parenteral administration and is associated with several side effects, including nephrotoxicity, ototoxicity, and hepatotoxicity [48]. Resistance was reported only in laboratory strains of *L. donovani* promastigotes.

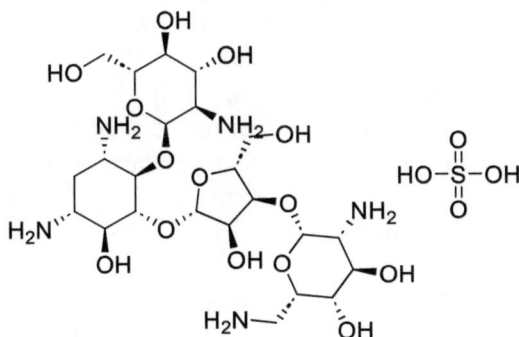

Paromomycin **5**

Fig. (5). Structure of paromomycin 5.

Pentamidine

Pentamidine **6** (Fig. **6**) is an aromatic diamine that is used in the treatment of visceral and cutaneous leishmaniasis [49, 50]. Originally, it was used to treat *Pneumocystis carinii* pneumonia [51]. High toxicity, emergence of resistance, and side effects, including myalgia, pain at the injection site, nausea, headache, hypotension, and irreversible insulin-dependent diabetes mellitus, resulted in limiting its clinical use [52, 53]. While the exact mode of action of the drug is still unknown, researchers hypothesize that the drug acts on the parasite´s mitochondria [54].

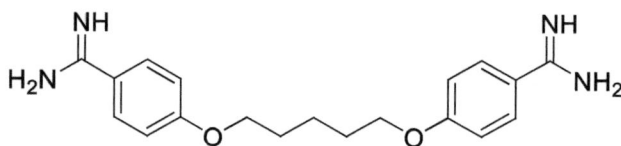

Pentamidine **6**

Fig. (6). Structure of pentamidine 6.

HERBAL ANTILEISHMANIAL AGENTS

Flavonoids and Chalcones

Chalcones, which are the precursors of flavonoids and isoflavonoids, are secondary plant metabolites. From the chemical point of view, the chalcone skeleton consists of two aryl rings joined together by an enone linker. Compound **7** (Fig. **7**) was extracted from the leaves of *Piper hispidum*. Ruiz *et al.* [55] tested it against *L. amazonensis* axenic amastigotes. The compound exhibited antileishmanial activity with an IC_{50} 0.8 mM (amphotericin B IC_{50} 0.2 mM) but was shown to display mild cytotoxicity. Another group tested compound **7** against extracellular promastigotes of *L. donovani, L. infantum, L. enrietii,* and *L. major* and against intracellular amastigote *L. donovani* occupying murine macrophages. Compound **7** was active against extracellular promastigotes of *L. major, L. donovani, L. infantum,* and *L. enrietii* with EC_{50} 0.10 µg/mL, EC_{50} 0.07 µg/mL, EC_{50} 0.18 µg/mL, and EC_{50} 0.08 µg/mL, respectively, compared to amphotericin B EC_{50} 0.03 µg/mL, EC_{50} 0.03 µg/mL, EC_{50} 0.04 µg/mL, and EC_{50} 0.02 µg/mL, respectively. Moreover, it was able to inhibit the intracellular amastigote of *L. donovani* with EC_{50} 0.44 µg/mL (amphotericin B EC_{50} 0.03 µg/mL) [56].

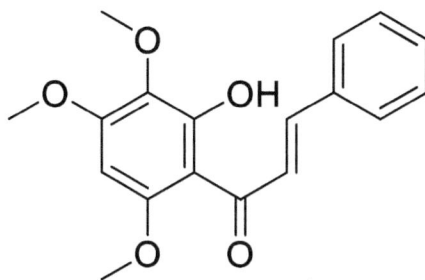

7

Fig. (7). Structure of compound 7 extracted from the leaves of *Piper hispidum.*.

Borges-Argàez *et al.* [57] isolated some flavonoids and chalcones from *Lonchocarpus spp.* and evaluated their antileishmanial activity against the promastigotes of *L. braziliensis*, *L. amazonensis,* and *L. donovani*. Among the compounds tested, flavone **8** (Fig. **8**) (IC_{50} 5.6 µg/mL for all 3 species) and chalcone **9** (IC_{50} 10-40 µg/mL) were the most active against the tested *Leishmania* parasites. The activity of flavone **8** was almost as that of pentamidine (IC_{50} 5 µg/mL).

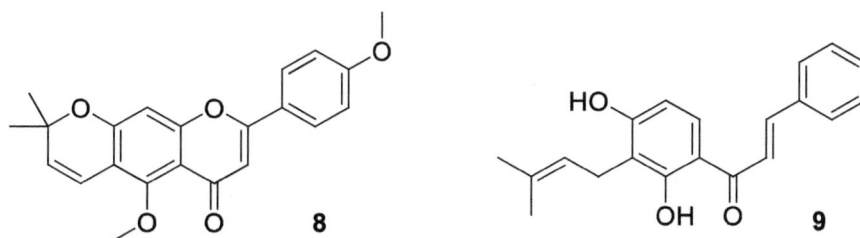

Fig. (8). Structures of flavone 8 and chalcone 9.

Naphthoquinones and Iridoids

2-Methyl-5-(3-methyl-but-2-enyloxy)-1,4-naphthoquinone **10** (Fig. **9**) was extracted from the roots of the plant *Plumbago zeylanica* and was tested against promastigote and amastigote forms of *L. donovani*. The prenyloxy-naphthoquinone exhibited an EC_{50} against promastigote (EC_{50} 0.573 mg/L) and amastigote (EC_{50} 1.045 mg/L) forms of *L. donovani,*which was significantly lower than the reference drug miltefosine (EC_{50} 1.697 mg/L and EC_{50} 3.053 mg/L) [58].

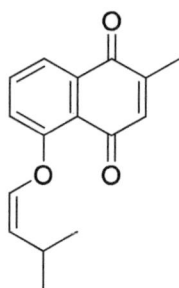

2-Methyl-5-(3-methyl-but-2-enyloxy)-1,4-naphthoquinone
10

Fig. (9). Structure of naphthoquinone derivative 10 extracted from the roots of the plant *Plumbago zeylanica*.

2-hydroxy-3-(3-methyl-2-butenyl)-1,4-naphthoquinone, known as lapachol **11** (Fig. **10**), is one of the components of the naphthoquinone group, isolated from some species of the plant family *Bignoniaceae*. In a study by Teixeira *et al.* [59], the leishmanicidal activity of this compound was evaluated *in vitro* against intracellular amastigotes of *L. braziliensis* and *in vivo* in an animal model and was compared to the reference drug sodium stibogluconate (Pentostam®). While the results demonstrated that lapachol exhibited marked antiamastigote activity *in vitro*, it seems that this activity is lost *in vivo*.

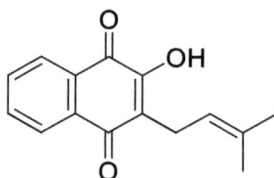

Lapachol **11**

Fig. (10). Structure of lapachol 11.

In the Madre de Dios region of Peru, extracts of seven medicinal plants are traditionally used for the treatment of cutaneous leishmaniasis. In the study by Castillo *et al.* [60], the antileishmanial activity of each of the extracts was evaluated against axenically grown amastigote forms of *L. amazonensis,* showing that the most active plant extract was obtained from the *Himatanthus sucuuba* barks. Further investigation showed the presence of the spirolactone iridoids plumericin **12** and isoplumericin **13** (Fig. **11**) in the extract. Both isolated compounds show strong activity against *L. amazonensis* axenic amastigotes (plumericin IC_{50} 0.21 µM, isoplumericin IC_{50} 0.28 µM, amphotericin B IC_{50} 0.52 µM). While isoplumericin showed toxicity against amastigotes infected macrophages, plumericin (IC_{50} 0.9 µM) resulted in a reduction of the macrophage infection comparable to amphotericin B (IC_{50} 1 µM).

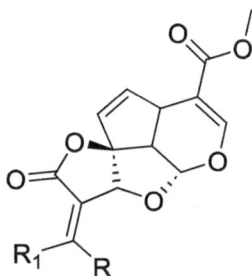

Plumericin **12**   R= CH₃   R₁= H
Isoplmericin **13**   R= H   R₁= CH₃

Fig. (11). Structures of the spirolactone iridoids plumericin 12 and isoplumericin 13.

Saponins

A plethora of plant-derived steroidal and triterpenoid saponins have been generally evaluated as antimicrobials. Of these, several natural and semi-synthetic saponins showed remarkable activities against *L. mexicana*, the causative agent of cutaneous leishmaniasis. In 2020, the triterpenoid sapogenin hederagenin **14** (Fig. **12**) which is readily extracted from *Hedera helix* (common ivy) in large quantities, was converted into 128 derivatives by Anderson and coworkers. These semisynthetic compounds, together with the isolated saponins, were subjected to a phenotypic screening approach for identification of the antileishmanial hits. Twelve compounds, including gypsogenin **15** (Fig. **12**), demonstrated high potency against axenic *L. mexicana* amastigotes (ED_{50} < 10.5 µM). Most importantly, the antileishmanial activities of hederagenin derivatives have been demonstrated. Hederagenin disuccinate was non-toxic to the macrophage host cell (SI> 10), highlighting the possibility of improving the selectivity of natural derivatives through chemical modification [61]. Previously, Delmas *et al.* [62] isolated hederacolchiside A1, α-hederin, and β-hederin from ivy and demonstrated their antileishmanial activities. All compounds inhibited *L. infantum* by affecting its membrane integrity, with hederacolchiside A1 **16** (Fig. **12**) at the top of the list. However, the tested saponins exhibited moderate cytotoxicity, where they inhibited DNA synthesis in human monocytes. Moreover, racemoside A **17** (Fig. **12**), a saponin isolated from *Asparagus racemosus*, inhibited *L. donovani* promastigotes (IC_{50} 1.31 µg/mL) with no toxic effects on human macrophages up to 10 µg/mL [63].

Hederagenin **14**   Gypsogenin **15**   Hederacolchiside A1 **16**

Racemoside A **17**

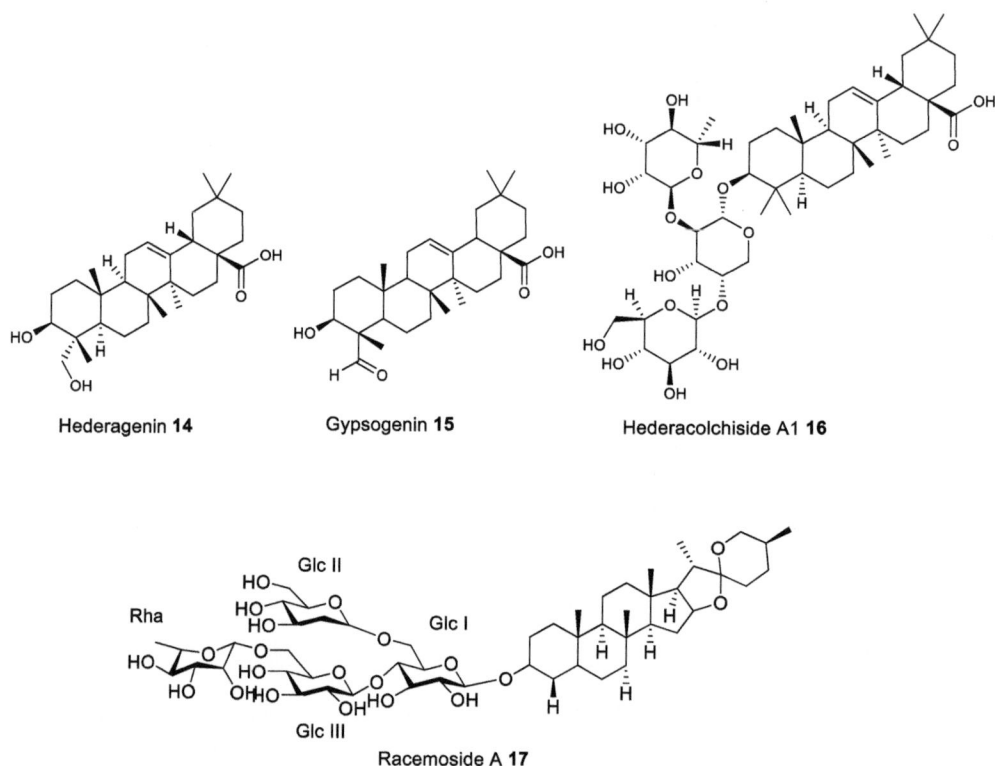

Fig. (12). Structures of saponins 14 – 17.

Valerino-Díaz and coworkers [64] developed an analytical method for the quantification of saponins extracted from the leaves of *Solanum paniculatum*, a species with a high content of steroidal saponins whose fruits are widely consumed as tonic beverage in Brazil. Spirostanic saponins were screened *in vitro* for antileishmanial activities against the amastigote and promastigote forms of *L. amazonensis*. The polyhydroxylated saponins **18**, **19**, and **20** (Fig. **13**) were the most active compounds, recording IC_{50} 8.51 ± 4.38, 10.75 ± 6.85, and 10.45 ± 4.21 µM, respectively, against promastigote forms and EC_{50} >25, 17.73 ± 0.99 and 19.57 ± 0.84 µM, respectively, against amastigote forms. The three saponins evidenced low toxicity in murine macrophage cells, thus promising the treatment of cutaneous leishmaniasis.

Quinolines

Quinolines have been historically known as the most effective antimalarial drugs [65]. However, attention has been devoted to repurposing antimalarials, including quinolines, for the management of leishmaniasis. Interestingly, chloroquine displayed considerable potency against *L. amazonensis* intracellular amastigotes [66]. In clinical trials, chloroquine was as effective as tetracycline for the treatment of cutaneous leishmaniasis [67].

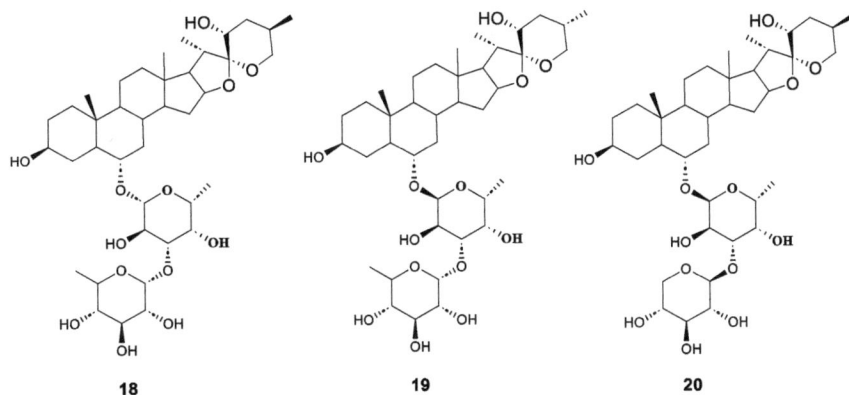

18   **19**   **20**

Fig. (13). Structures of polyhydroxylated saponins 18 – 20.

In a series of studies carried out by Alain Fournet and his group on *Galipea longiflora, it was shown that its* bark extracts led to the identification of 10 quinoline-based natural products [68, 69]. Of these compounds, 2-*n*-propylquinoline **21a**, 2-propenylquinoline **21b**, and 2-*trans*-epoxypropylquinoline **21c** (Fig. **14**) exhibited moderate *in vitro* activity against the promastigotes of several *Leishmania* species, with IC$_{50}$ ranging from 100 to 250 μM [69, 70]. 2-Pentylquinoline **21d** and 2-phenylquinoline **21e** (Fig. **14**) were also extracted from leaves and were then evaluated *in vivo* against *L. amazonensis* and *L. venezuelensis* [71]. Fournet *et al.* also reported that 2-propenylquinoline **21b** and 2-*trans*-epoxypropylquinoline **21c** (Fig. **14**) were comparable to the standard drug *N*-methylglucamine antimonate [69, 71].

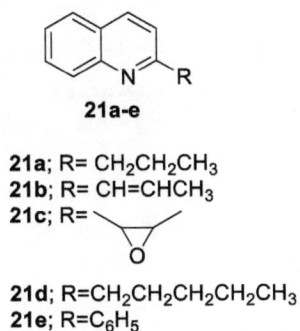

21a-e

21a; R= CH$_2$CH$_2$CH$_3$
21b; R= CH=CHCH$_3$
21c; R=
21d; R=CH$_2$CH$_2$CH$_2$CH$_2$CH$_3$
21e; R=C$_6$H$_5$

Fig. (14). Structures of five natural quinoline derivatives 21a-21e.

Lignans

Justicidone **22**, (Fig. **15**) isolated from *Justicia hyssopifolia*, was identified as a *C-5*, *C-8* dioxo-lignan of the arylnaphthalene type. The biological evaluation revealed that Justicidone **22** showed potential activity against *L. braziliensis* with an IC_{50} of 181.90 µM. The study was extended to investigate the activities of its synthetic precursors against *L. braziliensis* and *L. amazonensis* promastigotes. Interestingly, the diastereomeric mixture exhibited inhibitory activities against both parasite strains with IC_{50} 99.27 µM (*L. braziliensis*) and 181.75 µM (*L. amazonensis*) [72].

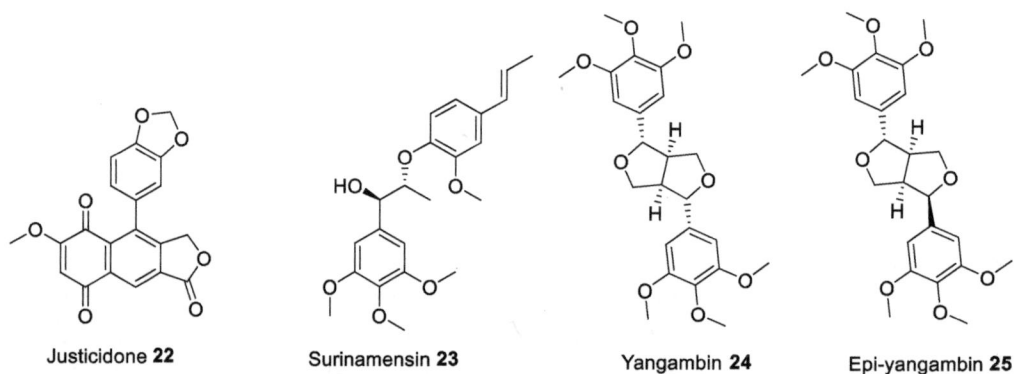

Fig. (15). Structures of lignans 22 – 25.

Surinamensin **23** (Fig. **15**), a neolignan isolated from *Virola Pavonis,* was found to be active against *L. donovani* at 100 µM. Twenty-five of its synthetic analogs with ether linkages and their corresponding *C-8* sulfur and nitrogen analogs were also evaluated. The highest selective activity was found in compounds with sulfur bridges [73].

Yangambin **24** and epi-yangambin **25** (Fig. **15**) are the major lignans extracted from a tree native to the Atlantic forests of Brazil called *Louro-de-Cheiro* [*Ocotea fasciculata (Nees) Mez*]. The leaves and bark of this tree are traditionally used in folk medicine. Jéssica Rebouças Silva *et al.* [74] investigated the immunomodulatory and leishmanicidal effects of both lignans against *L. amazonensis* and *L. braziliensis*. Yangambin **24** and epi-yangambin **25** reduced the intracellular viability of either species in a concentration-dependent manner, with IC_{50} 43.9 ± 5 and 22.6 ± 4.9 µM for *L. amazonensis*, compared to IC_{50} 76 ± 17 and 74.4 ± 9.8 µM for *L. braziliensis*. Epi-yangambin **25** thus proved to be more effective against *L. amazonensis*. Additionally, both lignans modulated the production of inflammatory mediators and cytokines by infected macrophages. Yangambin **24** increased IL-10 production by *L. braziliensis*-infected macrophages, whereas both lignans lowered the production of IL-6, NO, PGE2, and TNF-α in both species.

Terpenes and Terpenoids

Artemisia species have been extensively investigated for the management of various protozoal diseases, especially malaria and leishmaniasis [75]. Ethanolic extracts [76, 77] and essential oils [78 - 84] of some Artemisia species showed high antileishmanial activity. Artemisinin **26** (Fig. **16**) was reported to be active against amastigotes, alone or in combinations, as recommended by the WHO [85]. Several studies investigated the antileishmanial activities of synthetic Artemisinin derivatives. Avery *et al.* [75] modified artemisinin at various positions. It was found that among seventy artemisinin derivatives, the 10-deoxy 9*b*-[3,5-bis(trifluoromethyl)phenyl] artemisinin derivative **27** (Fig. **16**) showed IC$_{50}$of 0.3 mM with improved oral activity. *Taxus baccata* metabolites exhibited high potency against *L. donovani* amastigotes (IC$_{50}$ 70 nM). 10-Deacetylbaccatin III **28** (Fig. **16**), a taxol analog, was effective against *L. donovani* (200 nM - 1 mM) and safe on human macrophages at concentrations up to 5 mM [86].

Colares *et al.* [87] evaluated the essential oil of *Vanillosmopsis arborea* and its major component α-bisabolol **29** (Fig. **16**), a sesquiterpene alcohol, against promastigotes and amastigotes of *L. amazonensis*. Results showed their potency without any noticeable cytotoxicity. Morales-Yuste *et al.* [88] also studied the activity of bisabolol from *Chamomilla recutita*, which demonstrated an IC$_{50}$ of 10.99 mg/mL against *L. infantum* promastigote, with minimum cytotoxicity.

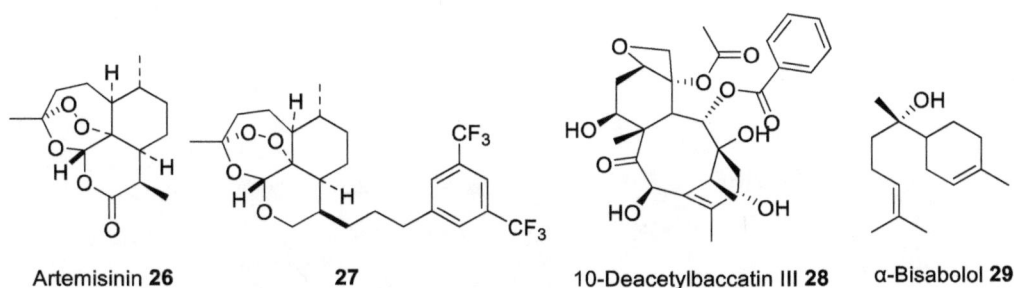

Artemisinin **26**   **27**   10-Deacetylbaccatin III **28**   α-Bisabolol **29**

Fig. (16).   Structures of artemisinin 26 and its derivative 27, in addition to the taxol analog 10-Deacetylbaccatin III 28 and the sesquiterpene alcohol α-bisabolol 29.

SYNTHESIZED ANTILEISHMANIAL AGENTS

Furans

Brendle *et al.* [89] synthesized a series of fifty-eight compounds and tested them for activity against *L. donovani* axenic amastigotes. The resulting activities were compared to the activity of pentamidine. While compound 2,4-bis--4-amidinophenyl)furan **30** (Fig. **17**) was twice as active as pentamidine (IC$_{50}$ 1.30 ± 0.21 μM), compound 2,5-bis-(4-amidinophenyl)furan **31** (IC$_{50}$, 2.76 ± 0.60 μM) (Fig. **17**) showed almost equal antileishmanial activity to pentamidine. In addition, compound **30** was selective towards the parasites, showing 19-fold more activity against the parasites than against the J774.G8 macrophage cell line.

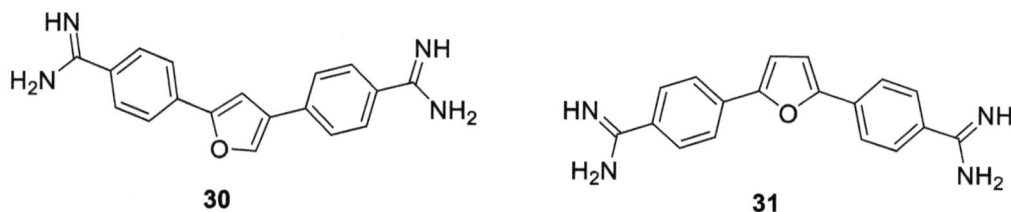

Fig. (17). Structures of furan derivatives 30 and 31.

In another study, Rezaei *et al.* [90] synthesized novel bis-arylimidamide derivatives with terminal catechol moieties as dihydrobromide salts. All developed compounds were examined for *in vitro* antiparasitic activity against the promastigotes of *L. major* and *L. infantum,* in addition to axenic amastigotes of *L. major*. Among the synthesized compounds, the furan-containing compound **32** (Fig. **18**) demonstrated the highest activity with submicromolar IC$_{50}$ values ranging from 0.29 to 0.36 μM. This activity is equipotent to the reference drug amphotericin B (IC$_{50}$ 0.28 − 0.33 μM).

Combining a chelating catechol functionality with an arylimidamide moiety resulted in the improvement of the cytotoxicity profile compared to the parent compounds, as shown by the results for the toxicity against human fibroblast cells.

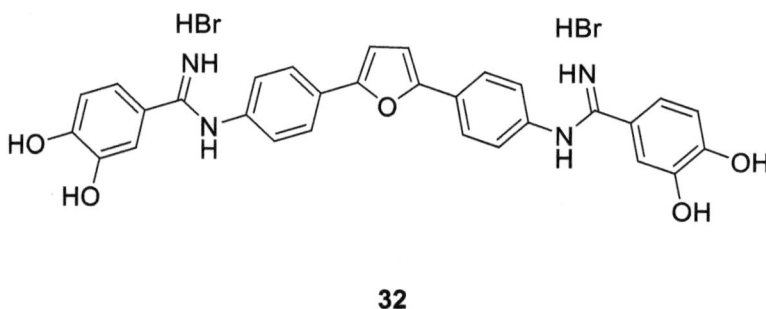

32

Fig. (18). Structure of furan-containing compound 32.

A series of compounds, including 5-nitrofuran nitrones, were developed by Pacheco *et al.* [91]. Among the synthesized molecules, the 5-nitrofuran nitrones **33a-c** (Fig. **19**) demonstrated the most potent leishmanicidal activity against intracellular amastigote forms of *L. amazonensis* and *L. infantum,* ranging from 0.019 to 2.76 µM, with excellent selectivity. Tests showed that compared to miltefosine, the developed molecule **33a** (Fig. **19**) was less toxic. In addition, the oral administration of **33b** to mice infected by *L. infantum* resulted in the reduction of the parasite load on the spleen by 76.6 and 95.0% and in the liver by more than 75% with doses of 50 and 100 mg/kg, respectively, administered twice a day, for 5 days.

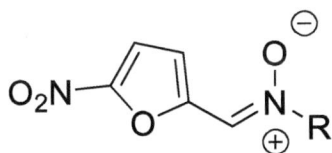

33

33a; R= -t-Bu
33b; R= -CH$_3$
33c; R= -Bn

Fig. (19). Structures of 5-nitrofuran nitrones 33a-c.

Pyrazoles

The research group of Dardari *et al.* [92] was able to develop a pyrazole derivative, 4-[2-(1-(ethylamino)-2-methylpropyl)phenyl]-3-(4-methyphenyl)-1-phenyl-pyrazole **34**, (Fig. **20**) that showed inhibitory ability against three species of *Leishmania,* namely *L. tropica, L. major,* and *L. infantum,* comparable to amphotericin B. The IC$_{50}$ values reported for the new compound against *L. tropica, L. major,* and *L. infantum* promastigotes were 0.48 µg/mL, 0.63 µg/mL, and 0.40 µg/mL, respectively. While that for amphotericin B were 0.23 µg/mL, 0.29 µg/mL, and 0.24 µg/mL, respectively.

In 2015, a series of compounds were synthesized by hybridization of pyrazole with five-membered heterocyclic moieties such as thiazoles, thiazolidinones, 1,3,4-thiadiazoles, and pyrazolines. The developed derivatives were evaluated for their *in vitro* antileishmanial activity against *Leishmania* aethiopica promastigotes and amastigotes. Their activities were compared to those of amphotericin B and miltefosine. Among the tested compounds, compound **35** (Fig. **21**), which is a result of the hybridization between pyrazole and 1,3,4-thiadiazole, displayed the highest antileishmanial activity. The *in vitro* antipromastigote activity demonstrated that compound **35** had an IC_{50} 0.0142 µg/mL better than both standard drugs miltefosine (IC_{50} 3.1921 µg/mL) and amphotericin B deoxycholate (IC_{50} 0.0472 µg/mL). Moreover, compound **35** (IC_{50} 0.13 µg/mL) showed lower IC_{50} values than amphotericin B deoxycholate (IC_{50} 0.2 µg/mL) and miltefosine (IC_{50} 0.3 µg/mL) against *L. aethiopica* amastigotes [93].

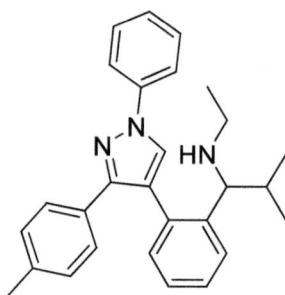

4-[2-(1-(Ethylamino)-2-methylpropyl)phenyl]-3-(4-methyphenyl)-1-phenylpyrazole
34

Fig. (20). Structure of pyrazole derivative 34.

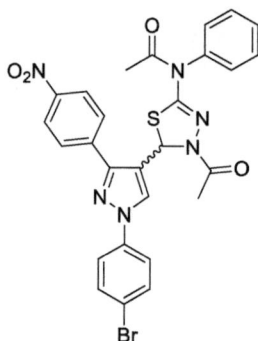

35

Fig. (21). Structure of pyrazole- and 1,3,4-thiadiazole-containing compound 35.

In another study, a series of aminopyrazole ureas were developed and evaluated for their activity against intracellular *L. infantum* amastigotes. Among the synthesized compounds, compound **36** (Fig. **22**) (IC_{50} 2.37 µM) exhibited very good *in vitro* potency against *L. infantum* compared with miltefosine (IC_{50} 7.26 µM). In addition, it showed high *in vivo* efficacy (>90%) against *L. infantum* [94].

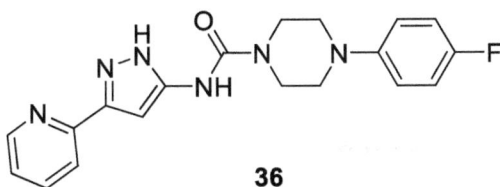

36

Fig. (22). Structure of aminopyrazole urea-based compound 36.

Chromenes and Coumarins

In natural products, coumarins (2*H*-chromene-2-ones) are among the common structural motifs that can be found. Several derivatives of these oxygenated heterocycles were isolated from plants and were found to have an inhibitory effect against the *Leishmania* parasite. However, several synthetic coumarins were synthesized and demonstrated potent activity against the parasite [95, 96].

Pierson *et al.* [97] synthetically developed a series of 4-arylcoumarins and tested their antileishmanial activity against extracellular promastigotes and intracellular amastigotes of the reference strain *L. donovani* (MHOM/IN/80/DD8). 4-(3`,4--Dimethoxyphenyl)-6,7-dimethoxycoumarin **37** (Fig. **23**) demonstrated potent activity (IC$_{50}$ 1.1 μM) and good selectivity toward *L. donovani* amastigote forms with an index twice than the reference amphotericin B.

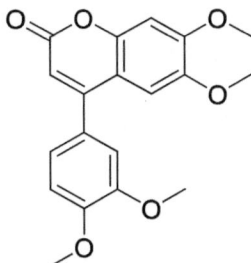

4-(3',4'-Dimethoxyphenyl)-6,7-dimethoxycoumarin
37

Fig. (23). Structure of 4-arylcoumarin derivative 37.

In another study, the development of a series of chromene-2-thione derivatives was reported. The synthesized compounds were screened against promastigote, axenic amastigote, and intracellular amastigote stages of *L. donovani*. Among the tested compounds, **38** and **39** (Fig. **24**) were found to be the most active. In addition, they showed minimal toxicity to human peripheral blood mononuclear cells [98].

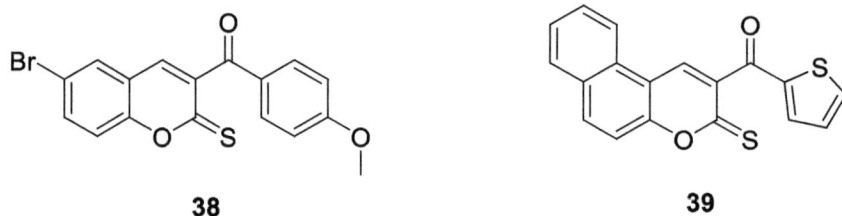

Fig. (24). Structures of chromene-2-thione derivatives 38 and 39.

Zaheer *et al.* [99] reported the synthesis of a series of novel 3-substituted-4-hydroxycoumarin derivatives. These compounds were screened for their antileishmanial activity against *L.donovani* promastigotes in addition to their antioxidant activity. Compounds **40** and **41** (Fig. **25**) demonstrated potent antileishmanial activity, *i.e.*, IC_{50} 9.90 $\pm$ 0.33 μM and IC_{50} 6.90 $\pm$ 0.12 μM, respectively, when compared with pentamidine and miltefosine. Moreover, the two compounds showed significant antioxidant activity.

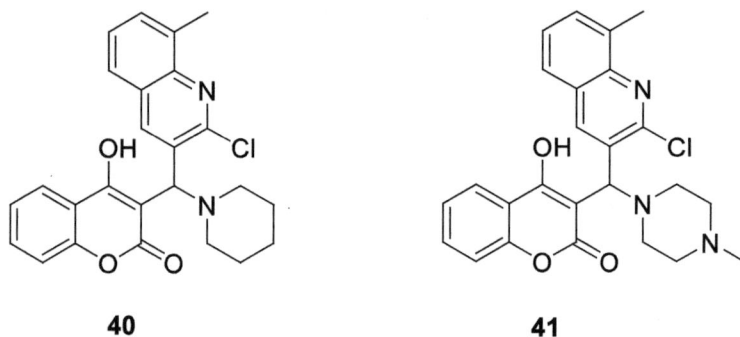

Fig. (25). Structures of 3-substituted-4-hydroxycoumarin derivatives 40 and 41.

Pyridines

In 2020, Nandikolla *et al.* [100] designed and synthesized novel 1,2,3-triazole analogs of imidazo-[1,2-*a*]pyridine-3-carboxamides and evaluated their antileishmanial inhibitory activity against the promastigotes of *L. major*. Compound **42** (Fig. **26**) exhibited comparable inhibitory activity (IC_{50} 15.1 μM) to miltefosine. Moreover, compound **42** was non-toxic to HeLa cells at 100 μM by an Alamar blue assay.

Fig. (26). Structure of pyridine- containing compound 42.

The synthesis of a new series of bis(indolyl)-pyridine derivatives that were screened *in vitro* for their antileishmanial activity against *L. donovani* promastigotes was reported. The results showed that most of the synthesized compounds displayed significant inhibitory activities on the growth of the parasite. Most of the synthesized compounds, mainly compound **43** (IC$_{50}$ 102.47 μM) and compound **44** (IC$_{50}$ 99.49 μM) (Fig. **27**), exhibited better activity against *L. donovani* promastigotes compared with sodium stibogluconate [101].

Fig. (27). Structures of bis(indolyl)-pyridine derivatives 43 and 44.

Indoles

Indole has proven to be one of the most privileged chemotypes for developing new efficient antiparasitic agents, especially antileishmanials [102]. Singh *et al.* [103] synthesized a series of 3,3-diaryl-4-(1-methyl-1*H*-indol-3-yl)azetid-n-2-ones and *N*-(1-methyl-1*H*-indol-3-yl)methyleneamines and evaluated their antileishmanial activity against *Leishmania* major promastigotes. The 3,3-diary-
-4-(1-methyl-1*H*-indol-3-yl)azetidin-2-ones were synthesized by the Staudinger's ketene-imine cycloaddition of *N*-(1-methyl-1*H*-indol-3-yl)methyleneamines

utilizing 2-diazo-1,2-diarylethanones as precursors of diarylketenes. Generally, the transformation of the methyleneamines to azetidin-2-ones showed improvement in anti-parasitic activity. Among the synthesized derivatives, compounds **45** and **46** (Fig. **28**) exhibited inhibitory activities comparable to that of the standard drug amphotericin B against *L. major* (IC$_{50}$ 0.56 ± 0.06 µg/mL).

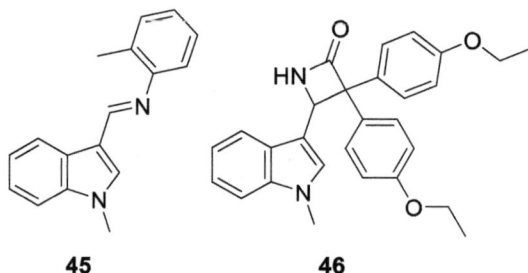

45   **46**

Fig. (28). Structures of indole-containing compounds 45 and 46.

Taha *et al.* [104] evaluated a series of indole-2-hydrazones as antileishmanials. Among the evaluated derivatives, *N'*-(1-(2-hydroxyphenyl) ethylidene)-1-meth-l-1*H*-indole-2-carbohydrazide **47** (Fig. **29**) was found to be superior to the standard drug pentamidine against *L. major* promastigotes, recording IC$_{50}$ 1.86 mM. In further studies [105], a new series of bisindole derivatives bearing substituted thiadiazolyl moieties were synthesized and evaluated for their antileishmanial activities. All derivatives exhibited outstanding potency with IC$_{50}$ ranging from 13.30 ± 0.50 to 0.7 ± 0.01 µM when compared to the standard pentamidine (IC$_{50}$ 7.20 ± 0.20 µM). The 3-((5-(4-(di(1*H*-indol-3-yl)methyl)phenyl)-1,3,4-thiadiazol-2-yl)amino) benzene-1,2-diol **48** (Fig. **29**) was found to be the most potent (IC$_{50}$ 0.7 ± 0.01 µM) among the series.

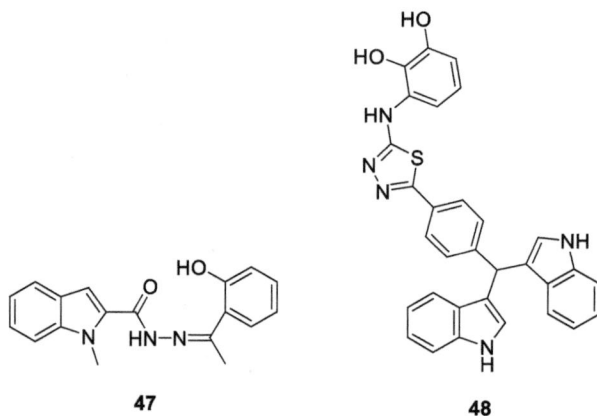

47   **48**

Fig. (29). Structures of indole-containing compounds 47 and 48.

Similarly, Bharate *et al.* [106] synthesized a series of diindolylmethane derivatives with promising antileishmanial activities against *L. donovani* promastigotes and axenic amastigotes. Structure-activity relationship analysis demonstrated that the nitroaryl-substituted diindolylmethanes were potent antileishmanials. The 4-Nitrophenyl-linked 3,3'-diindolylmethane **49** (Fig. **30**) was the most potent derivative, recording IC_{50} 7.88 and 8.37 µM against *L. donovani* promastigotes and amastigotes, respectively.

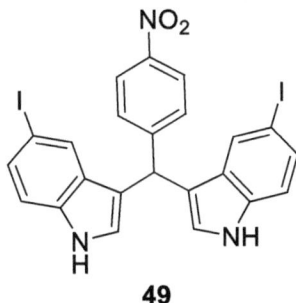

49

Fig. (30). Structure of compound 49.

Diotallevi and coworkers [107] evaluated the antileishmanial potential of a library of azole-bisindoles against *L. infantum* promastigotes and intracellular amastigotes. Most compounds showed good activity, recording IC_{50} ranging from 4 to 10 µM against the promastigotes. URB1483 **50** (Fig. **31**), a pyrrole-bisindole derivative, was selected as the most active derivative with no quantifiable cytotoxicity in THP-1, DH82, HEPG2, HaCaT, and HPF cells. It was comparable to pentamidine and significantly reduced the infection index of human and canine macrophages. Biochemical studies ruled out topoisomerase IB inhibition as the main mechanism of action for URB1483.

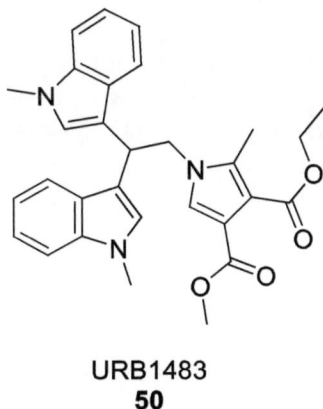

URB1483
50

Fig. (31). Structure of the pyrrole-bisindole derivative URB1483 50.

Quinolines

Sabt *et al.* [108] introduced a series of 7-chloroquinoline derivatives conjugated with isatin moieties **51a-c** (Fig. **32**) and evaluated their antileishmanial activities. The most active hybrids bearing 5-bromoindoline **51a**, 5-flouroindoline **51b**, and 5-trifluoromethoxy indoline **51c** exhibited significant antipromastigote and antiamastigote activities with IC_{50} values of 0.5084 and 0.60442 μM, 0.5572 and 0.72175 μM, and 0.6680 and 0.9446 μM, respectively, and were superior to the standard miltefosine. Folic and folinic acids reversed their antileishmanial effects in a similar manner to trimethoprim, confirming their antifolate mechanism.

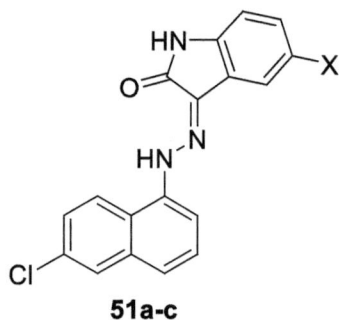

51a-c

51a; X=Br
51b; X=F
51c; X=CF$_3$

Fig. (32). Structures of compounds 51a-c.

Tejería *et al.* [109] utilized Povarov reaction conditions to synthesize hybrid phosphorated tetrahydroquinoline and quinoline and evaluated the target products for their antileishmanial activity against promastigotes and amastigote-infected splenocytes of *L. infantum*. Remarkably, the tetrahydroquinolylphosphine sulfide derivative **52** (Fig. **33**) bearing a para methoxy phenyl group showed promising antileishmanial activity (EC_{50} 0.61 ± 0.18 μM) compared to amphotericin B (EC_{50} 0.32 ± 0.05 μM) and similar selective index (SI = 56.87). In addition, the tetrahydroquinolinylphosphine with *p*-tolyl at position 4 of the heterocyclic core **53** (Fig. **33**) remarkably inhibited *Leishmania* topoisomerase IB.

Almandil *et al.* [110] synthesized and evaluated the antileishmanial potential of a series of quinoline-based thiadiazole derivatives. Most compounds were remarkably potent against *L. major* promastigote with IC_{50} ranging from 0.04 ± 0.01 to 5.60 ± 0.21 μM compared to the standard pentamidine (IC_{50} 7.02 ± 0.09 μM). The structure-activity relationship among the evaluated series was based on the substitution pattern on the phenyl group attached to the thiadiazole ring. It was noticed that the analogs bearing two phenolic groups **54a-d** (Fig. **34**) showed the highest inhibitory activities, recording submicromolar IC_{50} values.

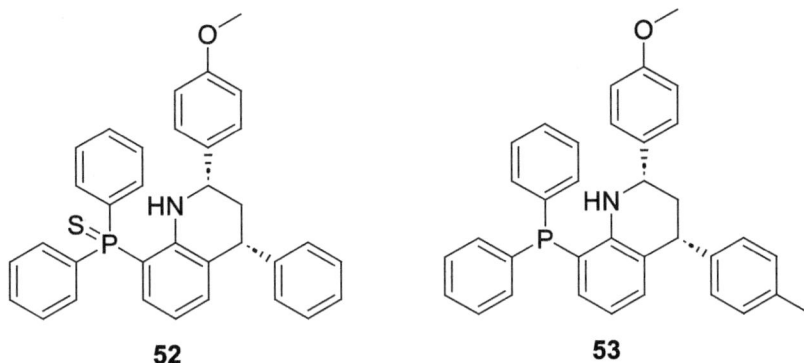

Fig. (33). Structures of tetrahydroquinolylphosphine derivatives 52 and 53.

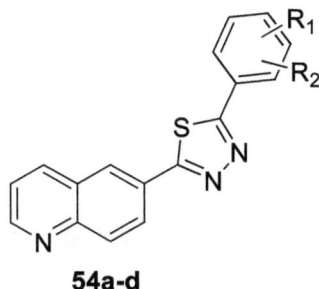

54a-d

54a; R₁=2-OH, R₂=3-OH
54b; R₁=2-OH, R₂=4-OH
54c; R₁=3-OH, R₂=4-OH
54d; R₁=2-OH, R₂=5-OH

Fig. (34). Structures of quinoline-based thiadiazole derivatives 54a-d.

New selective antileishmanial nitroquinoline derivatives **55a,b** (Fig. **35**) were introduced by Paloque *et al.* [111]. The 8-nitroquinolin-2-ol **55a** was comparable to the reference drugs miltefosine and pentamidine with considerable activities against *L. infantum* promastigotes (IC_{50} 7.6 mM), as well as *L. donovani* amastigotes and promastigotes (IC_{50} 6.5 mM and 6.6 mM, respectively). Interestingly, no *in vitro* toxicity was found. Further investigation of the nitroquinoline scaffold by Kieffer *et al.* [112] led to a relatively more potent 4-(- -bromophenyl)-8-nitroquinolin-2-ol derivative **55b**, which recorded an IC_{50} value of 3.3 mM against promastigotes of *L. donovani*. Results highlighted that the substitution of the quinoline ring by a substituted phenyl group influenced the antileishmanial activities.

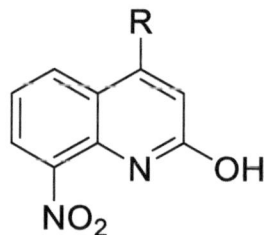

55a,b

55a; R$_1$=H
55b; R$_1$=*p*-BrC$_6$H$_4$

Fig. (35). Structures of nitroquinoline derivatives 55a,b.

Isoquinolines and Oxoisoaporphines

Barbolla and coworkers [113] utilized pyrrolo [1,2-*b*]isoquinoline as a starting point and developed palladium-catalyzed Heck-initiated cascade reactions for synthesizing a new series of *C-10* substituted derivatives. Their leishmanicidal activities were evaluated against *L. donovani* and *L. amazonensis*. The highest potency and selectivity were generally found for the 10-arylmethyl-substituted pyrroloisoquinolines **56a-c** (Fig. **36**). In particular, the derivative bearing dimethoxy phenyl group **56b** (IC$_{50}$ 3.30 μM, SI > 77.01) and the fluorinated derivative substituted with nitrophenyl group **56c** (IC$_{50}$ 3.93 μM, SI > 58.77) were approximately 10-fold more potent and selective than miltefosine against *L. amazonensis* in promastigote *in vitro* assays, while the derivative with unsubstituted phenyl **56a** was the most active derivative in the amastigote assays (IC$_{50}$ 33.59 μM, SI > 8.93). Almost all compounds did not show cytotoxicity in J774 cells (CC$_{50}$ > 100 μg/mL). Additionally, the authors developed the first Perturbation Theory Machine Learning (PTML) algorithm to predict multiple parameters (IC$_{50}$, K$_i$, *etc.*) *vs.* any *Leishmania* species and target protein, with high specificity (>98%) and sensitivity (>90%) in training and validation series.

Ponte-Sucre *et al.* [114] synthesized the isoquinolinium salts **57** and **58** (Fig. **37**), which were effective against intracellular amastigotes of *L. major* at low submicromolar concentrations. Toxicity against mammalian cells was observed at higher concentrations, where the antileishmanial activity was not associated with stimulation of the host macrophages to secrete cytokines or produce nitric oxide relevant to the leishmanicidal effects. These findings support the theory of the significance of quaternary nitrogen atom and its counter-ion in enhancing antileishmanial activity.

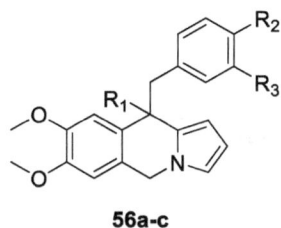

56a-c

56a; R$_1$=CH$_3$, R$_2$=H, R$_3$=H
56b; R$_1$=CH$_3$, R$_2$=OCH$_3$, R$_3$=OCH$_3$
56c; R$_1$=CF$_3$, R$_2$=NO$_2$, R$_3$=H

Fig. (36). Structures of pyrroloisoquinolines 56a-c.

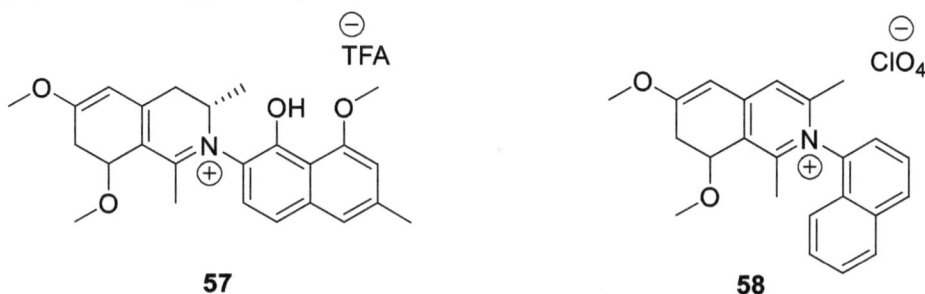

57

58

Fig. (37). Structures of isoquinolinium salts 57 and 58.

Sobarzo-Sanchez *et al.* [115] reported promising antileishmanial activities of the oxoisoaporphine derivatives **59a,b** (Fig. **38**) against *L. amazonensis* axenic amastigotes (IC$_{50}$ < 0.05 mM and 0.025 mM, respectively). The compounds were also active against *L. braziliensis, L. infantum,* and *L. guyanensis.* The benzo derivative **59a** led to a 99% *in vivo* reduction in the parasite burden when administered to BALB/c mice infected with *L. infantum* at a dose of 10 mg/kg without considerable cytotoxicity.

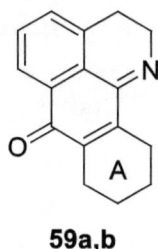

59a,b

59a; A=benzene
59b; A=cyclohexane

Fig. (38). Structures of oxoisoaporphine derivatives 59a,b.

Quinazolines and its Derivatives

Prinsloo and coworkers [116] synthesized a new series of mono- and bis-quinazolinones and then investigated their potential antileishmanial activities against *L. donovani* and *L. major* species. Their cytotoxicity profiles were assessed on Vero cells. The compounds were found to be safer than the reference halofuginone on the mammalian cells. The mono quinazolinone **60** and bisquinazolinone **61** (Fig. **39**) were the most active derivatives with growth inhibitory efficacies of 35% and 29% for *L. major* and *L. donovani* promastigotes, respectively. These outcomes suggested the inclusion of polar groups on the quinazolinone ring to potentially generate novel quinazolinone derivatives endowed with effective antileishmanial potential.

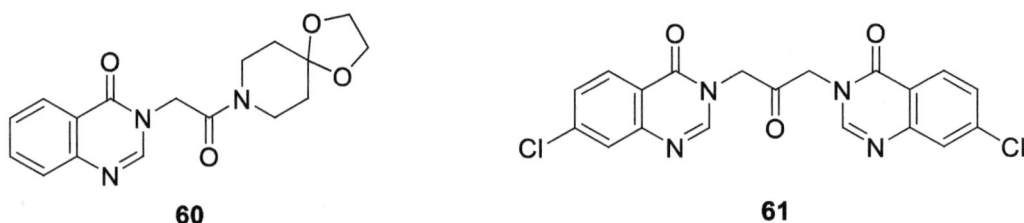

60   **61**

Fig. (39). Structures of mono quinazolinone 60 and bisquinazolinone 61.

Mendoza-Martínez and coworkers [117] synthesized a series of quinazoline-2,4,--triamine derivatives and evaluated their *in vitro* activities against *L. mexicana*. N^6-(ferrocenmethyl)quinazolin-2,4,6-triamine **62** (Fig. **40**) was the most active derivative (IC_{50} 0.93 µM) against promastigotes and intracellular amastigotes with low cytotoxicity in mammalian cells. Inhibition of DHFR was also explored, where the parasites were exposed at concentrations above LC_{50} (a concentration that shows an effect but does not kill all the parasites) after exposure to folic acid, folinic acid, and ferulic acid. Results revealed that the mechanism of its antileishmanial activity occurred partially *via* DHFR, but other mechanisms, such as the redox mechanism, could simultaneously occur owing to the presence of ferrocene, as indicated by electrochemical studies.

Van Horn *et al.* [118] evaluated the antileishmanial activity of a library of diverse compounds, including N^2,N^4-disubstituted quinazolines, originally designed as anticancer probes. The quinazolines **63a,b** (Fig. **41**) exhibiting EC_{50} values in the single-digit micromolar range against *L. mexicana* axenic amastigotes motivated the group to invest more in quest of potent antileishmanial agents. A detailed structure-activity relationship study focusing on the 2-and 4-positions as well as the quinazoline's benzenoid ring led to the discovery of the quinazoline-2,4-diamine **63c** (Fig. **41**) that recorded EC_{50} values of 0.83 and 4.1 µM against *L.*

donovani and L. amazonensis with promising selectivity. Moreover, it displayed efficacy in a murine model of visceral leishmaniasis, reducing liver parasitemia by 37% when given by the intraperitoneal route at 15 mg kg^{-1} day^{-1} for 5 consecutive days.

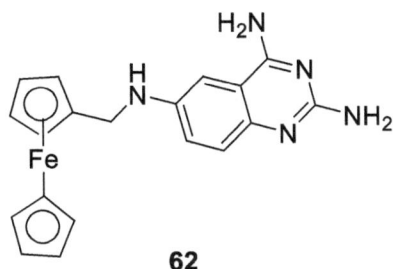

Fig. (40). Structure of compound 62.

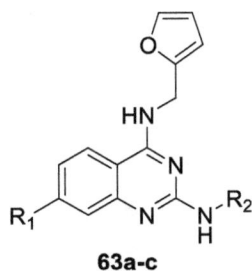

63a; R$_1$=H, R$_2$=CH(CH$_3$)$_2$
63b; R$_1$=H, R$_2$=p-C$_2$H$_5$OC$_6$H$_4$
63c; R$_1$=CH$_3$, R$_2$=CH(CH$_3$)$_2$

Fig. (41). Structures of quinazolines 63a-c.

Bekhit *et al.* [119] studied the antileishmanial activities of some quinazolinone derivatives and studied their structure-activity relationship. Results showed that 4-chlorostyryl-3-*p*-methylphenyl-4(3*H*)-quinazolinone **64** (Fig. **42**) was more active than miltefosine and amphotericin B in terms of IC$_{50}$. SAR studies highlighted the contribution of the styryl moiety and the aromatic group at positions 2 and 3, respectively, to the activity.

Khattab *et al.* [120] synthesized a small library of 2-aminobenzoylamino acid hydrazide derivatives and quinazolinones as antileishmanial agents. Compounds **65a-c** and **66** (Fig. **43**) exhibited higher antipromastigote activities against L. aethiopica than the standard drug miltefosine. Among the hit derivatives, 2-amino-**N**-(6- hydrazinyl-6-oxohexyl)benzamide **65c** was the most potent (IC$_{50}$

0.051 µM), being 154 folds more active than miltefosine (IC_{50} 7.832 µM) and half fold the activity of amphotericin B (IC_{50} 0.035 µM). Interestingly, this compound was safe and well tolerated in experimental animals, parenterally up to 100 mg/kg and orally up to 250 mg/kg.

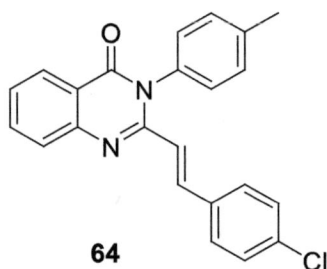

64

Fig. (42). Structure of quinazolinone derivative 64.

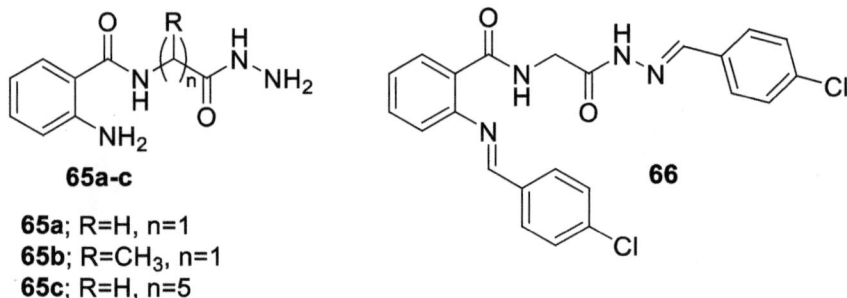

65a-c   **66**

65a; R=H, n=1
65b; R=CH₃, n=1
65c; R=H, n=5

Fig. (43). Structures of compounds 65a-c and compound 66.

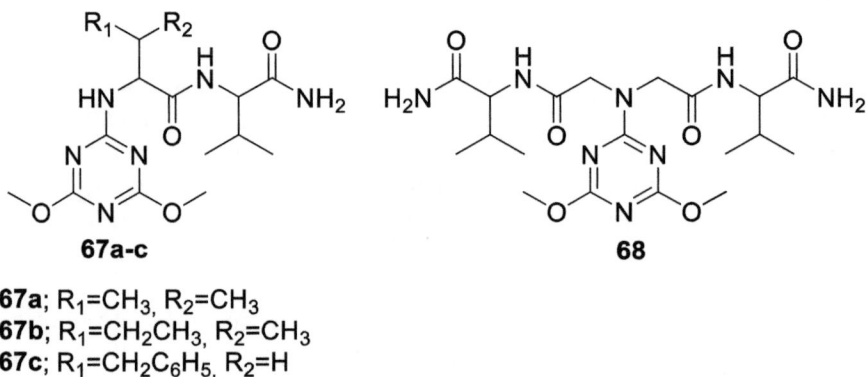

67a-c   **68**

67a; R₁=CH₃, R₂=CH₃
67b; R₁=CH₂CH₃, R₂=CH₃
67c; R₁=CH₂C₆H₅, R₂=H

Fig. (44). Structures of dimethoxytriazine derivatives 67a-c and 68.

Triazine

Khattab and coworkers [121] prepared a series of di-, tri-, and tetrapeptides bearing disubstituted s-triazine rings at the *N*-terminus and evaluated their antileishmanial activity. Among the screened series, four dimethoxytriazine derivatives **67a-c** and **68** (Fig. **44**) surpassed the antileishmanial potency of the reference drug miltefosine with no significance acute toxicity.

DRUG CANDIDATES TARGETING METABOLIC PATHWAYS OF *LEISHMANIA*

The metabolic pathways of *Leishmania* play a crucial role in the parasitic growth and proliferation during various stages of its life cycle. Based on the available genomics/proteomics information, known pathways-based (sterol, GPI, and folate biosynthesis pathways, purine salvage system, trypanothione, and hypusine pathways) *Leishmania*-specific proteins can be considered druggable targets for various repurposed and known drugs. Nevertheless, research is actively introducing lead compounds targeting these pathways as new promising antileishmanial therapeutics [122]. Herein, most of the currently utilized drugs, including the repurposed ones and lead compounds, are listed with their mechanism of action and relevant pathways (Table **1**).

Table 1. Main scaffolds and explored mechanisms of action of antileishmanial drugs.

Drugs/leads and their Chemical classes	Chemical Structure	The Target Metabolic Pathway	Mechanism of Action	Remarks	Refs.
Amphotericin; a polyene antifungal agent		Sterol biosynthetic pathway	Amphotericin B causes leishmanial promastigote cell lysis due to osmotic changes and the formation of aqueous pores.	Expensive. Kidneys' toxicity.	[123, 124]
Miltefosine; an alkylphospho-choline derivative		Sterol biosynthetic pathway	Miltefosine induces apoptosis in *L. donovani* and decreases parasite proliferation.	Teratogenicity.	[125, 126]
JS87; spiro[indoline-3,2-quinolin]-2-one derivative		Sterol biosynthetic pathway	JS87 impacts sterol biosynthesis at the SE enzyme level together with modifying the internal parasite control by interrupting the regulatory volume decline.	-	[127, 128]

(Table 1) cont.....

Drugs/leads and their Chemical classes	Chemical Structure	The Target Metabolic Pathway	Mechanism of Action	Remarks	Refs.
Mevastatin; a polyketide		Sterol biosynthetic pathway	Mevastatin interferes with sterol metabolism.	Neurotoxicity	[129, 130]
Ketanserin; a quinzoline derivative		Sterol biosynthetic pathway	Ketanserin inhibits the HMGR enzyme of *L. donovani*.	Dizziness, edema, dry mouth, weight gain, and prolonged QT interval in a dose-related manner.	[131, 132]
5-Fluorouracil; a pyrimidine nucleoside analogue		Purine salvage pathway	5-Fluorouracil is transformed *in vivo* to the active metabolite 5-fluoroxyuridine monophosphate, which binds to RNA and inhibits cell development. *Leishmania* are able to salvage pyrimidines from their host environment. However, *L. donovani* mutants lacking the pyrimidine salvage LdUPRT enzyme are hypersensitive to 5-fluorouracil at high doses.	Cytotoxicity.	[133]
Suramin; a polyanionic benzanilide derivative		Purine salvage pathway	Suramin significantly reduced the (splenic/hepatic) parasitic burden in BALB/c mice infected with *L. donovani*. It switched the immune response in the infected mice from TH2 to a TH1 type. Suramin inhibited the parasitic phosphoglycerate kinase (LmPGK). Therefore, suramin could be included in the repertoire of drugs used to treat VL.	Nephrotoxicity, hypersensitivity reactions, anemia, bone marrow toxicity, and lack of bioavailability.	[134, 135]
N-ethylmaleimide; a suphydryl alkylating agent		Glycosyl Phosphatidyl Inositol (GPI) biosynthesis	*N*-ethylmaleimide blocks glycosyl phosphatidyl inositol (GPI) biosynthesis by irreversible inhibition of the enzymatic multi-protein complex, the UDP-GlcNAc:PI α1-6 GlcNAc transferase (GPI-GnT).	-	[136]
Phenylmethylsulph-onyl fluoride; an alkylating agent		Glycosyl Phosphatidyl Inositol (GPI) biosynthesis	Phenylmethylsulphonyl fluoride is a serine esterase inhibitor that inhibits inositol acylation and diacylation steps and blocks GPI biosynthesis	-	[137]
Trimethoprim; a diaminopyrimidine derivative		Folate biosynthesis	Trimethoprim inhibits DHFR	-	[138]

(Table 1) cont.....

Drugs/leads and their Chemical classes	Chemical Structure	The Target Metabolic Pathway	Mechanism of Action	Remarks	Refs.
Cycloguanil; a 2,4-diaminotriazine derivative		Folate biosynthesis	Cycloguanil inhibits DHFR	-	[138]
RDS 777; an aminopyrimidine derivative		Trypanothi-one pathway	RDS 777 binds to trypanothione reductase and forms hydrogen bonds with the catalytic residues Glu466', Cys57, and Cys52, limiting Trypanothione binding and preventing its reduction.	-	[139]
Ammonium trichloro [1,2-ethanediolato-O,O']-tellurate (AS101); a tellurium-based compound		Trypanothi-one pathway	AS101 forms thiol bonds with cysteine residues of trypanothione reductase in *Leishmania* promastigotes, inducing ROS-mediated apoptosis *via* increased Ca^{2+} levels, loss of ATP, and mitochondrial membrane potential, as well as metacaspase activation. AS101 also blocks integrin-dependent PI3K/Akt signaling and activates host MAPKs and nuclear factor (NF)-κB in *L. donovani* infected macrophages, inhibiting the IL-10/STAT3 pathway.	Non-toxic immunomodulator.	[140]

RESISTANCE

Although leishmaniasis is treatable, resistance has developed almost for all drugs. Table **2** describes the ingenious mechanisms evolved by *Leishmania* to survive the toxic effects of the first-line drugs. With the limited antileishmanial agents in clinical use, combination therapy, good practices in drug supply, better compliance of patients, and hopefully developing efficient reversal agents can expand the lifespan of existing medications and halt drug resistance. Concerted efforts are thus required from the whole scientific community in partnership with the pharmaceutical industry to introduce new clinically suitable antiparasitics.

VACCINATION

Despite the efforts over the past years, till now, licenced vaccines against human leishmaniasis are unavailable. Leishmanization has been applied in endemic areas in Asia and Africa in a trial to achieve active immunization against *Leishmania* parasites. During this practice, exudates from active lesions are inoculated into a hidden part of the body of healthy individuals, resulting in the production of self-healing lesions in addition to the induction of a protective response against future infections. However, this practice presents several limitations, including the lack of standardization and the several adverse effects. Considering the different limitations, ongoing attempts aim at developing a safe and effective *Leishmania* vaccine for humans.

Table 2. Main mechanisms of drug resistance in clinical practice.

Drug	Resistance Mechanism	Refs.
Pentavalent antimonials	• The use of counterfeit medications with nonoptimal efficacy in endemic countries. • Arsenic, a metal related to antimony, contamination in drinking water. • Antimonials are prodrugs that require reduction to their trivalent form to acquire antileishmanial activity. This may occur in the host cell and parasites. The reduced form in macrophages enters the parasite through the aquaglyceroporin AQP1 localized at the parasite surface. A lower activity of AQP1 by gene deletion of reduced expression resulted in SbIII increased resistance. • The ABC transporter MRPA (ABCC3 alias PgpA) also confers resistance by sequestering drug-trypanothione conjugates within an intracellular organelle near the flagellar pocket, where the antimonial target(s) is probably absent. It is thought that the sequestered drugs are then expelled from the parasite through exocytosis occurring at the flagellar pocket. Finally, a protein localized at the parasite cell surface was reported to be responsible for the active efflux of TSH-conjugated-antimonial compounds outside the parasite. • Particular glycans at the parasite cell surface outwit the immune system of the host and allow resistance to the toxic effect of antimonial drugs by making the human host cell expel antimony drugs through the ATP-binding cassette (ABC) transporter MDR1 localized at the macrophage cell surface.	[141]
Amphotericin B	• Resistance in *L. promastigotes* was caused by a change in plasma membrane sterols, with ergosterol being replaced by a precursor, cholesta-5,7,24-trien-3β-ol. • Efflux, possibly by the parasite ABC transporter MDR1.	[141, 142]
Paromomycin	• Modulation of the parasitic translation rate, interactions with vesicle-mediated trafficking, also increased metabolism through glycolysis, and effective protection of important key players in parasitic resistance and survival by chaperone/stress-related proteins are all critical features of paromomycin resistance.	[141, 143]
Miltefosine	• Miltefosine interacts with the mitochondrion, either directly or indirectly, leading to its depolarization. Mutations in the drug translocation machinery have been detected in resistant parasitic mutants. • Changes in the expression level of ABC transporters involved in the efflux or sequestration of miltefosine have been incriminated in resistance. • Other factors, such as the calpain-like protein SKCRP14.1 and the HSP83, may also confer miltefosine resistance by interference with the parasite apoptosis.	[141]

First-generation vaccines consist of whole-killed parasites or partially purified fraction(s) of the parasite; therefore, they can mimic natural infections. Several methods were applied to kill the parasites, such as long-term *in vitro* culture, temperature, pressure, γ-radiation, and chemicals. These vaccines were very attractive due to the simplicity and low cost of their production, which is essential for wide distribution in developing countries. Nonetheless, these vaccines failed to achieve an adequate level of protection.

Multiple studies have focused on the development of second-generation vaccines that employ purified or recombinant proteins as vaccine antigens. These vaccines offer advantages such as purity and ease of large-scale and cost-effective production. Several second-generation vaccines, including LEISH-F1, LEISH-F2, and LEISH-F3, have reached clinical trials.

Third-generation vaccines or DNA vaccines consist of naked plasmid DNA or DNA encapsulated in a viral vector. They are considered safe due to the absence of the pathogenic organisms that evert virulence. Although DNA vaccines offer many advantages, including efficiency and immunogenic potential, only one candidate, namely ChAd63-KH, reached the clinical trials stage. Although the results are encouraging, further studies must be conducted to improve the effectiveness of DNA of third-generation vaccines [144, 145].

CONCLUDING REMARKS

Leishmaniasis is a complex disease caused by several species of the genus *Leishmania*. It affects people in several parts of the world. The disease presents itself in four clinical forms: Visceral leishmaniasis (VL), Cutaneous leishmaniasis (CL), Mucocutaneous leishmaniasis (MCL), and post kala-azar dermal leishmaniasis (PKDL). According to the *Leishmania* species involved, differences in the clinical manifestations and their severity are observed.

Many drugs, such as miltefosine, paromomycin, pentamidine, and amphotericin B, are currently employed in the treatment of the disease. However, toxicities and the emergence of resistance generated great interest in discovering and developing new effective molecules and vaccines.

Studies report the screening of natural products that possess antileishmanial activity, leading to the discovery of natural compounds that can serve as lead compounds for the development of new antileishmanial drugs. Over the years, efforts of the scientific community reported the discovery of new synthetic molecules with interesting antileishmanial profiles. Interestingly, derivatives of various chemical cores, such as furans, coumarins, and quinoline, presented antileishmanial activity.

Several druggable targets in the different metabolic pathways, such as sterol, GPI, and folate biosynthesis pathways, purine salvage system, trypanothione, and hypusine pathways, differ from their mammalian counterparts and were proposed for various repurposed and known drugs, in addition to new lead compounds.

REFERENCES

[1]   Torres-Guerrero E, Quintanilla-Cedillo MR, Ruiz-Esmenjaud J, Arenas R. Leishmaniasis: a review. F1000 Res 2017; 6(750): 750.
[http://dx.doi.org/10.12688/f1000research.11120.1] [PMID: 28649370]

[2]   Sangshetti JN, Kalam Khan FA, Kulkarni AA, Arote R, Patil RH. Antileishmanial drug discovery: comprehensive review of the last 10 years. RSC Advances 2015; 5(41): 32376-415.
[http://dx.doi.org/10.1039/C5RA02669E]

[3]   Kaufer A, Ellis J, Stark D, Barratt J. The evolution of trypanosomatid taxonomy. Parasit Vectors 2017; 10(1): 287.
[http://dx.doi.org/10.1186/s13071-017-2204-7] [PMID: 28595622]

[4]   Marcili A, Sperança MA, da Costa AP, *et al.* Phylogenetic relationships of *Leishmania* species based on trypanosomatid barcode (SSU rDNA) and gGAPDH genes: Taxonomic revision of *Leishmania* (L.) infantum chagasi in South America. Infect Genet Evol 2014; 25: 44-51.
[http://dx.doi.org/10.1016/j.meegid.2014.04.001] [PMID: 24747606]

[5]   Leishmaniasis [Internet]. World Health Organization. 2023. Available from: https://www.who.int/news-room/fact-sheets/detail/leishmaniasis

[6]   Gupta AK, Das S, Kamran M, Ejazi SA, Ali N. The pathogenicity and virulence of *Leishmania* - interplay of virulence factors with host defenses. Virulence 2022; 13(1): 903-35.
[http://dx.doi.org/10.1080/21505594.2022.2074130] [PMID: 35531875]

[7]   Leishmaniasis [Internet]. Centers for Disease Control and Prevention. 2017. Available from: https://www.cdc.gov/dpdx/leishmaniasis/index.html

[8]   Pearson RD, Sousa AQ. Clinical spectrum of Leishmaniasis. Clin Infect Dis 1996; 22(1): 1-13.
[http://dx.doi.org/10.1093/clinids/22.1.1] [PMID: 8824958]

[9]   Herwaldt BL. Leishmaniasis. Lancet 1999; 354(9185): 1191-9.
[http://dx.doi.org/10.1016/S0140-6736(98)10178-2] [PMID: 10513726]

[10]   Mukhopadhyay D, Dalton JE, Kaye PM, Chatterjee M. Post kala-azar dermal leishmaniasis: an unresolved mystery. Trends Parasitol 2014; 30(2): 65-74.
[http://dx.doi.org/10.1016/j.pt.2013.12.004] [PMID: 24388776]

[11]   Aronson N, Herwaldt BL, Libman M, *et al.* Diagnosis and treatment of leishmaniasis: Clinical practice guidelines by the infectious diseases society of america (IDSA) and the american sof tropical medicine and hygiene (ASTMH). Am J Trop Med Hyg 2017; 96(1): 24-45.
[http://dx.doi.org/10.4269/ajtmh.16-84256] [PMID: 27927991]

[12]   De Oliveira Rios É, Albino SL, Olimpio de Moura R, Nascimento IJ dos S. Targeting cysteine protease B to discover antileishmanial drugs: Directions and advances. Eur J Med Chem 2025; 289: 117500.
[http://dx.doi.org/10.1016/j.ejmech.2025.117500]

[13]   Hepburn NC. Cutaneous leishmaniasis: an overview. J Postgrad Med 2003; 49(1): 50-4.
[http://dx.doi.org/10.4103/0022-3859.928] [PMID: 12865571]

[14]   Baiocco P, Colotti G, Franceschini S, Ilari A. Molecular basis of antimony treatment in leishmaniasis. J Med Chem 2009; 52(8): 2603-12.
[http://dx.doi.org/10.1021/jm900185q] [PMID: 19317451]

[15]   Wyllie S, Cunningham ML, Fairlamb AH. Dual action of antimonial drugs on thiol redox metabolism in the human pathogen *Leishmania* donovani. J Biol Chem 2004; 279(38): 39925-32.

[http://dx.doi.org/10.1074/jbc.M405635200] [PMID: 15252045]

[16]   Frézard F, Demicheli C, Ribeiro RR. Pentavalent antimonials: new perspectives for old drugs. Molecules 2009; 14(7): 2317-36.
[http://dx.doi.org/10.3390/molecules14072317] [PMID: 19633606]

[17]   Gasser RA Jr, Magill AJ, Oster CN, Franke ED, Grögl M, Berman JD. Pancreatitis induced by pentavalent antimonial agents during treatment of leishmaniasis. Clin Infect Dis 1994; 18(1): 83-90.
[http://dx.doi.org/10.1093/clinids/18.1.83] [PMID: 7519887]

[18]   Brummitt CF, Porter JAH, Herwaldt BL. Reversible peripheral neuropathy associated with sodium stibogluconate therapy for American cutaneous leishmaniasis. Clin Infect Dis 1996; 22(5): 878-9.
[http://dx.doi.org/10.1093/clinids/22.5.878] [PMID: 8722966]

[19]   Rai US, Kumar H, Kumar U. Renal dysfunction in patients of kala azar treated with sodium antimony gluconate. J Assoc Physicians India 1994; 42(5): 383.
[PMID: 7829438]

[20]   Maheshwari A, Seth A, Kaur S, *et al.* Cumulative cardiac toxicity of sodium stibogluconate and amphotericin B in treatment of kala-azar. Pediatr Infect Dis J 2011; 30(2): 180-1.
[http://dx.doi.org/10.1097/INF.0b013e3181f55843] [PMID: 20823781]

[21]   Maristany Bosch M, Cuervo G, Matas Martín E, *et al.* Neurological toxicity due to antimonial treatment for refractory visceral leishmaniasis. Clin Neurophysiol Pract 2021; 6: 164-7.
[http://dx.doi.org/10.1016/j.cnp.2021.03.008] [PMID: 35112035]

[22]   Oliveira LF, Schubach AO, Martins MM, *et al.* Systematic review of the adverse effects of cutaneous leishmaniasis treatment in the New World. Acta Trop 2011; 118(2): 87-96.
[http://dx.doi.org/10.1016/j.actatropica.2011.02.007] [PMID: 21420925]

[23]   Kumar Saha A, Mukherjee T, Bhaduri A. Mechanism of action of amphotericin B on *Leishmania* donovani promastigotes. Mol Biochem Parasitol 1986; 19(3): 195-200.
[http://dx.doi.org/10.1016/0166-6851(86)90001-0] [PMID: 3736592]

[24]   Golenser J, Domb A. New formulations and derivatives of amphotericin B for treatment of leishmaniasis. Mini Rev Med Chem 2006; 6(2): 153-62.
[http://dx.doi.org/10.2174/138955706775476037] [PMID: 16472184]

[25]   Bern C, Adler-Moore J, Berenguer J, *et al.* Liposomal amphotericin B for the treatment of visceral leishmaniasis. Clin Infect Dis 2006; 43(7): 917-24.
[http://dx.doi.org/10.1086/507530] [PMID: 16941377]

[26]   Chattopadhyay A, Jafurulla M. A novel mechanism for an old drug: Amphotericin B in the treatment of visceral leishmaniasis. Biochem Biophys Res Commun 2011; 416(1-2): 7-12.
[http://dx.doi.org/10.1016/j.bbrc.2011.11.023] [PMID: 22100811]

[27]   Thakur CP, Narain S, Kumar N, Hassan SM, Jha DK, Kumar A. Amphotericin B is superior to sodium antimony gluconate in the treatment of Indian post-kala-azar dermal leishmaniasis. Ann Trop Med Parasitol 1997; 91(6): 611-6.
[http://dx.doi.org/10.1080/00034983.1997.11813179] [PMID: 9425363]

[28]   Wortmann G, Zapor M, Ressner R, *et al.* Lipsosomal amphotericin B for treatment of cutaneous leishmaniasis. Am J Trop Med Hyg 2010; 83(5): 1028-33.
[http://dx.doi.org/10.4269/ajtmh.2010.10-0171] [PMID: 21036832]

[29]   Pucadyil TJ, Tewary P, Madhubala R, Chattopadhyay A. Cholesterol is required for *Leishmania* donovani infection: implications in leishmaniasis. Mol Biochem Parasitol 2004; 133(2): 145-52.
[http://dx.doi.org/10.1016/j.molbiopara.2003.10.002] [PMID: 14698427]

[30]   Tewary P, Veena K, Pucadyil TJ, Chattopadhyay A, Madhubala R. The sterol-binding antibiotic nystatin inhibits entry of non-opsonized *Leishmania* donovani into macrophages. Biochem Biophys Res Commun 2006; 339(2): 661-6.
[http://dx.doi.org/10.1016/j.bbrc.2005.11.062] [PMID: 16310160]

[31]   Rodríguez NE, Gaur U, Wilson ME. Role of caveolae in *Leishmania* chagasi phagocytosis and intracellular survival in macrophages. Cell Microbiol 2006; 8(7): 1106-20.
[http://dx.doi.org/10.1111/j.1462-5822.2006.00695.x] [PMID: 16819964]

[32]   Ramos H, Valdivieso E, Gamargo M, Dagger F, Cohen BE, Amphotericin B. Amphotericin B kills unicellular leishmanias by forming aqueous pores permeable to small cations and anions. J Membr Biol 1996; 152(1): 65-75.
[http://dx.doi.org/10.1007/s002329900086] [PMID: 8660406]

[33]   Petit C, Yardley V, Gaboriau F, Bolard J, Croft SL. Activity of a heat-induced reformulation of amphotericin B deoxycholate (fungizone) against *Leishmania* donovani. Antimicrob Agents Chemother 1999; 43(2): 390-2.
[http://dx.doi.org/10.1128/AAC.43.2.390] [PMID: 9925541]

[34]   Meyerhoff A. U.S. Food and Drug Administration approval of AmBisome (liposomal amphotericin B) for treatment of visceral leishmaniasis. Clin Infect Dis 1999; 28(1): 42-8.
[http://dx.doi.org/10.1086/515085] [PMID: 10028069]

[35]   Berman JD, Badaro R, Thakur CP, *et al.* Efficacy and safety of liposomal amphotericin B (AmBisome) for visceral leishmaniasis in endemic developing countries. Bull World Health Organ 1998; 76(1): 25-32.
[PMID: 9615494]

[36]   Adler-Moore J, Proffitt RT. AmBisome: liposomal formulation, structure, mechanism of action and pre-clinical experience. J Antimicrob Chemother 2002; 49 (Suppl. 1): 21-30.
[http://dx.doi.org/10.1093/jac/49.suppl_1.21] [PMID: 11801577]

[37]   Gangneux JP, Sulahian A, Garin YJ, Farinotti R, Derouin F. Therapy of visceral leishmaniasis due to *Leishmania* infantum: experimental assessment of efficacy of AmBisome. Antimicrob Agents Chemother 1996; 40(5): 1214-8.
[http://dx.doi.org/10.1128/AAC.40.5.1214] [PMID: 8723469]

[38]   Unger C, Peukert M, Sindermann H, Hilgard P, Nagel G, Eibl H. Hexadecylphosphocholine in the topical treatment of skin metastases in breast cancer patients. Cancer Treat Rev 1990; 17(2-3): 243-6.
[http://dx.doi.org/10.1016/0305-7372(90)90054-J] [PMID: 2272039]

[39]   Soto J, Soto P. Miltefosine: oral treatment of leishmaniasis. Expert Rev Anti Infect Ther 2006; 4(2): 177-85.
[http://dx.doi.org/10.1586/14787210.4.2.177] [PMID: 16597200]

[40]   Monge-Maillo B, López-Vélez R. Miltefosine for visceral and cutaneous leishmaniasis: drug characteristics and evidence-based treatment recommendations. Clin Infect Dis 2015; 60(9): 1398-404.
[http://dx.doi.org/10.1093/cid/civ004] [PMID: 25601455]

[41]   Pinto-Martinez AK, Rodriguez-Durán J, Serrano-Martin X, Hernandez-Rodriguez V, Benaim G. Mechanism of action of miltefosine on *leishmania* donovani involves the impairment of acidocalcisome function and the activation of the sphingosine-dependent plasma membrane Ca^{2+} channel. Antimicrob Agents Chemother 2018; 62(1): e01614-17.
[http://dx.doi.org/10.1128/AAC.01614-17] [PMID: 29061745]

[42]   Dorlo TPC, Balasegaram M, Beijnen JH, de Vries PJ. Miltefosine: a review of its pharmacology and therapeutic efficacy in the treatment of leishmaniasis. J Antimicrob Chemother 2012; 67(11): 2576-97.
[http://dx.doi.org/10.1093/jac/dks275] [PMID: 22833634]

[43]   Valicherla GR, Tripathi P, Singh SK, *et al.* Pharmacokinetics and bioavailability assessment of Miltefosine in rats using high performance liquid chromatography tandem mass spectrometry. J Chromatogr B Analyt Technol Biomed Life Sci 2016; 1031: 123-30.
[http://dx.doi.org/10.1016/j.jchromb.2016.07.042] [PMID: 27475453]

[44]   Rai K, Cuypers B, Bhattarai NR, *et al.* Relapse after treatment with miltefosine for visceral leishmaniasis is associated with increased infectivity of the infecting *Leishmania* donovani strain.

MBio 2013; 4(5): e00611-13.
[http://dx.doi.org/10.1128/mBio.00611-13] [PMID: 24105765]

[45]   Palić S, Beijnen JH, Dorlo TPC. An update on the clinical pharmacology of miltefosine in the treatment of leishmaniasis. Int J Antimicrob Agents 2022; 59(1): 106459.
[http://dx.doi.org/10.1016/j.ijantimicag.2021.106459] [PMID: 34695563]

[46]   Sundar S, Chakravarty J. Paromomycin in the treatment of leishmaniasis. Expert Opin Investig Drugs 2008; 17(5): 787-94.
[http://dx.doi.org/10.1517/13543784.17.5.787] [PMID: 18447603]

[47]   Matos APS, Viçosa AL, Ré MI, Ricci-Júnior E, Holandino C. A review of current treatments strategies based on paromomycin for leishmaniasis. J Drug Deliv Sci Technol 2020; 57: 101664.
[http://dx.doi.org/10.1016/j.jddst.2020.101664]

[48]   Musa AM, Mbui J, Mohammed R, *et al.* Paromomycin and miltefosine combination as an alternative to treat patients with visceral leishmaniasis in eastern africa: A randomized, controlled, multicountry trial. Clin Infect Dis 2023; 76(3): e1177-85.
[http://dx.doi.org/10.1093/cid/ciac643] [PMID: 36164254]

[49]   Soto-Mancipe J, Grogl M, Berman JD. Evaluation of pentamidine for the treatment of cutaneous leishmaniasis in Colombia. Clin Infect Dis 1993; 16(3): 417-25.
[http://dx.doi.org/10.1093/clind/16.3.417] [PMID: 8384011]

[50]   Piccica M, Lagi F, Bartoloni A, Zammarchi L. Efficacy and safety of pentamidine isethionate for tegumentary and visceral human leishmaniasis: a systematic review. J Travel Med 2021; 28(6): taab065.
[http://dx.doi.org/10.1093/jtm/taab065] [PMID: 33890115]

[51]   Pearson RD, Hewlett EL. Pentamidine for the treatment of Pneumocystis carinii pneumonia and other protozoal diseases. Ann Intern Med 1985; 103(5): 782-6.
[http://dx.doi.org/10.7326/0003-4819-103-5-782] [PMID: 3901852]

[52]   Lai A Fat EJSK, Vrede MA, Soetosenojo RM, Lai A Fat RFM. Pentamidine, the drug of choice for the treatment of cutaneous leishmaniasis in Surinam. Int J Dermatol 2002; 41(11): 796-800.
[http://dx.doi.org/10.1046/j.1365-4362.2002.01633.x] [PMID: 12453009]

[53]   Gadelha EPN, Talhari S, Guerra JAO, *et al.* Efficacy and safety of a single dose pentamidine (7mg/kg) for patients with cutaneous leishmaniasis caused by L. guyanensis: a pilot study. An Bras Dermatol 2015; 90(6): 807-13.
[http://dx.doi.org/10.1590/abd1806-4841.20153956] [PMID: 26734860]

[54]   Sands M, Kron MA, Brown RB. Pentamidine: a review. Clin Infect Dis 1985; 7(5): 625-6344.
[http://dx.doi.org/10.1093/clinids/7.5.625] [PMID: 3903942]

[55]   Ruiz C, Haddad M, Alban J, *et al.* Activity-guided isolation of antileishmanial compounds from Piper hispidum. Phytochem Lett 2011; 4(3): 363-6.
[http://dx.doi.org/10.1016/j.phytol.2011.08.001]

[56]   Kayser O, Kiderlen AF. *in vitro* Leishmanicidal activity of naturally occurring chalcones. Phytother Res 2001; 15(2): 148-52.
[http://dx.doi.org/10.1002/ptr.701] [PMID: 11268116]

[57]   Borges-Argáez R, Balnbury L, Flowers A, *et al.* Cytotoxic and antiprotozoal activity of flavonoids from Lonchocarpus spp. Phytomedicine 2007; 14(7-8): 530-3.
[http://dx.doi.org/10.1016/j.phymed.2006.11.027] [PMID: 17291734]

[58]   Mishra BB, Gour JK, Kishore N, Singh RK, Tripathi V, Tiwari VK. An antileishmanial prenyloxy-naphthoquinone from roots of *Plumbago zeylanica*. Nat Prod Res 2013; 27(4-5): 480-5.
[http://dx.doi.org/10.1080/14786419.2012.696254] [PMID: 22708724]

[59]   Teixeira MJ, de Almeida YM, Viana JR, *et al. in vitro* and *in vivo* Leishmanicidal activity of 2-hydroxy-3-(3-methyl-2-butenyl)-1,4-naphthoquinone (lapachol). Phytother Res 2001; 15(1): 44-8.

[http://dx.doi.org/10.1002/1099-1573(200102)15:1<44::AID-PTR685>3.0.CO;2-1]   [PMID: 11180522]

[60] Castillo D, Arevalo J, Herrera F, *et al.* Spirolactone iridoids might be responsible for the antileishmanial activity of a Peruvian traditional remedy made with Himatanthus sucuuba (Apocynaceae). J Ethnopharmacol 2007; 112(2): 410-4.
[http://dx.doi.org/10.1016/j.jep.2007.03.025] [PMID: 17459622]

[61] Anderson O, Beckett J, Briggs CC, *et al.* An investigation of the antileishmanial properties of semi-synthetic saponins RSC Med Chem 2020; 11(7): 833-42.
[http://dx.doi.org/10.1039/D0MD00123F]

[62] Delmas F, Di Giorgio C, Elias R, *et al.* Antileishmanial activity of three saponins isolated from ivy, α-hederin, β-hederin and hederacolchiside A1, as compared to their action on mammalian cells cultured *in vitro*. Planta Med 2000; 66(4): 343-7.
[http://dx.doi.org/10.1055/s-2000-8541] [PMID: 10865451]

[63] Dutta A, Ghoshal A, Mandal D, *et al.* Racemoside A, an anti-leishmanial, water-soluble, natural steroidal saponin, induces programmed cell death in *Leishmania* donovani. J Med Microbiol 2007; 56(9): 1196-204.
[http://dx.doi.org/10.1099/jmm.0.47114-0] [PMID: 17761483]

[64] Valerino-Díaz AB, Zanatta AC, Gamiotea-Turro D, *et al.* An enquiry into antileishmanial activity and quantitative analysis of polyhydroxylated steroidal saponins from Solanum paniculatum L. leaves. J Pharm Biomed Anal 2020; 191: 113635.
[http://dx.doi.org/10.1016/j.jpba.2020.113635] [PMID: 32998105]

[65] Kaur K, Jain M, Reddy RP, Jain R. Quinolines and structurally related heterocycles as antimalarials. Eur J Med Chem 2010; 45(8): 3245-64.
[http://dx.doi.org/10.1016/j.ejmech.2010.04.011] [PMID: 20466465]

[66] Rocha VPC, Nonato FR, Guimarães ET, Rodrigues de Freitas LA, Soares MBP. Activity of antimalarial drugs *in vitro* and in a murine model of cutaneous leishmaniasis. J Med Microbiol 2013; 62(7): 1001-10.
[http://dx.doi.org/10.1099/jmm.0.058115-0] [PMID: 23538561]

[67] Malik F, Hanif M, Mustafa G. Comparing the efficacy of oral chloroquine versus oral tetracycline in the treatment of cutaneous leishmaniasis. J Coll Physicians Surg Pak 2019; 29(5): 403-5.
[http://dx.doi.org/10.29271/jcpsp.2019.05.403] [PMID: 31036105]

[68] Fournet A, Vagneur B, Richomme P, Bruneton J. Aryl-2 *et al*kyl-2 quinoléines nouvelles isolées d'une Rutacée bolivienne: *Galipea longiflora*. Can J Chem 1989; 67(12): 2116-8.
[http://dx.doi.org/10.1139/v89-329]

[69] Fournet A, Barrios AA, Muñoz V, Hocquemiller R, Cavé A, Bruneton J. 2-substituted quinoline alkaloids as potential antileishmanial drugs. Antimicrob Agents Chemother 1993; 37(4): 859-63.
[http://dx.doi.org/10.1128/AAC.37.4.859] [PMID: 8494383]

[70] Fournet A, Hocquemiller R, Roblot F, Cave A, Richomme P, Bruneton J. The chamanines, new 2-substituted quinolines isolated from a Bolivian antiparasitic plant (Galipea longiflora). J Nat Prod 1993.
[http://dx.doi.org/10.1021/np50099a013]

[71] Fournet A, Ferreira ME, Rojas De Arias A, *et al. in vivo* efficacy of oral and intralesional administration of 2-substituted quinolines in experimental treatment of new world cutaneous leishmaniasis caused by *Leishmania* amazonensis. Antimicrob Agents Chemother 1996; 40(11): 2447-51.
[http://dx.doi.org/10.1128/AAC.40.11.2447] [PMID: 8913444]

[72] Boluda CJ, Piñero J, Romero M, *et al.* Anti-leishmanial activity of justicidone and its synthetic precursors Nat Prod Commun 2007; 2(2): 1934578X0700200212.
[http://dx.doi.org/10.1177/1934578X0700200212]

[73]   Barata LES, Santos LS, Ferri PH, Phillipson JD, Paine A, Croft SL. Anti-leishmanial activity of neolignans from Virola species and synthetic analogues. Phytochemistry 2000; 55(6): 589-95.
[http://dx.doi.org/10.1016/S0031-9422(00)00240-5] [PMID: 11130669]

[74]   Rebouças-Silva J, Santos GF, Filho JMB, Berretta AA, Marquele-Oliveira F, Borges VM. *in vitro* leishmanicidal effect of Yangambin and Epi-yangambin lignans isolated from *Ocotea fasciculata* (Nees) Mez. Front Cell Infect Microbiol 2023; 12: 1045732.
[http://dx.doi.org/10.3389/fcimb.2022.1045732] [PMID: 36704104]

[75]   Avery MA, Muraleedharan KM, Desai PV, Bandyopadhyaya AK, Furtado MM, Tekwani BL. Structure-activity relationships of the antimalarial agent artemisinin. 8. design, synthesis, and CoMFA studies toward the development of artemisinin-based drugs against leishmaniasis and malaria. J Med Chem 2003; 46(20): 4244-58.
[http://dx.doi.org/10.1021/jm030181q] [PMID: 13678403]

[76]   Moghaddas E, Abouhosseini Tabari M, Youssefi MR, Ebrahimi MA, Nabavi Mousavi N, Naseri A. Antileashmanial activity of Artemisia sieberi essential oil against *Leishmania* infantum *in vitro*. Adv Herb Med 2017; 3(2): 40-6.

[77]   Emami SA, Zamanai Taghizadeh Rabe S, Ahi A, Mahmoudi M. Inhibitory activity of eleven Artemisia species from Iran against *Leishmania* major parasites. Iran J Basic Med Sci 2012; 15(2): 807-11.
[PMID: 23493354]

[78]   Ebrahimi-Sadr P, Ghaffarifar F, Hassan-Saraf ZM, Beheshti N. Effect of artemether on the recovery of lesions caused by *Leishmania* major Feyz Med Sci J 2013; 16(6).

[79]   Islamuddin M, Chouhan G, Tyagi M, Abdin MZ, Sahal D, Afrin F. Leishmanicidal activities of Artemisia annua leaf essential oil against Visceral Leishmaniasis. Front Microbiol 2014; 5: 626.
[http://dx.doi.org/10.3389/fmicb.2014.00626] [PMID: 25505453]

[80]   Babaee Khou L, Mohebali M, Lahiji N, Mehrabi Tavana A. The therapeutic effects of Eucalyptus, Myrtus, Ferula, Aretmisia, Allium and Urtica extracts against cutaneous leishmaniasis caused by Leishmanaia major in small white mice (out-bred). Hakim Res 2007; 10(2): 21-7.

[81]   Aloui Z, Messaoud C, Haoues M, *et al.* Asteraceae Artemisia campestris and Artemisia herba-alba essential oils trigger apoptosis and cell cycle arrest in *Leishmania* infantum promastigotes Evid Based Complement Alternat Med 2016; 2016.
[http://dx.doi.org/10.1155/2016/9147096]

[82]   Tariku Y, Hymete A, Hailu A, Rohloff J. Essential-oil composition, antileishmanial, and toxicity study of Artemisia abyssinica and Satureja punctata ssp. punctata from Ethiopia. Chem Biodivers 2010; 7(4): 1009-18.
[http://dx.doi.org/10.1002/cbdv.200900375] [PMID: 20397218]

[83]   Tariku Y, Hymete A, Hailu A, Rohloff J. *in vitro* evaluation of antileishmanial activity and toxicity of essential oils of Artemisia absinthium and Echinops kebericho. Chem Biodivers 2011; 8(4): 614-23.
[http://dx.doi.org/10.1002/cbdv.201000331] [PMID: 21480507]

[84]   Mirzaei F, Bafghi AF, Mohaghegh MA, Jaliani HZ, Faridnia R, Kalani H. *in vitro* anti-leishmanial activity of *Satureja hortensis* and *Artemisia dracunculus* extracts on *Leishmania* major promastigotes. J Parasit Dis 2016; 40(4): 1571-4.
[http://dx.doi.org/10.1007/s12639-015-0730-9] [PMID: 27876985]

[85]   Cortes S, Albuquerque A, Cabral LIL, Lopes L, Campino L, Cristiano MLS. *in vitro* susceptibility of *Leishmania* infantum to artemisinin derivatives and selected trioxolanes. Antimicrob Agents Chemother 2015; 59(8): 5032-5.
[http://dx.doi.org/10.1128/AAC.00298-15] [PMID: 26014947]

[86]   Georgopoulou K, Smirlis D, Bisti S, Xingi E, Skaltsounis L, Soteriadou K. *in vitro* activity of 10-deacetylbaccatin III against *Leishmania* donovani promastigotes and intracellular amastigotes. Planta

Med 2007; 73(10): 1081-8.
[http://dx.doi.org/10.1055/s-2007-981579] [PMID: 17691059]

[87]   Colares AV, Almeida-Souza F, Taniwaki NN, *et al. In vitro* antileishmanial activity of essential oil of Vanillosmopsis arborea (Asteraceae) baker Evid Based Complement Alternat Med 2013; 2013

[88]   Morales-Yuste M, Morillas-Márquez F, Martín-Sánchez J, Valero-López A, Navarro-Moll MC. Activity of (-)α-bisabolol against *Leishmania* infantum promastigotes. Phytomedicine 2010; 17(3-4): 279-81.
[http://dx.doi.org/10.1016/j.phymed.2009.05.019] [PMID: 19577452]

[89]   Brendle JJ, Outlaw A, Kumar A, *et al.* Antileishmanial activities of several classes of aromatic dications. Antimicrob Agents Chemother 2002; 46(3): 797-807.
[http://dx.doi.org/10.1128/AAC.46.3.797-807.2002] [PMID: 11850264]

[90]   Rezaei F, Saghaie L, Sabet R, Fassihi A, Hatam G. Novel catechol derivatives of arylimidamides as antileishmanial agents. Chem Biodivers 2018; 15(10): e1800228.
[http://dx.doi.org/10.1002/cbdv.201800228] [PMID: 29999602]

[91]   Pacheco JS, Costa DS, Cunha-Júnior EF, *et al.* Monocyclic nitro-heteroaryl nitrones with dual mechanism of activation: Synthesis and antileishmanial activity. ACS Med Chem Lett 2021; 12(9): 1405-12.
[http://dx.doi.org/10.1021/acsmedchemlett.1c00193] [PMID: 34531949]

[92]   Dardari Z, Lemrani M, Sebban A, *et al.* Antileishmanial and antibacterial activity of a new pyrazole derivative designated 4-[2-(1-(ethylamino)-2-methyl- propyl)phenyl]-3-(4-methypheny-)-1-phenylpyrazole. Arch Pharm (Weinheim) 2006; 339(6): 291-8.
[http://dx.doi.org/10.1002/ardp.200500266] [PMID: 16619283]

[93]   Bekhit AA, Hassan AMM, Abd El Razik HA, El-Miligy MMM, El-Agroudy EJ, Bekhit AEDA. New heterocyclic hybrids of pyrazole and its bioisosteres: Design, synthesis and biological evaluation as dual acting antimalarial-antileishmanial agents. Eur J Med Chem 2015; 94: 30-44.
[http://dx.doi.org/10.1016/j.ejmech.2015.02.038] [PMID: 25768697]

[94]   Mowbray CE, Braillard S, Speed W, *et al.* Novel amino-pyrazole ureas with potent *in vitro* and *in vivo* antileishmanial activity. J Med Chem 2015; 58(24): 9615-24.
[http://dx.doi.org/10.1021/acs.jmedchem.5b01456] [PMID: 26571076]

[95]   Arango V, Robledo S, Séon-Méniel B, *et al.* Coumarins from *Galipea panamensis* and Their Activity against *Leishmania* panamensis. J Nat Prod 2010; 73(5): 1012-4.
[http://dx.doi.org/10.1021/np100146y] [PMID: 20423106]

[96]   Ferreira ME, Rojas de Arias A, Yaluff G, *et al.* Antileishmanial activity of furoquinolines and coumarins from Helietta apiculata. Phytomedicine 2010; 17(5): 375-8.
[http://dx.doi.org/10.1016/j.phymed.2009.09.009] [PMID: 19879121]

[97]   Pierson JT, Dumètre A, Hutter S, *et al.* Synthesis and antiprotozoal activity of 4-arylcoumarins. Eur J Med Chem 2010; 45(3): 864-9.
[http://dx.doi.org/10.1016/j.ejmech.2009.10.022] [PMID: 19914747]

[98]   Verma RK, Prajapati VK, Verma GK, *et al.* Molecular docking and *in vitro* antileishmanial eEvaluation of chromene-2-thione analogues. ACS Med Chem Lett 2012; 3(3): 243-7.
[http://dx.doi.org/10.1021/ml200280r] [PMID: 24936236]

[99]   Zaheer Z, Khan FAK, Sangshetti JN, Patil RH. Expeditious synthesis, antileishmanial and antioxidant activities of novel 3-substituted-4-hydroxycoumarin derivatives. Chin Chem Lett 2016; 27(2): 287-94.
[http://dx.doi.org/10.1016/j.cclet.2015.10.028]

[100]   Nandikolla A, Srinivasarao S, Karan Kumar B, *et al.* Synthesis, study of antileishmanial and antitrypanosomal activity of imidazo pyridine fused triazole analogues. RSC Advances 2020; 10(63): 38328-43.
[http://dx.doi.org/10.1039/D0RA07881F] [PMID: 35517538]

[101] Khan FAK, Zaheer Z, Sangshetti JN, Patil RH, Farooqui M. Antileishmanial evaluation of clubbed bis(indolyl)-pyridine derivatives: One-pot synthesis, *in vitro* biological evaluations and in silico ADME prediction. Bioorg Med Chem Lett 2017; 27(3): 567-73.
[http://dx.doi.org/10.1016/j.bmcl.2016.12.018] [PMID: 28003139]

[102] Pacheco PAF, Santos MMM. Recent progress in the development of indole-based compounds active against malaria, trypanosomiasis and leishmaniasis. Molecules 2022; 27(1): 319.
[http://dx.doi.org/10.3390/molecules27010319] [PMID: 35011552]

[103] Singh GS, Al-kahraman YMSA, Mpadi D, Yasinzai M. Synthesis of N-(1-methyl-1H-indol-3-yl)methyleneamines and 3,3-diaryl-4-(1-methyl-1H-indol-3-yl)azetidin-2-ones as potential antileishmanial agents. Bioorg Med Chem Lett 2012; 22(17): 5704-6.
[http://dx.doi.org/10.1016/j.bmcl.2012.06.081] [PMID: 22832310]

[104] Taha M, Ismail NH, Ali M, *et al.* Synthesis of indole-2-hydrazones in search of potential leishmanicidal agents. Med Chem Res 2014; 23(12): 5282-93.
[http://dx.doi.org/10.1007/s00044-014-1082-1]

[105] Taha M, Uddin I, Gollapalli M, *et al.* Synthesis, anti-leishmanial and molecular docking study of bis-indole derivatives. BMC Chem 2019; 13(1): 102.
[http://dx.doi.org/10.1186/s13065-019-0617-4] [PMID: 31410413]

[106] Bharate SB, Bharate JB, Khan SI, *et al.* Discovery of 3,3′-diindolylmethanes as potent antileishmanial agents. Eur J Med Chem 2013; 63: 435-43.
[http://dx.doi.org/10.1016/j.ejmech.2013.02.024] [PMID: 23517732]

[107] Diotallevi A, Scalvini L, Buffi G, *et al.* Phenotype screening of an azole-bisindole chemical library identifies URB1483 as a new antileishmanial agent devoid of toxicity on human cells. ACS Omega 2021; 6(51): 35699-710.
[http://dx.doi.org/10.1021/acsomega.1c05611] [PMID: 34984300]

[108] Sabt A, Eldehna WM, Ibrahim TM, Bekhit AA, Batran RZ. New antileishmanial quinoline linked isatin derivatives targeting DHFR-TS and PTR1: Design, synthesis, and molecular modeling studies. Eur J Med Chem 2023; 246: 114959.
[http://dx.doi.org/10.1016/j.ejmech.2022.114959] [PMID: 36493614]

[109] Tejería A, Pérez-Pertejo Y, Reguera RM, *et al.* Antileishmanial activity of new hybrid tetrahydroquinoline and quinoline derivatives with phosphorus substituents. Eur J Med Chem 2019; 162: 18-31.
[http://dx.doi.org/10.1016/j.ejmech.2018.10.065] [PMID: 30408746]

[110] Almandil NB, Taha M, Rahim F, *et al.* Synthesis of novel quinoline-based thiadiazole, evaluation of their antileishmanial potential and molecular docking studies. Bioorg Chem 2019; 85: 109-16.
[http://dx.doi.org/10.1016/j.bioorg.2018.12.025] [PMID: 30605884]

[111] Paloque L, Verhaeghe P, Casanova M, *et al.* Discovery of a new antileishmanial hit in 8-nitroquinoline series. Eur J Med Chem 2012; 54: 75-86.
[http://dx.doi.org/10.1016/j.ejmech.2012.04.029] [PMID: 22608675]

[112] Kieffer C, Cohen A, Verhaeghe P, *et al.* Antileishmanial pharmacomodulation in 8-nitroquinoli-2(1H)-one series. Bioorg Med Chem 2015; 23(10): 2377-86.
[http://dx.doi.org/10.1016/j.bmc.2015.03.064] [PMID: 25846065]

[113] Barbolla I, Hernández-Suárez L, Quevedo-Tumailli V, *et al.* Palladium-mediated synthesis and biological evaluation of C-10b substituted Dihydropyrrolo[1,2-b]isoquinolines as antileishmanial agents. Eur J Med Chem 2021; 220: 113458.
[http://dx.doi.org/10.1016/j.ejmech.2021.113458] [PMID: 33901901]

[114] Ponte-Sucre A, Faber JH, Gulder T, *et al.* Activities of naphthylisoquinoline alkaloids and synthetic analogs against *Leishmania* major. Antimicrob Agents Chemother 2007; 51(1): 188-94.
[http://dx.doi.org/10.1128/AAC.00936-06] [PMID: 17088484]

[115] Sobarzo-Sánchez E, Bilbao-Ramos P, Dea-Ayuela M, *et al.* Synthetic oxoisoaporphine alkaloids: *in vitro*, *in vivo* and in silico assessment of antileishmanial activities. PLoS One 2013; 8(10): e77560.
[http://dx.doi.org/10.1371/journal.pone.0077560] [PMID: 24204870]

[116] Prinsloo IF, Zuma NH, Aucamp J, N'Da DD. Synthesis and *in vitro* antileishmanial efficacy of novel quinazolinone derivatives. Chem Biol Drug Des 2021; 97(2): 383-98.
[http://dx.doi.org/10.1111/cbdd.13790] [PMID: 32914553]

[117] Mendoza-Martíncz C, Galindo-Sevilla N, Correa-Basurto J, *et al.* Antileishmanial activity of quinazoline derivatives: Synthesis, docking screens, molecular dynamic simulations and electrochemical studies. Eur J Med Chem 2015; 92: 314-31.
[http://dx.doi.org/10.1016/j.ejmech.2014.12.051] [PMID: 25576738]

[118] Van Horn KS, Zhu X, Pandharkar T, *et al.* Antileishmanial activity of a series of N^2,N^4-disubstituted quinazoline-2,4-diamines. J Med Chem 2014; 57(12): 5141-56.
[http://dx.doi.org/10.1021/jm5000408] [PMID: 24874647]

[119] Birhan YS, Bekhit AA, Hymete A. Synthesis and antileishmanial evaluation of some 2,3-disubstitute--4(3H)-quinazolinone derivatives. Org Med Chem Lett 2014; 4(1): 10.
[http://dx.doi.org/10.1186/s13588-014-0010-1] [PMID: 26548988]

[120] Khattab SN, Haiba NS, Asal AM, *et al.* Study of antileishmanial activity of 2-aminobenzoyl amino acid hydrazides and their quinazoline derivatives. Bioorg Med Chem Lett 2017; 27(4): 918-21.
[http://dx.doi.org/10.1016/j.bmcl.2017.01.003] [PMID: 28087274]

[121] Khattab SN, Khalil HH, Bekhit AA, *et al.* 1,3,5-Triazino Peptide Derivatives: Synthesis, Characterization, and Preliminary Antileishmanial Activity. ChemMedChem 2018; 13(7): 725-35.
[http://dx.doi.org/10.1002/cmdc.201700770] [PMID: 29388337]

[122] Jain S, Sahu U, Kumar A, Khare P. Metabolic pathways of *Leishmania* parasite: source of pertinent drug targets and potent drug candidates. Pharmaceutics 2022; 14(8): 1590.
[http://dx.doi.org/10.3390/pharmaceutics14081590] [PMID: 36015216]

[123] Marcondes M, Biondo AW, Gomes AAD, *et al.* Validation of a *Leishmania* infantum ELISA rapid test for serological diagnosis of *Leishmania* chagasi in dogs. Vet Parasitol 2011; 175(1-2): 15-9.
[http://dx.doi.org/10.1016/j.vetpar.2010.09.036] [PMID: 21030153]

[124] Nascimento IJ dos S. Cavalcanti M de AT, de Moura RO. Exploring N-myristoyl transferase as a promising drug target against parasitic neglected tropical diseases. Eur J Med Chem 2023; 258: 115550.
[http://dx.doi.org/10.1016/j.ejmech.2023.115550] [PMID: 37336067]

[125] Croft SL, Coombs GH. Leishmaniasis– current chemotherapy and recent advances in the search for novel drugs. Trends Parasitol 2003; 19(11): 502-8.
[http://dx.doi.org/10.1016/j.pt.2003.09.008] [PMID: 14580961]

[126] Paris C, Loiseau PM, Bories C, Bréard J. Miltefosine induces apoptosis-like death in *Leishmania* donovani promastigotes. Antimicrob Agents Chemother 2004; 48(3): 852-9.
[http://dx.doi.org/10.1128/AAC.48.3.852-859.2004] [PMID: 14982775]

[127] Leañez J, Nuñez J, García-Marchan Y, *et al.* Anti-leishmanial effect of spiro dihydroquinoline-oxindoles on volume regulation decrease and sterol biosynthesis of *Leishmania* braziliensis. Exp Parasitol 2019; 198: 31-8.
[http://dx.doi.org/10.1016/j.exppara.2019.01.011] [PMID: 30690024]

[128] Moghaddam FM, Saberi V, Karimi A. Highly diastereoselective cascade [5 + 1] double Michael reaction, a route for the synthesis of spiro(thio)oxindoles. Sci Rep 2021; 11(1): 22834.
[http://dx.doi.org/10.1038/s41598-021-01766-6] [PMID: 34819540]

[129] Dinesh N, Soumya N, Singh S. Antileishmanial effect of mevastatin is due to interference with sterol metabolism. Parasitol Res 2015; 114(10): 3873-83.
[http://dx.doi.org/10.1007/s00436-015-4618-5] [PMID: 26183607]

[130]   Vural K, Tuğlu MI. Neurotoxic effect of statins on mouse neuroblastoma NB2a cell line. Eur Rev Med Pharmacol Sci 2011; 15(9): 985-91.
[PMID: 22013720]

[131]   Brogden RN, Sorkin EM. Ketanserin. Drugs 1990; 40(6): 903-49.
[http://dx.doi.org/10.2165/00003495-199040060-00010] [PMID: 2079001]

[132]   Singh S, Dinesh N, Kaur PK, Shamiulla B. Ketanserin, an antidepressant, exerts its antileishmanial action *via* inhibition of 3-hydroxy-3-methylglutaryl coenzyme A reductase (HMGR) enzyme of *Leishmania* donovani. Parasitol Res 2014; 113(6): 2161-8.
[http://dx.doi.org/10.1007/s00436-014-3868-y] [PMID: 24728519]

[133]   Azzouz S, Lawton P. *in vitro* effects of purine and pyrimidine analogues on *Leishmania* donovani and *Leishmania* infantum promastigotes and intracellular amastigotes. Acta Parasitol 2017; 62(3): 582-8.
[http://dx.doi.org/10.1515/ap-2017-0070] [PMID: 28682767]

[134]   Khanra S, Juin SK, Jawed JJ, *et al*. *in vivo* experiments demonstrate the potent antileishmanial efficacy of repurposed suramin in visceral leishmaniasis. PLoS Negl Trop Dis 2020; 14(8): e0008575.
[http://dx.doi.org/10.1371/journal.pntd.0008575] [PMID: 32866156]

[135]   Wiedemar N, Hauser DA, Mäser P. 100 years of suramin. Antimicrob Agents Chemother 2020; 64(3): e01168-19.
[http://dx.doi.org/10.1128/AAC.01168-19] [PMID: 31844000]

[136]   de Macedo CS, Shams-Eldin H, Smith TK, Schwarz RT, Azzouz N. Inhibitors of glycosyl-phosphatidylinositol anchor biosynthesis. Biochimie 2003; 85(3-4): 465-72.
[http://dx.doi.org/10.1016/S0300-9084(03)00065-8] [PMID: 12770785]

[137]   Masterson WJ, Ferguson MA. Phenylmethanesulphonyl fluoride inhibits GPI anchor biosynthesis in the African trypanosome. EMBO J 1991; 10(8): 2041-5.
[http://dx.doi.org/10.1002/j.1460-2075.1991.tb07734.x] [PMID: 1829674]

[138]   Wróbel A, Arciszewska K, Maliszewski D, Drozdowska D. Trimethoprim and other nonclassical antifolates an excellent template for searching modifications of dihydrofolate reductase enzyme inhibitors. J Antibiot (Tokyo) 2020; 73(1): 5-27.
[http://dx.doi.org/10.1038/s41429-019-0240-6] [PMID: 31578455]

[139]   Saccoliti F, Di Santo R, Costi R. Recent advancement in the search of innovative antiprotozoal agents targeting trypanothione metabolism. ChemMedChem 2020; 15(24): 2420-35.
[http://dx.doi.org/10.1002/cmdc.202000325] [PMID: 32805075]

[140]   Vishwakarma P, Parmar N, Chandrakar P, *et al*. Ammonium trichloro [1,2-ethanediolato-O,O-]-tellurate cures experimental visceral leishmaniasis by redox modulation of *Leishmania* donovani trypanothione reductase and inhibiting host integrin linked PI3K/Akt pathway. Cell Mol Life Sci 2018; 75(3): 563-88.
[http://dx.doi.org/10.1007/s00018-017-2653-3] [PMID: 28900667]

[141]   Légaré D, Ouellette M. Drug resistance in leishmania. In: Gotte M, Berghuis A, Matlashewski G, Wainberg M, Sheppard D, Eds. Handbook of Antimicrobial Resistance. New York, NY: Springer New York 2014; pp. 1-24.
[http://dx.doi.org/10.1007/978-1-4939-0667-3_17-1]

[142]   Mbongo N, Loiseau PM, Billion MA, Robert-Gero M. Mechanism of amphotericin B resistance in *Leishmania* donovani promastigotes. Antimicrob Agents Chemother 1998; 42(2): 352-7.
[http://dx.doi.org/10.1128/AAC.42.2.352] [PMID: 9527785]

[143]   Chawla B, Jhingran A, Panigrahi A, Stuart KD, Madhubala R. Paromomycin affects translation and vesicle-mediated trafficking as revealed by proteomics of paromomycin -susceptible -resistant *Leishmania* donovani. PLoS One 2011; 6(10): e26660.
[http://dx.doi.org/10.1371/journal.pone.0026660] [PMID: 22046323]

[144]   Dinc R. *Leishmania* vaccines: the current situation with its promising aspect for the future. Korean J

Parasitol 2022; 60(6): 379-91.
[http://dx.doi.org/10.3347/kjp.2022.60.6.379] [PMID: 36588414]

[145]   de Carvalho Clímaco M, Kraemer L, Fujiwara RT. Vaccine development for human leishmaniasis. In: Christodoulides M, Ed. Vaccines for neglected pathogens: Strategies, achievements and challenges: Focus on leprosy, leishmaniasis, melioidosis and tuberculosis. Cham: Springer International Publishing 2023; pp. 307-26.
[http://dx.doi.org/10.1007/978-3-031-24355-4_14]

CHAPTER 3

Chagas Diseases: State of the Art and New Perspectives

Gioele Renzi[1,*], Silvia Selleri[1], Claudiu T. Supuran[1] and Fabrizio Carta[1,*]

[1] *Neurofarba Department, Pharmaceutical and Nutraceutical Section, University of Florence, Firenze FI, Sesto Fiorentino, Italy*

Abstract: American trypanosomiasis, also known as Chagas Disease (CD), is a Neglected Tropical Disease (NTD) of the infectious type, having the protozoan parasite *Trypanosoma cruzi* (*T. cruzi*) as the etiologic agent. The CD is usually transmitted to human hosts by means of the Triatomine bug bites, and it is endemic in regions characterized by substandard environmental conditions, such as Central and South America. The globalization of goods and people significantly contributed to spreading CD to regions not previously affected and/or not adequate for the proliferation of transmitting bugs. This chapter reviews the main features of the disease, its main symptoms, the actual therapies, and the most advanced, although not for clinical use and currently considered for further development.

Keywords: Chagas Disease (CD), Chronic Chagas Cardiomyopathy (CCC), Benznidazole, Fosravuconazole Llysine ethanolate (E1224), *Trypanosoma cruzi* (*T. cruzi*), Nifurtimox, Neglected Tropical Disease (NTD), Posaconazole, Ravuconazole.

INTRODUCTION

Neglected tropical diseases (NTDs) account for almost 20 diverse conditions, which are mostly present as endemic within the tropical areas of the planet. They usually spread amongst the lowest social classes and disproportionately affect women and children over males. Such diseases primarily impact individuals' health and have significant effects at social and economic levels. Overall, the epidemiology of NTDs is quite complex as it is usually associated with multistep life cycles, and it is often strictly related to environmental circumstances. For instance, the majority of NTDs are vector-borne and nourished from animal reservoirs [1]. Among the NTDs is the American trypanosomiasis, also named

* **Corresponding authors Gioele Renzi and Fabrizio Cart:** Neurofarba Department, Pharmaceutical and Nutraceutical Section, University of Florence, Firenze FI, Sesto Fiorentino, Italy;
E-mails: gioele.renzi@unifi.it, fabrizio.carta@unifi.it

Igor Jose dos Santos Nascimento & Ricardo Olimpio de Moura (Eds.)

Chagas Disease (CD) after the Brazilian physician and researcher Carlos Ribeiro Justiniano Chagas, who discovered the disease in 1909 and demonstrated its etiological agent being the protozoan parasite *Trypanosoma cruzi* (*T. cruzi*) [2, 3].

To date, about 7 million people worldwide are estimated to be infected with *T. cruzi*. Usually, the transmission of such a parasite occurs by means of the Triatomine insect bites, or alternatively through the ingestion of foods and beverages or organ transplantation contaminated with the bug excrements. Some clinical cases of infections were reported to occur through the maternal-fetal route [4, 5].

The CD was traditionally endemic in Central and South America, specifically in regions characterized by substandard environmental conditions that are ideal for the proliferation of Triatomines. In the modern era, the globalization of goods and people highly contributed to the spread of CD to regions not previously affected [6 - 10].

Many actions are considered to control CD, and among others are insecticide spraying to eliminate vector bugs and educational programs for the exposed population to raise awareness of the pathology and the vectors. Besides such activities, research activities focused on the development of efficient diagnostic tools and treatment options are continuously pursued. As a result, a significative reduction of new infections is reported, which, however, does not impede CD from being considered a public health priority [6, 11 - 17].

T. cruzi Transmission

The life cycle of *T. cruzi* involves an invertebrate vector, such as the Triatomine insects, which include members of the *Reduviidae* family and a vertebrate host (*i.e.*, humans). It evolves through developmental stages associated with the three distinct morphological forms of trypomastigote, amastigote, and epimastigotes, as reported in Fig. (**1A-C**) [3].

The amastigote and epimastigote forms of *T. cruzi* both replicate through binary fission, respectively, within the hindgut and mammalian cells of the triatomine vector, while trypomastigote stages are not endowed with replicative ability. Areas of exposed mucous membranes (*i.e.*, eyes or lips) or skin are usually bitten by triatomine bugs, which subsequently defecate or urinate close to the bite sites. As a result, the infecting parasite enters the body through any skin break and invades the closest tissues before spreading deeper up to the heart and gastro-intestinal system [3]. Thus host blood results rich in circulating trypomastigotes, hence turning the vectors into infected ones by sucking blood. Moreover, such infectious stages may develop within the insect gut, where they multiply into epimastigotes [14 - 16].

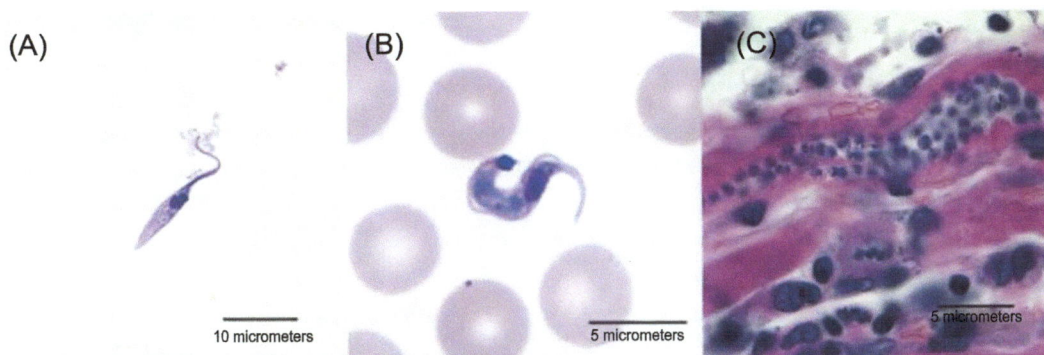

Fig. (1). *Trypanosoma cruzi* and its morphological forms. (**A**) Epimastigotes form and are capable of replication in culture (Giemsa-stain). (**B**) A smear of peripheral blood with trypomastigote within an acute Chagas disease-affected patient (Giemsa-stain). (**C**) Patients with chronic Chagas disease, view of a cardiac myocyte with amastigotes inside (hematoxylin and eosin stain) [3].

Besides the classical diffusion by triatomine bites, *T. cruzi* can also be transmitted to human hosts by means of:

• Oral transmission is due to the consumption of food contaminated with *T. cruzi* and/or water. Such transmission is associated with a higher incidence of more severe case outbreaks and mortality than vector-borne disease [17].
• Vertical or congenital transmission from an infected mother (especially with high parasitic load) to newborns during pregnancy or childbirth [18].
• Transfusion of whole blood or platelets [19, 20], solid organs, and bone marrow transplants from infected donors [21]. Specific accidents that occurred in biologic laboratories have been identified as an unintentional source of *T. cruzi* transmission [4, 22].

Pathogenesis of Chagas Disease

Since *T. cruzi* inoculation occurs, the pathogenesis and the symptomatology of CD have evolved over time, with the protozoan load increasing within the host. As a result, the disease slowly becomes relevant symptomatology and is associated with higher degrees of health risks (Fig. **2**).

Organ dysfunction or damage is mainly associated with the acute phase of the disease due to the host's strong inflammatory response and the action of the parasite itself. Hence, tissues such as skeletal, cardiac, and smooth muscles may present *T. cruzi* as a nest of amastigote form. Moreover, the central nervous system (CNS), gonads, and mononuclear phagocytes may also be infected [24,

25]. Once the acute phase is settled, the host triggers an intense inflammatory response with the aim of controlling the parasite efficiently. Such response is assured by activation of the innate immune response, such as macrophages and natural cell killers by antibody production (Table **1**) [26].

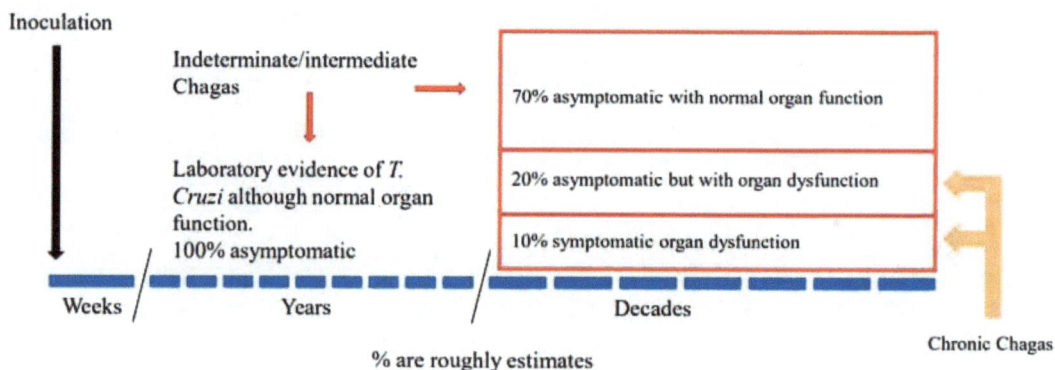

Fig. (2). Pathogenesis of CD over the time [23].

Table 1. Pathogenetic mechanisms proposed for CD [27].

-	Proposed Mechanism	Description
Parasite persistence	Parasite immunity (*i.e.*, specific one)	Whether in animal models and acute (and occasionally chronic) human infections, the co-occurrence of parasites and parasite antigens is accompanied by inflammation, characterized by the presence of mononuclear cells and sometimes eosinophils. The parasite triggers both humoral and cellular immunity responses, and notably, the latter demonstrates a more pronounced protective effect than the former in animal models with secondary infections.
-	Cell lysis induced by parasite	Parasites are capable of interacting with Toll-like receptors (TLRs), developing an early inflammatory response, thus triggering the production of cytokines and chemokines, which allow the recruitment of inflammatory cells and their response. In the initial inflammatory response against the parasites, neutrophils, and eosinophils are involved, playing a crucial role, although causing destruction of both infected and uninfected cells, leading to tissue damage. In the Chagas chronic phase, the reshaping of cardiac tissue is caused by acute infection, *i.e.*, by TLR involved. Cell invasion by *T. cruzi* is supported by findings such as cross-reactivity with some complex aiming membrane attack (C9).

(Table 1) cont.....

-	Proposed Mechanism	Description
Neurogenic	Primary neuronal damage	Chagasic megacolon and megaesophagus are considered the primary processes leading to neuronal loss and damage. Such damage can be a contributing factor, thus suggested by patients often presenting dysautonomia, although the impact on heart issues has not been proved yet due to complex analysis. Parasite neurotoxin secretion is suggested as the main actor in neuronal damage occurrence, although opinions are controversial.
Autoimmune or immune	Microvasculature damage	*T. cruzi* prompts the production of different substances, either directly or indirectly, affecting microcirculation. Such substances include prostaglandins, thromboxane, endothelin-1, and others, which can induce microinfarcts and vasoconstriction, contributing to heart fibrosis.
-	Eosinophils and antibodies cytotoxicity	Eosinophils and neutrophils represent the parasite's initial inflammatory response. Myocytes are destroyed by these cells in their attempt to clear the infection (surrounding damage to tissue). As the infection progresses chronically, antibody production leads to toxicity towards various cells by cytotoxicity, which is antibody-dependent and cell-mediated.
-	Parasite induced Autoimmunity	*T. cruzi* infection may strongly activate both B and T cells, resulting in a polyclonal immune response. This evidence, such as autoimmunity of B-cells, is confirmed by the occurrence of antibodies targeting muscarinic cholinergic and beta-adrenergic receptors. Autoimmunity shown by T-cells is evidenced by the appearance of T-lymphocytes involved in the myocytes and other cells destruction, leading such response spread to ongoing tissue damage.
-	Host cells DNA integration	Inflammation may be induced by cells presenting parasite DNA, in particular influencing immune response due to kinetoplast DNA integration within multiple genome areas. In germ cells, vertical transmission concerning integrated kinetoplast was proved to cause myocarditis onset in animal models. Such an effect turns out to be stronger for the first generation, while it decreases for succeeding generations.

To the best of our knowledge, the pathogenesis of chronic chagasic cardiomyopathies is not entirely understood, and the effects on the organ were assumed to be the autoimmune type. So far, several autoantigens that cross-react with *T. cruzi* antigens and autoantibodies have been identified [26]. However, such evidence does not complete the gaps in the knowledge on the role of autoimmunity in CD pathogenesis [26]. The establishment and progression of cardiomyopathies associated with Chagas disease turned out to be finely regulated by the balance between the active immune response by the host and the persistence of infection [27 - 30].

Signs and Symptoms

During the acute stages of the infection, the CD is asymptomatic in almost all affected patients, and it manifests multiple symptoms at cardiovascular and gastroenteric levels only when it turns into chronic. Table **2** summarizes the main clinical signs and symptoms associated with CD at various stages [31].

Table 2. Clinical features and diagnoses of CD. ECG=electrocardiogram [31].

-	Geographical Distribution	Clinical Signs and Symptoms	Diagnosis
Acute forms, which include reactivation in immunosuppressed patients			
Vectorial	Endemic countries	1–2 weeks of incubation period. Common signs indicating the portal of entry: cutaneous lesion known as chagoma or palpebral edema, recognized as the Romaña sign. The majority of cases (95-99%) present with mild symptoms such as persistent fever, fatigue, hepatomegaly, splenomegaly, and lymphadenopathy. Only in rare cases, complications such as meningoencephalitis or myocarditis may arise. The risk of mortality ranges from 0.2% to 0.5%.	Detection of patient parasitemia up to 90 days is involved as a direct parasitological method. Such methods include Giemsa-stained thick and thin blood films, fresh blood examination, and buffy coats. Strout method and PCR techniques are also employed.
Congenital	Endemic and non-endemic countries	From birth to several weeks of the incubation period. Most cases either exhibit no symptoms or present with mild ones. Complications may include abortion, prematurity, low birth weight, and neonatal death. Common symptoms include edema, jaundice, fever, splenomegaly, hepatomegaly, myocarditis, respiratory distress syndrome, and meningoencephalitis. The risk of mortality is less than 2%.	Strout method, microhaematocrit, and concentration methods are employed. PCR techniques are also employed, resulting in the most sensitive technique.
Oral	Restricted areas of endemic countries	3-22 days of incubation period. Symptoms may manifest as dyspnea, fever, periocular edema, vomiting, cough, myalgia, abdominal pain, chest pain, hepatomegaly, and splenomegaly. The risk of mortality ranges from 1% to 35%.	Same as vectorial

(Table 2) cont.....

-	Geographical Distribution	Clinical Signs and Symptoms	Diagnosis
Transplant and/or transfusion	Same as congenital geographic distribution	8-160 days of incubation period with persistent fever. The same clinical features are observed in vector-borne cases. Variable risk of mortality, depending on the severity of the disease.	Same as vectorial. PCR techniques give positive results, especially days to weeks before trypomastigotes become detectable in the blood.
HIV patients with reactivated infection	Same as congenital geographic distribution	Infection which shares characteristics with other opportunistic ones. Predominantly affecting CNS, it presents in 75-90% of cases as either single or multiple space-occupying lesions. Cardiac involvement, such as pericardial effusion, myocarditis, or exacerbation of previous cardiomyopathy, is also common, occurring in 10-55% of cases. The associated risk of mortality is around 20%.	Direct parasitological methods. Identification of parasites may occur in tissue samples, CSF, or other bodily fluids, although PCR is not effective for diagnosis. Serological tests are a valuable solution for detecting chronic infection.
Reactivation in other immunosuppressed patients	Same as congenital geographic distribution	Reactivation arises after transplantation or in patients with hematological malignancies. Clinical presentations are mainly panniculitis and other skin disorders. The risk of mortality is influenced by the severity of the disease and prompting diagnosis.	Direct parasitological methods. The identification of parasites may occur in tissue samples using PCR. The real-time technique can indicate an escalating parasite load, leading to a higher risk of reactivation.
Chronic Form			
Indeterminate form	Same as congenital geographic distribution	Asymptomatic	Serology through detection of IgG. PCR: low sensitivity
Gastrointestinal and cardiac form	Same as congenital geographic distribution	Cardiac symptoms may present as palpitations, dizziness, syncope, fatigue, and even stroke. In advanced stages, edema, dyspnea, left ventricular dysfunction, atypical chest pain, and congestive heart failure are found. Gastrointestinal symptoms could include regurgitation, dysphagia, and severe constipation due to colonic or esophageal dilation.	Same as the indeterminate form

The initial acute phase of the infection lasts approximately 6 to 8 weeks, and even though a considerable amount of microscopically sensible parasitemia are detectable in blood specimens, such a phase is often associated with no clinical symptoms or unrecognized features due to very tame and non-specific symptoms. Less than 50% of people bitten by triatomine bugs clearly show the characteristic signs of skin lesions or purplish swelling on the eyelids. Romaña sign, described as unilateral painless edema of the palpebrae/periocular tissues, may occur when the entry portal for *T. cruzi* is represented by the conjunctiva. Alternatively, inflammation nodules (*Chagoma*) may appear if the infective agent is acquired *via* insect bite. These signs are accompanied by fever that may last for several weeks and locally enlarged lymph nodes. Other acute and non-specific manifestations include enlarged lymph glands, pallor, headache, difficulties in breathing, pains associated with muscles abdominal or chest regions, anorexia, oedemas, hepatosplenomegaly, and generalized lymphadenopathies. Around 5% of patients infected with *T. cruzi* are exposed to severe acute symptoms, including sinus infections of the bacterial and viral types. On some occasions, conjunctivitis and other infections to the closest tissues may also occur. Specifically, in children of < 5 years of age, elderly, and immunosuppressed patients, fulminant myocarditis, congestive heart failure (HF), pericardial effusion, and meningoencephalitis were registered [32 - 34].

The typical symptoms that arise from acute infections will usually resolve spontaneously over weeks or months without any pharmacological treatment. As a follow-up, an indeterminate chronic phase of CD takes place, which is mainly characterized by undetectable parasitemia since *protozoa* are hidden mainly within the heart and gastroenteric tissues. Usually, asymptomatic chronic infections may last for decades unless serious cardiac and gastrointestinal complications may arise, thus posing significant health risks if not pharmacologically treated [35 - 38].

Severe and frequently recognized symptoms of chronic CD usually develop to the cardiac level and account for almost 30% of all cases, while gastrointestinal-associated symptoms account for 5-20% of cases (typically enlargement of the esophagus or colon called megaesophagus and megacolon, respectively) and mixed in 5-10% [28, 39 - 44].

CD Associated Cardiomyopathies

Among the CD-affected organs, the heart is particularly exposed as various electrical dysfunctions are detected, such as left anterior fascicular block (LAFB), right bundle branch block (RBBB), sinus node dysfunction (leading to strong bradycardia), ventricular arrhythmias, as well as wall motion abnormalities in segmental left ventricular [6]. In addition, structural abnormalities to the cardiac tissue may also be present and include left ventricle aneurysms or, in worse cases, thrombus formation, causing secondary embolism, thus leading to progressive heart failure and death. Cardiocirculatory damages are present in CD-affected patients also, with either sustained or not ventricular tachycardia, multiple ventricular extra-systoles, and congestive heart failure due to progressive dilated cardiomyopathy. During the acute phase of the disease, myocytes and capillary endothelia may be damaged by cell-mediated immune features, such as necrosis of myocytes by coagulative damages, either including or not surrounding tissues, hyaline degeneration of muscle fibers, thus involving pericardium and epicardium. Quite interestingly, coronary arteries in epicardium do not seem to be affected [14, 35]. Prolonged tissue survival of *T. cruzi,* mainly when associated with asymptomatic CD, results in irreversible lesions at cardiac level neural cells, which involve either the nerves and muscles [34, 45 - 47]. CD-associated sudden deaths usually involve patients in early adulthood and account for mortality rates spanning between 55-65%. Usually, arrhythmias are mainly sustained by ventricular tachycardia (VT) degenerating into ventricular fibrillation (VF). Additional fatal events are reported, such as progressive degeneration of myocardial contraction functionality (occurring in 25-30% of patients), stroke (10-15%), and eventually left ventricular apical aneurysm or heart failure [15, 32]. Included are fulminant myocarditis with a wide range of electro and echocardiographic abnormalities, to congestive heart failure, pericardial effusion, and meningoencephalitis [40, 48, 49].

The earliest ECG signs of cardiomyopathies associated with CD reveal defects in the conduction systems, such as the RBBB and LAFB, membrane potential repolarization abnormalities, low QRS voltage, and multiform premature ventricular contractions [32, 34].

CD cardiomyopathies are highly arrhythmogenic and are quite often associated with ventricular tachycardias, atrioventricular block, sinus bradycardias, atrial fibrillation, and atrial flutter. The appearance of recurrent syncopes and/or anomalous cardiac abnormalities is better investigated by 24-hour Holter monitoring, which represents the most common and first-hand method to assess any Chronic Chagas Cardiomyopathy (CCC) [6, 39, 50 - 52]. Since CD is an inflammatory condition, a more profound and complete investigation of the organ is obtained correctly by using the echocardiography technique [53]. Sub-clinical signs typical of asymptomatic CD are usually associated with diastolic function [54] and are mainly located on the left ventricular apex and inferior and inferolateral walls [34]. As CCCs evolve, variations at the left ventricular diameter and ejection fraction are reliable predictors of mortality in analogy to other forms of cardiomyopathy, whilst the presence of ventricular aneurysms is a predictor of mural thrombus and stroke [49, 55]. Chronic CD infections include gastrointestinal symptoms mainly due to damage to the intramural neurons, which induce characteristic changes to the digestive tract, such as enlargement of the esophagus and/or colon. Such a condition may be asymptomatic at the earlier stages and include motility disorder with mild achalasia, which can evolve into esophageal reflux, odynophagia, cough, megaesophagus, dysphagia, abdominal and chest pain, and regurgitation during sleep. Volvulus, bowel ischemia, and fecaloma may occur after chronic constipation, being caused by the progression of CD-associated colonic dysruptions to megacolon [15, 32]. Early diagnoses followed by adequate pharmacological treatments, therefore, are crucial for managing CD.

Parasitological Diagnosis

Microscopic trypomastigotes visualization by screening peripheral blood or other body fluids (*i.e.*, cerebrospinal one) may be executed as an accurate diagnosis of CD, either of acute or congenital type (Fig. **3**) [41].

Direct techniques represent the most accurate methodologies for obtaining a correct evaluation of the parasite load or identifying *T. cruzi* in the trypomastigotes form as well [3]. They all need fresh blood samples or thin and thick blood smears, as in the Giemsa staining procedures. Indirect parasitological methods include PCR, a more sensitive technique than blood cultures or xenodiagnoses, and it has proven to be very useful and reliable for the diagnosis of CD transmitted by mother-to-child [56 - 60]. It should be considered that parasitemia is higher within the first few weeks of infection, thus allowing specific antibodies to develop, whereas chronic CD shows parasitaemic values low and intermittent, and that makes PCR-based diagnostics and direct parasitological/microscopic detections unreliable or too close to their detection limits [41, 61]. The data variability associated with the PCR may be ascribed to multiple factors such as used blood volumes, genetic diversity of *T. cruzi*, targeted genes, immunosuppression host events, CD infection stage, and, more specifically, laboratory-applied methodologies [61, 62].

Overall, serological techniques are all based on the use of recombinant antigens and synthetic peptides, which include 3 indirect techniques, *i.e.*, haemagglutination, fluorescent assay, and ELISA [41, 63]. On the other hand, rapid diagnostic tests (*i.e.*, immunochromatographic assays using recombinant proteins) are not sufficiently sensitive to be used as first-line diagnostic tools [62].

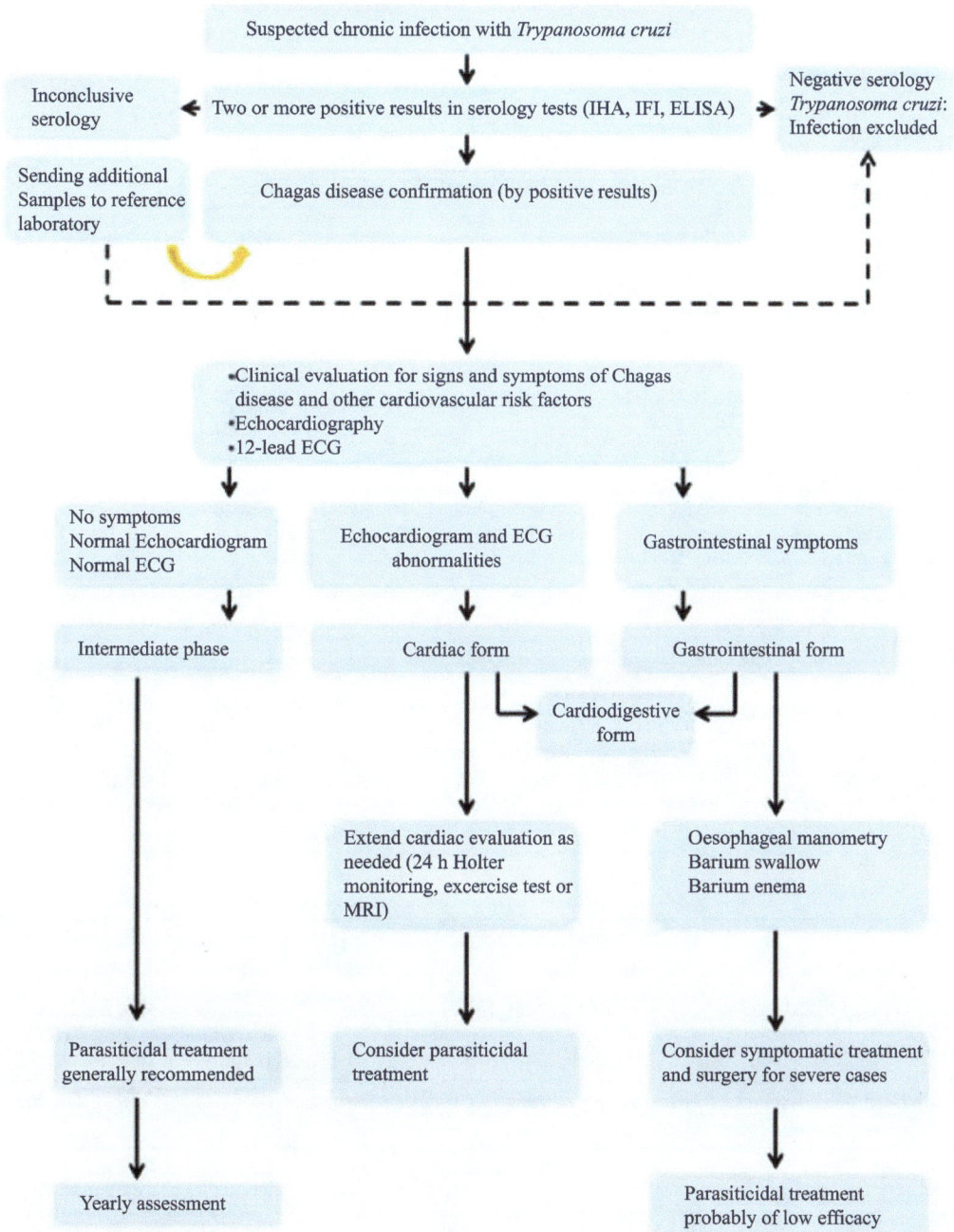

Fig. (3). Schematic workflow for the assessment of chronic CD in patients. IFAT=Indirect Fluorescent Antibody Test; HAI= Inhibition of Hemagglutination; ECG=Electrocardiogram; ECG=Echocardiogram [31].

Pharmacological Treatment of CD

Primary care on CD affected patients is gradually assuming an essential role since medical specialists apply the most appropriate treatment after careful evaluation of the disease. Post-treatment surveillance holds equal significance, especially for subjects particularly exposed to cardiovascular complications.

The main purpose of CD pharmacological approaches is to eradicate the parasite from infected individuals, as well as to decrease the probability of developing associated symptomatologies (Table **3**) [31].

Despite the importance of the global scale of CD, Nifurtimox, and Benznidazole are the only two drugs effectively used as antiinfectives for the management of *T. cruzi* since the 1970s. Usually, they are administered under monotherapy regimens for 60–90-day cycles (Fig. **4**).

Table 3. Treatment of CD according to disease stages. cART= Antiretroviral Combination Therapy; IRIS = Immune Inflammatory Reconstitution syndrome [31].

Chagas Disease Treatment	
Acute Infection	
Oral and/or vectorial infection	Treatment is based on starting with antiparasitic drugs as soon as possible. In particular, Benznidazole is administered at 5–10 mg/kg per day for 60 days, which may be swapped to Nifurtimox 10–15 mg/kg per day for 60–90 days. Among children below 12 years of age, Nifurtimox is administered at 15 mg/kg per day for 60 days, while Benznidazole is administered at 10 mg/kg per day for the same time.
Congenital	Treatment is based on using Nifurtimox 15–20 mg/kg per day for 60 days or Benznidazole 10 mg/kg per day for the same period.
Pregnant women	With other potentially teratogenic drugs, a risk-benefit ratio is considered in pregnant women. Moreover, neonatal abnormalities were not shown using Benznidazole, although experience was limited.
Laboratory accidents	Nifurtimox is administered at 8–10 mg/kg per day, and Benznidazole is administered at 5–7.5 mg/kg per day, both for 10–14 days.
Infected donor's transplant or post-transfusion	Nifurtimox 8–10 mg/kg per day or Benznidazole 5–7.5 mg/kg per day, both administered for 60 days.
Chronic Infection	
Treatment in children	Conversely to acute infection, Benznidazole is administered as 5–7.5 mg/kg per day for 60 days, whilst Nifurtimox is 8–10 mg/kg per day for 60–90 days.

Chagas Disease Treatment	
Adults therapy	Treatment is based on Nifurtimox 8–10 mg/kg per day for 60–90 days or administration of Benznidazole as 5–7.5 mg/kg per day for 60 days. Such dosages are strongly indicated for childbearing-age women, although it is discouraged concerning pregnant women. In advanced (moderated or not) visceral disease and in long-lasting infection, no planned benefits were demonstrated.
HIV-infected patients	Both in infected and non-HIV-infected patients, especially when presenting a CD4 count lower than 200 cells per μL, treatment combining cART and antiparasitic drugs is recommended.
Patients' treatment after transplant	No recommendations are given for antitrypanosomal drug prophylaxis in patients infected before transplantation by *T. cruzi*; alive donors, as well as potential patients receiving heart transplants, both infected with *Trypanosoma cruzi*, should consider pretransplant treatment. Among them, administration of Benznidazole (5 mg/kg per day) is preferred over Nifurtimox (8–10 mg/kg per day) for 60 days of treatment, constantly monitoring drug toxicity. In order to exclude reactivation in seropositive patients, or possibly infection acquired from a donor, for seronegative patients and seropositive donors, careful parasitological monitoring post-transplant is necessary.
Patients already being treated with immunosuppressive drugs	Further advantages for avoiding post-treatment reactivations were considered when treating all patients. Moreover, in patients not previously treated with trypanocidal drugs, parasitological screening is recommended and should be closely conducted.
Reactivation Cases	
HIV-infected patients	Treatment is based on starting with antiparasitic drugs as soon as possible. In particular, Benznidazole is administered as 5–7.5 mg/kg per day for 60 days, although in CNS involvement, higher doses should be considered (15 mg/kg per day), which may be swapped to Nifurtimox 8–10 mg/kg per day for the same time. Further treatment consists of cART (though without reports for *T. cruzi* IRIS) with early onset. Benznidazole represents follow-up prophylaxis by administering 5 mg/kg per day, with a dosage of three times per week. Nevertheless, 200 mg daily should be maintained until the CD4 count reaches values above 200–250 cells/μL for 6 months, alongside an undetectable HIV viral load.
Transplant patients	Although more extended periods are strongly recommended, actual therapy accounts for the administration of Nifurtimox, 8–10 mg/kg per day for 90 days, or Benznidazole, with 5–7.5 mg/kg per day for 60 days, with close toxicity monitoring.
Failure of Treatment	
Immunocompetent patients	Outcomes of positive PCR results are usually associated with treatment failure. Thus, unchanged outcomes concerning original therapy and indications should suggest retreatment with or without closer monitoring activity. Antiparasitic regimen including the same or different drug for 60-90 days may be used, while more extended drug regimens as well as combination treatments might be evaluated.

(Table 3) cont.....

Chagas Disease Treatment	
Patients with immunosuppression	Retreatment by using the same or different drug for 60-90 days should be initiated in such patients, while more extended drug regimens, as well as combination treatments, might be evaluated.

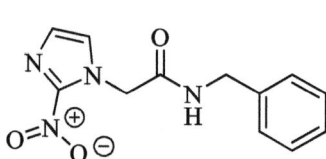

Benznidazole   **Nifurtimox**

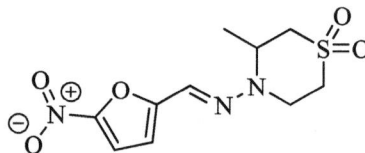

Fig. (4). Chemical structures of Benznidazole and Nifurtimox.

Nifurtimox turned out to be highly effective, especially when promptly administered at the beginning of the infectious process. For instance, metadata analysis accounts for the therapeutic efficacy of Nifurtimox spanning from 65-80% and reaching nearly 100% for individuals with early diagnosed acute and congenitally acquired CD. The incidence of adverse effects registered in patients treated with Nifurtimox is quite relevant (*i.e.*, 43.0% to 97.5%). The most prevalent are anorexia, abdominal pains, headache, dizziness, vertigo, weight loss, and generalized neurological disorders (*i.e.*, irritability, insomnia, disorientation, mood instability, paresthesias, peripheral neuropathies). In addition, gastroenteric effects such as nausea, occasionally associated with fever and rashes, were also reported [41, 47, 52, 64].

Nifurtimox undergoes within the parasite a process of reductive metabolism, which leads to the generation of highly toxic nitro radical species that determine oxidative stress and damage at DNA, protein, lipid levels, and mitochondrial dysfunction.

Benznidazole is the drug of choice for *T. cruzi*-affected patients' treatment as it reports superior tissue penetration features, safety, tolerability, and therapeutic efficacy profiles when compared to Nifurtimox [47]. A typical signature of benznidazole is its significant therapeutic efficacy, *i.e.*, in both the acute and the early phases of *T. cruzi* infection. For instance, almost all neonatal patients affected with congenital CD and subjected to Benznidazole treatment show no traces of the etiological agent in the serological specimens within their first year of life, whereas the efficacy percentage decreases to 76% in non-neonatal individuals with acute CD [65, 66]. Treatment for chronic CD by the administration of Benznidazole at indeterminate stages accounts for a success rate of 60-93% for children with age below 12 years old and 2-40% for adults presenting late chronic CD [42, 67 - 69]. Such observations are entirely consistent with various clinical cases that reported the development of Benznidazole persistent parasite strains associated with chronic forms of CD [70 - 75]. The trial conducted in 2015 and named BENEFIT (Benznidazole Evaluation for Interrupting Trypanosomiasis) included 2854 CCC-diagnosed patients treated by the administration of either Benznidazole or a placebo for 80 days and subsequently followed for 5.4 years. Although most of the patients underwent negative seroconversion, no significant reduction in signs associated with cardiac deterioration was registered. Such a trial was the most convincing clinical proof of the effectiveness of Benznidazole in parasite clearance [72]. The most frequent adverse reactions associated with Benznidazole include hypersensitivity, allergic dermatitis, primarily concerning skin rash (29–50%), gastroenteric intolerances (5–15%), and general symptoms such as anorexia, headache, asthenia, sleeping disorders (5-40%) [52, 73]. Rare occurrences of less than 1% of registered cases include neuropathies and bone marrow suppression. Peripheral neuropathies usually take place in the late period of the treatment and, although reversible events, may persist for months, thus necessitating immediate suspension of the drug [43, 72, 74, 75]. In this context, Nifurtimox appears as a safer alternative drug [76]. The exact mechanism of action of Benznidazole is believed to involve selectively an enzyme found in protozoan parasites but not in humans. *i.e.*, the trypanosomal type-I nitroreductase (NTRI) [77], thus leading to the generation of toxic intermediates of the nitro-radical type responsible for inducing lethal damages at the DNA and protein level as well as disruption of the trypanosomal red-ox homeostasis. Evidence for an alternative mode of action accounts for Benznidazole to affect the glutathione (and trypanothione) pathway [78].

Accumulating evidence primarily obtained from observational studies indicates that both Nifurtimox and Benznidazole reduce morbidity and mortality when administered to adults with chronic CD [39, 45, 72]. However, their administration to pregnant women and/or patients affected by severe renal or hepatic deficiencies is strongly discouraged [40]. Overall, the therapeutic effectiveness of both drugs is vastly diminished with long-lasting CDs, thus including individuals experiencing reactivation of the infection (*i.e.*, due to immunosuppression) and patients in the early chronic stages of CD [52].

The mild side effects associated with Nifurtimox and Benznidazole are usually reduced by the administration of antihistamines, corticosteroids, or their combination [79].

A timely and appropriate diagnosis of the disease remains highly vital for the identification of the most effective treatment against CD, as schematically reproduced in Fig. (**5**).

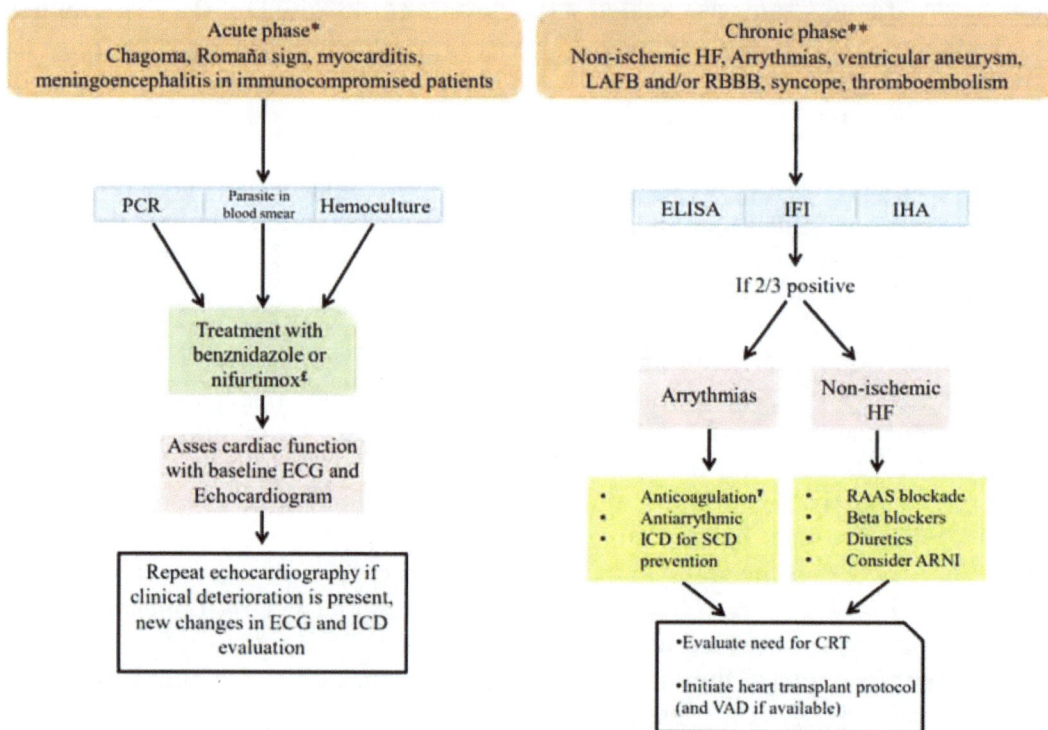

Fig. (5). Diagnosis and Treatment of Chagas Cardiomyopathy. Acute phase*: exposure time about 1-2 weeks, Patients living in endemic areas or patients who recently traveled to such regions; Chronic phase**: Patients who were born/lived in endemic areas for long periods or patients who obtained platelet or blood transfusions, *i.e.*, in regions that do include immigrant people from endemic areas. £ 60 days of monotherapy; ¥ Echocardiography for identifying cardiac thrombus anticoagulation evaluated in atrial fibrillation with previous degenerated events (*i.e.*, thromboembolic ones). PCR: Polymerase Chain Reaction; HF: Heart Failure; LAFB: Left Anterior Fascicular Block; RBBB: Right Bundle Branch Block; ELISA: Enzyme-Linked Immunosorbent Assay; IFI: Immunofluorescent Antibody Assay; IHA: Indirect Hemagglutination; CRT: Cardiac Resynchronization Therapy; VAD: Ventricular Assist Device; ARNI: Angiotensin Receptor Neprilysin Inhibitors; RAAS: Renin-Angiotensin-Aldosterone System; ECC: Electrocardiogram; SCD: Sudden Cardiac Death; ICD: Implantable Cardioverter Defibrillator [6].

Novel Therapeutic Approaches

Since Benznidazole and Nifurtimox were introduced for the clinical treatment of CD, allopurinol and some derivatives of the triazole type (*i.e.*, inhibitors of the ergosterol biosynthesis) were investigated in clinical trials, case reports, and observational studies. The administration of antifungal agents Posaconazole [80, 81] and Ravuconazole [82] in monotherapy proved effective in treating chronic *T. cruzi* sustained infections (Fig. **6**).

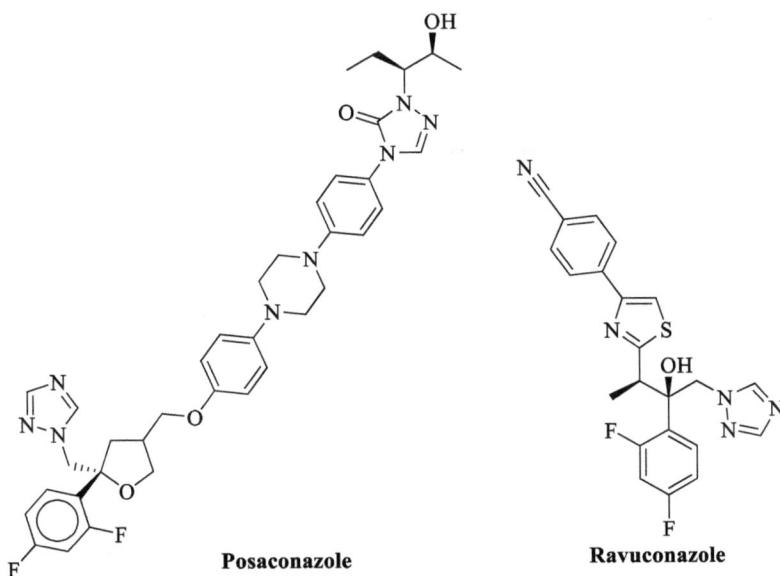

Fig. (6). Chemical structures of Posaconazole and Ravuconazole.

Quite interestingly, the optimization of Benznidazole monotherapy by intermittent dosing schedules [83], dose-reduced ones [84, 85], or other combinations [86] resulted in higher therapeutic effects. Such experimental findings, however, did not find any therapeutic application so far.

Trials involving Posaconazole for CCC treatment and the Ravuconazole L-lysine ethanolate derivative E1224 for chronic indeterminate CD demonstrated few benefits when compared to Benznidazole alone treatment, which showed failures in long-term treatment [82].

All the above-reported azole-containing compounds are known for their anti-fungal activity by inhibition of the sterol 14α-demethylase (CYP51) and thus interfere with the ergosterol biosynthesis. The same mechanism was reported for the inhibition of *T. cruzi* growth [87, 88].

The experimental bis triazole compound D0870 in Fig. (**7**) was reported to have superior activity either in acute and in chronic phase *in vivo* models of *T. cruzi* infection [89] acting *via* a dual mode of action, which involved either the sterol biosynthesis as well as blockade of cytokinesis [90, 91]. The *R*-(+) enantiomer was found to be the most potent one. Despite such promising data, the clinical development of D0870 was suspended due to adverse cardiac events [92]. TAK187 was evaluated in chronic and acute mouse models of CD, leading to better results and also providing enhanced protection against associated cardiac damages [93, 94] (Fig. **7**).

A plethora of azole-containing compounds as effective inhibitors of the *T. cruzi*-expressed CYP51 enzyme are reported in the literature, and almost all of them reported *in vitro* and *in vivo* effects of relevance [95 - 100]. Conversely, Fexinidazole in Fig. (**7**) is an exciting compound that retains a mode of action similar to previously reported azole-containing derivatives. Its structural features, however, heavily affect the *in situ* generation of metabolites as well as the toxicity profile of the drug itself [77, 101]. In particular, the real players in the observed pharmacological activity are sulphoxide and sulphone metabolites, originating from the metabolism of methyl sulfide [102]. Fexinidazole is currently in Phase II/III clinical trials for late-stage CD [103]. Besides CYP51, the squalene synthase (SQS; EC:2.5.1.2) enzyme is also implicated in sterol biosynthesis; hence, the first step in sterol synthesis is the conversion of farnesyl pyrophosphate to squalene. The aryl quinuclidines ER-119884 and E- 5700 were particularly potent in inhibiting *T. cruzi* SQS [104] (Fig. **7**).

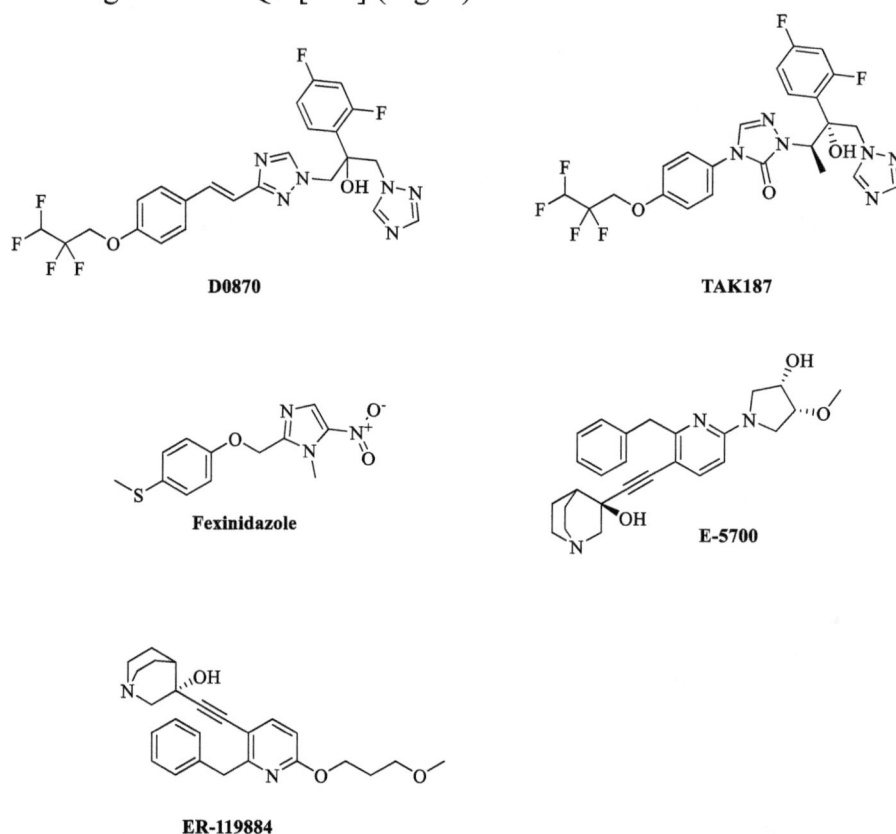

Fig. (7). Chemical structures of D0870, TAK187, Fexinidazole, E-5700 and ER-119884.

A potential new druggable target for the management of CD is represented by the *T. Cruzi* Carbonic Anhydrase (TcCA; 4.2.1.1) [105, 106]. This metalloenzyme is deeply associated with growth and virulence factors of the pathogen and is involved in breathing, CO_2 and bicarbonate transport, pH regulation, electrolyte secretions, as well as biosynthetic reactions [107]. Thus, various contributions in the literature account for intensive research intended to afford detailed structure-activity relation (SAR) on TcCA-directed inhibitors by means of screening primary sulfonamides, sulfamates, phenols, thiols, and hydroxamates [108 - 115].

The peptides Peptidyl nitrile and Peptidyl keto benzothiazoles are reversible and competitive inhibitors of enzyme prolyl oligopeptidase Tc80 (EC:3.4.21.26), which is secreted by the protozoan in its infective trypomastigote and replicative intracellular amastigote forms [116, 117]. Tc80 activity is necessary for the degradation of the extracellular collagens of the infected cell matrix, and thus, this enzyme is assumed essential for allowing the protozoan *T. cruzi* to invade non-phagocytic host cells [118, 119].

The derivative K777, a vinyl sulfone-containing compound, is the most potent inhibitor of the lysosomal cysteine peptidase enzyme Cruzipain (EC:3.4.22.51) expressed in all forms of *T. cruzi* parasite. Although such a compound was suspended from preclinical assessment, it still represents a valid reference for this class of inhibitors and the validation of Cruzipain as a druggable CD target, including natural-derived products such as Carvedilol [120] (Fig. **8**).

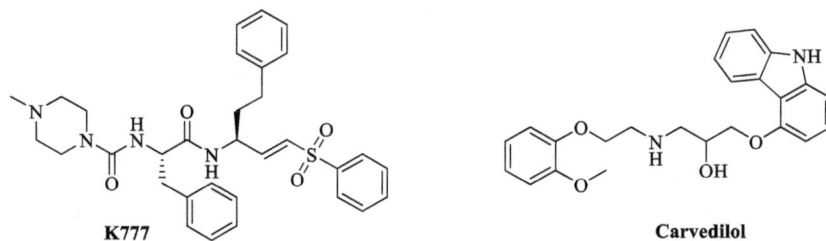

Fig. (8). Chemical structures of K777 and Carvedilol.

The main hurdle in CD drug development is represented by translation limitations concerning *in vivo* animal models and data for humans. Overall, current animal models showed scarce predictive values in preclinical stages [121 - 123]. Since cohort studies involving CD-affected patients bearing cardiac symptoms are limited, most of the available experimental clinical data make use of outcome studies on non-ischemic heart failure (HF) cases. Guideline-directed medical therapy (GDMT), incorporating the use of beta-blockers, renin-angiotensin-aldosterone (RAA) system blockade, as well as diuretics (*i.e.*, with higher diuretic doses for the treatment of systemic congestive manifestations), are commonly employed [40]. Therefore, due to elevated SCD, as well as high arrhythmogenic features and risks associated with CCC, early administration of amiodarone is recommended. Despite such studies demonstrating the effectiveness of Amiodarone in reducing ventricular arrhythmias, conclusive evidence on SCD is lacking. In analogy, the same findings were reported for non-ischemic HFs [124, 125]. Ivabradine treatment reported differences in baseline features with a clinical trend towards the improvement of heart rate in a small follow-up analysis on CCC-affected patients [126].

For individuals with ventricular fibrillation or ventricular tachycardia (VT), in particular, those defined as sustained, refractory, and hemodynamically unstable, and in order to prevent secondary SCD, the use of implantable cardioverter defibrillators (ICD), although in the absence of specific data for CCC, is strongly recommended [32, 39, 40, 127].

Bradyarrhythmias, as well as lower heart rates, are often exhibited by CD patients, and that makes the use of beta-blocker drugs challenging. Bradycardia may also periodically restrict the use of medications like amiodarone and digoxin [40, 45, 128].

Due to the considerable incidence of atrial fibrillation, atrial flutter, and systemic embolism, Ivabradine treatment reported differences in baseline features with a clinical trend toward the improvement of heart rate in a small follow-up analysis on CCC-affected patients [126].

Due to the considerable incidence of atrial fibrillation, atrial flutter, and systemic embolism associated with mural thrombus and apical aneurysms, anticoagulation therapy is strongly recommended for the management of the disease, especially when the stroke risk is higher than significant bleeding risk [45, 47, 129]. Criteria are generally similar to other etiologies, except for relative contraindications such as megacolon or megaesophagus [49, 130, 131]. Immunosuppressive therapies need careful monitoring and awareness of CD reactivation risk. For instance, meningoencephalitis is defined as the most frequent manifestation directly linked to poor prognosis [15, 45, 132].

Prevention

The first line of CD prevention involves controlling vector transmission as well as blood screening and organ donors, whilst antitrypanosomal therapy is being used as prophylaxis [133].

Sleeping in potentially triatomine-infested shacks or dirty mud dwellings should be avoided by travelers. Consuming possibly contaminated brown juices or fruits should also be avoided. Among the different strategies for preventing infection, mosquito nets and insect repellents are considered mainly because, unfortunately, there is no vaccine available yet to prevent *T. cruzi* transmission [134].

A secondary line of prevention involves timely screening tests for CD to tackle any infection progress. Screening is also recommended for children whose mothers were from endemic countries and, especially, for those presenting an indexed case as a family member [135].

Screening for *T. cruzi* infection should be conducted on pregnant women exposed to the parasite. In case of a new diagnosis in such patients, it is essential to follow an appropriate and proper protocol for evaluating visceral compartment involvement and determining post-delivery strategies of treatment [136].

During pregnancy, Nifurtimox or Benznidazole treatments are not recommended, although conclusive teratogenicity evidence is lacking [137] due to insufficient data concerning prenatal safety.

Fetal proteins bound with reactive metabolites in rats [138] and children's chromosomal aberrations were found to be linked with parasiticidal treatment [138, 139].

Thus, a careful evaluation should be conducted on the risk-benefit ratio, as well as potentially teratogenic drugs, both in acute infection cases or reactivation ones.

Mother-to-child risk of transmission during future pregnancies should be reduced by treating chronic infection after delivery [57].

However, no recommendation for chronic CD-affected mothers was given concerning interrupting or discontinuing breastfeeding. Concerning *T. cruzi* transmission through lactation in humans, only a few data were developed, and available reports bear significant limitations [140, 141].

Bleeding nipples or fissures in the mother may be useful to recommend discontinuation of breastfeeding (temporary), while milk thermal treatment (microwaving or pasteurization) before infant feeding can serve as a safer alternative [142].

Equally, infants may be exposed to risk with breastfeeding in mothers with acute infection or reactivations. Thus, mothers presenting CD diagnoses should be excluded as donors from human milk banks, with the aim of eliminating potential transmission. Moreover, according to the findings in which treatment with parasiticidal drugs showed to be not necessary for mothers presenting chronic infection, treatments with Nifurtimox or Benznidazole are generally discouraged during lactation. Hence, Nifurtimox was less safe than Benznidazole, as suggested by recent information [143, 144].

CONCLUSION

Manifestations of CD concerning heart level are described as the most critical clinical symptoms of such disease, characterized by distinctive signs and a high mortality rate. Thus, a significant challenge is represented by addressing organ disease and preventing new infections. At the same time, a key approach involves ensuring the accessibility of readily available diagnosis and treatment, particularly among women, mostly those of childbearing age, young adults, and children. Thus, the effectiveness of existing drugs should be optimized, despite their current limitations, with the aim of decreasing secondary transmission frequency. The implementation of such measures should be part of a global strategy, including improvements concerning conditions (*i.e.*, socioeconomic) of less fortunate populations, or instead, in Central and South America, increasing awareness of the disease in non-endemic countries and sustained vector control programs. Concurrently, efforts should be made to enhance medication access, as well as healthcare system programs for such susceptible communities, encouraging primary healthcare and promoting social participation [145]. Conducting active cohort studies using standardized methods is essential to establish Chagas disease epidemiology, whether in endemic or in non-endemic countries, hence, concerning cardiovascular diseases, concurrent risk factors should be considered. Proactive measures may provide benefits to the identification of individuals with elevated risk, thus, data will be useful for obtaining a more reliable prognosis. To date, long-term follow-up analysis should be implemented, although up to now, interruptions occur frequently; all of this serves to address such obstacles, particularly appropriate for migrants facing hurdles such as legal or bureaucratic obstacles to accessing diagnosis and treatment, such as lack of knowledge of diseases, illegal work, and limited access to services healthcare in the host country. The active search for patients becomes crucial to inserting them into the healthcare system. A crucial priority is represented by asymptomatic patients and their visceral participation, with the aim of investigating accurate predictive markers in order to minimize redundant auxiliary medical visits or tests by identifying low-risk individuals. Nevertheless, a significant challenge in clinical management is represented by the absence of early markers, which leads to prolonged follow-ups and numerous unnecessary tests and causes uncertainty about the effectiveness of treatment. Furthermore, the development of new treatments is hampered by the lack of early markers, as well as the impracticality of extended follow-up periods for efficacy assessment.

Prompt integration of laboratory data into clinical applications is an essential requirement for the development of effective, well-tolerated, and cost-effective drugs. In order to achieve this, improvements in the development process of novel drugs and the identification of new targets for therapeutic action are necessary. According to the disease stage, therapy may involve benznidazole in both indeterminate and acute phases (etiological treatment) or the so-called guideline-directed medical therapy (GDMT) for treating patients during advanced chronic phase with symptomatic features.

Additional therapeutic options include antiarrhythmic therapies for some specific indications, anticoagulation for mural thrombus, ICD, ventricular tachycardia ablation, and VAD concerning major ventricular dysfunction, as well as heart transplants in eligible patients.

To date, it is imperative to identify reliable biomarkers for diagnosis and subsequently drive treatment according to the stage of the disease and thus evaluate therapeutic responses.

Specific clinical trials are required to evaluate the effectiveness of antitrypanosomal treatment and optimize treatment guidelines. Enhanced animal models, reflecting chronic infection factors in humans more accurately, are needed.

Moreover, with the aim of removing the neglected tropical disease label associated with Chagas disease, international and very stable collaborations are essential to be established in order to address the substantial challenges concerning the discovery of new drugs, preferably through partnerships between public and private organizations. While remarkable progress has been made in preventing and controlling CD in recent decades, it has expanded globally, remaining a substantial public challenge in Central and South America and thus becoming a rising health issue in non-endemic countries, *i.e.*, in Europe or the United States. Few countries have implemented reporting and surveillance systems for both acute and chronic cases, as well as active transmission routes. Strong socioeconomic and environmental determinants influence the CD, and its interconnected dimensions underscore the necessity of multi-sectorial approaches.

REFERENCES

[1]   Available from: https://www.who.int/health-topics/neglected-tropical-diseases   (last   access 28/12/2023).

[2]   Hochberg NS, Montgomery SP. Chagas Disease. Ann Intern Med 2023; 176(2): ITC17-32.
[http://dx.doi.org/10.7326/AITC202302210] [PMID: 36780647]

[3]   Bern C, Messenger LA, Whitman JD, Maguire JH. Chagas disease in the united states: A public health approach. Clin Microbiol Rev 2019; 33(1): e00023-19.

[http://dx.doi.org/10.1128/CMR.00023-19] [PMID: 31776135]

[4]   Available from: https://www.who.int/en/news-room/fact-sheets/detail/chagas-disease-(american trypanosomiasis) (last access 28/12/2023).

[5]   Available from: https://www.cdc.gov/parasites/chagas/index.html (last access 28/12/2023).

[6]   Echavarría NG, Echeverría LE, Stewart M, Gallego C, Saldarriaga C. Chagas disease: Chronic chagas cardiomyopathy. Curr Probl Cardiol 2021; 46(3): 100507.
[http://dx.doi.org/10.1016/j.cpcardiol.2019.100507] [PMID: 31983471]

[7]   Carabarin-Lima A, González-Vázquez MC, Rodríguez-Morales O, *et al.* Chagas disease (American trypanosomiasis) in Mexico: An update. Acta Trop 2013; 127(2): 126-35.
[http://dx.doi.org/10.1016/j.actatropica.2013.04.007] [PMID: 23643518]

[8]   Antinori S, Galimberti L, Bianco R, Grande R, Galli M, Corbellino M. Chagas disease in Europe: A review for the internist in the globalized world. Eur J Intern Med 2017; 43: 6-15.
[http://dx.doi.org/10.1016/j.ejim.2017.05.001] [PMID: 28502864]

[9]   Basile L, Jansá JM, Carlier Y, *et al.* Chagas disease in European countries: the challenge of a surveillance system. Euro Surveill 2011; 16(37): 19968.
[http://dx.doi.org/10.2807/ese.16.37.19968-en] [PMID: 21944556]

[10]   Requena-Méndez A, Aldasoro E, de Lazzari E, *et al.* Prevalence of Chagas disease in Latin-American migrants living in Europe: a systematic review and meta-analysis. PLoS Negl Trop Dis 2015; 9(2): e0003540.
[http://dx.doi.org/10.1371/journal.pntd.0003540] [PMID: 25680190]

[11]   Chagas disease in Latin America: an epidemiological update based on 2010 estimates. Wkly Epidemiol Rec 2015; 90(6): 33-43.
[PMID: 25671846]

[12]   Dias JCP, Silveira AC, Schofield CJ. The impact of Chagas disease control in Latin America: a review. Mem Inst Oswaldo Cruz 2002; 97(5): 603-12.
[http://dx.doi.org/10.1590/S0074-02762002000500002] [PMID: 12219120]

[13]   Ribeiro I, Sevcsik AM, Alves F, *et al.* New, improved treatments for Chagas disease: from the R&D pipeline to the patients. PLoS Negl Trop Dis 2009; 3(7): e484.
[http://dx.doi.org/10.1371/journal.pntd.0000484] [PMID: 19582163]

[14]   Benziger CP, do Carmo GAL, Ribeiro ALP. Chagas Cardiomyopathy. Cardiol Clin 2017; 35(1): 31-47.
[http://dx.doi.org/10.1016/j.ccl.2016.08.013] [PMID: 27886788]

[15]   World Health Organization. Weekly Epidemiological Record (WER). WHO. 2015; 6: 33–44.

[16]   Kirchhoff LV. Trypanosoma species (american trypanosomiasis, chagas' disease): biology of trypanosomes. In: Bennett JE, Dolin R, Blaser MJ, Eds. Mandell, Douglas, and Bennett's Principles and Practice of Infectious Diseases. 8th ed. Elsevier 2015; pp. 3108-15.
[http://dx.doi.org/10.1016/B978-1-4557-4801-3.00278-2]

[17]   Noya BA, Díaz-Bello Z, Colmenares C, *et al.* Update on oral Chagas disease outbreaks in Venezuela: epidemiological, clinical and diagnostic approaches. Mem Inst Oswaldo Cruz 2015; 110(3): 377-86.
[http://dx.doi.org/10.1590/0074-02760140285] [PMID: 25946155]

[18]   Howard EJ, Xiong X, Carlier Y, Sosa-Estani S, Buekens P. Frequency of the congenital transmission of *Trypanosoma cruzi* : a systematic review and meta-analysis. BJOG 2014; 121(1): 22-33.
[http://dx.doi.org/10.1111/1471-0528.12396] [PMID: 23924273]

[19]   Cancino-Faure B, Fisa R, Riera C, Bula I, Girona-Llobera E, Jimenez-Marco T. Evidence of meaningful levels of *Trypanosoma cruzi* in platelet concentrates from seropositive blood donors. Transfusion 2015; 55(6): 1249-55.
[http://dx.doi.org/10.1111/trf.12989] [PMID: 25683267]

[20]   Bern C, Montgomery SP, Katz L, Caglioti S, Stramer SL. Chagas disease and the US blood supply. Curr Opin Infect Dis 2008; 21(5): 476-82.
[http://dx.doi.org/10.1097/QCO.0b013e32830ef5b6] [PMID: 18725796]

[21]   Pierrotti LC, Carvalho NB, Amorin JP, Pascual J, Kotton CN, López-Vélez R. Chagas disease recommendations for solid-organ transplant recipients and donors. Transplantation 2018; 102(2S) (Suppl. 2): S1-7.
[http://dx.doi.org/10.1097/TP.0000000000002019] [PMID: 29381572]

[22]   Hofflin JM, Sadler RH, Araujo FG, Page WE, Remington JS. Laboratory-acquired chagas disease. Trans R Soc Trop Med Hyg 1987; 81(3): 437-40.
[http://dx.doi.org/10.1016/0035-9203(87)90162-3] [PMID: 3120369]

[23]   Guarner J. Introduction: One health and emerging infectious diseases. Semin Diagn Pathol 2019; 36(3): 143-5.
[http://dx.doi.org/10.1053/j.semdp.2019.04.004] [PMID: 31005358]

[24]   Shikanai-Yasuda MA, Carvalho NB. Oral transmission of Chagas disease. Clin Infect Dis 2012; 54(6): 845-52.
[http://dx.doi.org/10.1093/cid/cir956] [PMID: 22238161]

[25]   Laranja FS, Dias E, Nobrega G, Miranda A. Chagas' Disease. Circulation 1956; 14(6): 1035-60.
[http://dx.doi.org/10.1161/01.CIR.14.6.1035] [PMID: 13383798]

[26]   Bonney K, Engman D. Chagas heart disease pathogenesis: one mechanism or many? Curr Mol Med 2008; 8(6): 510-8.
[http://dx.doi.org/10.2174/156652408785748004] [PMID: 18781958]

[27]   Poveda C, Fresno M, Gironès N, *et al.* Cytokine profiling in Chagas disease: towards understanding the association with infecting *Trypanosoma cruzi* discrete typing units (a BENEFIT TRIAL sub-study). PLoS One 2014; 9(3): e91154.
[http://dx.doi.org/10.1371/journal.pone.0091154] [PMID: 24608170]

[28]   Tarleton RL. Parasite persistence in the aetiology of Chagas disease. Int J Parasitol 2001; 31(5-6): 550-4.
[http://dx.doi.org/10.1016/S0020-7519(01)00158-8] [PMID: 11334941]

[29]   Dutra WO, Menezes CAS, Magalhães LMD, Gollob KJ. Immunoregulatory networks in human Chagas disease. Parasite Immunol 2014; 36(8): 377-87.
[http://dx.doi.org/10.1111/pim.12107] [PMID: 24611805]

[30]   Machado FS, Dutra WO, Esper L, *et al.* Current understanding of immunity to *Trypanosoma cruzi* infection and pathogenesis of Chagas disease. Semin Immunopathol 2012; 34(6): 753-70.
[http://dx.doi.org/10.1007/s00281-012-0351-7] [PMID: 23076807]

[31]   Pérez-Molina JA, Molina I. Chagas disease. Lancet 2018; 391(10115): 82-94.
[http://dx.doi.org/10.1016/S0140-6736(17)31612-4] [PMID: 28673423]

[32]   Bern C. Chagas' Disease. N Engl J Med 2015; 373(5): 456-66.
[http://dx.doi.org/10.1056/NEJMra1410150] [PMID: 26222561]

[33]   Laranja FS, Dias E, Nobrega G, Miranda A. Chagas' Disease. Circulation 1956; 14(6): 1035-60.
[http://dx.doi.org/10.1161/01.CIR.14.6.1035] [PMID: 13383798]

[34]   Acquatella H, Asch FM, Barbosa MM, *et al.* Recommendations for multimodality cardiac imaging in patients with chagas disease: A report from the american society of echocardiography in collaboration with the interamerican association of echocardiography (ecosiac) and the cardiovascular imaging department of the brazilian society of cardiology (DIC-SBC). J Am Soc Echocardiogr 2018; 31(1): 3-25.
[http://dx.doi.org/10.1016/j.echo.2017.10.019] [PMID: 29306364]

[35]   Dias JCP. The indeterminate form of human chronic Chagas' disease: a clinical epidemological

review. Rev Soc Bras Med Trop 1989; 22(3): 147-56.
[http://dx.doi.org/10.1590/S0037-86821989000300007] [PMID: 2486527]

[36]   Bittencourt AL, Sadigursky M, Barbosa HS. [Congenital Chagas' disease. Study of 29 cases]. Rev Inst Med Trop São Paulo 1975; 17(3): 146-59.
[PMID: 806110]

[37]   Coura JR, de Abreu LL, Pereira JB, Willcox HP. [Morbidity in Chagas' disease. IV. Longitudinal study of 10 years in Pains and Iguatama, Minas Gerais, Brazil]. Mem Inst Oswaldo Cruz 1985; 80(1): 73-80.
[http://dx.doi.org/10.1590/S0074-02761985000100011] [PMID: 3937015]

[38]   Espinosa R, Carrasco HA, Belandria F, *et al.* Life expectancy analysis in patients with Chagas' disease: prognosis after one decade (1973–1983). Int J Cardiol 1985; 8(1): 45-56.
[http://dx.doi.org/10.1016/0167-5273(85)90262-1] [PMID: 3997291]

[39]   Chappuis F, Jackson Y. Chagas disease and african trypanosomiasis. harri-son's principles of internal medicine, 20e. AccessPharmacy. McGraw-Hill medical. In: Jameson JL, Fauci AS, Kasper DL, Hauser SL, Longo DL, Loscalzo J, editors. Harrison's principles of internal medicine. 20th Ed. McGraw-Hill; 2018; 1601–1609.

[40]   Rassi A Jr, Rassi A, Marin-Neto JA. Chagas disease. Lancet 2010; 375(9723): 1388-402.
[http://dx.doi.org/10.1016/S0140-6736(10)60061-X] [PMID: 20399979]

[41]   WHO. Control of Chagas disease: second report of the WHO expert Commit-tee. WHO technical report series, 905. Geneva: World Health Organization, 2002.

[42]   Viotti R, Vigliano C, Lococo B, *et al.* Long-term cardiac outcomes of treating chronic Chagas disease with benznidazole versus no treatment: a nonrandomized trial. Ann Intern Med 2006; 144(10): 724-34.
[http://dx.doi.org/10.7326/0003-4819-144-10-200605160-00006] [PMID: 16702588]

[43]   Pérez-Ayala A, Pérez-Molina JA, Norman F, *et al.* Chagas disease in Latin American migrants: a Spanish challenge. Clin Microbiol Infect 2011; 17(7): 1108-13.
[http://dx.doi.org/10.1111/j.1469-0691.2010.03423.x] [PMID: 21073628]

[44]   Salvador F, Treviño B, Sulleiro E, *et al. Trypanosoma cruzi* infection in a non-endemic country: epidemiological and clinical profile. Clin Microbiol Infect 2014; 20(7): 706-12.
[http://dx.doi.org/10.1111/1469-0691.12443] [PMID: 24329884]

[45]   Echeverria LE, Morillo CA. American Trypanosomiasis (Chagas Disease). Infect Dis Clin North Am 2019; 33(1): 119-34.
[http://dx.doi.org/10.1016/j.idc.2018.10.015] [PMID: 30712757]

[46]   Andrade ZA. Immunopathology of Chagas disease. Mem Inst Oswaldo Cruz 1999; 94 (Suppl. 1): 71-80.
[http://dx.doi.org/10.1590/S0074-02761999000700007] [PMID: 10677693]

[47]   Andrade JP, Marin Neto JA, Paola AA, *et al.* I Latin American Guidelines for the diagnosis and treatment of Chagas' heart disease: executive summary. Arq Bras Cardiol 2011; 96(6): 434-42.
[http://dx.doi.org/10.1590/S0066-782X2011000600002] [PMID: 21789345]

[48]   Rassi A Jr, Rassi SG, Rassi A. Sudden death in Chagas' disease. Arq Bras Cardiol 2001; 76(1): 75-96.
[http://dx.doi.org/10.1590/S0066-782X2001000100008] [PMID: 11175486]

[49]   Nunes MCP, Beaton A, Acquatella H, *et al.* Chagas Cardiomyopathy: An Update of Current Clinical Knowledge and Management: A Scientific Statement From the American Heart Association. Circulation 2018; 138(12): e169-209.
[http://dx.doi.org/10.1161/CIR.0000000000000599] [PMID: 30354432]

[50]   Rochitte CE, Oliveira PF, Andrade JM, *et al.* Myocardial delayed enhancement by magnetic resonance imaging in patients with Chagas' disease: a marker of disease severity. J Am Coll Cardiol 2005; 46(8): 1553-8.
[http://dx.doi.org/10.1016/j.jacc.2005.06.067] [PMID: 16226184]

[51]   Sánchez-Montalvá A, Salvador F, Rodríguez-Palomares J, *et al.* Chagas cardiomyopathy: usefulness of ECG and echocardiogram in a non-endemic country. PLoS One 2016; 11(6): e0157597.
[http://dx.doi.org/10.1371/journal.pone.0157597] [PMID: 27308824]

[52]   Bern C, Montgomery SP, Herwaldt BL, *et al.* Evaluation and treatment of chagas disease in the United States: a systematic review. JAMA 2007; 298(18): 2171-81.
[http://dx.doi.org/10.1001/jama.298.18.2171] [PMID: 18000201]

[53]   Parada H, Carrasco HA, Añez N, Fuenmayor C, Inglessis I. Cardiac involvement is a constant finding in acute Chagas' disease: a clinical, parasitological and histopathological study. Int J Cardiol 1997; 60(1): 49-54.
[http://dx.doi.org/10.1016/S0167-5273(97)02952-5] [PMID: 9209939]

[54]   Cianciulli TF, Lax JA, Saccheri MC, *et al.* Early detection of left ventricular diastolic dysfunction in Chagas' disease. Cardiovasc Ultrasound 2006; 4(1): 18.
[http://dx.doi.org/10.1186/1476-7120-4-18] [PMID: 16573837]

[55]   Viotti RJ, Vigliano C, Laucella S, *et al.* Value of echocardiography for diagnosis and prognosis of chronic Chagas disease cardiomyopathy without heart failure. Br Heart J 2004; 90(6): 655-60.
[http://dx.doi.org/10.1136/hrt.2003.018960] [PMID: 15145872]

[56]   Nunes MCP, Dones W, Morillo CA, Encina JJ, Ribeiro AL. Chagas Disease. J Am Coll Cardiol 2013; 62(9): 767-76.
[http://dx.doi.org/10.1016/j.jacc.2013.05.046] [PMID: 23770163]

[57]   Murcia L, Carrilero B, Munoz-Davila MJ, Thomas MC, López MC, Segovia M. Risk factors and primary prevention of congenital Chagas disease in a nonendemic country. Clin Infect Dis 2013; 56(4): 496-502.
[http://dx.doi.org/10.1093/cid/cis910] [PMID: 23097582]

[58]   Bern C, Verastegui M, Gilman RH, *et al.* Congenital *Trypanosoma cruzi* transmission in Santa Cruz, Bolivia. Clin Infect Dis 2009; 49(11): 1667-74.
[http://dx.doi.org/10.1086/648070] [PMID: 19877966]

[59]   Bua J, Volta BJ, Perrone AE, *et al.* How to improve the early diagnosis of *Trypanosoma cruzi* infection: relationship between validated conventional diagnosis and quantitative DNA amplification in congenitally infected children. PLoS Negl Trop Dis 2013; 7(10): e2476.
[http://dx.doi.org/10.1371/journal.pntd.0002476] [PMID: 24147166]

[60]   Edwards MS, Stimpert KK, Bialek SR, Montgomery SP. Evaluation and management of congenital chagas disease in the united states. J Pediatric Infect Dis Soc 2019; 8(5): 461-9.
[http://dx.doi.org/10.1093/jpids/piz018] [PMID: 31016324]

[61]   Brasil PEAA, De Castro L, Hasslocher-Moreno AM, Sangenis LHC, Braga JU. ELISA versus PCR for diagnosis of chronic Chagas disease: systematic review and meta-analysis. BMC Infect Dis 2010; 10(1): 337.
[http://dx.doi.org/10.1186/1471-2334-10-337] [PMID: 21108793]

[62]   Schijman AG, Bisio M, Orellana L, *et al.* International study to evaluate PCR methods for detection of *Trypanosoma cruzi* DNA in blood samples from Chagas disease patients. PLoS Negl Trop Dis 2011; 5(1): e931.
[http://dx.doi.org/10.1371/journal.pntd.0000931] [PMID: 21264349]

[63]   Flores-Chávez M, Cruz I, Rodríguez M, *et al.* [Comparison of conventional and non-conventional serological tests for the diagnosis of imported Chagas disease in Spain]. Enferm Infecc Microbiol Clin 2010; 28(5): 284-93.
[PMID: 19962790]

[64]   Forsyth CJ, Hernandez S, Olmedo W, *et al.* Safety profile of nifurtimox for treatment of chagas disease in the United States. Clin Infect Dis 2016; 63(8): 1056-62.
[http://dx.doi.org/10.1093/cid/ciw477] [PMID: 27432838]

[65]   Russomando G, de Tomassone MM, de Guillen I, *et al.* Treatment of congenital Chagas' disease diagnosed and followed up by the polymerase chain reaction. Am J Trop Med Hyg 1998; 59(3): 487-91.
       [http://dx.doi.org/10.4269/ajtmh.1998.59.487] [PMID: 9749649]

[66]   Schijman AG, Altcheh J, Burgos JM, *et al.* Aetiological treatment of congenital Chagas' disease diagnosed and monitored by the polymerase chain reaction. J Antimicrob Chemother 2003; 52(3): 441-9.
       [http://dx.doi.org/10.1093/jac/dkg338] [PMID: 12917253]

[67]   Sosa Estani S, Segura EL, Ruiz AM, Velazquez E, Porcel BM, Yampotis C. Efficacy of chemotherapy with benznidazole in children in the indeterminate phase of Chagas' disease. Am J Trop Med Hyg 1998; 59(4): 526-9.
       [http://dx.doi.org/10.4269/ajtmh.1998.59.526] [PMID: 9790423]

[68]   Sgambatti de Andrade ALS, Zicker F, de Oliveira RM, *et al.* Randomised trial of efficacy of benznidazole in treatment of early *Trypanosoma cruzi* infection. Lancet 1996; 348(9039): 1407-13.
       [http://dx.doi.org/10.1016/S0140-6736(96)04128-1] [PMID: 8937280]

[69]   Fabbro DL, Streiger ML, Arias ED, Bizai ML, del Barco M, Amicone NA. Trypanocide treatment among adults with chronic Chagas disease living in Santa Fe city (Argentina), over a mean follow-up of 21 years: parasitological, serological and clinical evolution. Rev Soc Bras Med Trop 2007; 40(1): 1-10.
       [http://dx.doi.org/10.1590/S0037-86822007000100001] [PMID: 17486245]

[70]   Chatelain E. Chagas disease research and development: Is there light at the end of the tunnel? Comput Struct Biotechnol J 2017; 15: 98-103.
       [http://dx.doi.org/10.1016/j.csbj.2016.12.002] [PMID: 28066534]

[71]   Kratz JM. Drug discovery for chagas disease: A viewpoint. Acta Trop 2019; 198: 105107.
       [http://dx.doi.org/10.1016/j.actatropica.2019.105107] [PMID: 31351074]

[72]   Morillo CA, Marin-Neto JA, Avezum A, *et al.* BENEFIT Investigators. Randomized Trial of Benznidazole for Chronic Chagas'. Cardiomyopathy N Engl J Med 2015; 14: 1295-306.
       [http://dx.doi.org/10.1056/NEJMoa1507574] [PMID: 26323937]

[73]   Cançado JR. Criteria of Chagas disease cure. Mem Inst Oswaldo Cruz 1999; 94 (Suppl. 1): 331-5.
       [http://dx.doi.org/10.1590/S0074-02761999000700064] [PMID: 10677750]

[74]   Pinazo MJ, Muñoz J, Posada E, *et al.* Tolerance of benznidazole in treatment of Chagas' disease in adults. Antimicrob Agents Chemother 2010; 54(11): 4896-9.
       [http://dx.doi.org/10.1128/AAC.00537-10] [PMID: 20823286]

[75]   Molina I, Salvador F, Sánchez-Montalvá A, *et al.* Toxic profile of benznidazole in patients with chronic Chagas disease: risk factors and comparison of the product from two different manufacturers. Antimicrob Agents Chemother 2015; 59(10): 6125-31.
       [http://dx.doi.org/10.1128/AAC.04660-14] [PMID: 26195525]

[76]   Pérez-Molina JA, Sojo-Dorado J, Norman F, *et al.* Nifurtimox therapy for Chagas disease does not cause hypersensitivity reactions in patients with such previous adverse reactions during benznidazole treatment. Acta Trop 2013; 127(2): 101-4.
       [http://dx.doi.org/10.1016/j.actatropica.2013.04.003] [PMID: 23583863]

[77]   Hall BS, Wilkinson SR. Activation of benznidazole by trypanosomal type I nitroreductases results in glyoxal formation. Antimicrob Agents Chemother 2012; 56(1): 115-23.
       [http://dx.doi.org/10.1128/AAC.05135-11] [PMID: 22037852]

[78]   Trochine A, Creek DJ, Faral-Tello P, Barrett MP, Robello C. Benznidazole biotransformation and multiple targets in *Trypanosoma cruzi* revealed by metabolomics. PLoS Negl Trop Dis 2014; 8(5): e2844.
       [http://dx.doi.org/10.1371/journal.pntd.0002844] [PMID: 24853684]

[79]   Rassi A, Amato Neto V, de Siqueira AF, *et al.* [Treatment of chronic Chagas' disease with an association of nifurtimox and corticoid]. Rev Soc Bras Med Trop 2002; 35(6): 547-50.
[http://dx.doi.org/10.1590/S0037-86822002000600001] [PMID: 12612733]

[80]   Available from: www.clinicaltrials.gov # NCT01162967 (last access 28/12/2023).

[81]   Available from: www.clinicaltrials.gov # NCT01377480 (last access 28/12/2023).

[82]   Diniz LF, Caldas IS, Guedes PMM, *et al.* Effects of ravuconazole treatment on parasite load and immune response in dogs experimentally infected with *Trypanosoma cruzi.* Antimicrob Agents Chemother 2010; 54(7): 2979-86.
[http://dx.doi.org/10.1128/AAC.01742-09] [PMID: 20404124]

[83]   Morillo CA, Waskin H, Sosa-Estani S, *et al.* Benznidazole and posaconazole in eliminating parasites in asymptomatic T. cruzi carriers. J Am Coll Cardiol 2017; 69(8): 939-47.
[http://dx.doi.org/10.1016/j.jacc.2016.12.023] [PMID: 28231946]

[84]   Álvarez MG, Hernández Y, Bertocchi G, *et al.* New scheme of intermittent benznidazole administration in patients chronically infected with *Trypanosoma cruzi*: a pilot short-term follow-up study with adult patients. Antimicrob Agents Chemother 2016; 60(2): 833-7.
[http://dx.doi.org/10.1128/AAC.00745-15] [PMID: 26596935]

[85]   Soy D, Aldasoro E, Guerrero L, *et al.* Population pharmacokinetics of benznidazole in adult patients with Chagas disease. Antimicrob Agents Chemother 2015; 59(6): 3342-9.
[http://dx.doi.org/10.1128/AAC.05018-14] [PMID: 25824212]

[86]   Altcheh J, Moscatelli G, Mastrantonio G, *et al.* Population pharmacokinetic study of benznidazole in pediatric Chagas disease suggests efficacy despite lower plasma concentrations than in adults. PLoS Negl Trop Dis 2014; 8(5): e2907.
[http://dx.doi.org/10.1371/journal.pntd.0002907] [PMID: 24853169]

[87]   Lepesheva GI, Waterman MR. Structural basis for conservation in the CYP51 family. Biochim Biophys Acta Proteins Proteomics 2011; 1814(1): 88-93.
[http://dx.doi.org/10.1016/j.bbapap.2010.06.006] [PMID: 20547249]

[88]   Lepesheva GI, Ott RD, Hargrove TY, *et al.* Sterol 14α-demethylase as a potential target for antitrypanosomal therapy: enzyme inhibition and parasite cell growth. Chem Biol 2007; 14(11): 1283-93.
[http://dx.doi.org/10.1016/j.chembiol.2007.10.011] [PMID: 18022567]

[89]   Urbina JA, Payares G, Molina J, *et al.* Cure of short- and long-term experimental Chagas' disease using D0870. Science 1996; 273(5277): 969-71.
[http://dx.doi.org/10.1126/science.273.5277.969] [PMID: 8688084]

[90]   Urbina JA, Lazardi K, Aguirre T, Piras MM, Piras R. Antiproliferative effects and mechanism of action of ICI 195,739, a novel bis-triazole derivative, on epimastigotes and amastigotes of Trypanosoma (Schizotrypanum) cruzi. Antimicrob Agents Chemother 1991; 35(4): 730-5.
[http://dx.doi.org/10.1128/AAC.35.4.730] [PMID: 2069379]

[91]   Lazardi K, Urbina JA, de Souza W. Ultrastructural alterations induced by ICI 195,739, a bis-triazole derivative with strong antiproliferative action against Trypanosoma (Schizotrypanum) cruzi. Antimicrob Agents Chemother 1991; 35(4): 736-40.
[http://dx.doi.org/10.1128/AAC.35.4.736] [PMID: 2069380]

[92]   Williams KJ, Denning DW. Termination of development of D0870. J Antimicrob Chemother 2001; 47(5): 720-1.
[http://dx.doi.org/10.1093/oxfordjournals.jac.a002691] [PMID: 11328795]

[93]   Urbina JA, Payares G, Sanoja C, *et al.* Parasitological cure of acute and chronic experimental Chagas disease using the long-acting experimental triazole TAK-187. Activity against drug-resistant *Trypanosoma cruzi* strains. Int J Antimicrob Agents 2003; 21(1): 39-48.
[http://dx.doi.org/10.1016/S0924-8579(02)00274-1] [PMID: 12507836]

[94] Corrales M, Cardozo R, Segura MA, Urbina JA, Basombrío MA, Basombrı MA. Comparative efficacies of TAK-187, a long-lasting ergosterol biosynthesis inhibitor, and benznidazole in preventing cardiac damage in a murine model of Chagas' disease. Antimicrob Agents Chemother 2005; 49(4): 1556-60.
[http://dx.doi.org/10.1128/AAC.49.4.1556-1560.2005] [PMID: 15793138]

[95] Papadopoulou MV, Trunz BB, Bloomer WD, *et al.* Novel 3-nitro-1H-1,2,4-triazole-based aliphatic and aromatic amines as anti-chagasic agents. J Med Chem 2011; 54(23): 8214-23.
[http://dx.doi.org/10.1021/jm201215n] [PMID: 22023653]

[96] Papadopoulou MV, Bloomer WD, Rosenzweig HS, Kaiser M, Chatelain E, Ioset JR. Novel 3-nitr--1H-1,2,4-triazole-based piperazines and 2-amino-1,3-benzothiazoles as antichagasic agents. Bioorg Med Chem 2013; 21(21): 6600-7.
[http://dx.doi.org/10.1016/j.bmc.2013.08.022] [PMID: 24012457]

[97] Papadopoulou MV, Bloomer WD, Rosenzweig HS, *et al.* Novel 3-nitro-1H-1,2,4-triazole-based amides and sulfonamides as potential antitrypanosomal agents. J Med Chem 2012; 55(11): 5554-65.
[http://dx.doi.org/10.1021/jm300508n] [PMID: 22550999]

[98] Papadopoulou MV, Bloomer WD, Rosenzweig HS, *et al.* Novel 3-nitro-1H-1,2,4-triazole-based compounds as potential anti-Chagasic drugs: *in vivo* studies. Future Med Chem 2013; 5(15): 1763-76.
[http://dx.doi.org/10.4155/fmc.13.108] [PMID: 24144412]

[99] Davies C, Cardozo RM, Negrette OS, Mora MC, Chung MC, Basombrío MÁ. Hydroxymethylnitrofurazone is active in a murine model of Chagas' disease. Antimicrob Agents Chemother 2010; 54(9): 3584-9.
[http://dx.doi.org/10.1128/AAC.01451-09] [PMID: 20566772]

[100] Serafim EOP, Silva ATA, Moreno AH, *et al.* Pharmacokinetics of hydroxymethylnitrofurazone, a promising new prodrug for Chagas' disease treatment. Antimicrob Agents Chemother 2013; 57(12): 6106-9.
[http://dx.doi.org/10.1128/AAC.02522-12] [PMID: 24080661]

[101] Hall BS, Bot C, Wilkinson SR. Nifurtimox activation by trypanosomal type I nitroreductases generates cytotoxic nitrile metabolites. J Biol Chem 2011; 286(15): 13088-95.
[http://dx.doi.org/10.1074/jbc.M111.230847] [PMID: 21345801]

[102] Torreele E, Bourdin Trunz B, Tweats D, *et al.* Fexinidazole--a new oral nitroimidazole drug candidate entering clinical development for the treatment of sleeping sickness. PLoS Negl Trop Dis 2010; 4(12): e923.
[http://dx.doi.org/10.1371/journal.pntd.0000923] [PMID: 21200426]

[103] Bahia MT, Andrade IM, Martins TAF, *et al.* Fexinidazole: a potential new drug candidate for Chagas disease. PLoS Negl Trop Dis 2012; 6(11): e1870.
[http://dx.doi.org/10.1371/journal.pntd.0001870] [PMID: 23133682]

[104] Shang N, Li Q, Ko TP, *et al.* Squalene synthase as a target for Chagas disease therapeutics. PLoS Pathog 2014; 10(5): e1004114.
[http://dx.doi.org/10.1371/journal.ppat.1004114] [PMID: 24789335]

[105] Mansoldo FRP, Carta F, Angeli A, Cardoso VS, Supuran CT, Vermelho AB. Chagas disease: Perspectives on the past and present and challenges in drug discovery. Molecules 2020; 25(22): 5483.
[http://dx.doi.org/10.3390/molecules25225483] [PMID: 33238613]

[106] Beatriz Vermelho A, Rodrigues GC, Nocentini A, Mansoldo FRP, Supuran CT. Discovery of novel drugs for Chagas disease: is carbonic anhydrase a target for antiprotozoal drugs? Expert Opin Drug Discov 2022; 17(10): 1147-58.
[http://dx.doi.org/10.1080/17460441.2022.2117295] [PMID: 36039500]

[107] Supuran CT, Capasso C. Protozoan Carbonic Anhydrases. In zinc enzyme in-hibitors; springer: cham, Switzwerland, 2016; 111–133.

[http://dx.doi.org/10.1007/7355_2016_11]

[108] Bonardi A, Parkkila S, Supuran CT. Inhibition studies of the protozoan α-carbonic anhydrase from *Trypanosoma cruzi* with phenols. J Enzyme Inhib Med Chem 2022; 37(1): 2417-22.
[http://dx.doi.org/10.1080/14756366.2022.2119965] [PMID: 36065959]

[109] Llanos MA, Sbaraglini ML, Villalba ML, *et al.* A structure-based approach towards the identification of novel antichagasic compounds: *Trypanosoma cruzi* carbonic anhydrase inhibitors. J Enzyme Inhib Med Chem 2020; 35(1): 21-30.
[http://dx.doi.org/10.1080/14756366.2019.1677638] [PMID: 31619095]

[110] Bonardi A, Vermelho AB, da Silva Cardoso V, *et al.* N-Nitrosulfonamides as carbonic anhydrase inhibitors: A Promising chemotype for targeting chagas disease and leishmaniasis. ACS Med Chem Lett 2019; 10(4): 413-8.
[http://dx.doi.org/10.1021/acsmedchemlett.8b00430] [PMID: 30996772]

[111] Vermelho AB, Capaci GR, Rodrigues IA, Cardoso VS, Mazotto AM, Supuran CT. Carbonic anhydrases from Trypanosoma and Leishmania as anti-protozoan drug targets. Bioorg Med Chem 2017; 25(5): 1543-55.
[http://dx.doi.org/10.1016/j.bmc.2017.01.034] [PMID: 28161253]

[112] Alafeefy AM, Ceruso M, Al-Jaber NA, Parkkila S, Vermelho AB, Supuran CT. A new class of quinazoline-sulfonamides acting as efficient inhibitors against the α-carbonic anhydrase from *Trypanosoma cruzi*. J Enzyme Inhib Med Chem 2015; 30(4): 581-5.
[http://dx.doi.org/10.3109/14756366.2014.956309] [PMID: 25373503]

[113] Rodrigues GC, Feijó DF, Bozza MT, *et al.* Design, synthesis, and evaluation of hydroxamic acid derivatives as promising agents for the management of Chagas disease. J Med Chem 2014; 57(2): 298-308.
[http://dx.doi.org/10.1021/jm400902y] [PMID: 24299463]

[114] Güzel-Akdemir Ö, Akdemir A, Pan P, *et al.* A class of sulfonamides with strong inhibitory action against the α-carbonic anhydrase from *Trypanosoma cruzi*. J Med Chem 2013; 56(14): 5773-81.
[http://dx.doi.org/10.1021/jm400418p] [PMID: 23815159]

[115] Pan P, Vermelho AB, Capaci Rodrigues G, *et al.* Cloning, characterization, and sulfonamide and thiol inhibition studies of an α-carbonic anhydrase from *Trypanosoma cruzi*, the causative agent of Chagas disease. J Med Chem 2013; 56(4): 1761-71.
[http://dx.doi.org/10.1021/jm4000616] [PMID: 23391336]

[116] Joyeau R, Maoulida C, Guillet C, *et al.* Synthesis and activity of pyrrolidinyl- and thiazolidinyl-dipeptide derivatives as inhibitors of the Tc80 prolyl oligopeptidase from *Trypanosoma cruzi*. Eur J Med Chem 2000; 35(2): 257-66.
[http://dx.doi.org/10.1016/S0223-5234(00)00118-5] [PMID: 10758287]

[117] Silva JV, da Santos SS, Machini MT, Giarolla J. Neglected tropical diseases and infectious illnesses: Potential targeted peptides employed as hits compounds in drug design. J Drug Target 2020; 1-15.
[PMID: 33059502]

[118] Bourguignon SC, Cavalcanti DFB, de Souza AMT, *et al. Trypanosoma cruzi*: Insights into naphthoquinone effects on growth and proteinase activity. Exp Parasitol 2011; 127(1): 160-6.
[http://dx.doi.org/10.1016/j.exppara.2010.07.007] [PMID: 20647011]

[119] Bivona AE, Sánchez Alberti A, Matos MN, *et al. Trypanosoma cruzi* 80 kDa prolyl oligopeptidase (Tc80) as a novel immunogen for Chagas disease vaccine. PLoS Negl Trop Dis 2018; 12(3): e0006384.
[http://dx.doi.org/10.1371/journal.pntd.0006384] [PMID: 29601585]

[120] Salas-Sarduy E, Landaburu LU, Karpiak J, *et al.* Novel scaffolds for inhibition of Cruzipain identified from high-throughput screening of anti-kinetoplastid chemical boxes. Sci Rep 2017; 7(1): 12073.
[http://dx.doi.org/10.1038/s41598-017-12170-4] [PMID: 28935948]

[121]   Bustamante JM, Craft JM, Crowe BD, Ketchie SA, Tarleton RL. New, combined, and reduced dosing treatment protocols cure *Trypanosoma cruzi* infection in mice. J Infect Dis 2014; 209(1): 150-62.
[http://dx.doi.org/10.1093/infdis/jit420] [PMID: 23945371]

[122]   Francisco AF, Lewis MD, Jayawardhana S, Taylor MC, Chatelain E, Kelly JM. Limited ability of posaconazole to cure both acute and chronic *Trypanosoma cruzi* infections revealed by highly sensitive *in vivo* imaging. Antimicrob Agents Chemother 2015; 59(8): 4653-61.
[http://dx.doi.org/10.1128/AAC.00520-15] [PMID: 26014936]

[123]   Chatelain E, Konar N. Translational challenges of animal models in Chagas disease drug development: a review. Drug Des Devel Ther 2015; 9: 4807-23.
[http://dx.doi.org/10.2147/DDDT.S90208] [PMID: 26316715]

[124]   Stein C, Migliavaca CB, Colpani V, *et al.* Amiodarone for arrhythmia in patients with Chagas disease: A systematic review and individual patient data meta-analysis. PLoS Negl Trop Dis 2018; 12(8): e0006742.
[http://dx.doi.org/10.1371/journal.pntd.0006742] [PMID: 30125291]

[125]   Bocchi EA, Rassi S, Guimarães GV. Safety profile and efficacy of ivabradine in heart failure due to Chagas heart disease: a *post hoc* analysis of the SHIFT trial. ESC Heart Fail 2018; 5(3): 249-56.
[http://dx.doi.org/10.1002/ehf2.12240] [PMID: 29266804]

[126]   Cardinalli-Neto A, Bestetti RB, Cordeiro JA, Rodrigues VC. Predictors of all-cause mortality for patients with chronic Chagas' heart disease receiving implantable cardioverter defibrillator therapy. J Cardiovasc Electrophysiol 2007; 18(12): 1236-40.
[http://dx.doi.org/10.1111/j.1540-8167.2007.00954.x] [PMID: 17900257]

[127]   Benatti RD, Oliveira GH, Bacal F. Heart Transplantation for Chagas Cardiomyopathy. J Heart Lung Transplant 2017; 36(6): 597-603.
[http://dx.doi.org/10.1016/j.healun.2017.02.006] [PMID: 28284779]

[128]   Sousa AS, Xavier SS, Freitas GR, Hasslocher-Moreno A. Prevention strategies of cardioembolic ischemic stroke in Chagas' disease. Arq Bras Cardiol 2008; 91(5): 306-10.
[http://dx.doi.org/10.1590/S0066-782X2008001700004] [PMID: 19142374]

[129]   Fiorelli AI, Santos RHB, Oliveira JL Jr, *et al.* Heart transplantation in 107 cases of Chagas' disease. Transplant Proc 2011; 43(1): 220-4.
[http://dx.doi.org/10.1016/j.transproceed.2010.12.046] [PMID: 21335192]

[130]   Bacal F, Silva CP, Pires PV, *et al.* Transplantation for Chagas' disease: an overview of immunosuppression and reactivation in the last two decades. Clin Transplant 2010; 24(2): E29-34.
[http://dx.doi.org/10.1111/j.1399-0012.2009.01202.x] [PMID: 20088914]

[131]   Gray EB, La Hoz RM, Green JS, *et al.* Reactivation of chagas disease among heart transplant recipients in the United States, 2012-2016. Transpl Infect Dis 2018; 20(6): e12996.
[http://dx.doi.org/10.1111/tid.12996] [PMID: 30204269]

[132]   U.S. Department of Health and Human Services; U.S. Food and Drug Admin-istration; Center for Biologics Evaluation and Research. Use of Serological Tests to Reduce the Risk of Transmission of Trypanosoma cruzi Infection in Blood and Blood Components. Guidance for Industry. December 2017.

[133]   World Health Organization. Chagas disease (also known as American trypano-somiasis). World Health Organization; 2021.

[134]   Zulantay I, Apt W, Ramos D, *et al.* The epidemiological relevance of family study in Chagas disease. PLoS Negl Trop Dis 2013; 7(2): e1959.
[http://dx.doi.org/10.1371/journal.pntd.0001959] [PMID: 23457649]

[135]   González-Tomé MI, Rivera Cuello M, Camaño Gutierrez I, *et al.* Recommendations for the diagnosis, treatment and follow-up of the pregnant woman and child with Chagas disease. Sociedad Española de Infectología Pediátrica. Sociedad de Enfermedades Infecciosas y Microbiología Clínica. Enferm Infecc

Microbiol Clin 2013; 31(8): 535-42.
[PMID: 23374862]

[136] Lorke D. Embryotoxicity studies of nifurtimox in rats and mice and study of fertility and general reproductive performance. Arzneimittelforschung 1972; 22(9): 1603-7.
[PMID: 4678718]

[137] Gorla NB, Ledesma OS, Barbieri GP, Larripa IB. Assessment of cytogenetic damage in chagasic children treated with benznidazole. Mutat Res Genet Toxicol Test 1988; 206(2): 217-20.
[http://dx.doi.org/10.1016/0165-1218(88)90163-2] [PMID: 3140001]

[138] Norman FF, López-Vélez R. Chagas disease and breast-feeding. Emerg Infect Dis 2013; 19(10): 1561-6.
[http://dx.doi.org/10.3201/eid1910.130203] [PMID: 24050257]

[139] Gorla NB, Ledesma OS, Barbieri GP, Larripa IB. Thirteenfold increase of chromosomal aberrations non-randomly distributed in chagasic children treated with nifurtimox. Mutat Res Genet Toxicol Test 1989; 224(2): 263-7.
[http://dx.doi.org/10.1016/0165-1218(89)90165-1] [PMID: 2507913]

[140] de Toranzo EG, Masana M, Castro JA. Administration of benznidazole, a chemotherapeutic agent against Chagas disease, to pregnant rats. Covalent binding of reactive metabolites to fetal and maternal proteins. Arch Int Pharmacodyn Ther 1984; 272(1): 17-23.
[PMID: 6440493]

[141] Ferreira CS, Martinho PC, Amato Neto V, Cruz RRB. Pasteurization of human milk to prevent transmission of Chagas disease. Rev Inst Med Trop São Paulo 2001; 43(3): 161-2.
[http://dx.doi.org/10.1590/S0036-46652001000300008] [PMID: 11452325]

[142] García-Bournissen F, Moroni S, Marson ME, *et al.* Limited infant exposure to benznidazole through breast milk during maternal treatment for Chagas disease. Arch Dis Child 2015; 100(1): 90-4.
[http://dx.doi.org/10.1136/archdischild-2014-306358] [PMID: 25210104]

[143] Garcia-Bournissen F, Altcheh J, Panchaud A, Ito S. Is use of nifurtimox for the treatment of Chagas disease compatible with breast feeding? A population pharmacokinetics analysis. Arch Dis Child 2010; 95(3): 224-8.
[http://dx.doi.org/10.1136/adc.2008.157297] [PMID: 19948512]

[144] Sartor P, Colaianni I, Cardinal MV, Bua J, Freilij H, Gürtler RE. Improving access to Chagas disease diagnosis and etiologic treatment in remote rural communities of the Argentine Chaco through strengthened primary health care and broad social participation. PLoS Negl Trop Dis 2017; 11(2): e0005336.
[http://dx.doi.org/10.1371/journal.pntd.0005336] [PMID: 28192425]

[145] Navarro M, Berens-Riha N, Hohnerlein S, *et al.* Cross-sectional, descriptive study of Chagas disease among citizens of Bolivian origin living in Munich, Germany. BMJ Open 2017; 7(1): e013960.
[http://dx.doi.org/10.1136/bmjopen-2016-013960] [PMID: 28093440]

CHAPTER 4

Novel Agents against Human African Trypanosomiasis: Updates on Medicinal Chemistry and Target Identification

Evelyn Funjika[1], Godfrey Mayoka[2], Dickson Mambwe[1] and **Peter Mubanga Cheuka[1,*]**

[1] *Department of Chemistry, School of Natural Sciences, University of Zambia, Lusaka, Zambia*

[2] *Department of Pharmacology and Pharmacognosy, School of Pharmacy, Jomo Kenyatta University of Agriculture and Technology, Nairobi, Kenya*

Abstract: Also known as sleeping sickness, human African trypanosomiasis (HAT) is caused by protozoan parasites of the genus *Trypanosoma* transmitted between humans by the bites of tsetse flies (glossina). HAT is caused by two parasite subspecies - *Trypanosoma brucei gambiense* (accounting for 92% of reported cases and causes chronic illness) and *Trypanosoma brucei rhodesiense* (accounting for 8% of reported cases and is responsible for the acute form of the disease). The former can advance, affecting the central nervous system, while the latter can develop rapidly with multiple organs, including the brain, being invaded. If left untreated, HAT is generally fatal. According to the World Health Organization, in the period 2016 – 2020, about 55 million people were at risk of infection, with nearly 1000 cases reported in 2018. Current treatment options have limitations such as complex administration procedures, limited effectiveness, emergence of drug resistance, and undesirable side effects. Therefore, new drugs are required. In this book chapter, we summarize current efforts aimed at identifying new drug candidates and their corresponding mechanisms of action. We highlight medicinal chemistry optimization efforts for different candidates while giving detailed insights into the mechanism of function for the corresponding drug targets. Such information is of value as it equips drug discovery scientists with information about chemical modifications, which can lead to improvement in certain physicochemical and biological properties of new chemical entities.

Keywords: HSPs, HAT, MAPKs, Protein tyrosine kinases, Rhodesain, Sleeping sickness, T. b. gambiense, T. b. rhodesiense.

---

[*] **Corresponding author Peter Mubanga Cheuka:** Department of Chemistry, School of Natural Sciences, University of Zambia, Lusaka, Zambia; Tel: +260968930603; E-mail: peter.cheuka@unza.zm

Igor Jose dos Santos Nascimento & Ricardo Olimpio de Moura (Eds.)

INTRODUCTION

HAT, also known as sleeping sickness, is a devastating parasitic disease caused by the blood- and tissue-borne parasites of the genus *Trypanosoma* [1]. As of 2022, the estimated number of HAT cases globally was 799. This low number of HAT cases is a result of global control efforts by the World Health Organisation, national control programs, bilateral cooperation, and non-governmental organizations during the 1990s and 2000s [2, 3]. However, any relaxation in these efforts can cause a resurgence, as was observed in 1970. After 1970, the number of cases continued to increase, and by 1998, almost 40,000 cases were reported, with an estimated 300,000 undetected and untreated cases. Recent risk estimates for the period 2016 to 2020 were 55 million people, with only 3 million at moderate risk [3]. Unfortunately, the population with the highest risk of acquiring HAT mainly lives in rural and remote communities, which tend to have limited access to healthcare, thereby complicating its quick diagnosis and treatment [4].

Transmission of *Trypanosoma* parasites occurs when an infected tsetse fly bites a mammalian host, such as a human, introducing the parasites into the bloodstream [1]. In the mammalian host, the parasite proliferates as slender bloodstream forms (BFs), which rely solely on glycolysis for energy production. These slender BFs develop into non-replicating stumpy BFs, which then develop into procyclic forms (PFs) after transmission to the fly [5, 6]. As the parasites transition, they undergo morphological and metabolic changes, such as switching from glycolysis to oxidative phosphorylation and changing their surface coat from variant surface glycoproteins to procyclins [7]. The PFs then develop into epimastigotes and then to mammalian-infective metacyclic trypomastigotes [5].

There are two main forms of HAT, each with different epidemiological characteristics. Approximately 92% of HAT cases are caused by *Trypanosoma brucei gambiense,* which causes the slowly progressing form known as West African sleeping sickness [3]. This is normally found in countries such as Angola, the Central African Republic, the Democratic Republic of the Congo, and Sudan. It mainly affects rural and forested areas [2]. The primary vector responsible for transmitting *T. b. gambiense* is the tsetse fly belonging to the *Glossina palpalis* group. Humans are the primary reservoir host for *T. b. gambiense*, although it can also infect other mammals, including non-human primates [1, 8]. *T. b. rhodesiense* is responsible for 8% of HAT cases and causes the faster-progressing form known as East African sleeping sickness [3]. It is more prevalent in savannah and woodland areas occurring normally in countries such as Uganda, Kenya, Tanzania, and Zambia [2]. The primary vector responsible for transmitting *T. b. rhodesiense* is the tsetse fly belonging to the the *Glossina morsitans* group.

In addition to humans, a range of domestic and wild animals can serve as reservoir hosts for *T. b. rhodesiense* [1, 8].

In this book chapter, we discuss current diagnosis and treatment strategies against the *Trypanosoma* parasites. We also discuss the use of target-based drug discovery methods to identify HAT targets and provide a few examples of novel HAT targets where the structure-activity relationship has been used to identify small molecule inhibitors for these targets.

CURRENT DIAGNOSIS AND TREATMENT STRATEGIES FOR HAT

HAT is diagnosed using clinical examination, serological tests, and microscopic evaluation of body fluids [9]. There are two main stages of HAT. During the early stage, which is referred to as the hemolymphatic stage, symptoms include fever, headaches, joint pain, and lymphadenopathy. This stage is followed by a meningoencephalitic stage, when the parasite invades the central nervous system, causing personality changes, sleep disturbances, and neurological disorders [3]. It is important to identify the form and stage of the disease, as the treatment of HAT is dependent on this. The second stage of infection requires drugs that can cross the blood-brain barrier for them to be effective. Treatment for *gambiense*-HAT has relied on pentamidine, eflornithine, nifurtimox, and fexinidazole (Fig. **1**), whereas for *rhodesiense*-HAT, the main treatment options are suramin, melarsoprol, and eflornithine (Fig. **1**) [10]. Early treatment is recommended as it improves treatment outcomes. Treatment outcome is monitored by follow-up for up to 24 months and involves clinical as well as laboratory assessments. Some assessments require cerebrospinal fluid as the parasites may remain viable and reproductive [10].

Management of HAT in resource-limited health facilities poses a challenge for the patient and carers [11]. Most of the HAT medications need complex methods of administration and strict adherence to the treatment course, with some necessitating prolonged hospitalization. For drugs such as fexinidazole, patients need to have consumed a meal to ensure the drug absorption is sufficient and that the active metabolites reach therapeutic levels [12]. HAT medications are also known to cause adverse reactions in some patients, such as nausea, vomiting, and decreased appetite. Nifurtimox–eflornithine combination therapy, or NECT, may cause side effects such as abdominal pain, nausea, and vomiting but may also trigger seizures and occasional psychotic reactions and hallucinations [12]. The drive for new drugs against neglected diseases such as HAT is driven by the medical need for improved drugs that are easier to administer, with improved efficacy, and are more tolerable.

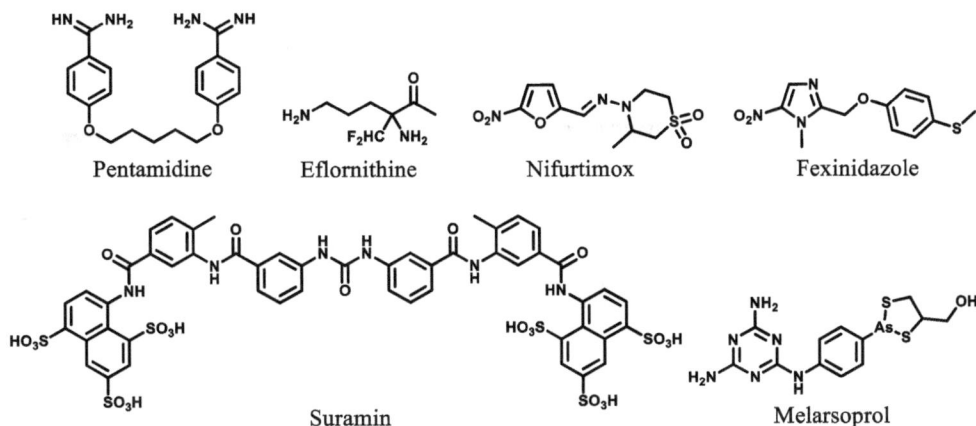

Fig. (1). Chemical structures of anti-HAT drugs in clinical use.

TARGET-BASED DRUG DESIGN STRATEGIES FOR HAT

The process of drug discovery is long and expensive with no guarantee that the identified drug candidates will be approved for clinical use. Target-based screening using purified proteins provides a great opportunity to generate structural information to guide the chemistry design of inhibitory compounds. This approach gives a better understanding of the structure-activity relationship (SAR) as well as the relationship between compound affinity and target inhibition or binding [13, 14]. To minimize the cost and resources used in the anti-HAT drug discovery process, target product profiles (TPPs) also help to ensure that drug discovery projects address the requirements of patients and healthcare providers [13, 15]. Table **1** presents an example of a TPP produced by the organization Drugs for Neglected Diseases initiative (DNDi) for the development of new anti-HAT drugs that target stages 1 and 2 of the disease [16].

The lifecycle of *Trypanosoma* parasites between the mammalian host and tsetse fly vector involves complex changes in gene expression, cell morphology, surface coat composition, and metabolism. Targets can be identified based on their role in the parasite lifecycle. As an example, nitroreductase (NTR) enzymes are a class of enzymes found in trypanosomes that play a crucial role in the metabolism of nitro compounds. NTRs can reduce nitrated compounds, including certain drugs, converting them into toxic intermediates, which can be detrimental to the parasite [17]. There are 2 classes of NTRs. Type I (oxygen-insensitive) NTRs carry out two-electron reductions, whereas type II (oxygen-sensitive) carry out one-electron reductions. The reduction of the nitro group produces amines *via* nitroso and hydroxylamine intermediates. These intermediates can potentially react with biomolecules to exert toxic and mutagenic effects [17, 18]. Drugs such as nifurtimox exploit this vulnerability in the trypanosome's metabolism. Nifurtimox undergoes metabolic activation by the parasite's NTRs, generating toxic intermediates that can kill the trypanosome [12].

Table 1. Example of a TPP for the development of new treatment for stages 1 and 2 of HAT (produced by DNDi).

-	Ideal	Acceptable
Target population	• Effective against stages 1 and 2. • Effective in melarsoprol-refractory patients. • All patients, including pregnant and lactating women.	• Effective against stages 1 and 2.
Target species	• Efficacy against both *T. b. gambiense* and *T. b. rhodesiense.*	• Efficacy against *T. b. gambiense* only.
Efficacy	• Clinical efficacy > 95% at 18-month follow-up.	• Clinical efficacy determined by expert consultation.
Safety/tolerability	• < 0.1% drug-related mortality. • No monitoring for adverse events (AEs).	• < 1% possibly related mortality. • Weekly simple lab testing (field testing) for AEs.
Formulation	• Adult and pediatric formulations.	
Treatment regimen	• < 7 days oral once daily or • < 7 days intramuscular injection once daily.	• 10 days oral or • < 10 days intramuscular injection.
Stability	• Stability in climatic zone 4 for > 3 years.	• Stability in climatic zone 4 for > 12 months.
Cost	• < EUR 30/course (drug cost only).	• < EUR 100/course. • < EUR 200/course OK if very good on other criteria.

Another example is pafuramidine, which is a prodrug of furamidine and has benzamidine moieties in the chemical structure, connected *via* a furan center. Incorporating methoxy moieties is a vital strategy to improve the bioavailability of pafuramidine as it enhances permeability across biological barriers [19]. The mitochondrion membrane potential is also an important feature that drives accumulation of the drug within the organelle and a decrease in the membrane potential of *T. brucei* mitochondrion has been reported upon exposure to pafuramidine. The unique accumulation profile of pafuramidine, as supported by other studies, implicates variations in cellular uptake mechanisms or inhibition of mitochondrion accumulation as being most significant in the resistance phenomena [20, 21]. Typical of diamidines, pafuramidine binds to the minor groove of the DNA double helix with a preponderance to target the AT-rich sequences [22, 23]. The compound can bind to both mitochondrial and nuclear DNA and has demonstrated impeccable affinity for these targets, being able to accumulate to high levels even when exposed to low concentrations [24]. Consequently, DNA replication and transcription are compromised. DNA binding has been demonstrated to correlate with trypanocidal activity, providing validation for drug discovery efforts [25].

NOVEL ANTI-HAT TARGETS

Over the past decade, researchers have used technological advancements and new insights into the mechanism of parasite's biochemical pathways to identify potential drug candidates for HAT treatment. In this section, we discuss some novel HAT targets, outlining their role in the parasite's life cycle. The structures of small molecule inhibitors that have been identified for these targets are shown in Fig. (**2**).

Protein Tyrosine Kinases (PTKs)

PTKs catalyze protein phosphorylation on tyrosine amino acid residues [26, 27] [28 - 30]. Kinases that phosphorylate both tyrosine and serine/threonine are essential for cell signaling networks that regulate various processes [27]. In vertebrates, PTKs take two general forms - receptor tyrosine kinases (RTKs) and non-receptor tyrosine kinases (NRTKs). RTKs (*e.g.*, the epidermal growth factor receptor (EGFR) or vascular endothelial growth factor receptor (VEGFR)) are transmembrane proteins activated by binding of hormones to their extracellular domains. NRTKs (*e.g.*, Src-family protein kinases), on the other hand, are cytosolic and can be activated by cytokine receptors or RTKs. Trypanosomes lack RTKs and do not encode classical phosphotyrosine binding domains such as SH2 [31, 32]. The divergent nature of the tyrosine phosphorylation system in trypanosomes, compared to that of humans, can be exploited in the design of inhibitors devoid of toxicity.

Eukaryotic protein kinases catalyze the transfer of a phosphate group from MgATP to serine/threonine and tyrosine residues in protein substrates to produce phosphoproteins and MgADP. There is a large volume of published studies that have suggested that tyrosine kinases catalyze phosphorylation *via* a dissociative mechanism – one in which the γ-phosphate detaches from ATP to form a metaphosphate-like intermediate, which is then intercepted by the nucleophilic hydroxyl of the tyrosine residue in the protein substrate [33]. In order to trigger the initial detachment of the γ-phosphate from ATP, the enzyme is thought to concentrate a positive charge on the anionic oxygens of the departing ADP, which weakens the P – O bond between the γ-phosphorous atom and the bridging oxygen. The positive charges are provided by a conserved lysine side chain and a Mg^{2+} ion, which point towards the β-phosphate.

PTKs have been identified as targets in trypanosomes by employing inhibitors known to be tyrosine kinase inhibitors, some of which are shown in Fig. (**2**). For instance, genistein has been found to block trypanosome replication [34], while tyrphostin A47 inhibits tyrosine phosphorylation of proteins [35]. In a drug repurposing effort, the anticancer drugs canertinib and lapatinib (Fig. **2**) (both inhibitors of human EGFR) have been shown to be vital against bloodstream *T. brucei* [36]. When orally administered in a mouse model of HAT, lapatinib suppressed parasitemia, prolonged the survival of all treated mice, and cured 25% of infected mice [37]. Further experiments using affinity chromatography, which involved eluting proteins with drugs, demonstrated that they bind to kinases (*e.g.*, *T. brucei* lapatinib-binding protein kinase-1 (*Tb*LBPK1) in the case of lapatinib). Lapatinib binding to four kinase targets was also corroborated by *in silico* binding efforts employing homology modeling and molecular docking [36].

Mitogen-activated Protein Kinases (MAPKs)

MAPKs are protein kinases that phosphorylate their own threonine and serine residues (auto-phosphorylation) or those located on their substrates to activate or deactivate their targets [38]. MAPKs regulate essential cellular processes such as proliferation, stress responses, apoptosis, and immune defense [39 - 41]. The MAPK cascade comprises a module of consecutive phosphorylations, *i.e.*, after an initial stimulus, an upstream MAPK phosphorylates the one downstream. For instance, a MAP kinase kinase kinase kinase (MAP4K) phosphorylates and activates a MAP kinase kinase kinase (MAP3K). In turn, MAP3K phosphorylates and activates MAP kinase kinase (MAP2K), which then phosphorylates the conserved threonine and tyrosine residues found in the activation loop of a MAP kinase (MAPK) [42, 43]. Studies on *T. brucei* have identified 7 MAPKs, which are involved in a variety of cellular functions such as response to interferon-ɣ in the bloodstream forms (MAPKKFR1) [44], differentiation into procyclic forms (MAPK2) [45], modulation of cell growth in procyclic forms (*Tb*ECK1) [46], control of virulence and differentiation of bloodstream forms (*Tb*MAPK5) [47], conferring resistance to temperature-related stress in procyclic forms (*Tb*MAPK4) [48], cell growth in bloodstream forms (*Tb*ERK8) [49], and proliferation in procyclic forms (MAPKLK1) [50].

Studies aimed at understanding the detailed molecular events characterizing the transfer of a phosphate group in phosphorylations catalyzed by MAPKs are scanty. However, using a quantum mechanics/molecular mechanics (QM/MM) approach, Turjanski *et al*. have shed some light on the understanding of the mechanistic details of such a reaction in MAPKs [51]. The catalytic site of ERK2 (extracellular activated protein kinase 2), a kinase belonging to one subfamily of MAPKs, was constructed and used to study the phosphate transfer event. The

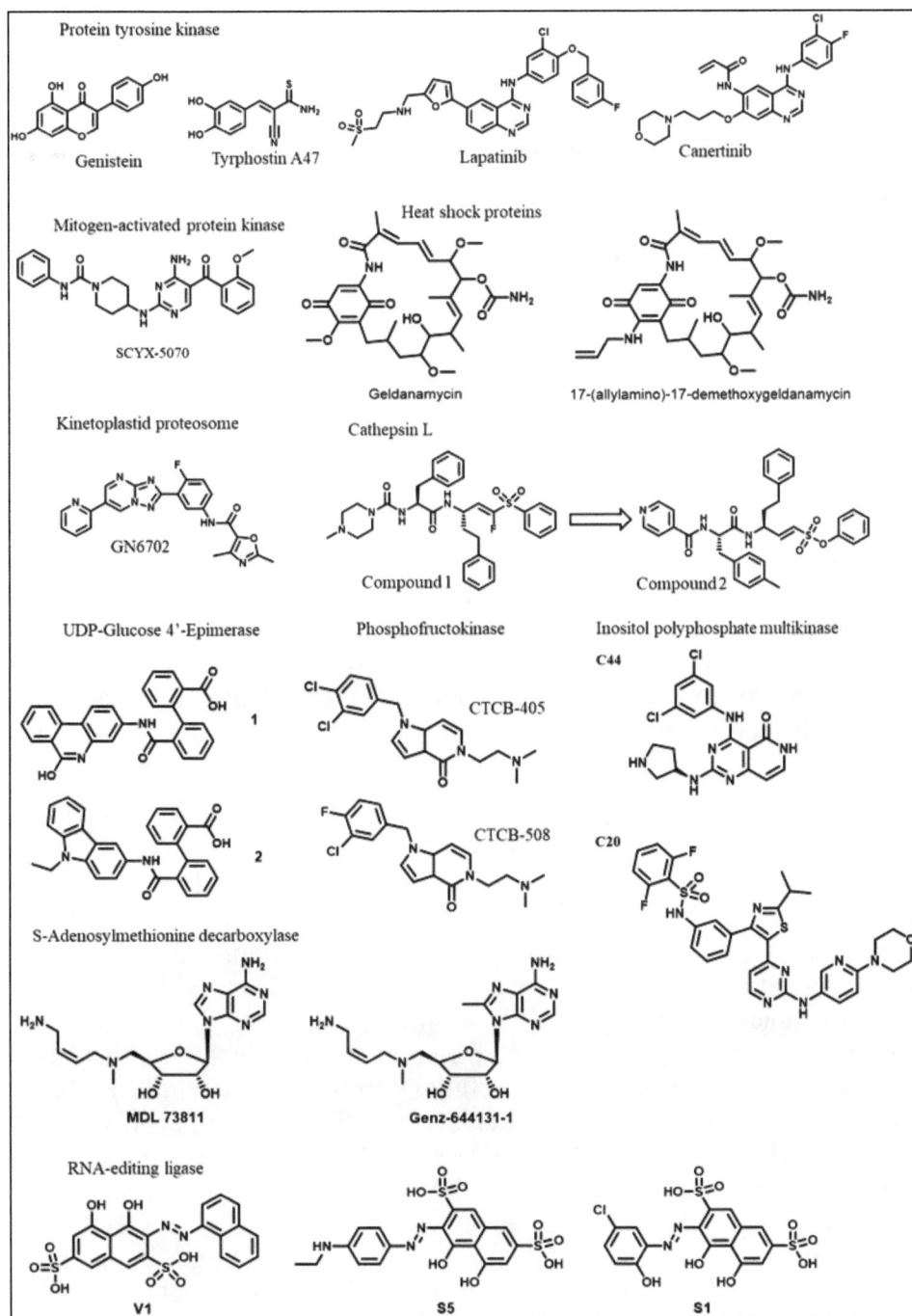

Fig. (2). Example of small molecule inhibitors for novel HAT targets.

proposed catalytic reaction is said to possess a ~ 90% dissociative character, with the γ-phosphate almost dissociating completely from ATP before being intercepted by the OH group of the threonine residue in the protein substrate. Like the mechanisms for PFK and PTKs, a conserved aspartate residue acts as a base, deprotonating the OH of the threonine residue as it attacks the metaphosphate-like intermediate.

The 2,4-diaminopyrimidine compound **SCYX-5070** Fig. (**2**) is an example of a compound that exerts its trypanocidal activity partly *via* inhibition of MAPKs [52]. *in vitro*, it was found to trigger irreversible effects on parasite survival or kill the *T. brucei* parasites within a short period of exposure (10 – 12 hours). The compound also cured mice with an acute infection of trypanosomiasis with no evidence of compound-related chronic or acute toxicity. A derivative of **SCYX-5070** was later immobilized on a sepharose matrix, followed by incubation of the immobilized compound with total parasite extracts. The 2,4-diaminopyrimidine derivative was found to bind to MAPK2 and MAPK9, among other proteins, thereby partly validating MAPKs as targets from a chemoproteomics perspective. In another study by Pfister and colleagues, the importance of *Tb*MAPK5 to trypanosomes was also demonstrated with knockout procyclic forms of the parasites differentiating prematurely in mice and culture. Infection of immunocompromised mice with the knockout mutants also resulted in a peak parasitemia level that was 16 times lower than that in mice with wild-type infection [53].

Heat Shock Proteins (HSPs)

HSPs assist newly synthesized proteins in folding and also contribute to the regulation of gene expression and signal transduction events [54]. These proteins perform various functions, including mediation of protein-protein interactions, protein stabilization, and protein modification. In addition, HSPs are known for their stress adaptation role, and their ubiquitous presence in the cytosolic network ensures that cells can navigate through different assaults, including thermo-related stresses, making them essential for cellular proliferation [55]. HSPs have been best described as drug targets in other therapeutic areas, especially cancer and neurodegenerative disorders. Among them, HSP-90 has been widely studied. HSP-90's action is dependent on ATP hydrolysis and interacts with co-chaperones through its *N*-terminal nucleotide-binding domain (NBD) or middle client protein-binding domain. Validation of HSP-90 as a target in parasites such as *Plasmodium falciparum* has been done using the inhibitor geldanamycin (GA) through an *in vitro* [^{3}H]hypoxanthine incorporation assay. The derivative 17-(allyamino)-17-demethoxygeldanamycin (17AAG) has lower potency than GA; however, it is a more preferred drug candidate as it exhibits lesser hepatotoxicity.

The ability to inhibit *P. falciparum* prompted the investigation of GA and its derivatives on other parasites, including *Trypanosoma evansi*. Swiss female mice infected with *T. evansi* were treated with 17AAG intraperitoneally at a dose of 30 mg/kg of body weight. Plots of the number of parasites against the number of days showed that untreated mice had an elevated number of parasites, resulting in death by the 9th day post-infection. Percentage viability analysis showed a 60% survival rate of the 17AAG-treated mice [56]. In a separate study, several compounds were screened using differential scanning fluorimetry and isothermal measurement to identify potential inhibitors for *T. brucei* that target HSP-83, the homolog of human HSP-90. A number of molecules were shown to interact primarily with the *N*-terminal ATPase domain, suggesting that this domain can be a focus for identifying and optimizing inhibitors of HSP-83. In kinetoplastid parasites, HSP-83 has been identified as a promising target for which selective hit compounds have been profiled [56, 57].

Kinetoplastid Proteasome

The kinetoplastid proteasome is a large multi-subunit protein complex that regulates numerous cellular functions, including normal protein turnover and degradation of misfolded proteins. It is generally located in the cytoplasm and nucleus of cells. The proteasome consists of a proteolytic 20S core, which is divided into two subunits, α and β. The β subunit is sub-divided into $\beta 1$, $\beta 2$, and $\beta 5$, which are responsible for cleaving negatively charged amino acids, positively charged amino acids, and hydrophobic amino acids, respectively [58]. The proteasome can act dependent or independently of ubiquitination. The enzymes in the ubiquitin-proteasome pathway have received much interest as drug targets in trypanosomatid diseases, as reviewed elsewhere [58, 59]. The importance of the proteasome in kinetoplastid parasites is shown by an increased level of ubiquitinated protein when *T. cruzi* trypomastigotes are transformed into amastigotes [60, 61]. During this transition, the cytoskeletal proteins associated with flagella are shown to be degraded by the ubiquitin-proteasome pathway; hence, inhibition with lactacytin and **MG132** targets this pathway and interferes with the formation of amastigotes [61].

In a study by Khare and colleagues, **GNF6702** was identified as a selective inhibitor of the kinetoplastid proteasome, and it was shown to clear parasites in murine models of leishmaniasis, Chagas disease, and HAT [62]. **GNF6702** was derived from an azabenzoxazole, **GNF5343**, which was identified in initial proliferation assays with 3 million other compounds. Further modifications to improve bioavailability and potency included the replacement of the azabenzoxazole center with C6-substituted imidazo- and triazolopyrimidine cores, the furan group for a dimethyloxazole ring, and further substitutions at the C6 position, resulting in **GNF6702. GNF6702** inhibits the kinetoplastid proteasome through a non-competitive mechanism, does not inhibit the mammalian proteasome or growth of mammalian cells, and is well-tolerated in mice [62]. However, its progression into clinical testing was hampered by solubility-limited oral absorption [63].

Tb Cathepsin L (*Tb*CatL)

*Tb*CatL (also commonly called rhodesain) is the major cysteine protease expressed by *T. b. rhodesiense* and is considered an attractive target for anti-HAT drug discovery because of its essential biological functions in the parasite. In the lysosomes, it plays an essential role in the proteolysis of both parasite and host proteins transported within the parasite [64]. It is also involved in immune system evasion by degrading the host immunoglobulins [65] and by turning over the variant surface glycoproteins of the *Trypanosoma* coat [66]. Additionally, due to its capability to degrade the blood-brain barrier (BBB) components, rhodesain is also responsible for the onset of the neurological stage of the disease. Rhodesain is a clan CA, family C1 (papain family) cathepsin L-like cysteine protease, which is a single polypeptide chain consisting of 215 amino acid residues. It adopts the typical papain-like fold with a left and right domain and a catalytic triad (Cys25, His162, and Asn182) located in a cleft between the two domains. The catalytic mechanism involves the generation of the strongly nucleophilic thiolate ion in a deprotonation step facilitated by a basic imidazole ring of His162. The Cys25 thiolate ion then attacks the carbonyl carbon in the peptide bond forming a tetrahedral intermediate, which subsequently eliminates the amino portion of the cleaved protein. A water molecule, activated by a basic imidazole of His162, then, hydrolyzes the thioester bond generating the carboxyl portion of the cleaved protein while the catalytic amino acid residues are restored [67, 68].

Rhodesain has been chemically validated as an appropriate drug target after it was shown that its specific inhibitor killed the parasites [64]. A recent report has also described a medicinal chemistry optimization of compound **1** aimed at improving inhibition potency (against rhodesain) and selectivity against human cathepsins B and L [69]. This effort led to the identification of compound **2,** which demonstrated single-digit nanomolar affinity on rhodesain with high selectivity over mammalian cathepsin B. The compound was also shown to accumulate in mice brain tissue following intraperitoneal and oral administration in addition to its favorable metabolism. Other inhibitors of rhodesain have exhibited *in vivo* efficacy in an acute mouse HAT-infection model [70].

Tb UDP-Glucose 4'-Epimerase (*Tb*GalE)

*Tb*GalE (also known as UDP-glucose 4'-epimerase) is a short-chain dehydrogenase and reductase enzyme of the Leloir pathway of galactose metabolism. It catalyzes the final step in normal galactose metabolism by regenerating UDP-glucose [71]. In the bloodstream form, the parasite uses a dense cell-surface coat of variant surface glycoprotein to escape the innate and adaptive immune responses of the mammalian host and a highly glycosylated transferrin receptor to take up host transferrin, an essential growth factor [72, 73]. Galactose is known to be present in these glycoproteins, as well as other flagellar pockets and endosomal and lysosomal glycoproteins. The fact that the parasite cannot take up galactose indicates that it might be dependent on the action of UDP-glucose 4'-epimerase to convert UDP-Galactose to UDP-Gal, which is then incorporated into glycoconjugates *via* UDP-Gal-dependent galactosyltransferases. Roper and colleagues described the cloning of *T. brucei* GalE, encoding *T. brucei* UDP-Glc-4'-epimerase, and reported on the functional characterization by complementation of a GalE-deficient *Escherichia coli* mutant and an enzymatic assay of recombinant protein [74]. Using a transgenic parasite expressing the TETR tetracycline repressor protein gene, a tetracycline-inducible conditional GalE null mutant of T. *brucei* was produced. When tetracycline was stopped, cell division stopped, and a significant amount of cells died, indicating that galactose metabolism in *T. brucei* occurs through UDP-Galactose-4'-epimerase and is necessary for the proliferation of the parasite [74]. Consequently, identifying compounds that inhibit this key step of trypanosomal galactose synthesis may serve as useful scaffolds for future drug design and optimization.

In 2010, Durrant and colleagues employed computer-aided drug design using AutoDock Vina software to perform the relaxed complex scheme (RCS) docking protocol [75]. They identified 14 low micromolar inhibitors of *Tb*GalE. The promising molecules belonged to a series containing the 2'-carbamoyl-[1,1'-biphenyl]-2-carboxylate core scaffold and the 2'-(phenylcarbamoyl)-[1,1'-biphenyl]-2-carboxylic acid core scaffold in a subsequent screen such as compounds **1** and **2**. These are believed to participate in many of the same hydrogen bonds that characterize UDP-glucose binding. The addition of different groups to the fused ring system, such as electronegative moieties, may exploit other interactions to enhance the potency. However, when whole cell assays were carried out using the identified molecules, except for a few, most of the molecules performed poorly, which was attributed to their hydrophobic nature, making it difficult to transverse the membrane to the intracellular targets [75]. To date, there is little evidence of further efforts to develop/optimize most of these compounds for HAT.

Phosphofructokinase (PFK)

PFK catalyzes the third step in glycolysis, phosphorylating fructose 6-phosphate (F6P) to fructose 1,6-bisphosphate (F16BP). The bloodstream form of *T. brucei* depends on the high concentration (5 mM) of glucose in the host's blood for fuel. The parasite mitochondria, at this life cycle stage, are significantly compromised, unable to carry out oxidative phosphorylation, which makes it exclusively reliant on glycolysis as the sole source of ATP, located in organelles called glycosomes [76]. The corresponding three human isoforms (*h*PFK-M, *h*PFK-L, and *h*PFK-P) have low sequence identity (~ 20%) to *T. brucei* PFK despite sharing very similar active sites, raising hopes for the prospect of designing inhibitors with high selectivity [77]. A crystal structure of *T. brucei* PFK in complex with ATP, with F6P modeled into the crystal structure, has revealed binding interactions in the binding site [78]. Based on simulations carried out on PFK-2 from *E. coli*, it appears the phosphoryl transfer occurs *via* a dissociative mechanism similar to the one for PTKs [79]. After the detachment of the γ-phosphate from ATP, the hydroxyl at position 1 of F6P attacks this metaphosphate-like intermediate with the Asp229 assisting in the deprotonation of the hydroxyl [79].

CTCB-405 Fig. (**2**) is an example of a recently reported inhibitor of PFK that potently inhibits *Tb*PFK (IC_{50} = 0.18 µM) while retaining sub-micromolar potency on *T. b. gambiense* (EC_{50} = 0.19 µM) and *T. b. rhodesiense* (EC_{50} = 0.25 µM). It was also found to reduce parasitemia in the body and blood of an infected mouse model of stage 1 disease. Another analog, **CTCB-508** (Fig. **2**), exhibited a rapid reduction of parasitemia in a stage 2 mouse infection model with a clear reduction in parasitemia in the brains of mice, albeit a sterile parasitological cure was not achieved [80].

Inositol Polyphosphate Multikinase (IPMK)

IPMK is an enzyme in the inositol phosphate (IP) pathway comprising diverse phosphate intermediates. Having a ubiquitous distribution among eukaryotes, inositol phosphates are vital signaling molecules mediating indispensable roles for cellular survival, including regulating DNA transcription, mRNA export, and DNA repair. Of the inositol phosphates, perhaps the most well-known are the second messengers IP3 and DAG, formed from the hydrolysis of PIP2. Other polyphosphates include IP4, IP5, IP6, and IP7, which are essential for diverse cellular functions revealing their druggability [81]. IPs play a crucial role in the development stages of trypanosomes as they traverse between the mammalian host and the insect vector [82]. IPMK phosphorylates Ins(1,4,5)P3 produced by PI-specific phospholipase C (PLC) to generate Ins(1,3,4,5)P4 and Ins(1,3,4,5,6)P5. Proteins that interact with Ins(1,4,5)P3 or Ins(1,3,4,5)P4 carry out functions that are linked with processes that differ between stages, suggesting that these intermediates may be involved in regulating these processes [5]. The knockdown of IPMK resulted in developmental changes of bloodstream forms of the parasites, such as expression of procyclic surface coat, up-regulation of RNA-binding proteins, and a metabolic shift from glycolysis to oxidative phosphorylation, which shows the important role that IPs play in regulating the shift from BF to PF stage in trypanosomes [81, 83, 84].

Cestari and colleagues screened a library of 520 compounds from a GlaxoSmithKline library against *T. brucei* and identified 48 compounds with EC_{50} values between 1 and 3 µM. They further used a chemogenomics approach to identify compounds that target the IP pathway using cell lines in which the expression of genes in specific pathways was knocked down, eliminated, or overexpressed [82]. Compounds **C44** and **C20** were shown to inhibit *T. brucei* IPMK with EC_{50} values of 0.83 and 0.28 µM. They compared compound structure similarities of **C44** and **C20** with other molecules. Differences in the pyridopyrimidine group and phenyl groups of compounds **C44** and **C20,** respectively, were suggested to have an effect on the activity of the molecules. Furthermore, the **C44** and **C20** series of compounds could inhibit intracellular amastigote growth by more than 50%, which suggests that the inhibition of IPMK is lethal to amastigotes [82]. These results imply that these molecules are promising candidates for the development of clinical inhibitors against kinetoplastid IPMKs.

RNA-editing Ligase (REL1)

REL1 plays a key role during post-transcriptional modification, which is an essential step in protein synthesis after DNA replication and transcription events. In the case of kinetoplastid protozoa such as *Trypanosoma* parasites, mitochondrial gene expression features a unique RNA editing phase involving insertion or deletion of uridyl moieties, a process that requires the enzyme RNA editing ligase 1 [85]. The products of this modification step are vital for parasite viability, as proven by knockdown and knockout studies of the REL1 gene [86, 87]. Crystal structures of REL1 from *Trypanosoma* parasites reveal a high degree of conservation within species. Mitochondrial DNA encodes components of the oxidative phosphorylation system (subunits of NADH dehydrogenase, cytochrome oxidase, and ATP synthase, as well as apocytochrome b), and most of the respective transcripts undergo RNA editing. BFs lack cytochromes and rely on glycolysis for ATP production, whereas insect forms produce most ATP by cytochrome-mediated oxidative phosphorylation. The ability of dyskinetoplastic (dk) mutants to grow as BFs but not as insect forms is consistent with this view. However, BFs have rotenone-sensitive NADH dehydrogenase activity and preferentially edit mRNAs for this complex [88]. Thus, the loss of editing of NADH dehydrogenase subunits would be lethal to cells that require this activity. REL1 is a particularly attractive drug target because there are no known close human homologs, hence providing the prospects of selective toxicity against the parasite. Using a virtual screen of the REL1 crystal structure against the National Cancer Institute (NCI) Diversity Set, Amaros *et al.* selected the top 30 compounds predicted to interact with REL1's ATP-binding pocket. The relaxed complex scheme (RCS), which redocks the chemicals to receptor structures taken from an explicitly solvated molecular dynamics trajectory, was used to further refine these. After the ligands were rearranged and filtered according to their drug-like characteristics, an initial group of eight ligands was suggested; two of these showed micromolar action against REL1. Following RCS rescoring and a hierarchical similarity search using the most active compound throughout the entire NCI database, an additional set of 6 ligands was found, 2 of which were verified as REL1 inhibitors ($IC_{50} \sim 1 \mu M$). Three closely related 4,5-dihydrox--2,7-naphthalenedisulfonic acid scaffold-containing compounds, **V1, S1,** and **S5** (Fig. **2**), were revealed as the most promising compounds against the most closely related bacteriophage T4 RNA ligase 2 (REL2), as well as against human DNA ligase III, indicated a considerable degree of selectivity for RNA ligases [85].

S-Adenosylmethionine Decarboxylase (AdoMetDC)

AdoMetDC is a key enzyme in the pathway leading to polyamines, which are small organic cations crucial for cellular growth with important roles in various cellular processes including replication, transcription, and translation [89 - 91]. The pyruvoyl-dependent AdoMetDC catalyzes the decarboxylation of *S*-adenosylmethionine (AdoMet) to form decarboxy AdoMet, which then donates the aminopropyl group to one of the amino groups of putrescine, leading to the formation of spermidine [92]. The human AdoMetDC (*h*AdoMetDC) has active sites with covalently bound pyruvate cofactor. An auto-processing reaction generates the pyruvate and also leads to the cleavage of a peptide bond into the α and β subunits [93, 94]. The auto-processing and decarboxylation events in the mammalian enzyme are both stimulated by putrescine. In trypanosomatids, polyamine metabolism is unique, which is thought to contribute to selectivity [95 - 98]. Differences between the parasite and human forms of AdoMetDC include protein turnover rates and the conjugation of spermidine to glutathione to form trypanothione, which is required for redox chemistry in the trypanosome parasite. The parasite AdoMetDC is also activated by binding the catalytically dead paralog called prozyme, which is present only in trypanosomatids [99], while putrescine, which activates *h*AdoMetDC, does not affect the activity of the *T. brucei* heterodimer [100].

Literature has no information on the exact mechanistic steps associated with the *Tb*AdoMetDC-mediated decarboxylation. The proposed mechanism is based on AdoMetDC isolated from *Thermotoga maritima*. Since AdoMetDC is synthesized as a proenzyme, it undergoes auto-processing by serinolysis (cleavage using a serine amino acid residue), forming a pyruvate functionality at the *C*-terminus of the α chain. The amino functionality of AdoMet condenses with the pyruvoyl, forming a Schiff base intermediate. This then undergoes decarboxylation followed by protonation from a cysteine amino acid residue. A water molecule finally hydrolyzes the resulting Schiff base, forming decarboxy AdoMet while restoring the pyruvoyl functional group [101 - 103].

RNA interference and gene knockout experiments have indicated that suppression of AdoMetDC or its regulatory subunit prozyme is lethal to the parasite [104]. **Genz-644131** is one of the most advanced examples of AdoMetDC inhibitors [105]. It was discovered from a lead optimization program of **MDL 73811**, an irreversible inhibitor of AdoMetDC and a structural mimetic of decarboxy AdoMet. **Genz-644131** has been found to be highly potent against *T. brucei rhodesiense in vitro*, with enzyme kinetic studies showing it to be roughly 5 times more potent than **MDL 73811** on *T. brucei brucei* AdoMetDC-prozyme complex. Apart from exhibiting good PK parameters compared to **MDL 73811, Genz-644131** exhibited a 4.3-fold higher brain penetration. It also cured mice infected with *T. b. brucei* strain LAB 110 EATRO, thereby validating AdoMetDC as an important parasite target [105].

CONCLUSION

There have been significant advances in understanding the biology of trypanosomal parasites, including genome sequencing of three major *Trypanosoma* pathogen groups. This information can be exploited to develop more effective drugs against these parasites. For example, acoziborole was identified as a pre-clinical candidate in 2009 by the Anacor chemical library. Acoziborole is now a drug candidate under clinical trial that is being developed as a single-dose oral treatment for *T. b. gambiense* sleeping sickness by DNDi. Researchers can continue to make use of advances in computer systems and algorithms that can significantly reduce the expenses needed to carry out screens of biological targets and chemical libraries using ensemble-based approaches. There is a need for more studies that examine the mechanism of parasite clearance for identified compounds and use structure-activity relationships to optimize the molecules in the hopes of improving plasma levels and brain penetration. The ultimate goal of these research efforts is to develop more effective and less toxic drugs for HAT treatment. More cooperative efforts between academia and the pharmaceutical industry can ensure that this goal is achieved, and this will enable the provision of affordable and reliable drugs to the communities that need them.

REFERENCES

[1] Barrett MP, Burchmore RJS, Stich A, *et al.* The trypanosomiases. Lancet 2003; 362(9394): 1469-80.
[http://dx.doi.org/10.1016/S0140-6736(03)14694-6] [PMID: 14602444]

[2] Franco JR, Cecchi G, Priotto G, *et al.* Monitoring the elimination of human African trypanosomiasis at continental and country level: Update to 2018. PLoS Negl Trop Dis 2020; 14(5): e0008261.
[http://dx.doi.org/10.1371/journal.pntd.0008261] [PMID: 32437391]

[3] WHO. Trypanosomiasis, human African (sleeping sickness). 2023. Available from: https://www.who.int/news-room/fact-sheets/detail/trypanosomiasis-human-african-(sleeping-sickness)

[4] Elenga VA, Lissom A, Elion DOA, *et al.* Risk factors and prevalence of human African trypanosomiasis in individuals living in remote areas of the republic of Congo. BMC Public Health 2022; 22(1): 2322.
[http://dx.doi.org/10.1186/s12889-022-14577-9] [PMID: 36510162]

[5] MacGregor P, Szöőr B, Savill NJ, Matthews KR. Trypanosomal immune evasion, chronicity and transmission: an elegant balancing act. Nat Rev Microbiol 2012; 10(6): 431-8.
[http://dx.doi.org/10.1038/nrmicro2779] [PMID: 22543519]

[6] Roditi I, Schwarz H, Pearson TW, *et al.* Procyclin gene expression and loss of the variant surface glycoprotein during differentiation of Trypanosoma brucei. J Cell Biol 1989; 108(2): 737-46.
[http://dx.doi.org/10.1083/jcb.108.2.737] [PMID: 2645304]

[7] Batram C, Jones NG, Janzen CJ, Markert SM, Engstler M. Expression site attenuation mechanistically links antigenic variation and development in Trypanosoma brucei. eLife 2014; 3: e02324.
[http://dx.doi.org/10.7554/eLife.02324] [PMID: 24844706]

[8] N'Djetchi MK, Ilboudo H, Koffi M, *et al.* The study of trypanosome species circulating in domestic animals in two human African trypanosomiasis foci of Côte d'Ivoire identifies pigs and cattle as potential reservoirs of Trypanosoma brucei gambiense. PLoS Negl Trop Dis 2017; 11(10): e0005993.
[http://dx.doi.org/10.1371/journal.pntd.0005993] [PMID: 29045405]

[9] CDC. Parasites - African Trypanosomiasis (also known as Sleeping Sickness). 2023. Available from: https://www.cdc.gov/parasites/sleepingsickness/health_professionals/index.html

[10] Lindner AK, Lejon V, Chappuis F, *et al.* New WHO guidelines for treatment of gambiense human African trypanosomiasis including fexinidazole: substantial changes for clinical practice. Lancet Infect Dis 2020; 20(2): e38-46.
[http://dx.doi.org/10.1016/S1473-3099(19)30612-7] [PMID: 31879061]

[11] Mulenga P, Chenge F, Boelaert M, *et al.* Integration of human african trypanosomiasis control activities into primary healthcare services: A scoping review. Am J Trop Med Hyg 2019; 101(5): 1114-25.
[http://dx.doi.org/10.4269/ajtmh.19-0232] [PMID: 31482788]

[12] Venturelli A, Tagliazucchi L, Lima C, *et al.* Current treatments to control african trypanosomiasis and one health perspective. Microorganisms 2022; 10(7): 1298.
[http://dx.doi.org/10.3390/microorganisms10071298] [PMID: 35889018]

[13] Gilbert IH. Target-based drug discovery for human African trypanosomiasis: selection of molecular target and chemical matter. Parasitology 2014; 141(1): 28-36.
[http://dx.doi.org/10.1017/S0031182013001017] [PMID: 23931634]

[14] Frearson JA, Wyatt PG, Gilbert IH, Fairlamb AH. Target assessment for antiparasitic drug discovery. Trends Parasitol 2007; 23(12): 589-95.
[http://dx.doi.org/10.1016/j.pt.2007.08.019] [PMID: 17962072]

[15]   Wyatt PG, Gilbert IH, Read KD, Fairlamb AH. Target validation: linking target and chemical properties to desired product profile. Curr Top Med Chem 2011; 11(10): 1275-83.
[http://dx.doi.org/10.2174/156802611795429185] [PMID: 21401506]

[16]   DNDi. Target product profile for sleeping sickness.. Available from: https://dndi.org/diseases/sleeping-sickness/target-product-profile/

[17]   Hall BS, Wilkinson SR. Activation of benznidazole by trypanosomal type I nitroreductases results in glyoxal formation. Antimicrob Agents Chemother 2012; 56(1): 115-23.
[http://dx.doi.org/10.1128/AAC.05135-11] [PMID: 22037852]

[18]   Whitmore GF, Varghese AJ. The biological properties of reduced nitroheterocyclics and possible underlying biochemical mechanisms. Biochem Pharmacol 1986; 35(1): 97-103.
[http://dx.doi.org/10.1016/0006-2952(86)90565-4] [PMID: 3510061]

[19]   Yan GZ, Generaux CN, Yoon M, *et al.* A semiphysiologically based pharmacokinetic modeling approach to predict the dose-exposure relationship of an antiparasitic prodrug/active metabolite pair. Drug Metab Dispos 2012; 40(1): 6-17.
[http://dx.doi.org/10.1124/dmd.111.040063] [PMID: 21953913]

[20]   Basselin M, Denise H, Coombs GH, Barrett MP. Resistance to pentamidine in Leishmania mexicana involves exclusion of the drug from the mitochondrion. Antimicrob Agents Chemother 2002; 46(12): 3731-8.
[http://dx.doi.org/10.1128/AAC.46.12.3731-3738.2002] [PMID: 12435669]

[21]   Baker N, de Koning HP, Mäser P, Horn D. Drug resistance in African trypanosomiasis: the melarsoprol and pentamidine story. Trends Parasitol 2013; 29(3): 110-8.
[http://dx.doi.org/10.1016/j.pt.2012.12.005] [PMID: 23375541]

[22]   Mathis AM, Bridges AS, Ismail MA, *et al.* Diphenyl furans and aza analogs: effects of structural modification on *in vitro* activity, DNA binding, and accumulation and distribution in trypanosomes. Antimicrob Agents Chemother 2007; 51(8): 2801-10.
[http://dx.doi.org/10.1128/AAC.00005-07] [PMID: 17517831]

[23]   Wilson WD, Tanious FA, Mathis A, Tevis D, Hall JE, Boykin DW. Antiparasitic compounds that target DNA. Biochimie 2008; 90(7): 999-1014.
[http://dx.doi.org/10.1016/j.biochi.2008.02.017] [PMID: 18343228]

[24]   Mathis AM, Holman JL, Sturk LM, *et al.* Accumulation and intracellular distribution of antitrypanosomal diamidine compounds DB75 and DB820 in African trypanosomes. Antimicrob Agents Chemother 2006; 50(6): 2185-91.
[http://dx.doi.org/10.1128/AAC.00192-06] [PMID: 16723581]

[25]   Barrett MP, Gemmell CG, Suckling CJ. Minor groove binders as anti-infective agents. Pharmacol Ther 2013; 139(1): 12-23.
[http://dx.doi.org/10.1016/j.pharmthera.2013.03.002] [PMID: 23507040]

[26]   Kentrup H, Becker W, Heukelbach J, *et al.* Dyrk, a dual specificity protein kinase with unique structural features whose activity is dependent on tyrosine residues between subdomains VII and VIII. J Biol Chem 1996; 271(7): 3488-95.
[http://dx.doi.org/10.1074/jbc.271.7.3488] [PMID: 8631952]

[27]   Lemmon MA, Schlessinger J. Cell signaling by receptor tyrosine kinases. Cell 2010; 141(7): 1117-34.
[http://dx.doi.org/10.1016/j.cell.2010.06.011] [PMID: 20602996]

[28]   Sessa G, Raz V, Savaldi S, Fluhr R. PK12, a plant dual-specificity protein kinase of the LAMMER family, is regulated by the hormone ethylene. Plant Cell 1996; 8(12): 2223-34.
[PMID: 8989879]

[29]   Letwin K. Mizzen L, Motro B, Ben-David Y, Bernstein A, Pawson T. A mammalian dual specificity protein kinase, Nek1, is related to the NIMA cell cycle regulator and highly expressed in meiotic germ cells The EMBO Journal 1992; 11(10): 3521-31.

[http://dx.doi.org/10.1002/j.1460-2075.1992.tb05435.x]

[30] Parker LL, Atherton-Fessler S, Piwnica-Worms H. p107wee1 is a dual-specificity kinase that phosphorylates p34cdc2 on tyrosine 15. Proc Natl Acad Sci USA 1992; 89(7): 2917-21.
[http://dx.doi.org/10.1073/pnas.89.7.2917] [PMID: 1372994]

[31] Parsons M, Worthey EA, Ward PN, Mottram JC. Comparative analysis of the kinomes of three pathogenic trypanosomatids: Leishmania major, Trypanosoma brucei and Trypanosoma cruzi. BMC Genomics 2005; 6(1): 127.
[http://dx.doi.org/10.1186/1471-2164-6-127] [PMID: 16164760]

[32] Lim WA, Pawson T. Phosphotyrosine signaling: evolving a new cellular communication system. Cell 2010; 142(5): 661-7.
[http://dx.doi.org/10.1016/j.cell.2010.08.023] [PMID: 20813250]

[33] Wang Z, Cole PA. Chapter one - Catalytic mechanisms and regulation of protein kinases. In: Shokat KM, Ed. Methods in Enzymology. Academic Press 2014; pp. 1-21.

[34] Wheeler-Alm E, Shapiro SZ. Evidence of tyrosine kinase activity in the protozoan parasite Trypanosoma brucei. J Protozool 1992; 39(3): 413-6.
[http://dx.doi.org/10.1111/j.1550-7408.1992.tb01473.x] [PMID: 1640387]

[35] Hamadien M, Bakhiet M, Harris RA. Interferon-γ induces secretion of trypanosome lymphocyte triggering factor *via* tyrosine protein kinases. Parasitology 2000; 120(3): 281-7.
[http://dx.doi.org/10.1017/S0031182099005521] [PMID: 10759086]

[36] Katiyar S, Kufareva I, Behera R, *et al*. Lapatinib-binding protein kinases in the African trypanosome: identification of cellular targets for kinase-directed chemical scaffolds. PLoS One 2013; 8(2): e56150.
[http://dx.doi.org/10.1371/journal.pone.0056150] [PMID: 23437089]

[37] Behera R, Thomas SM, Mensa-Wilmot K. New chemical scaffolds for human african trypanosomiasis lead discovery from a screen of tyrosine kinase inhibitor drugs. Antimicrob Agents Chemother 2014; 58(4): 2202-10.
[http://dx.doi.org/10.1128/AAC.01691-13] [PMID: 24468788]

[38] Johnson GL, Lapadat R. Mitogen-activated protein kinase pathways mediated by ERK, JNK, and p38 protein kinases. Science 2002; 298(5600): 1911-2.
[http://dx.doi.org/10.1126/science.1072682] [PMID: 12471242]

[39] Dong C, Davis RJ, Flavell RA. MAP kinases in the immune response. Annu Rev Immunol 2002; 20(1): 55-72.
[http://dx.doi.org/10.1146/annurev.immunol.20.091301.131133] [PMID: 11861597]

[40] Liu Y, Shepherd eg, Nelin LD. MAPK phosphatases — regulating the immune response. Nat Rev Immunol 2007; 7(3): 202-12.
[http://dx.doi.org/10.1038/nri2035] [PMID: 17318231]

[41] Arthur JSC, Ley SC. Mitogen-activated protein kinases in innate immunity. Nat Rev Immunol 2013; 13(9): 679-92.
[http://dx.doi.org/10.1038/nri3495] [PMID: 23954936]

[42] Qi M, Elion EA. MAP kinase pathways. J Cell Sci 2005; 118(16): 3569-72.
[http://dx.doi.org/10.1242/jcs.02470] [PMID: 16105880]

[43] Songyang Z, Lu KP, Kwon YT, *et al*. A structural basis for substrate specificities of protein Ser/Thr kinases: primary sequence preference of casein kinases I and II, NIMA, phosphorylase kinase, calmodulin-dependent kinase II, CDK5, and Erk1. Mol Cell Biol 1996; 16(11): 6486-93.
[http://dx.doi.org/10.1128/MCB.16.11.6486] [PMID: 8887677]

[44] Hua SB, Wang CC. Interferon-gamma activation of a mitogen-activated protein kinase, KFR1, in the bloodstream form of Trypanosoma brucei. J Biol Chem 1997; 272(16): 10797-803.
[http://dx.doi.org/10.1074/jbc.272.16.10797] [PMID: 9099733]

[45] Müller IB, Domenicali-Pfister D, Roditi I, Vassella E. Stage-specific requirement of a mitogen-activated protein kinase by Trypanosoma brucei. Mol Biol Cell 2002; 13(11): 3787-99.
[http://dx.doi.org/10.1091/mbc.e02-02-0093] [PMID: 12429824]

[46] Ellis J, Sarkar M, Hendriks E, Matthews K. A novel ERK-like, CRK-like protein kinase that modulates growth in *Trypanosoma brucei via* an autoregulatory C-terminal extension. Mol Microbiol 2004; 53(5): 1487-99.
[http://dx.doi.org/10.1111/j.1365-2958.2004.04218.x] [PMID: 15387824]

[47] Wang MH, Wen YZ, Wei Y, *et al.* Mitogen-activated protein kinase 5, a novel molecular marker for the identification and detection of Trypanozoon species. Acta Trop 2012; 122: 183-8.
[http://dx.doi.org/10.1016/j.actatropica.2012.01.009]

[48] Güttinger A, Schwab C, Morand S, Roditi I, Vassella E. A mitogen-activated protein kinase of Trypanosoma brucei confers resistance to temperature stress. Mol Biochem Parasitol 2007; 153(2): 203-6.
[http://dx.doi.org/10.1016/j.molbiopara.2007.02.001] [PMID: 17368580]

[49] Mackey ZB, Koupparis K, Nishino M, McKerrow JH. High-throughput analysis of an RNAi library identifies novel kinase targets in Trypanosoma brucei. Chem Biol Drug Des 2011; 78(3): 454-63.
[http://dx.doi.org/10.1111/j.1747-0285.2011.01156.x] [PMID: 21668652]

[50] Batista M, Kugeratski FG, de Paula Lima CV, *et al.* The MAP kinase MAPKLK1 is essential to Trypanosoma brucei proliferation and regulates proteins involved in mRNA metabolism. J Proteomics 2017; 154: 118-27.
[http://dx.doi.org/10.1016/j.jprot.2016.12.011] [PMID: 28039027]

[51] Turjanski AG, Hummer G, Gutkind JS. How mitogen-activated protein kinases recognize and phosphorylate their targets: A QM/MM study. J Am Chem Soc 2009; 131(17): 6141-8.
[http://dx.doi.org/10.1021/ja8071995] [PMID: 19361221]

[52] Mercer L, Bowling T, Perales J, *et al.* 2,4-Diaminopyrimidines as potent inhibitors of Trypanosoma brucei and identification of molecular targets by a chemical proteomics approach. PLoS Negl Trop Dis 2011; 5(2): e956.
[http://dx.doi.org/10.1371/journal.pntd.0000956] [PMID: 21347454]

[53] Domenicali Pfister D, Burkard G, Morand S, Renggli CK, Roditi I, Vassella E. A Mitogen-activated protein kinase controls differentiation of bloodstream forms of Trypanosoma brucei. Eukaryot Cell 2006; 5(7): 1126-35.
[http://dx.doi.org/10.1128/EC.00094-06] [PMID: 16835456]

[54] Folgueira C, Requena JM. A postgenomic view of the heat shock proteins in kinetoplastids. FEMS Microbiol Rev 2007; 31(4): 359-77.
[http://dx.doi.org/10.1111/j.1574-6976.2007.00069.x] [PMID: 17459115]

[55] Droll D, Minia I, Fadda A, *et al.* Post-transcriptional regulation of the trypanosome heat shock response by a zinc finger protein. PLoS Pathog 2013; 9(4): e1003286.
[http://dx.doi.org/10.1371/journal.ppat.1003286] [PMID: 23592996]

[56] Pallavi R, Roy N, Nageshan RK, *et al.* Heat shock protein 90 as a drug target against protozoan infections: biochemical characterization of HSP90 from Plasmodium falciparum and Trypanosoma evansi and evaluation of its inhibitor as a candidate drug. J Biol Chem 2010; 285(49): 37964-75.
[http://dx.doi.org/10.1074/jbc.M110.155317] [PMID: 20837488]

[57] Pizarro JC, Hills T, Senisterra G, *et al.* Exploring the Trypanosoma brucei Hsp83 potential as a target for structure guided drug design. PLoS Negl Trop Dis 2013; 7(10): e2492.
[http://dx.doi.org/10.1371/journal.pntd.0002492] [PMID: 24147171]

[58] Silva ML, de Santiago-Silva KM, Fabris M, Camargo PG, de Lima Ferreira Bispo M. Proteasome as a drug target in trypanosomatid diseases. Curr Drug Targets 2023; 24(10): 781-9.
[http://dx.doi.org/10.2174/1389450124666230719104147] [PMID: 37469152]

[59] Bijlmakers MJ. Ubiquitination and the proteasome as drug targets in trypanosomatid diseases. Front Chem 2021; 8: 630888.
[http://dx.doi.org/10.3389/fchem.2020.630888] [PMID: 33732684]

[60] Kurup SP, Tarleton RL. The Trypanosoma cruzi flagellum is discarded *via* asymmetric cell division following invasion and provides early targets for protective CD8⁺ T cells. Cell Host Microbe 2014; 16(4): 439-49.
[http://dx.doi.org/10.1016/j.chom.2014.09.003] [PMID: 25299330]

[61] González J, Ramalho-Pinto FJ, Frevert U, *et al.* Proteasome activity is required for the stage-specific transformation of a protozoan parasite. J Exp Med 1996; 184(5): 1909-18.
[http://dx.doi.org/10.1084/jem.184.5.1909] [PMID: 8920878]

[62] Khare S, Nagle AS, Biggart A, *et al.* Proteasome inhibition for treatment of leishmaniasis, Chagas disease and sleeping sickness. Nature 2016; 537(7619): 229-33.
[http://dx.doi.org/10.1038/nature19339] [PMID: 27501246]

[63] Nagle A, Biggart A, Be C, *et al.* Discovery and characterization of clinical candidate LXE408 as a kinetoplastid-selective proteasome inhibitor for the treatment of leishmaniases. J Med Chem 2020; 63(19): 10773-81.
[http://dx.doi.org/10.1021/acs.jmedchem.0c00499] [PMID: 32667203]

[64] Steverding D, Sexton DW, Wang X, Gehrke SS, Wagner GK, Caffrey CR. Trypanosoma brucei: Chemical evidence that cathepsin L is essential for survival and a relevant drug target. Int J Parasitol 2012; 42(5): 481-8.
[http://dx.doi.org/10.1016/j.ijpara.2012.03.009] [PMID: 22549023]

[65] Lalmanach G, Boulangé A, Serveau C, *et al.* Congopain from Trypanosoma congolense: drug target and vaccine candidate. Biol Chem 2002; 383(5): 739-49.
[http://dx.doi.org/10.1515/BC.2002.077] [PMID: 12108538]

[66] Overath P, Chaudhri M, Steverding D, Ziegelbauer K. Invariant surface proteins in bloodstream forms of Trypanosoma brucei. Parasitol Today 1994; 10(2): 53-8.
[http://dx.doi.org/10.1016/0169-4758(94)90393-X] [PMID: 15275499]

[67] Zhai X, Meek TD. Catalytic mechanism of cruzain from *Trypanosoma cruzi* as determined from solvent kinetic isotope effects of steady-state and pre-steady-state kinetics. Biochemistry 2018; 57(22): 3176-90.
[http://dx.doi.org/10.1021/acs.biochem.7b01250] [PMID: 29336553]

[68] Ettari R, Tamborini L, Angelo IC, *et al.* Inhibition of rhodesain as a novel therapeutic modality for human African trypanosomiasis. J Med Chem 2013; 56(14): 5637-58.
[http://dx.doi.org/10.1021/jm301424d] [PMID: 23611656]

[69] Jung S, Fuchs N, Johe P, *et al.* Fluorovinylsulfones and -sulfonates as potent covalent reversible inhibitors of the trypanosomal cysteine protease rhodesain: Structure–activity relationship, inhibition mechanism, metabolism, and *in vivo* studies. J Med Chem 2021; 64(16): 12322-58.
[http://dx.doi.org/10.1021/acs.jmedchem.1c01002] [PMID: 34378914]

[70] Giroud M, Dietzel U, Anselm L, *et al.* Repurposing a library of human cathepsin L Ligands: Identification of macrocyclic lactams as potent rhodesain and *Trypanosoma brucei* inhibitors. J Med Chem 2018; 61(8): 3350-69.
[http://dx.doi.org/10.1021/acs.jmedchem.7b01869] [PMID: 29590750]

[71] Song HB, He M, Cai ZP, *et al.* UDP-Glucose 4-Epimerase and β-1,4-Galactosyltransferase from the Oyster *Magallana gigas* as Valuable Biocatalysts for the Production of Galactosylated Products. Int J Mol Sci 2018; 19(6): 1600.
[http://dx.doi.org/10.3390/ijms19061600] [PMID: 29844279]

[72] Pinger J, Nešić D, Ali L, *et al.* African trypanosomes evade immune clearance by O-glycosylation of the VSG surface coat. Nat Microbiol 2018; 3(8): 932-8.

[http://dx.doi.org/10.1038/s41564-018-0187-6] [PMID: 29988048]

[73]   Mehlert A, Wormald MR, Ferguson MAJ. Modeling of the N-glycosylated transferrin receptor suggests how transferrin binding can occur within the surface coat of Trypanosoma brucei. PLoS Pathog 2012; 8(4): e1002618.
[http://dx.doi.org/10.1371/journal.ppat.1002618] [PMID: 22496646]

[74]   Roper JR, Güther MLS, Milne KG, Ferguson MAJ. Galactose metabolism is essential for the African sleeping sickness parasite *Trypanosoma brucei*. Proc Natl Acad Sci USA 2002; 99(9): 5884-9.
[http://dx.doi.org/10.1073/pnas.092669999] [PMID: 11983889]

[75]   Durrant JD, Urbaniak MD, Ferguson MAJ, McCammon JA. Computer-aided identification of Trypanosoma brucei uridine diphosphate galactose 4′-epimerase inhibitors: toward the development of novel therapies for African sleeping sickness. J Med Chem 2010; 53(13): 5025-32.
[http://dx.doi.org/10.1021/jm100456a] [PMID: 20527952]

[76]   Haanstra JR, González-Marcano EB, Gualdrón-López M, Michels PAM. Biogenesis, maintenance and dynamics of glycosomes in trypanosomatid parasites. Biochim Biophys Acta Mol Cell Res 2016; 1863(5): 1038-48.
[http://dx.doi.org/10.1016/j.bbamcr.2015.09.015] [PMID: 26384872]

[77]   Martinez-Oyanedel J, McNae IW, Nowicki MW, *et al.* The first crystal structure of phosphofructokinase from a eukaryote: Trypanosoma brucei. J Mol Biol 2007; 366(4): 1185-98.
[http://dx.doi.org/10.1016/j.jmb.2006.10.019] [PMID: 17207816]

[78]   McNae IW, Martinez-Oyanedel J, Keillor JW, Michels PAM, Fothergill-Gilmore LA, Walkinshaw MD. The crystal structure of ATP-bound phosphofructokinase from Trypanosoma brucei reveals conformational transitions different from those of other phosphofructokinases. J Mol Biol 2009; 385(5): 1519-33.
[http://dx.doi.org/10.1016/j.jmb.2008.11.047] [PMID: 19084537]

[79]   Murillo-López J, Zinovjev K, Pereira H, *et al.* Studying the phosphoryl transfer mechanism of the E. coli phosphofructokinase-2: from X-ray structure to quantum mechanics/molecular mechanics simulations. Chem Sci (Camb) 2019; 10(10): 2882-92.
[http://dx.doi.org/10.1039/C9SC00094A] [PMID: 30996866]

[80]   McNae IW, Kinkead J, Malik D, *et al.* Fast acting allosteric phosphofructokinase inhibitors block trypanosome glycolysis and cure acute African trypanosomiasis in mice. Nat Commun 2021; 12(1): 1052.
[http://dx.doi.org/10.1038/s41467-021-21273-6] [PMID: 33594070]

[81]   Cestari I, Haas P, Moretti NS, Schenkman S, Stuart K. Chemogenetic characterization of inositol phosphate metabolic pathway reveals druggable enzymes for targeting kinetoplastid parasites. Cell Chem Biol 2016; 23(5): 608-17.
[http://dx.doi.org/10.1016/j.chembiol.2016.03.015] [PMID: 27133314]

[82]   Cestari I, Anupama A, Stuart K. Inositol polyphosphate multikinase regulation of *Trypanosoma brucei* life stage development. Mol Biol Cell 2018; 29(9): 1137-52.
[http://dx.doi.org/10.1091/mbc.E17-08-0515] [PMID: 29514930]

[83]   Haanstra JR, van Tuijl A, Kessler P, *et al.* Compartmentation prevents a lethal turbo-explosion of glycolysis in trypanosomes. Proc Natl Acad Sci USA 2008; 105(46): 17718-23.
[http://dx.doi.org/10.1073/pnas.0806664105] [PMID: 19008351]

[84]   Furuya T, Kessler P, Jardim A, Schnaufer A, Crudder C, Parsons M. Glucose is toxic to glycosome-deficient trypanosomes. Proc Natl Acad Sci USA 2002; 99(22): 14177-82.
[http://dx.doi.org/10.1073/pnas.222454899] [PMID: 12386344]

[85]   Amaro RE, Schnaufer A, Interthal H, Hol W, Stuart KD, McCammon JA. Discovery of drug-like inhibitors of an essential RNA-editing ligase in *Trypanosoma brucei*. Proc Natl Acad Sci USA 2008; 105(45): 17278-83.
[http://dx.doi.org/10.1073/pnas.0805820105] [PMID: 18981420]

[86]   Rusché LN, Huang CE, Piller KJ, Hemann M, Wirtz E, Sollner-Webb B. The two RNA ligases of the Trypanosoma brucei RNA editing complex: cloning the essential band IV gene and identifying the band V gene. Mol Cell Biol 2001; 21(4): 979-89.
[http://dx.doi.org/10.1128/MCB.21.4.979-989.2001] [PMID: 11158286]

[87]   Gao G, Simpson L. Is the Trypanosoma brucei REL1 RNA ligase specific for U-deletion RNA editing, and is the REL2 RNA ligase specific for U-insertion editing? J Biol Chem 2003; 278(30): 27570-4.
[http://dx.doi.org/10.1074/jbc.M303317200] [PMID: 12748175]

[88]   Surve S, Heestand M, Panicucci B, Schnaufer A, Parsons M. Enigmatic presence of mitochondrial complex I in Trypanosoma brucei bloodstream forms. Eukaryot Cell 2012; 11(2): 183-93.
[http://dx.doi.org/10.1128/EC.05282-11] [PMID: 22158713]

[89]   Pegg AE. Mammalian polyamine metabolism and function. IUBMB Life 2009; 61(9): 880-94.
[http://dx.doi.org/10.1002/iub.230] [PMID: 19603518]

[90]   Childs AC, Mehta DJ, Gerner EW. Polyamine-dependent gene expression. Cell Mol Life Sci 2003; 60(7): 1394-406.
[http://dx.doi.org/10.1007/s00018-003-2332-4] [PMID: 12943227]

[91]   Wickner RB. Herbert Tabor, 1918–2020: Polyamines, NIH, and the *JBC*. Proc Natl Acad Sci USA 2021; 118(5): e2023986118.
[http://dx.doi.org/10.1073/pnas.2023986118]

[92]   Pegg AE. S-Adenosylmethionine decarboxylase. Essays Biochem 2009; 46: 25-46.
[http://dx.doi.org/10.1042/bse0460003] [PMID: 20095968]

[93]   Tolbert WD, Zhang Y, Cottet SE, *et al.* Mechanism of human S-adenosylmethionine decarboxylase proenzyme processing as revealed by the structure of the S68A mutant. Biochemistry 2003; 42(8): 2386-95.
[http://dx.doi.org/10.1021/bi0268854] [PMID: 12600205]

[94]   Bale S, Ealick SE. Structural biology of S-adenosylmethionine decarboxylase. Amino Acids 2010; 38(2): 451-60.
[http://dx.doi.org/10.1007/s00726-009-0404-y] [PMID: 19997761]

[95]   Fairlamb AH, Blackburn P, Ulrich P, Chait BT, Cerami A. Trypanothione: a novel bis(glutathionyl)spermidine cofactor for glutathione reductase in trypanosomatids. Science 1985; 227(4693): 1485-7.
[http://dx.doi.org/10.1126/science.3883489] [PMID: 3883489]

[96]   Willert E, Phillips MA. Regulation and function of polyamines in African trypanosomes. Trends Parasitol 2012; 28(2): 66-72.
[http://dx.doi.org/10.1016/j.pt.2011.11.001] [PMID: 22192816]

[97]   Casero RA Jr, Marton LJ. Targeting polyamine metabolism and function in cancer and other hyperproliferative diseases. Nat Rev Drug Discov 2007; 6(5): 373-90.
[http://dx.doi.org/10.1038/nrd2243] [PMID: 17464296]

[98]   Bacchi CJ, Nathan HC, Hutner SH, McCann PP, Sjoerdsma A. Polyamine metabolism: a potential therapeutic target in trypanosomes. Science 1980; 210(4467): 332-4.
[http://dx.doi.org/10.1126/science.6775372] [PMID: 6775372]

[99]   Willert EK, Fitzpatrick R, Phillips MA. Allosteric regulation of an essential trypanosome polyamine biosynthetic enzyme by a catalytically dead homolog. Proc Natl Acad Sci USA 2007; 104(20): 8275-80.
[http://dx.doi.org/10.1073/pnas.0701111104] [PMID: 17485680]

[100]   Ekstrom JL, Mathews II, Stanley BA, Pegg AE, Ealick SE. The crystal structure of human S-adenosylmethionine decarboxylase at 2.25 Å resolution reveals a novel fold. Structure 1999; 7(5): 583-95.
[http://dx.doi.org/10.1016/S0969-2126(99)80074-4] [PMID: 10378277]

[101] Xiong H, Stanley BA, Pegg AE. Role of cysteine-82 in the catalytic mechanism of human S-adenosylmethionine decarboxylase. Biochemistry 1999; 38(8): 2462-70.
[http://dx.doi.org/10.1021/bi9825201] [PMID: 10029540]

[102] Toms AV, Kinsland C, McCloskey DE, Pegg AE, Ealick SE. Evolutionary links as revealed by the structure of Thermotoga maritima S-adenosylmethionine decarboxylase. J Biol Chem 2004; 279(32): 33837-46.
[http://dx.doi.org/10.1074/jbc.M403369200] [PMID: 15150268]

[103] Lee BI, Suh SW. Crystal structure of the schiff base intermediate prior to decarboxylation in the catalytic cycle of aspartate α-decarboxylase. J Mol Biol 2004; 340(1): 1-7.
[http://dx.doi.org/10.1016/j.jmb.2004.04.049] [PMID: 15184017]

[104] Willert EK, Phillips MA. Regulated expression of an essential allosteric activator of polyamine biosynthesis in African trypanosomes. PLoS Pathog 2008; 4(10): e1000183.
[http://dx.doi.org/10.1371/journal.ppat.1000183] [PMID: 18949025]

[105] Barker RH Jr, Liu H, Hirth B, *et al.* Novel S-adenosylmethionine decarboxylase inhibitors for the treatment of human African trypanosomiasis. Antimicrob Agents Chemother 2009; 53(5): 2052-8.
[http://dx.doi.org/10.1128/AAC.01674-08] [PMID: 19289530]

CHAPTER 5

Schistosomiasis: State of the Art and New Perspectives

Salma Darwish[1], Mohamed Teleb[1], Sherine N. Khattab[2] and Adnan A. Bekhit[1,3,*]

[1] *Department of Pharmaceutical Chemistry, Faculty of Pharmacy, Alexandria University, Alexandria 21521, Egypt*

[2] *Chemistry Department, Faculty of Science, Alexandria University, Alexandria 21321, Egypt*

[3] *Pharmacy Program, Allied Health Department, College of Health and Sport Sciences, University of Bahrain, Sakhir 32038, Kingdom of Bahrain*

Abstract: Schistosomiasis, a neglected tropical disease, affects millions worldwide. Treatment and control strategies rely entirely on the single drug praziquantel (PZQ), making the prospect of resistance emergence worrisome. The pressing need to introduce new antischistosomal agents necessitates exploring and repurposing chemotherapeutic history besides designing novel leads. In this context, this chapter summarizes the parasite life cycle, its clinical manifestations, and the progress in schistosomiasis chemotherapy with an overview of the validated drug targets, the emergence of drug resistance, and vaccination trials.

Keywords: Current schistosomiasis treatment, Neglected tropical diseases, Repurposed antischistosomal agents, Resistance, Schistosomiasis, Specific schistosomal targets, Vaccination.

INTRODUCTION

Schistosomiasis is one of the most important neglected tropical diseases (NTD) that is caused by blood flukes of the genus Schistosoma. Nearly 250 million humans are affected by this disease, which is associated with poverty as its transmission is connected with a lack of hygiene, poor access to safe water, and lack of adequate sanitation. Among the five species that can infect humans, the three most common are *Schistosoma haematobium*, *Schistosoma japonicum*, and *Schistosoma mansoni* [1, 2]. As controlling the disease is currently based on the

* **Corresponding author Adnan A. Bekhit:** Department of Pharmaceutical Chemistry, Faculty of Pharmacy, Alexandria University, Alexandria 21521, Egypt; Pharmacy Program, Allied Health Department, College of Health and Sport Sciences, University of Bahrain, Sakhir 32038, Kingdom of Bahrain; E-mails: adnbekhit@hotmail.com; adnbekhit@pharmacy.alexu.edu.eg

Igor Jose dos Santos Nascimento & Ricardo Olimpio de Moura (Eds.)
All rights reserved-© 2025 Bentham Science Publishers

use of praziquantel, scientists are working on the identification and characterisation of potential new targets and drug repurposing to develop new treatment methods. In addition, researchers are working to develop a vaccine to help control the disease in combination with the drug of choice employed.

THE LIFE CYCLE OF SCHISTOSOMA

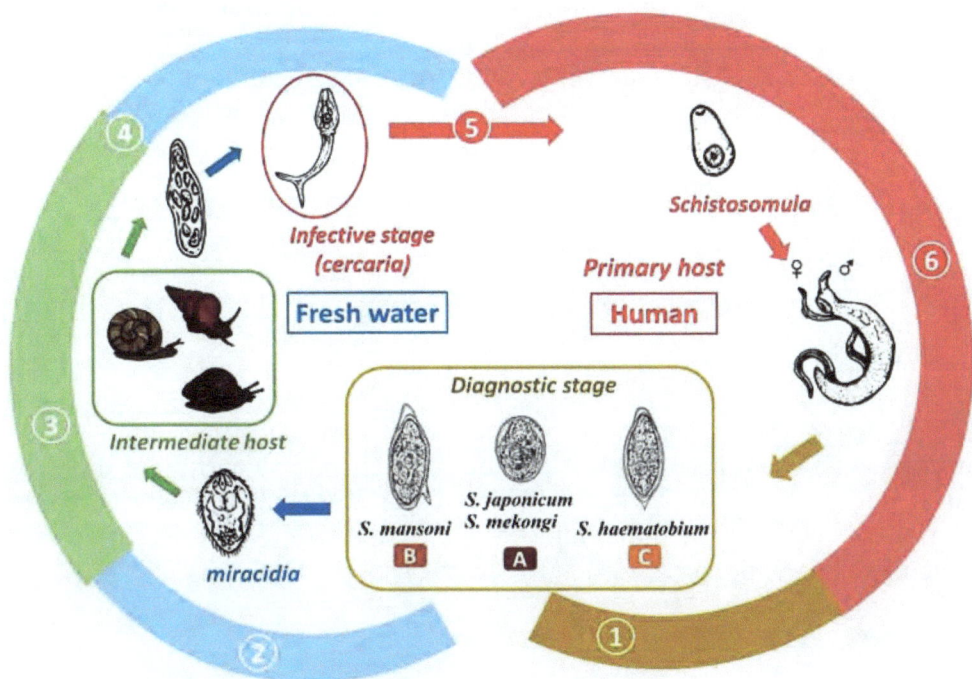

Fig. (1). Schematic representation of the life cycle of Schistosoma.

The life cycle of Schistosoma follow the following steps (Fig **1**): 1. Depending on the species of the parasite, the eggs are released through faeces or urine of infected patients contaminating fresh water. 2. In appropriate conditions, the released eggs hatch setting free larvae called miracidia which infect snails. 3. Each species of Schistosoma parasite infects a certain genus of the snail. While **S. haematobium** infects snails of the genus *Bulinus*, the intermediate hosts of **S. japonicum** are snails of the genus *Oncomelania*. However, **S. mekongi** larvae infect snails of the genus *Neutricula* and the miracidia of **S. mansoni** infect snails of the genus *Biomphalaria*. 4. After entering the intermediate host, the miracidium loses its ciliated plates, thereby turning into a mother sporocyst, which produces daughter sporocysts. The latter either produces the next larval stage known as cercaria or produces more daughter sporocysts. 5. When the cercariae penetrate the human skin, they shed their forked tails turning into another larval form called the schistosomula. These migrate throughout the body's tissues through the blood circulation. 6. The liver is the location where the schistosomula mature into male and female adult worms. After copulation, the pair migrates and resides in the mesenteric venules, the locations of which are determined according to the species of the parasite. While the copulated worms of **S. haematobium** often exist in the bladder and ureters, they can be found in the rectal venules. However, the adult worm pairs of **S. japonicum** occur more frequently in the small intestine. The worms of **S. mansoni** reside in either large or small intestines. After reaching their different destinations they deposit numerous eggs which are eliminated in urine or faeces so that the cycle can continue [3 - 5].

CLINICAL MANIFESTATIONS OF HUMAN SCHISTOSOMIASIS

Clinically, schistosomiasis consists of two phases namely (i) acute schistosomiasis and (ii) chronic schistosomiasis.

Acute Schistosomiasis

It is a systemic hypersensitivity induced by the penetrating, migrating, and maturing larvae as well as eggs. It can be divided into two clinical pictures: (i) cercarial dermatitis or swimmer's itch and (ii) Katayama fever or syndrome. Generally, the severity of the symptoms is related to the larval burden and the immune response to the presented antigens [6, 7].

Cercarial Dermatitis or Swimmer's Itch

Within 24 hours after contact with the infective cercariae, the affected person develops an itch and a rash that can last for up to 3 weeks. The rash that is provoked by the penetration of the cercariae, develops with papules and vesicles and is usually self-limiting unless a secondary infection takes place [6, 8].

Katayama Fever or Syndrome

The Katayama fever currently known as Katayama syndrome is a symptom complex resulting from the hypersensitivity reaction to the migrating eggs and schistosomula. The symptoms start 2 to 12 weeks post-infection during the maturation of the schistosomula into the adult form which then mates and lays eggs. The severity of the symptoms is related to the infecting species. The symptoms start suddenly and include fatigue, fever, malaise, myalgia, urticaria, eosinophilia, and non-productive cough. Other pulmonary, abdominal, and neurological symptoms can also take place [6, 9].

Chronic Schistosomiasis

Nearly half of the produced eggs get trapped in the different host tissues leading to inflammation and fibrosis. The accumulated eggs induce an eosinophilic granulomatous reaction. The focal areas of fibrosis in the affected organs can develop into organ failure leading to clinical morbidity. While intestinal schistosomiasis is caused by infection with *S. mansoni, S. japonicum, S. intercalatum, S. mekongi,* and occasionally, *S. haematobium,* urinary schistosomiasis is most frequently implicated by *S. haematobium.* Neuroschistosomiasis on the other hand, affects any region of the central nervous system. While the smaller *S. japonicum* eggs are capable of reaching the brain, the larger eggs of other species (such as *S. mansoni* and *S. haematobium*) are usually found in the lower spinal cord. Additionally, infection by *S. mansoni* and *S. japonicum* are connected to the development of pulmonary hypertension [6, 10].

CURRENT ANTISCHISTOSOMAL DRUGS

Praziquantel

Praziquantel (PZQ) **1** (Fig. **2**), the generic name of 2-[cyclohexylcarbonyl--3,6,7,11*b*-tetrahydro-1*H*-pyrazino [2,1-*a*]isoquinolin-4-one, was initially created as a tranquilizer. In the mid-1970s, the drug gained importance after the discovery of its anthelminthic properties against cestodes and all schistosome species. It then became the cornerstone of all schistosome treatments [11 - 13]. For more than 50 years, PZQ has been available in the market in the form of 600 mg tablets. The prescribed dose is 40 mg/kg for *S. haematobium* and *S. mansoni* infections, and 60 mg/kg for *S. japonicum* and *S. mekongi* infections [14]. PZQ is considered the best antischistosomal monotherapy owing to its safety, accessibility, and efficacy against all schistosome species affecting humans [11]. Among the mild adverse effects attributed to the drug are diarrhea and vomiting. The anthelminthic mechanism of PZQ encompasses three major actions: (1) rapid influx of calcium ions, (2) adult worm teguments vacuolation and blebbing, and (3) muscle contractions [12, 13]. The increase in intracellular calcium ions, followed by sodium and potassium ions slows down influx resulting in muscle contraction of the worm and alterations of the tegument. Although the exact target responsible for calcium homeostasis disruption is not well defined, these alterations expose the worm surface antigens to the host immune system defences [15 - 17]. Various studies hypothesized that voltage-operated calcium channels are the major targets accountable for the accumulation of calcium ions [15, 18].

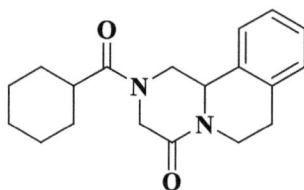

Praziquantel 1

Fig. (2). Chemical structure of the Praziquantel.

Oxamniquine

Oxamniquine **2** (Fig. **3**) is a tetrahydroquinoline derivative primarily used when the parasitic disease is caused by *S. mansoni* species [11, 19]. The compound was produced during the 1940s and was not widely marketable owing to toxicity. Oxamniquine's ineffectiveness against the worms of *S. japonicum* and *S. haematobium* is related to its mechanism of action, as the drug should be activated by sulfotransferase, which is an esterifying enzyme only expressed in *S. mansoni* worm [11, 20]. In the active sulfate ester form, it dissociates into electrophilic reactants that can alkylate, irreversibly damage schistosomal DNA, inhibit protein synthesis, and lead to death. Despite its effectiveness, the drug is associated with a set of side effects including seizures, orange-red urine, and sleep induction. The drug also may be prone to acquired resistance due to genetic alterations of the esterifying enzyme [11, 21].

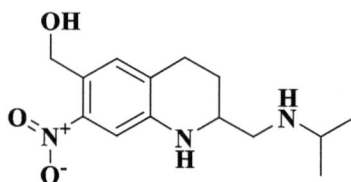

Oxamniquine 2

Fig. (3). Chemical structure of the Oxamniquine.

DRUG REPURPOSING AND TREATMENT OF SCHISTOSOMIASIS

While the development of a vaccine against schistosomiasis is difficult, expensive, and of long duration, and currently the treatment of the neglected disease depends mainly on a single drug namely praziquantel, which is ineffective against the juvenile form, there is a necessity to develop new antischistosomal drugs. Drug repositioning or drug repurposing is a promising strategy to obtain new antischistosomal drugs. This approach involves finding new indications/ targets for compounds that are either validated for use or are still in the development stage for other human diseases. Lower costs, reduced risk, and decreased time to market because of the availability of preclinical data facilitates and helps fasten the process of drug approval, therefore this strategy is quite appealing [22].

Antimalarial Agents

Mefloquine **3** (Fig. **4**) is a marketed drug for the prevention and treatment of malaria infection. In 2009, Keiser *et al.* [23] reported the encouraging antischistosomal effect following oral administration as a single dose of 400 mg/kg to mice infected with either juvenile or adult stages of *S. mansoni* and *S. japonicum*. Results showed that worm burden reductions approached or exceeded the benchmark criteria defined by the World Health Organization (WHO) for possible antischistosomal lead compounds by approaching or exceeding 80% worm burden reduction.

In 2014, another research group continued the work and recovered the worms from the liver of infected mice, for two to seven days, following treatment to examine modifications on the tegumental surface of juvenile and adult schistosome worms by electron microscopy. The electron microscopy examination displayed variable levels of tegumental changes in the form of retracted ventral sucker and oral sucker, a fusion of tegumental ridges, pitting of the tegument and corrugations with swelling of the tegument in parts, and shrinkage in the other parts with the formation of deep furrows, disruption and peeling of the tegument with loss of spines and blebbing. These results confirm the promising effect of mefloquine in the treatment of schistosomiasis [24].

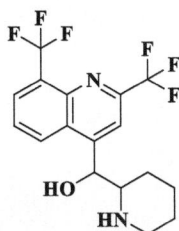

Mefloquine 3

Fig. (4). Chemical Structure of the Mefloquine.

In 2017, Krieg *et al.* [25] synthesised and characterised a series of aryl methylamino steroids and tested their antiparasitic activity against the asexual blood stages of the malaria parasite *P. falciparum* (strain 3D7) and *S. mansoni* adult worms. Compound **4** (Fig. **5**) exerted strong antiplasmodial activity against *P. falciparum* 3D7 (IC_{50} 6.6 nM). Surprisingly, the steroid compounds displayed remarkable physiological and morphological effects on adult *S. mansoni* worms *in vitro* which led to the death of the trematode parasite. At a concentration of 1 mM, compound **4** resulted in reduced motility and viability, while at a concentration of 10 mM, the compound induced the death of the parasites within a week. These effects were accompanied by tegumental invaginations and oedema-like swellings of the body. Moreover, the use of confocal laser scanning microscopy (CLSM) showed the presence of an enlarged gut lumen and degradation of the gastrodermis. Additionally, disorganization of oocytes within the ovary and reduced sizes of testicular lobes in males were noted. It must be mentioned that the steroid compounds display low cytotoxicity in mammalian cells and do not induce acute toxicity symptoms in mice.

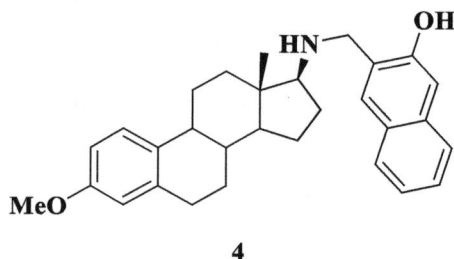

4

Fig. (5). Chemical structure of compound 4.

Antibiotics

The oral nitrofuran antibiotic nifuroxazide **5** (Fig. **6**) is used in several countries worldwide to treat diarrhoea and infectious colitis. As it has proved to be well tolerated and safe, several studies investigated its potential as an anticancer agent [26 - 29], and as an inhibitor in inflammatory diseases [30]. Additionally, it was reported to inhibit and reverse pulmonary fibrosis [31]. Moreover, its reprofiling as antiprotozoal has been reported [32].

In 2023, Roquini *et al.* [33] disclosed the antischistosomal properties of nifuroxazide against the flatworm *S. mansoni in vitro* and in an animal model of schistosomiasis, for both prepatent and patent schistosome infections. The *in vitro* results obtained after 72hrs incubation showed that the nitrofuran antibiotic induced deleterious effects on *S. mansoni* adult worms in a concentration-dependant manner. Like praziquantel, male worms were more susceptible to nifuroxazide than female worms (EC_{50} 8.28 and 13.79 µM against male and female worms, respectively). Additionally, phenotypic studies revealed that nifuroxazide induced morphological alterations in the tegument of the adult worms. These were more notable in male worms than in female worms.

In vivo experiments in both prepatent (juvenile parasite form) and patent (adult parasite form) murine infection models using a single oral dose of 400 mg/kg were conducted and evaluated. Results indicate that the drug in the administered dose was capable of significantly reducing the worm burden by around 40% in both infection forms compared to the control model. Additionally, the applied dose of nifuroxazide resulted in comparable reductions of egg burden in patent infection as praziquantel (~80%). The data suggests that the drug interferes directly with egg production. Target fishing studies were carried out to analyse the mechanism of action of nifuroxazide. Serine/threonine kinases and matrix metallopeptidase-7 are among the predicted protein targets.

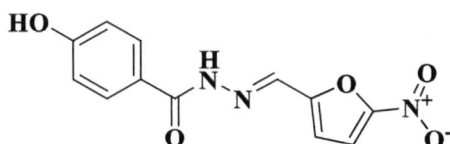

Nifuroxazide 5

Fig. (6). Chemical structure of the Nifuroxazide.

Anti-inflammatory Agents

In 2014, Carvalho *et al.* [34] investigated the *in vitro* effect of diclofenac **6** (Fig. 7) against both juvenile and adult *S. mansoni* worms, using praziquantel as a reference. The obtained results indicated the ability of diclofenac to kill both juvenile and adult stages of the parasite at concentrations of ≥3.25 and ≥6.5 µg/ml, respectively. It is worth mentioning that as to the effect on the juvenile stage, diclofenac was more potent than praziquantel. However, the mechanism by which the schistosomicidal effect of diclofenac takes place is still unknown.

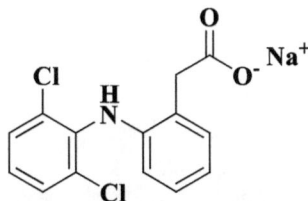

Diclofenac sodium 6

Fig. (7). Chemical structure of Diclofenac sodium.

In another study conducted by Lago *et al.* [35] the antischistosomal effects of 73 nonsteroidal anti-inflammatory drugs (NSAIDs) commonly used in medical and veterinary fields were assessed. Among these, five compounds effectively killed adult stages of the worm at 50 µM. The most effective NSAID was mefenamic acid (Fig. **8**) with a 50% lethal concentration (LC_{50}) value of 11.01 µM. Additionally, it influenced parasite motility and viability, and it induced severe tegumental damage in schistosomes. Based on the *in vitro* results, the five compounds with promising antischistosomal effects were tested *in vivo* using a patent and a prepatent *S. mansoni* infection in a mouse model.

Two treatment regimens were applied. In the first treatment plan, the mice harbouring adult *S. mansoni* (patent infection) were orally administered 400 mg/kg body weight as a single dose 42 days post-infection. Mefenamic acid **7** displayed the highest schistosomicidal properties, with a worm burden reduction of 75.5%. Because mefenamic acid is rapidly absorbed after oral administration and possesses a short half-life of 2hrs, the second treatment regimen was applied. This plan included administering the drug once a day for five consecutive days in a dose of 100 mg/kg/day, 21 days (prepatent infection) or 42 days (patent infection) postinfection with *S. mansoni*. Under this treatment, the drug achieved a high total worm burden reduction of 82.1% and 67.2% in mice harbouring adult and juvenile schistosomes, respectively. Additionally, mefenamic acid decreased the immature eggs in patent and prepatent infection by 92% and 78% respectively. Furthermore, the anthelminthic activity of mefenamic acid in both *in vitro* and *in vivo* experiments exceeds the criteria specified by the World Health Organization (WHO) for schistosomiasis potential compounds. Moreover, mefenamic acid highly reduced hepato-, and splenomegaly evident in *S. mansoni*-infected animals.

It is worth highlighting that the doses used were within the range in which the drug has been used in clinical practice, therefore it is eligible for clinical repurposing in the treatment of schistosomiasis.

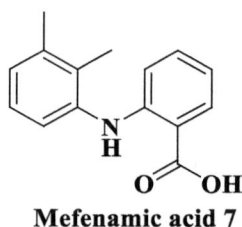

Mefenamic acid 7

Fig. (8). Chemical structure of the Mefenamic acid.

Among the NSAIDs tested by Lago and his group was celecoxib **8** (Fig. **9**). However, using the single dose regimen of 400 mg/kg body weight as a single dose 42 days post-infection achieved only a 45.3% reduction in worm burden. Additionally, *in vitro* results displayed moderate schistosomicidal activity against adult worms ($LC_{50} > 25$ µM).

In 2021, Abou-El-Naga *et al.* [36] decided to further investigate the *in vivo* activity of celecoxib against the different developmental stages of *S. mansoni* infection using another dosing regimen aiming to improve its antischistosomal activity. In the applied treatment regimen, the drug was administered in multiple oral doses of 20 mg/kg/day for five days against the invasive, juvenile, and adult stages. On the contrary to praziquantel, results confirmed the highly potent schistosomicidal activity of celecoxib against both juvenile and the invasive stages of the parasite.

As of now, the exact mechanism by which celecoxib exerts its schistosomicidal effects is not known, the group suggested several possible pathways from which a few will be discussed.

Although the parasite does not possess COX-2 enzymes, it is able to synthesise prostaglandins. PG-E$_2$ synthesised by both the host and the cercariae aids in the skin penetration of the invading larvae and its transformation. As a COX-2 inhibitor, celecoxib decreases the cercarial penetration by reducing the host-derived PG-E$_2$ thereby decreasing the number of adult worms.

Celecoxib is highly lipophilic, consequently, it can dissolve in the lipid bilayer of the tegument leading to the modification of the membrane lipid physical properties, high membrane fluidity, and alteration of the membrane permeability. Disarrangement of the tegument can affect the worm's nutrition, development, and maturation. Electron microscopic studies performed confirmed that the tegument might be a candidate target of the drug.

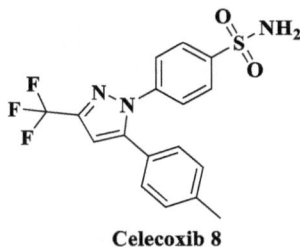

Celecoxib 8

Fig. (9). Chemical structure of the Celecoxib.

Anticancer Drugs

114 FDA-approved anticancer agents were screened for their possible antischistosomal activities. 11 Drugs, almost kinase inhibitors, were identified with high *in vitro* antiparasitic activity against both larval and adult stages of *S. mansoni* [37]. Trametinib **9** and vandetanib **10** (Fig. **10**) exhibited promising activities against larval (IC$_{50}$ 4.6 and 0.9 μM) and adult (IC$_{50}$ 4.1 and 9.5 μM) *S. mansoni*, respectively. Additionally, both were moderately active in chronic *S. mansoni*-infected mice when administered as a single dose (63.6% and 48.1% reduction of worm burden, respectively).

Other studies were conducted to explore the activity of 5-azacytidine **11** (Fig. **10**) with in-depth analysis at the molecular level. 5-Azacytidine is an FDA-approved ribonucleoside analogue utilized for the treatment of myelodysplastic syndrome [38]. Results revealed that 5-azacytidine inhibited schistosome egg production, modulated schistosome transcription and translation, and affected schistosome stem cell proliferation and maintenance [39].

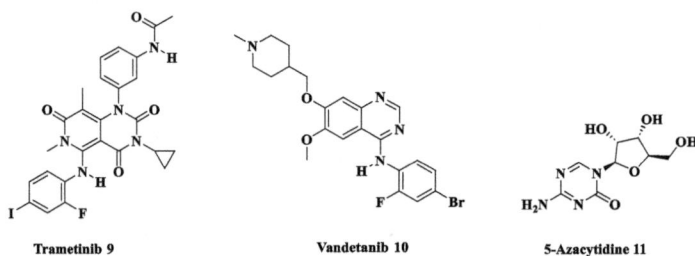

Fig. (10). Chemical structure od Trametinib, Vandetanib, and 5-Azacytidine.

Alkylphospholipid analogues *e.g.*, miltefosine **12** and edelfosine **13** (Fig. **11**) were repurposed for schistosomiasis treatment. Miltefosine, initially developed as an anticancer agent [40], was the first oral drug licensed for leishmaniasis treatment [41]. Edelfosine has been also identified as an antitumor [42] and antileishmanial agent [43]. In the second decade of the 21st century, it was reported that oral miltefosine administration as a daily dose of 20 mg/kg for 5 successive days to mice infected with invasive, juvenile, or adult stages of *S. mansoni* significantly reduced the worm burden and the hepatic granulomata size [44]. Edelfosine also resulted in a reduction of female (29.1%) and male (46.84%) worm burdens in the murine model of *S. mansoni* and decreased the total number of eggs recovered in livers (54.2% reduction) [45].

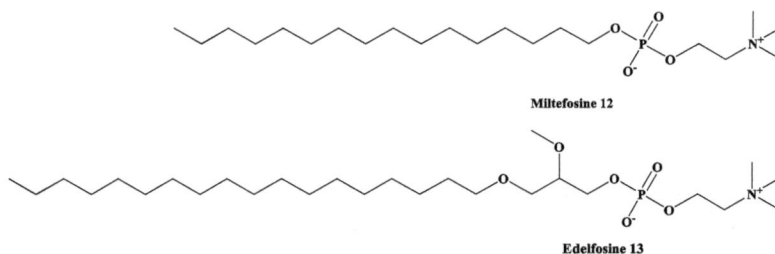

Fig. (11). Chemical structure of Miltefosine and Edelfosine.

Chlorambucil **14** (Fig. **12**) is mainly used to treat chronic lymphocytic leukaemia, as well as Hodgkin and non-Hodgkin lymphomas. Recently, it has been shown to be active *in vivo* against *S. mansoni* in mouse models of various stages, especially the juvenile stage of infection in oral doses of 2.5 mg/kg/day for 5 successive days. It induced 76% total worm burden reduction, and up to 89% intestinal and hepatic egg count reduction, along with oogram alterations. Besides, it promoted amelioration of the hepatic histopathology and induced significant shortening of male and female worms [46].

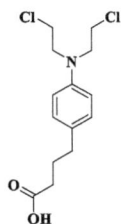

Chlorambucil 14

Fig. (12). Chemical structure of Chlorambucil.

Less selective anticancer chemotherapy such as hydroxyurea **15** and cisplatin **16** (Fig. **13**) were also shown to be effective, as they affected schistosoma viability *in vitro* and *in vivo*. Results showed that these drugs exhibited praziquantel-like effects on *S. mansoni* worms and host mouse liver. However, the actual application of these drugs for antischistosomal therapy is questionable due to toxicity issues [47].

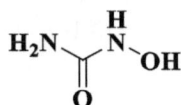

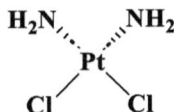

Hydroxurea 15   **Cisplatin 16**

Fig. (13). Chemical structure of Hydroxurea and Cisplatin.

Statins

HMG-CoA reductase, the rate-limiting enzyme of the cholesterol synthesis pathway in humans, was found to be crucial for schistosome survival. In the 1980s, studies conducted by Vandewaa *et al.* [48] showed that egg production by schistosomes is associated with HMG-CoA reductase activity. Cholesterol precursors such as mevalonate and farnesol were also found to stimulate egg production. The inhibitors of cholesterol synthesis lovastatin **17** and atorvastatin **18** (Fig. **14**) reduced egg laying by schistosome females. Chen *et al.* [49] showed that mevalonate not only plays a vital role in egg production, but also in the parasite survival. Regarding the effect on parasite load, moderate activities were observed with atorvastatin (46% worm burden reduction in *S. haematobium-*

infected hamsters) [50] and lovastatin (30% worm burden reduction in *S. mansoni*-infected mice) [51]. It is worth mentioning that Schistosoma death either by specific RNAi of HMG-CoA or statins is related to caspase activation. Schistosomes HMG-CoA reductase is thus considered a validated target for combating the parasite on chemical and genetic bases [52].

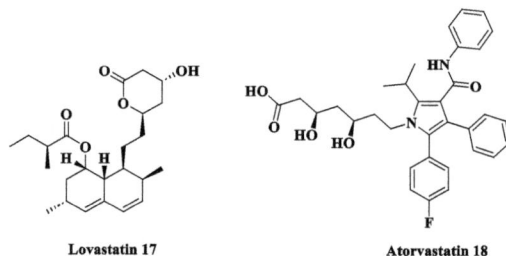

Fig. (14). Chemical structure of Lovastatin and Atorvastatin.

Organometallics

In 2017, Hess *et al.* [53] synthesised benzyl, ferrocenyl, and ruthenocenyl oxamniquine derivatives **19-21** (Fig. **15**) aiming specifically at modulating the drug's properties and selectivity. In this study, ferrocenyl compounds were subjected to *in vitro* screening on adult and juvenile worms followed by *in vivo* evaluation on *S. mansoni*-infected mice. The promising compounds accomplished more than 75% worm killing surpassing oxamniquine which showed 67% effectiveness. Mild toxicity was observed for all compounds in L6 rats´ skeletal myoblast cells after 72hrs, showing IC_{50} values of 57.9-100.3 µM being close to that of the reference ($IC_{50} > 90µM$).

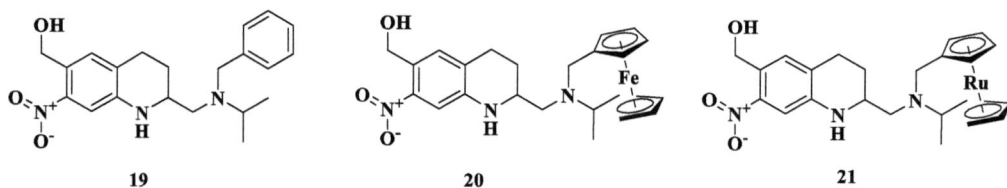

Fig. (15). Chemical structure of the compounds **19**, **20** and **21**.

In 2014, Keiser *et al.* [54] evaluated various chloroquine derivatives including ferroquine (FQ) **22**, ruthenoquine (RQ) **23,** and hydroxyl ferroquine (FQ-OH) **24** (Fig. **16**) against the newly transformed schistosomula (NTS) and *S. mansoni* adult worms. Inhibition of hemozoin formation and generation of OH radicals in oxidizing conditions were studied as the principal mechanisms of action. FQ was shown to be able to permeate membranes and accumulate in the parasite's digestive vacuole [55], preventing biomineralization of hemozoin leading to death. The OH radicals' generation enabled the breakdown of the digestive vacuole membrane by FQ, but not by RQ or chloroquine. Such radicals may also oxidize glutathione, which is crucial for heme detoxification. FQ-OH also produced radicals with lower cytotoxicity compared to FQ. Unfortunately, none of the tested compounds displayed *in vivo* activity in *S. mansoni*-infected mice as indicated by the observed low total worm reductions (0-36%), following the administration of oral doses up to 800 mg/kg. All the studied metallocenes showed moderate cytotoxicity against MRC-5 cells [54].

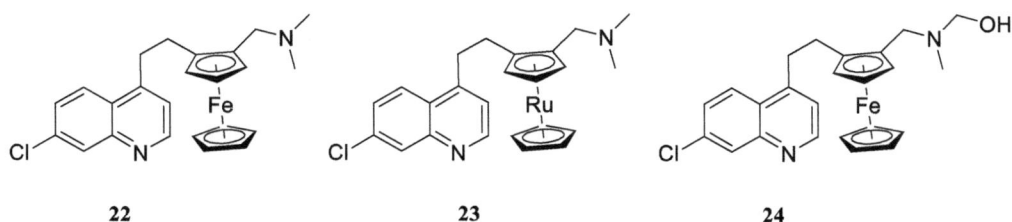

Fig. (16). Chemical structure of compounds **22**, **23** and **24**.

In 2016, Khan and his research team [56] expanded the investigation of their synthetic library of side- and cross-bridged tetraazamacrocyclic ligands beyond anti-HIV and antimalarial drug discovery programs to include antischistosomal research. The tetraazamacrocyclic derivatives as represented by compounds **25-27** (Fig. **17**), and their metal complexes **25a,b-27a, b** (Fig. **17**) were screened for their potential *in vitro* and *in vivo* anthelminthic activity against *S. mansoni*. Incubation of the studied compounds at 33 µM caused 62-100% mortality of NTS. **27, 27a,** and **27b,** exhibiting 100% inhibition of viability of NTS at 10 µM, were further evaluated for IC_{50} values against both NTS and adult worms. All compounds screened against NTS showed IC_{50} values comparable to the standard PZQ IC_{50}.

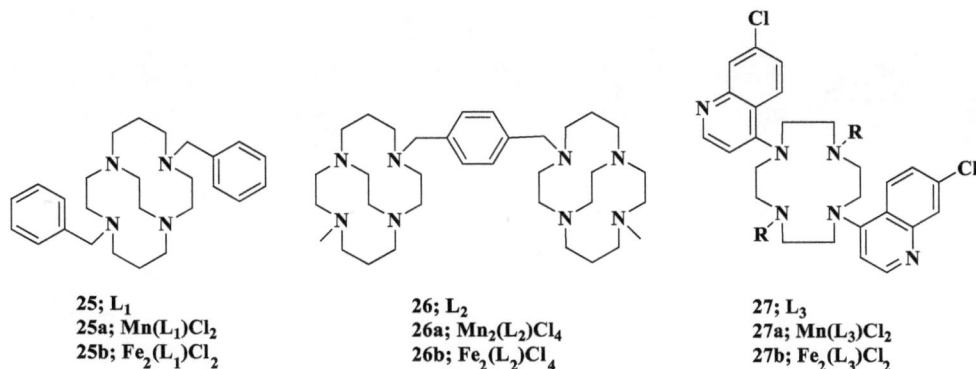

25; L₁
25a; Mn(L₁)Cl₂
25b; Fe₂(L₁)Cl₂

26; L₂
26a; Mn₂(L₂)Cl₄
26b; Fe₂(L₂)Cl₄

27; L₃
27a; Mn(L₃)Cl₂
27b; Fe₂(L₃)Cl₂

Fig. (17). Chemical structure of tetraazamacrocyclic derivatives.

Hess and his group studied modification of PZQ based on the inclusion of a ferrocene moiety as represented by **28** and **29** (Fig. **18**). In their study [57], modification of the cyclohexyl and aromatic rings was rationalized. Compounds without the cyclohexyl ring avoided hydroxylation to the corresponding metabolite with less activity, while modifications of the aromatic ring did not alter the schistosomicidal activities.

Subsequent studies led to the synthesis of diastereomeric chromium-tricarbony--PZQ derivatives **30, 31** (Fig. **18**). These chromium-based derivatives were selected for the ability of chromium moieties to increase lipophilicity and metabolic stability. The Cr-PZQ racemates were screened on *S. mansoni* worms and showed IC_{50} values of 0.25 and 0.27 µM, which are highly comparable to that of PZQ alone. These compounds also showed no toxicity towards MRC-5 human fibroblast cells, thus exhibiting some selective antiparasitic effect [55].

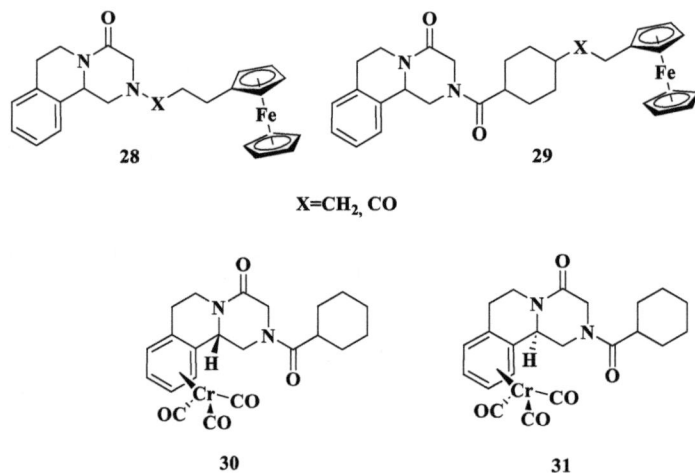

Fig. (18). Chemical structure of compounds **28, 29, 30**, and **31**.

In a study by Portes and colleagues [58], Epiisopiloturine (EPI) **32** (Fig. **19**), an imidazole alkaloid, was complexed with copper and zinc salts to improve its antiparasitic properties. Results showed that coordination with copper (II) in $[Cu(EPI)_4](ClO_4)_2$ enhanced the antiparasitic activity of EPI, whereas the zinc (II) complex $Zn(EPI)_2Cl_2$ was less active than the free drug. None of the evaluated complexes was toxic to mammalian cells. Approximately 60% of tegumental disruptions were observed after 24 hours of incubation with 250 µM of $[Cu(EPI)_4](ClO_4)_2$. Oviposition was observed in experiments utilizing both complexes in the 60-250 µM range, with a major egg-laying reduction of below 25% at a 62.5 µM concentration of the Cu-EPI complex. The bioactivity of the studied copper complex was proposed to be due to the redox activity of copper.

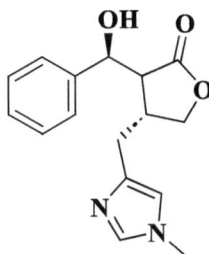

Epiisopiloturine 32

Fig. (19). Chemical structure of Epiisopiloturine (EPI).

POTENTIAL MOLECULAR TARGETS IN SCHISTOSOMIASIS

Epigenetic Regulators

The complex development and differentiation of the schistosome parasite suggest that the gene transcription at the different life cycle stages is strictly controlled through different epigenetic mechanisms including DNA methylation, and post-translational reversible modifications of histones among others.

Histone Modifying Enzymes

HDAC Inhibitors

Histone deacetylases (HDACs) are enzymes responsible for the catalysis of the removal of the acetyl mark from the lysine residues of different substrates including histones and non-histone regulatory proteins *e.g.* transcription factors (p53), nuclear import factors, and cytoskeletal proteins (α-tubulin) affecting a wide array of physiological processes. These enzymes are divided into two major categories; the classical Zn^{2+}-dependent HDACs and sirtuins [59].

The schistosomal genome encodes HDAC isoforms that are orthologous to their human counterparts. The characterised parasitic HDACs belong to classes I (smHDAC1, 3, and 8), II (smHDAC4, 5, and 6), and III (smSirt1, 2, 5, 6, and 7) [60, 61].

In all life- cycle stages of *S. mansoni*, the expression of class I HDACs has been recorded [62]. While the expression of the hHDAC8 transcript in normal human tissues is much less compared to those of hHDAC1 and hHDAC3 [63], the parasitic orthologue smHDAC8 is highly expressed compared to smHDAC1 and smHDAC3 at all stages of the Schistosoma life-cycle except schistosomula suggesting the vital functional role of the isoform in the different developmental stages of the parasite [62]. As a result, smHDAC8 represents an interesting target for developing new antischistosomal drug candidates. It must be noted that the design of a selective inhibitor against smHDAC8 is challenging because of the strong similarity between smHDAC8 and its human counterpart [62, 64].

Compound **33** (Fig. **20**) is one of the 3-amidobenzohydroxamates that were synthesised by Heimburg *et al.* [65], which displayed significant *in vitro* dose-dependent killing of the schistosomula, as well as a pronounced reduction in egg laying in addition to the separation of the adult worm pairs. While selectivity towards the human orthologue requires improvement, these chemical compounds were highly selective over hHDAC1 and hHDAC6.

Further investigation of the structure-activity relationship of benzhydroxamates as inhibitors of smHDAC8 and the chemical optimization of the **33** resulted in the development of novel benzhydroxamate inhibitors. When tested *in vitro* against the different enzymes, the developed compounds showed inhibition of both sm- and hHDAC8 in the nanomolar range. Most of them displayed lower inhibitory activity towards HDAC1 and HDAC6. Moreover, generated inhibitors displayed a good safety profile against human HEK293 cells.

The Alamar Blue-based viability assay utilising parasites cultured *in vitro* was applied to synthesised compounds to test for their toxicity towards the larval schistosome, along with the lead compound **33**, the reported HDAC8 selective inhibitor PCI-34051 and praziquantel.

Results show that the synthesised inhibitor **34** (Fig. **20**) exhibited the most noticeable dose-dependent decrease in the larvae viability, killing almost 98% of the parasite larvae. The compound **34** could not be further tested *in vivo* because of its lipophilicity and poor solubility. To overcome the latter, the more soluble analogous compound **35** (Fig. **20**) was synthesised as a hydrochloride salt. The analogue was able to display almost the same activity as **34** towards smHDAC8, however, it did not succeed in exhibiting toxicity towards the larval form of the schistosoma [66].

It is worth mentioning that studies connected hydroxamic acid-based inhibitors with different pharmacokinetic and pharmacodynamic problems, in addition to various off-target side effects limiting their use [67 - 69], therefore attempts to develop non-hydroxamic acid inhibitors that display the same inhibitory activity as hydroxamates are of great interest.

In 2018, Guidi *et al.* [70] screened a library containing class I HDAC inhibitors against the larval stage of Schistosoma and obtained several hit compounds with the ability to reduce the ability of survival of *S. mansoni* larval and adult forms. From the obtained compounds, SmI-148 **36** and SmI-558 **37** (Fig. **20**) affected the reproductive system of the mature female worms and decreased the number of eggs laid *in vitro*.

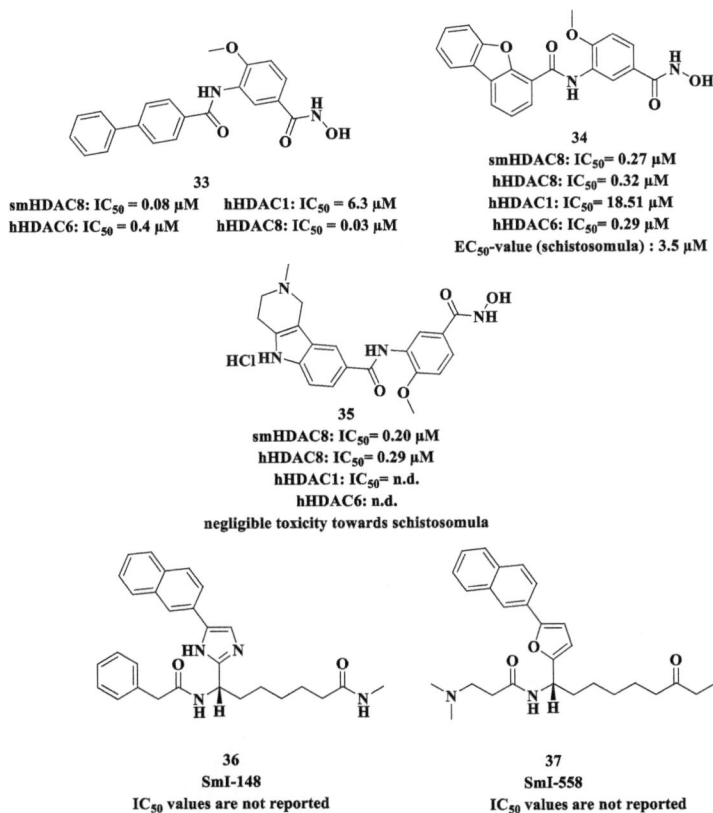

33
smHDAC8: IC$_{50}$ = 0.08 µM   hHDAC1: IC$_{50}$ = 6.3 µM
hHDAC6: IC$_{50}$ = 0.4 µM   hHDAC8: IC$_{50}$ = 0.03 µM

34
smHDAC8: IC$_{50}$= 0.27 µM
hHDAC8: IC$_{50}$= 0.32 µM
hHDAC1: IC$_{50}$= 18.51 µM
hHDAC6: IC$_{50}$= 0.29 µM
EC$_{50}$-value (schistosomula) : 3.5 µM

35
smHDAC8: IC$_{50}$= 0.20 µM
hHDAC8: IC$_{50}$= 0.29 µM
hHDAC1: IC$_{50}$= n.d.
hHDAC6: n.d.
negligible toxicity towards schistosomula

36
SmI-148
IC$_{50}$ values are not reported

37
SmI-558
IC$_{50}$ values are not reported

Fig. (20). Chemical structure of the compounds **33-37**.

Sirtuin Inhibitors

In 2013, a research group was able to characterise all sirtuins encoded in the schistosome genome *Sm*Sirt1-5. They reported that inhibiting these NAD$^+$ dependent lysine deacetylases, which are produced throughout the lifetime of the parasite, leads to the death of the schistosomula, the adult worm pairs separation, in addition to damage to the worm reproductive organs. Consequently, targeting schistosome sirtuins in drug discovery is valid [61].

Mondali *et al.* [71] conducted an *in vitro* screening of the GSK Kinetobox library and studied the structure-activity relationships of the identified hits. The hit compound TCMDC-143295 **38** (Fig. **21**) presented good selectivity for *Sm*SIRT2 over *h*SIRT2, therefore it was useful to develop some analogues **39**, **40**, and **41** (Fig. **21**). These compounds exhibited improved potency and selectivity for *Sm*Sirt2 over the human isotype, resulting in reduced viability in schistosomula, in addition to reduced adult worms' pairing and egg laying with no general toxicity to human cells.

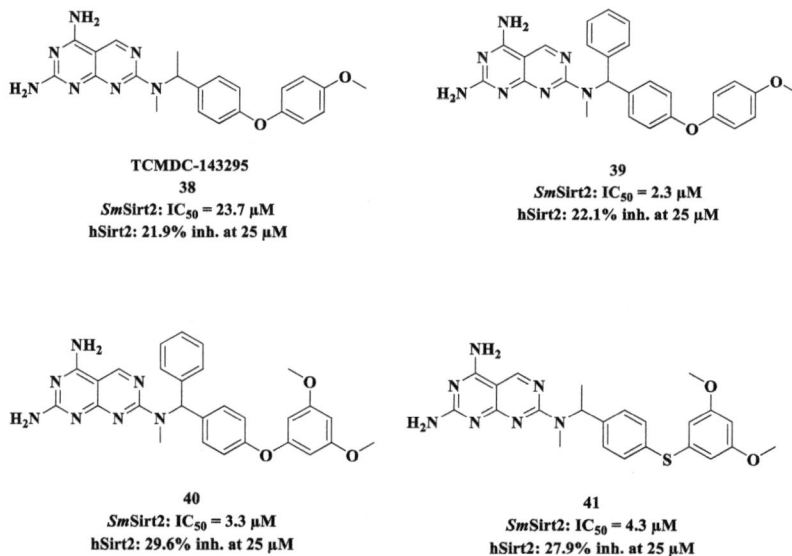

TCMDC-143295
38
*Sm*Sirt2: IC_{50} = 23.7 μM
hSirt2: 21.9% inh. at 25 μM

39
*Sm*Sirt2: IC_{50} = 2.3 μM
hSirt2: 22.1% inh. at 25 μM

40
*Sm*Sirt2: IC_{50} = 3.3 μM
hSirt2: 29.6% inh. at 25 μM

41
*Sm*Sirt2: IC_{50} = 4.3 μM
hSirt2: 27.9% inh. at 25 μM

Fig. (21). Chemical structure of compounds **38-41**.

Histone Methylation

According to Goll *et al.* [72] Dnmt2, which possesses only weak DNA methyltransferase activity while it exercises strong methyltransferase activity toward tRNA[Asp] and other tRNAs, is the only DNA methyltransferase encoded in the schistosome genome.

In 2018, Roquis *et al.* [73] revealed that the H3K27 histone methyltransferase inhibitor GSK343 **42** (Fig. **22**), a selective inhibitor of EZH2 histone H3K27 methyltransferase in human cells, was able to efficiently block the transition of the parasite from the stage of miracidium to sporocyst suggesting that H3K27 trimethylation is essential for life cycle progression. Afterward, the research group of Pereira [74] conducted a study to test the effects of GKS343, on varied developmental stages of *S. mansoni in vitro*.

Based on the results of a previous study [75], which determined that the median lethal dose LD_{50} for the inhibitor GSK343 in schistosomula was 24.5 μM, the doses of the drug that were administered by Pereira *et al.* were 20 μM and 50 μM. The effects on adult female and male worms and schistosomula were observed at different time intervals (3, 6, 12, 24, and 48 hours).

Upon exposure to GSK343 the *S. mansoni* adult worms exhibited reduced motility depending on the concentration and incubation time. Results indicate that a 40% reduction in motility was observed 48 hours after exposure to the sublethal dose of 20 μM. At a dose of 50 μM, the motility was affected after 12hrs and decreased to 50% after 24hrs. At the latter time interval, some dead worms could be detected. However, after 48 hours of incubation, all worms were considered dead.

Pairing of the worm couples decreased to around 50% upon exposure to 20 μM of the drug for 48 hours. On the other hand, the dose of 50 μM was capable of reducing the worm pairing to almost zero after only 3 hours of exposure.

Additionally, GSK343 at 20 μM resulted in tegumental damage that could be detected using scanning electron microscopy. Moreover, a reduction of the egg-laying of the drug-treated female worms compared to the control was noted.

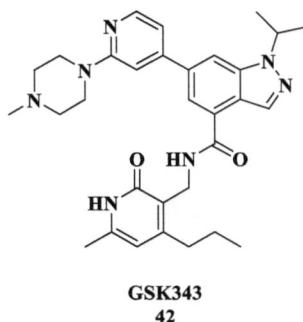

GSK343
42

Fig. (22). Chemical structure of compound GSK343 **42**.

Protein kinases Inhibitors

An extensive RNA interference analysis was conducted along with an experimental phenotypic study to recognize the functions of the different *S. mansoni* genes. About 10% (250 genes) were found to be necessary for the parasite's existence. Upon ranking drugs that display potent inhibitory activity against these gene targets, genes encoding protein kinases (PKs) namely, serine-threonine PK (STK25), and TAO were identified as promising epigenetic targets [76]. The name of the latter is based on its composition of a thousand and one amino acids.

In *S. mansoni*, tyrosine kinases (TKs) recognized as Abelson murine leukemia (Abl) SmAbl1 and SmAbl2 have been identified. Imatinib **43** (Fig. **23**) a potent inhibitor of human Abl-kinase, was suggested as a novel antischistosomal drug. However, the outcomes were disappointing since the imatinib binding affinity was negatively influenced by the host albumin and α-1 acid glycoprotein [77].

Computer-aided drug design approach alongside an experimental *ex vivo* phenotypic screening was conducted to validate several TKs as potential antischistosomal drug targets. Several anticancer agents besides Imatinib such as Nilotinib **44,** Bosutinib **45**, Vandetanib **46**, and Crizotinib **47** (Fig. **23**) showed promising activities. Kinomics analyses of the three Schistosoma species showed that calcium/calmodulin-regulated kinase (CAMK) could be also a potential PK target. Some PKs in *S. japonicum* and *S. mansoni* were recorded as validated drug targets for 16 FDA-approved drugs [78].

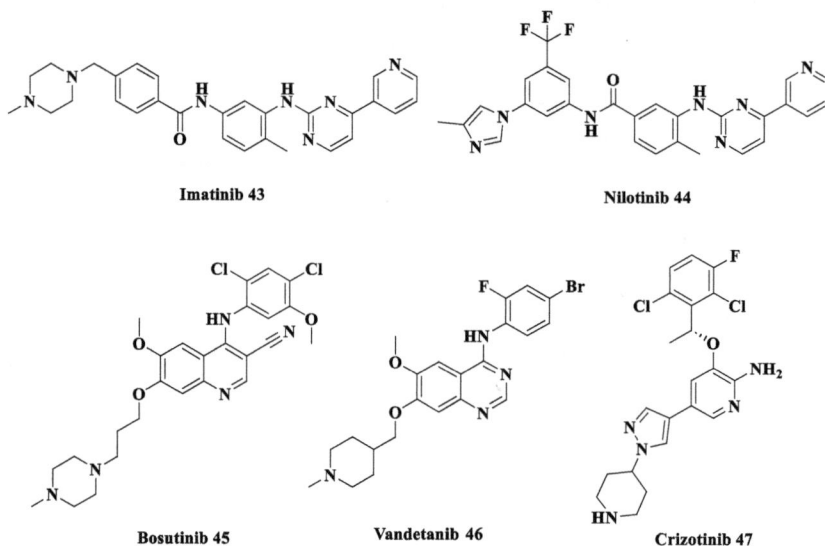

Imatinib 43

Nilotinib 44

Bosutinib 45

Vandetanib 46

Crizotinib 47

Fig. (23). Chemical structure of compounds **43-47**.

During cercarial shedding, high expression of Smp38 mitogen-activated PK (MAPK) was detected, pointing out its important role in host skin penetration. Therefore, Smp38 MAPK was considered a potential therapeutic target for the treatment and control of schistosomiasis [79].

Cyclic adenosine, guanine, and cytosine MP-dependent PK (PKA, PKG, and PKC, respectively) are classified among the cyclin-dependent kinases (AGC group) that were recognized but could not be associated with specific functions. Further studies are still in progress for exploring AGC signalling functions.

In addition to RNA biogenesis, atypical PK Riok-2 is involved in various cellular processes. Its location is in the vitellarium and ovary. Bioinformatics analysis revealed its high potential as a drug target. *S. mansoni* polo-like kinase 1 (SmPLK1) displayed high expression in adults and sporocysts. Selective human PLK1 inhibitors led to decreased production of oocysts and spermatocytes in female and male reproductive organs, respectively. SAR-guided studies introduced BI2536 **48** (Fig. **24**) as a highly efficient benzimidazole thiophene inhibitor against schistosomula and juveniles [80]. Other PKs inhibitors including Nilotinib **44**, Bosutinib **45**, Crizotinib **47**, Genistein **49**, Sorafenib **50,** and Dasatinib **51** (Fig. **24**) were recommended for investigation in the treatment of *S. japonicum* [81].

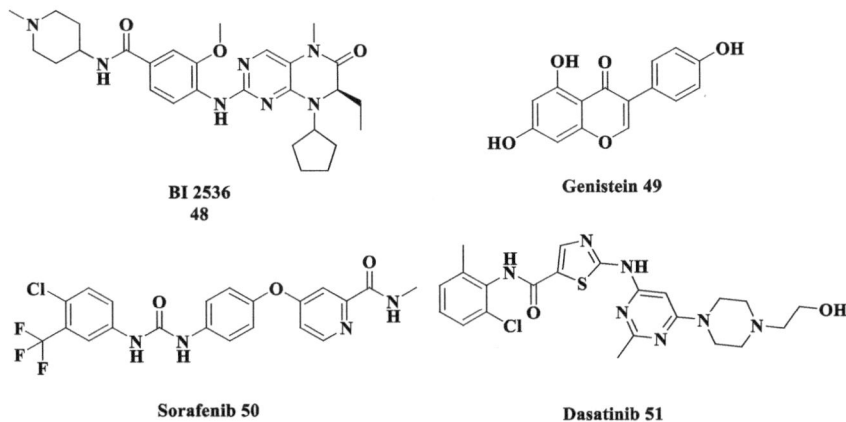

Fig. (24). Chemical structure of compounds **48-51**.

Protease Inhibitors

For schistosomes to survive, proteases are necessary. These are proteolytic enzymes that facilitate nutrient uptake, hatching, host invasion, and evasion of host immunity [82]. Several studies focused on cysteine (thiol) and aspartic (pepsin, cathepsin, rennin) proteases; however, high attention was paid to serine proteases (trypsin/chymotrypsin-like). The cercarial elastase (SmCE), which plays a great role in skin invasion by the infective larval stage of the parasite, was the most broadly studied serine protease [83]. The role of protease inhibitors is to prevent potentially harmful effects resulting from excess proteolytic activity by proteases.

Based on the class of protease targeted, inhibitors could be categorized into serine protease inhibitors (serpins, Kunitz-type, Kazal-type), cysteine protease inhibitors (cystatins), alpha-2-macroglobulin and metalloproteinase inhibitors. These inhibitors can interact with the substrate in several ways, therefore they are classified into four categories: (i) blockers of the protease active site (canonical inhibitors) [84]; (ii) compounds that occupy a secondary binding site adjacent to the active site (exosite inhibitors); (3) mixed canonical and exosite inhibitors; and (4) allosteric inhibitors that can bind to the enzyme in any place other than the active site [85]. Table **1** lists the most common inhibitors, their respective molecular targets, the location of target expression, and species.

CYP450 Inhibitors

Analyzing the gene sequence of *S. mansoni* disclosed a 22% sequence identity of the CYP450 gene with that identified in humans. CYP450s are heme-containing monooxygenases that normally interact with cellular oxygen and related substrates. They are crucial to producing cholesterol and ergosterol, as well as the metabolism of fatty acids and prostaglandins involved in cell signalling. Double-stranded RNA silencing study was performed in schistosomula to confirm the essentiality of CYP450 for parasite survival. Results showed that these experiments led to the complete death of the worms. Treatment of adults and developing eggs with miconazole **52**, (Fig. **25**) a CYP450 inhibitor led to *S. mansoni* death, and arrest of embryonic development, respectively [98].

Table 1. The most common protease inhibitors and their molecular targets, location of expression, and species.

Species	Protease	Location of Expression	Protease Inhibitor	Refs.
S. mansoni	Chymotrypsin, Neutrophil elastase	Head gland of schistosomules, spines of adults	*S. mansoni* serpin isoform 3 (SmSPI)	[86]
S. mansoni	Neutrophil elastase	Adult worms	*S. mansoni* protease inhibitor, 56 kDa (SmPi56)	[87 - 89]
S. mansoni	SmCE	Cercariae	SmSrpQ (Smp_062080)	[90]
S. mansoni	Trypsin, chymotrypsin, Neutrophil elastase	Adults, schistosomula, eggs	*S. mansoni* Kunitz-type protease inhibitor (SmKI-1)	[91, 92]
S. mansoni	Cysteine	Worm	Phenyl vinyl sulfone (K11777) and valproic acid	[93, 94]
S. japonicum	Trypsin, chymotrypsin, pancreatic elastase	Cercariae, schistosomula, eggs, adult male worms	SjB10	[95]
S. japonicum	Trypsin	Eggs	SjB6	[96]
S. japonicum	Trypsin, chymotrypsin, Neutrophil elastase	Eggs, adult worms	*S. japonicum* Kunitz type protease inhibitor (SjKI-1)	[92]
S. haematobium	Thrombin	Surface of adult worms	ShSPI	[96, 97]

In further studies, different fluconazole **53** (Fig. **25**) treatment regimens were evaluated in experimentally *S. mansoni*-infected mice. Results showed that early or late administration resulted in significant inhibition of *S. mansoni* CYP450 expression in the adult stage. Early exposure to fluconazole during the first week of infection decreased the number of schistosomula reaching the adult stage and resulted in the inhibition of *S. mansoni* CYP450 expression. In the early treatment group, the fewest number of eggs per liver tissue gram was recorded. Results highlighted that fluconazole is an *S. mansoni* CYP450 gene expression inhibitor with a greater effect on the schistosomula stage [99].

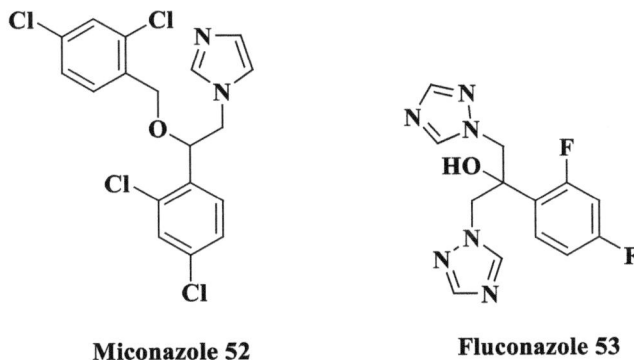

Miconazole 52   **Fluconazole 53**

Fig. (25). Chemical structure of the Miconazole and Fluconazole.

Transporters Inhibitors

ABC multidrug transporters are members of the efflux transporters of the ATP binding cassette (ABC) protein superfamily, which comprises one of the largest groups of transmembrane proteins [100, 101]. Multidrug resistance results from increased efflux of original drugs as well as other unrelated compounds *via* overexpression, amplification, or modification of a subset of these ABC transporters. P-glycoprotein (Pgp) is considered the prototypical eukaryotic ABC multidrug transporter [102]. Being important regulators of drug susceptibility, ABC transporters are viewed as excellent candidate targets for inhibitors that can act as adjuncts to current anthelmintics to enhance their potency. Several laboratories have explored overcoming drug resistance mainly by repurposing available drugs as ABC transporter inhibitors [102 - 107]. A 2003 patent reported that verapamil **54** and nifedipine **55** (Fig. **26**) reduced egg production in *S. mansoni* [108]. In addition to their activity, both drugs are relatively potent inhibitors of *S. mansoni* Pgp. A combination of molecular genetics and pharmacological approaches later confirmed the reported results on egg production reduction and showed that these effects were attributable to interference with schistosome ABC transporters [109, 110]. Other Pgp inhibitors including dexverapamil **56**, tariquidar **57**, cyclosporin A **58,** and C-4 **59** (Fig. **26**), a derivative of curcumin, were studied *in vitro* and in mice harbouring adult *S. mansoni*. Intraperitoneal doses of dexverapamil (60 mg/kg), tariquidar (15 mg/kg), cyclosporin A (60 mg/kg) and C-4 (50 mg/kg) decreased liver egg burden by approximately 65, 55, 50, and 80%, respectively, and reduced the granuloma size. *in vitro*, these Pgp inhibitors resulted in a concentration-dependent reduction in parasite egg production [111].

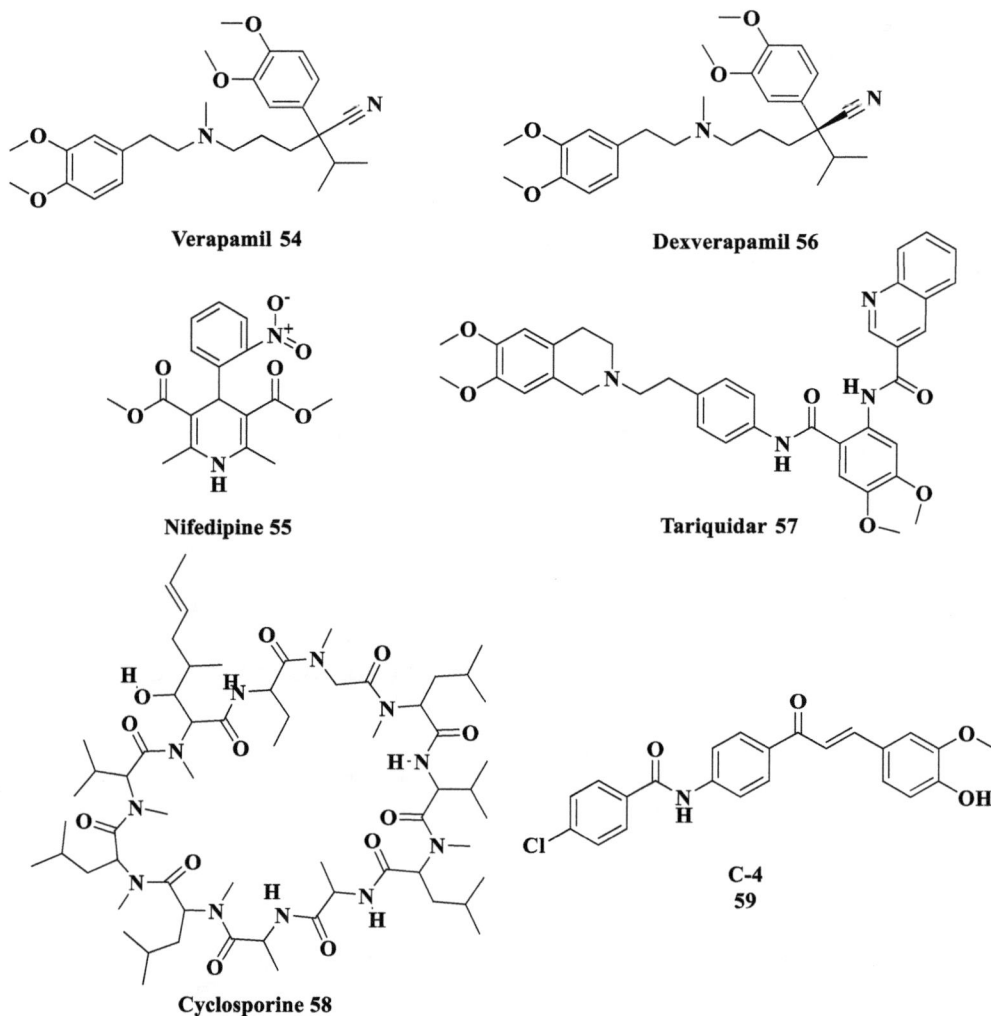

Fig. (26). Chemical structure of compounds 54-59.

Specific Targets

Based on how schistosomes obtain nutrients, several emerging targets are expected to be suitable to disrupt their nutrient intake besides altering their gut and intestinal normal morphology. The distribution, functions, and expected consequences of inhibition of these key targets are summarized in Table 2.

Table 2. Specific antischistosomal targets distribution, functions, and consequences of inhibition.

Target	Species	Location of Expression	Functions	Inhibition Consequences	Refs.
VAMP2	*S. japonicum*	Tegument	Maintains the normal morphology of the tegument and mediates membrane fusion.	Tegument shedding.	[112, 113]
TSP-2	*S.mansoni, S. japonicum* and *S. haematobium*	Tegument	Scaffold for the formation of protein complexes.	Thinner tegument and formation of vacuoles.	[114 - 117]
MEG-4.1	*S.mansoni* and *S. japonicum*	Oesophagus	Processing of host cells.	Disable to evade the host immune response.	[118, 119]
FoxA	*S.mansoni*	Oesophagus	Maintains expression of MEG-4.1 and differentiation of oesophageal gland cells.	Oesophageal gland ablation.	[120]
FTZ-F1 and MEG-8.3	*S.mansoni*	Oesophagus	Maintains oesophageal gland and head integrity.	Loss of the ability to accumulate nutrients.	[121]
HNF4	*S.mansoni, S. japonicum,* and *S. haematobium*	Intestine	Renewal of intestinal stem cells and formation of microvilli-like structures.	Feeding disorders, impairment of gut processes.	[122 - 125]

DRUG RESISTANCE

Although several lead antischistosomal agents have been identified, no drugs other than the repurposed antimalarials have been marketed since the introduction of PZQ. Furthermore, the success of PZQ led to the unavailability of other antischistosomal drugs in most countries. Thus, the control of this prevalent disease almost relies entirely on a single drug. For any disease, reliance on a single drug leads to resistance. The uncertainty of the exact molecular target of PZQ makes it difficult to study and surmount the mechanism of resistance. Although substantial evidence suggests that PZQ interacts with voltage-gated calcium channels, other molecular targets have also been proposed [12, 17, 126]. There are also several non-target-based changes that could influence the effectiveness of PZQ including changes in worm maturation rates [127] and sex ratios. Since PZQ-action appears to be immune-dependent, another possible resistance mechanism is based on the loss or modulation of parasitic antigens that become exposed following PZQ treatment. There are further studies that indicate that multidrug transporters are involved in modulating PZQ susceptibility [128], where the chronic exposure of worms to sub-lethal doses of PZQ leads to upregulation of SMDR2 and schistosome MRP1 [129, 130]. However, genomic and post-genomic strategies could lead to insights into the drug's mode of action and provide markers for monitoring the emergence of resistance [106].

VACCINATION

In parasitic diseases as schistosomiasis, several protein interactions between the human host and the parasite take place. The identification and characterisation of these interactions are essential for the development of new therapeutic methods and vaccines. Nowadays, researchers aim to develop a prophylactic schistosomiasis vaccine which would be a good and lasting way to control the disease whether it is used alone or with praziquantel. Sm14, SmTSP-2, and Sm-p80 are three potential vaccine candidates for *S. mansoni* that have shown promising results and are in different clinical trial phases. In addition, there are other schistosomal antigens considered as vaccine candidates such as Sm97, Sj97, Sm29, and SmKI1 that are evaluated in several pre-clinical studies [131, 132]. In the following paragraphs, some of the mentioned candidates will be discussed.

Schistosoma mansoni 14-kDa Fatty Acid-Binding Protein (Sm14)

Schistosomes lack oxygen-dependent synthetic pathways required for the synthesis of sterols and fatty acids needed for membrane formation, protein anchoring, maturation, and egg production [133]. Sm14 is one of the fatty acid-binding proteins (FABPs), which are expressed in all lifecycle stages of the parasite where they play an important role in absorbance, and transport, in addition to compartmentalization of fatty acids from the host. Therefore, Sm14 is considered a good candidate for vaccine development [134].

When tested in mice without an adjuvant, recombinant Sm14 (rSm14) provided up to 67% host protection against cercariae challenge observable as reduced *S. mansoni* worm burden. In addition, no notable autoimmune response was elicited [135].

In 2016, a study was conducted to evaluate the safety and immunogenicity of rSm14 in 20 male volunteers from a non-endemic area for schistosomiasis in brazil. The administered vaccine was formulated with glucopyranosyl lipid A (GLA) adjuvant in an oil-in-water emulsion. Results obtained showed that the rSm14/GLA-SE vaccine was highly immunogenic and safe [136].

In continuation of the work, a phase IIa trial was conducted in which the formulated vaccine was administered intramuscularly in two doses (2.5 µg and 5 µg/dose) to 30 male adults living in a highly endemic area for both *S. mansoni* and *S. haematobium* at the Senegal River Basin. Results confirmed safety and strong and long-lasting immunogenicity. Based on the results of the phase IIa trial, a phase 2b study in school-aged children living in the same endemic area of Senegal was designed and initiated. Results are not published yet [137].

Schistosoma mansoni 29 Kilodalton Protein Sm29

Sm29 is an antigen highly expressed on the outer tegument of *S. mansoni,* in lung-stage schistosoluma and adult worms. In 2008, Cardoso *et al.* [138] demonstrated that Sm29 is a valuable candidate for the development of a vaccine. Studies confirmed that high levels of IgG1 and IgG3 antibodies against Sm29 can be identified in naturally resistant people and patients showing resistance to re-infection living in endemic areas for schistosomiasis in Brazil. Furthermore, administration of recombinant Sm29 (rSm29) elicited high levels of protection in mice through induction of Th1 immune response and reduction of worm burden, liver granulomas, and intestinal eggs.

In another study by Alves *et al.* [139] the effect of using alum or monophosphoryl lipid A (MPLA) as an adjuvant with rSm29 in the vaccine formulation used in an animal model of *S. mansoni* reinfection was assessed. Results show that vaccine formulation containing alum is more effective as it was able to elicit partial protection against reinfection, and a 29-37% reduction of parasite burden in immunized mice. On the other hand, the formulation containing MPLA was not able to reduce the worm burden.

While most studies test different antigens separately to test their efficiency as candidates for vaccine development, Mossallam *et al.* [140] decided to produce a recombinant fusion protein comprised of the two promising schistosomal antigens Sm14 and Sm29 and named it FSm14/29. The latter was administered to Swiss albino mice in two formulations either unadjuvanted or adjuvanted with polyinosinic-polycytidylic acid adjuvant. Afterwards, the mice were challenged with cercariae, and the different parameters whether parasitological or immunological were assessed seven weeks post-infection. Results show that mice vaccinated with unadjuvanted and adjuvanted FSm14/29 displayed a decrease in adult worm burden by 44.7 and 48.4%, respectively. Significant reductions in the hepatic and intestinal egg burden after the administration of both formulations containing FSm14/29 were observed. Moreover, adult worms recovered from the groups immunized with both vaccine formulations containing the fusion protein exhibited structural deformities that were undetectable in adult worms recovered from all other experimental groups including the infected unvaccinated negative control group, the adjuvant group and groups immunized with the individual antigens.

CONCLUDING REMARKS

Schistosomes are parasites with a complex life cycle composed of several developmental stages, taking place in two different hosts: snail host (intermediate host) and human host (definitive host). To eradicate the parasitic disease, new treatment methods to support the currently used drug, Praziquantel must be developed.

Drug repurposing is a rapid, cost-effective, and reduced-risk approach currently used to discover the antischistosomal activity of validated drugs whether in use or still in development. Additionally, new potential targets are being identified and characterised to use in the process of antischistosomal drug discovery. Although the development procedure of a vaccine is costly, slow, and difficult, important steps have been taken to develop a prophylactic vaccine. Presently, three vaccine candidates for *S. mansoni* have demonstrated encouraging results and are in different clinical trial phases. Moreover, there are additional candidates that are investigated in several pre-clinical studies.

REFERENCES

[1]   Gemma S, Federico S, Brogi S, Brindisi M, Butini S, Campiani G. Chapter Four - Dealing with schistosomiasis: Current drug discovery strategies. In: Chibale K, Ed. Annu Rep Med Chem 53. Academic Press 2019; pp. 107-38.

[2]   (WHO) WHO. Schistosomiasis 2023. Available from: https://www.who.int/news-room/fact sheets/detail /schistosomiasis

[3]   DPDx-CfDCaP-Schistosomiasis 2019. Available from: https://www.cdc.gov/dpdx/schistosomiasis/index.html

[4]   yourgenome.org. Available from: https://www.yourgenome.org/facts/what-is-schistosomiasis/

[5]   Nelwan ML. Schistosomiasis: Life cycle, diagnosis, and control. Curr Ther Res Clin Exp 2019; 91: 5-9.
        [http://dx.doi.org/10.1016/j.curtheres.2019.06.001] [PMID: 31372189]

[6]   Carbonell C, Rodríguez-Alonso B, López-Bernús A, *et al.* Clinical spectrum of schistosomiasis: An update. J Clin Med 2021; 10(23): 5521.
        [http://dx.doi.org/10.3390/jcm10235521] [PMID: 34884223]

[7]   Jauréguiberry S, Paris L, Caumes E. Acute schistosomiasis, a diagnostic and therapeutic challenge. Clin Microbiol Infect 2010; 16(3): 225-31.
        [http://dx.doi.org/10.1111/j.1469-0691.2009.03131.x] [PMID: 20222897]

[8]   Lambertucci JR. Acute schistosomiasis mansoni: revisited and reconsidered. Mem Inst Oswaldo Cruz 2010; 105(4): 422-35.
        [http://dx.doi.org/10.1590/S0074-02762010000400012] [PMID: 20721485]

[9]   Ross AG, Vickers D, Olds GR, Shah SM, McManus DP. Katayama syndrome. Lancet Infect Dis 2007; 7(3): 218-24.
        [http://dx.doi.org/10.1016/S1473-3099(07)70053-1] [PMID: 17317603]

[10]   King CH, Dangerfield-Cha M. The unacknowledged impact of chronic schistosomiasis. Chronic Illn 2008; 4(1): 65-79.
        [http://dx.doi.org/10.1177/1742395307084407] [PMID: 18322031]

[11]   Aruleba RT, Adekiya TA, Oyinloye BE, *et al.* PZQ therapy: how close are we in the development of effective alternative anti-schistosomal drugs? Infect Disord Drug Targets 2019; 19(4): 337-49.
[http://dx.doi.org/10.2174/1871526519666181231153139] [PMID: 30599112]

[12]   Doenhoff MJ, Cioli D, Utzinger J. Praziquantel: mechanisms of action, resistance and new derivatives for schistosomiasis. Curr Opin Infect Dis 2008; 21(6): 659-67.
[http://dx.doi.org/10.1097/QCO.0b013e328318978f] [PMID: 18978535]

[13]   Cioli D, Pica-Mattoccia L, Archer S. Antischistosomal drugs: Past, present ... and future? Pharmacol Ther 1995; 68(1): 35-85.
[http://dx.doi.org/10.1016/0163-7258(95)00026-7] [PMID: 8604437]

[14]   Colley DG, Bustinduy AL, Secor WE, King CH. Human schistosomiasis. Lancet 2014; 383(9936): 2253-64.
[http://dx.doi.org/10.1016/S0140-6736(13)61949-2] [PMID: 24698483]

[15]   Vale N, Gouveia MJ, Rinaldi G, Brindley PJ, Gärtner F, Correia da Costa JM. Praziquantel for schistosomiasis: single-drug metabolism revisited, mode of action, and resistance. Antimicrob Agents Chemother 2017; 61(5): e02582-16.
[http://dx.doi.org/10.1128/AAC.02582-16] [PMID: 28264841]

[16]   Cupit PM, Cunningham C. What is the mechanism of action of praziquantel and how might resistance strike? Future Med Chem 2015; 7(6): 701-5.
[http://dx.doi.org/10.4155/fmc.15.11] [PMID: 25996063]

[17]   Greenberg RM. Are Ca^{2+} channels targets of praziquantel action? Int J Parasitol 2005; 35(1): 1-9.
[http://dx.doi.org/10.1016/j.ijpara.2004.09.004] [PMID: 15619510]

[18]   Jeziorski MC, Greenberg RM. Voltage-gated calcium channel subunits from platyhelminths: Potential role in praziquantel action. Int J Parasitol 2006; 36(6): 625-32.
[http://dx.doi.org/10.1016/j.ijpara.2006.02.002] [PMID: 16545816]

[19]   Gryseels B, Polman K, Clerinx J, Kestens L. Human schistosomiasis. Lancet 2006; 368(9541): 1106-18.
[http://dx.doi.org/10.1016/S0140-6736(06)69440-3] [PMID: 16997665]

[20]   Doenhoff MJ, Wheatcroft-Francklow K. Schistosome drug resistance: praziquantel Management of Multiple Drug-Resistant Infections. Springer 2004; pp. 341-52.
[http://dx.doi.org/10.1007/978-1-59259-738-3_19]

[21]   Gouveia MJ, Brindley PJ, Gärtner F, Costa JMC, Vale N. Costa JMCd, Vale N. Drug repurposing for schistosomiasis: combinations of drugs or biomolecules. Pharmaceuticals (Basel) 2018; 11(1): 15.
[http://dx.doi.org/10.3390/ph11010015] [PMID: 29401734]

[22]   Moreira-Filho JT, Silva AC, Dantas RF, *et al.* Schistosomiasis drug discovery in the era of automation and artificial intelligence. Front Immunol 2021; 12: 642383.
[http://dx.doi.org/10.3389/fimmu.2021.642383] [PMID: 34135888]

[23]   Keiser J, Chollet J, Xiao SH, *et al.* Mefloquine--an aminoalcohol with promising antischistosomal properties in mice. PLoS Negl Trop Dis 2009; 3(1): e350.
[http://dx.doi.org/10.1371/journal.pntd.0000350] [PMID: 19125172]

[24]   Fouad MAH, Fakahany AF, Younis MS, El Hamshary AMS, Hassan ME, Ali HM. Effect of mefloquine on worm burden and tegumental changes in experimental Schistosoma mansoni infection. J Microsc Ultrastruct 2014; 2(1): 7-11.
[http://dx.doi.org/10.1016/j.jmau.2014.03.001]

[25]   Krieg R, Jortzik E, Goetz AA, *et al.* Arylmethylamino steroids as antiparasitic agents. Nat Commun 2017; 8(1): 14478.
[http://dx.doi.org/10.1038/ncomms14478] [PMID: 28211535]

[26]   Yang F, Hu M, Lei Q, *et al.* Nifuroxazide induces apoptosis and impairs pulmonary metastasis in

breast cancer model. Cell Death Dis 2015; 6(3): e1701.
[http://dx.doi.org/10.1038/cddis.2015.63] [PMID: 25811798]

[27]   Nelson EA, Walker SR, Kepich A, *et al.* Nifuroxazide inhibits survival of multiple myeloma cells by directly inhibiting STAT3. Blood 2008; 112(13): 5095-102.
[http://dx.doi.org/10.1182/blood-2007-12-129718] [PMID: 18824601]

[28]   Zhao T, Jia H, Cheng Q, *et al.* Nifuroxazide prompts antitumor immune response of TCL-loaded DC in mice with orthotopically-implanted hepatocarcinoma. Oncol Rep 2017; 37(6): 3405-14.
[http://dx.doi.org/10.3892/or.2017.5629] [PMID: 28498414]

[29]   Bailly C. Toward a repositioning of the antibacterial drug nifuroxazide for cancer treatment. Drug Discov Today 2019; 24(9): 1930-6.
[http://dx.doi.org/10.1016/j.drudis.2019.06.017] [PMID: 31260646]

[30]   Elsherbiny NM, Zaitone SA, Mohammad HMF, El-Sherbiny M. Renoprotective effect of nifuroxazide in diabetes-induced nephropathy: impact on NFκB, oxidative stress, and apoptosis. Toxicol Mech Methods 2018; 28(6): 467-73.
[http://dx.doi.org/10.1080/15376516.2018.1459995] [PMID: 29606028]

[31]   Gan C, Zhang Q, Liu H, *et al.* Nifuroxazide ameliorates pulmonary fibrosis by blocking myofibroblast genesis: a drug repurposing study. Respir Res 2022; 23(1): 32.
[http://dx.doi.org/10.1186/s12931-022-01946-6] [PMID: 35172837]

[32]   Kaiser M, Mäser P, Tadoori LP, Ioset JR, Brun R. Antiprotozoal activity profiling of approved drugs: A starting point toward drug repositioning. PLoS One 2015; 10(8): e0135556.
[http://dx.doi.org/10.1371/journal.pone.0135556] [PMID: 26270335]

[33]   Roquini V, Mengarda AC, Cajas RA, *et al.* The existing drug nifuroxazide as an antischistosomal agent: *In vitro, in vivo,* and *in silico* Studies of Macromolecular Targets. Microbiol Spectr 2023; 11(4): e01393-23.
[http://dx.doi.org/10.1128/spectrum.01393-23] [PMID: 37409934]

[34]   Carvalho AAL, Mafud AC, Pinto PLS, Mascarenhas YP, de Moraes J. Schistosomicidal effect of the anti-inflammatory drug diclofenac and its structural correlation with praziquantel. Int J Antimicrob Agents 2014; 44(4): 372-4.
[http://dx.doi.org/10.1016/j.ijantimicag.2014.06.018] [PMID: 25178921]

[35]   Lago EM, Silva MP, Queiroz TG, *et al.* Phenotypic screening of nonsteroidal anti-inflammatory drugs identified mefenamic acid as a drug for the treatment of schistosomiasis. EBioMedicine 2019; 43: 370-9.
[http://dx.doi.org/10.1016/j.ebiom.2019.04.029] [PMID: 31027918]

[36]   Abou-El-Naga IF, El-Temsahy MM, Mogahed NMFH, Sheta E, Makled S, Ibrahim EI. Effect of celecoxib against different developmental stages of experimental Schistosoma mansoni infection. Acta Trop 2021; 218: 105891.
[http://dx.doi.org/10.1016/j.actatropica.2021.105891] [PMID: 33773944]

[37]   Cowan N, Keiser J. Repurposing of anticancer drugs: *in vitro* and *in vivo* activities against Schistosoma mansoni. Parasit Vectors 2015; 8(1): 417.
[http://dx.doi.org/10.1186/s13071-015-1023-y] [PMID: 26265386]

[38]   Drug Approval Package: Vidaza (Azacitidine) NDA 2004.

[39]   Geyer KK, Munshi SE, Vickers M, *et al.* The anti-fecundity effect of 5-azacytidine (5-AzaC) on Schistosoma mansoni is linked to dis-regulated transcription, translation and stem cell activities. Int J Parasitol Drugs Drug Resist 2018; 8(2): 213-22.
[http://dx.doi.org/10.1016/j.ijpddr.2018.03.006] [PMID: 29649665]

[40]   Hilgard P, Klenner T, Stekar J, Unger C. Alkylphosphocholines: a new class of membrane-active anticancer agents. Cancer Chemother Pharmacol 1993; 32(2): 90-5.
[http://dx.doi.org/10.1007/BF00685608] [PMID: 8485813]

[41] Soto J, Toledo J, Gutierrez P, *et al.* Treatment of American cutaneous leishmaniasis with miltefosine, an oral agent. Clin Infect Dis 2001; 33(7): e57-61.
[http://dx.doi.org/10.1086/322689] [PMID: 11528586]

[42] Mollinedo F, de la Iglesia-Vicente J, Gajate C, *et al. in vitro* and *in vivo* selective antitumor activity of Edelfosine against mantle cell lymphoma and chronic lymphocytic leukemia involving lipid rafts. Clin Cancer Res 2010; 16(7): 2046-54.
[http://dx.doi.org/10.1158/1078-0432.CCR-09-2456] [PMID: 20233887]

[43] Varela-M RE, Villa-Pulgarin JA, Yepes E, *et al. in vitro* and *in vivo* efficacy of ether lipid edelfosine against Leishmania spp. and SbV-resistant parasites. PLoS Negl Trop Dis 2012; 6(4): e1612.
[http://dx.doi.org/10.1371/journal.pntd.0001612] [PMID: 22506086]

[44] Eissa MM, El-Azzouni MZ, Amer EI, Baddour NM. Miltefosine, a promising novel agent for schistosomiasis mansoni. Int J Parasitol 2011; 41(2): 235-42.
[http://dx.doi.org/10.1016/j.ijpara.2010.09.010] [PMID: 21055404]

[45] Yepes E, Varela-M RE, López-Abán J, Dakir ELH, Mollinedo F, Muro A. *in vitro* and *in vivo* anti-schistosomal activity of the alkylphospholipid analog edelfosine. PLoS One 2014; 9(10): e109431.
[http://dx.doi.org/10.1371/journal.pone.0109431] [PMID: 25302497]

[46] Eissa MM, Mossallam SF, Amer EI, Younis LK, Rashed HA. Repositioning of chlorambucil as a potential anti-schistosomal agent. Acta Trop 2017; 166: 58-66.
[http://dx.doi.org/10.1016/j.actatropica.2016.11.006] [PMID: 27836498]

[47] Eldeeb E, Fahmy S, Elbakry K, Hyder A. A single dose of the antineoplastics hydroxyurea or cisplatin has praziquantel-like effects on Schistosoma mansoni worms and host mouse liver. Biomed Pharmacother 2018; 99: 570-5.
[http://dx.doi.org/10.1016/j.biopha.2018.01.098] [PMID: 29902867]

[48] Vandewaa EA, Mills G, Chen G-Z, Foster LA, Bennett JL. Physiological role of HMG-CoA reductase in regulating egg production by Schistosoma mansoni. Am J Physiol 1989; 257(3 Pt 2): R618-25.
[PMID: 2782464]

[49] Chen GZ, Foster L, Bennett J. Antischistosomal action of mevinolin: evidence that 3-hydrox--methylglutaryl-coenzyme a reductase activity in Schistosoma mansoni is vital for parasite survival. Naunyn Schmiedebergs Arch Pharmacol 1990; 342(4): 477-82.
[http://dx.doi.org/10.1007/BF00169467] [PMID: 2123968]

[50] Soliman MFM, Ibrahim MM. Antischistosomal action of atorvastatin alone and concurrently with medroxyprogesterone acetate on Schistosoma haematobium harboured in hamster: surface ultrastructure and parasitological study. Acta Trop 2005; 93(1): 1-9.
[http://dx.doi.org/10.1016/j.actatropica.2004.08.006] [PMID: 15589792]

[51] Araújo N, Kohn A, Oliveira ÁA, Katz N. Schistosoma mansoni: ação da lovastatina no modelo murino. Rev Soc Bras Med Trop 2002; 35(1): 35-8.
[http://dx.doi.org/10.1590/S0037-86822002000100007] [PMID: 11873259]

[52] Rojo-Arreola L, Long T, Asarnow D, Suzuki BM, Singh R, Caffrey CR. Chemical and genetic validation of the statin drug target to treat the helminth disease, schistosomiasis. PLoS One 2014; 9(1): e87594.
[http://dx.doi.org/10.1371/journal.pone.0087594] [PMID: 24489942]

[53] Hess J, Panic G, Patra M, *et al.* Ferrocenyl, ruthenocenyl, and benzyl oxamniquine derivatives with cross-species activity against Schistosoma mansoni and Schistosoma haematobium. ACS Infect Dis 2017; 3(9): 645-52.
[http://dx.doi.org/10.1021/acsinfecdis.7b00054] [PMID: 28686009]

[54] Keiser J, Vargas M, Rubbiani R, Gasser G, Biot C. *in vitro* and *in vivo* antischistosomal activity of ferroquine derivatives. Parasit Vectors 2014; 7(1): 424.
[http://dx.doi.org/10.1186/1756-3305-7-424] [PMID: 25190030]

[55]   Ong YC, Roy S, Andrews PC, Gasser G. Metal compounds against neglected tropical diseases. Chem Rev 2019; 119(2): 730-96.
[http://dx.doi.org/10.1021/acs.chemrev.8b00338] [PMID: 30507157]

[56]   Khan MOF, Keiser J, Amoyaw PNA, *et al.* Discovery of antischistosomal drug leads based on tetraazamacrocyclic derivatives and their metal complexes. Antimicrob Agents Chemother 2016; 60(9): 5331-6.
[http://dx.doi.org/10.1128/AAC.00778-16] [PMID: 27324765]

[57]   Hess J, Keiser J, Gasser G. Toward organometallic antischistosomal drug candidates. Future Med Chem 2015; 7(6): 821-30.
[http://dx.doi.org/10.4155/fmc.15.22] [PMID: 25996072]

[58]   Portes MC, De Moraes J, Véras LMC, *et al.* Structural and spectroscopic characterization of epiisopiloturine-metal complexes, and anthelmintic activity *vs. S. mansoni.* J Coord Chem 2016; 69(10): 1663-83.
[http://dx.doi.org/10.1080/00958972.2016.1182162]

[59]   Seto E, Yoshida M. Erasers of histone acetylation: the histone deacetylase enzymes. Cold Spring Harb Perspect Biol 2014; 6(4): a018713.
[http://dx.doi.org/10.1101/cshperspect.a018713] [PMID: 24691964]

[60]   Scholte LLS, Mourão MM, Pais FSM, *et al.* Evolutionary relationships among protein lysine deacetylases of parasites causing neglected diseases. Infect Genet Evol 2017; 53: 175-88.
[http://dx.doi.org/10.1016/j.meegid.2017.05.011] [PMID: 28506839]

[61]   Lancelot J, Caby S, Dubois-Abdesselem F, *et al.* Schistosoma mansoni Sirtuins: characterization and potential as chemotherapeutic targets. PLoS Negl Trop Dis 2013; 7(9): e2428.
[http://dx.doi.org/10.1371/journal.pntd.0002428] [PMID: 24069483]

[62]   Oger F, Dubois F, Caby S, *et al.* The class I histone deacetylases of the platyhelminth parasite Schistosoma mansoni. Biochem Biophys Res Commun 2008; 377(4): 1079-84.
[http://dx.doi.org/10.1016/j.bbrc.2008.10.090] [PMID: 18977200]

[63]   Nakagawa M, Oda Y, Eguchi T, *et al.* Expression profile of class I histone deacetylases in human cancer tissues. Oncol Rep 2007; 18(4): 769-74.
[http://dx.doi.org/10.3892/or.18.4.769] [PMID: 17786334]

[64]   Marek M, Kannan S, Hauser AT, *et al.* Structural basis for the inhibition of histone deacetylase 8 (HDAC8), a key epigenetic player in the blood fluke Schistosoma mansoni. PLoS Pathog 2013; 9(9): e1003645.
[http://dx.doi.org/10.1371/journal.ppat.1003645] [PMID: 24086136]

[65]   Heimburg T, Chakrabarti A, Lancelot J, *et al.* Structure-based design and synthesis of novel inhibitors targeting HDAC8 from *Schistosoma mansoni* for the treatment of schistosomiasis. J Med Chem 2016; 59(6): 2423-35.
[http://dx.doi.org/10.1021/acs.jmedchem.5b01478] [PMID: 26937828]

[66]   Ghazy E, Heimburg T, Lancelot J, *et al.* Synthesis, structure-activity relationships, cocrystallization and cellular characterization of novel smHDAC8 inhibitors for the treatment of schistosomiasis. Eur J Med Chem 2021; 225: 113745.
[http://dx.doi.org/10.1016/j.ejmech.2021.113745] [PMID: 34392190]

[67]   Codd R. Traversing the coordination chemistry and chemical biology of hydroxamic acids. Coord Chem Rev 2008; 252(12-14): 1387-408.
[http://dx.doi.org/10.1016/j.ccr.2007.08.001]

[68]   Marmion CJ, Griffith D, Nolan KB. Hydroxamic acids − An intriguing family of enzyme inhibitors and biomedical ligands. Eur J Inorg Chem 2004; 2004(15): 3003-16.
[http://dx.doi.org/10.1002/ejic.200400221]

[69]   Shen S, Kozikowski AP. Why hydroxamates may not be the best histone deacetylase inhibitors—what

some may have forgotten or would rather forget? ChemMedChem 2016; 11(1): 15-21.
[http://dx.doi.org/10.1002/cmdc.201500486] [PMID: 26603496]

[70]   Guidi A, Saccoccia F, Gennari N, *et al*. Identification of novel multi-stage histone deacetylase (HDAC) inhibitors that impair Schistosoma mansoni viability and egg production. Parasit Vectors 2018; 11(1): 668.
[http://dx.doi.org/10.1186/s13071-018-3268-8] [PMID: 30587243]

[71]   Monaldi D, Rotili D, Lancelot J, *et al*. Structure–reactivity relationships on substrates and inhibitors of the lysine deacylase sirtuin 2 from *Schistosoma mansoni* (*Sm* sirt2). J Med Chem 2019; 62(19): 8733-59.
[http://dx.doi.org/10.1021/acs.jmedchem.9b00638] [PMID: 31496251]

[72]   Goll MG, Kirpekar F, Maggert KA, *et al*. Methylation of tRNAAsp by the DNA methyltransferase homolog Dnmt2. Science 2006; 311(5759): 395-8.
[http://dx.doi.org/10.1126/science.1120976] [PMID: 16424344]

[73]   Roquis D, Taudt A, Geyer KK, *et al*. Histone methylation changes are required for life cycle progression in the human parasite Schistosoma mansoni. PLoS Pathog 2018; 14(5): e1007066.
[http://dx.doi.org/10.1371/journal.ppat.1007066] [PMID: 29782530]

[74]   Pereira ASA, Amaral MS, Vasconcelos EJR, *et al*. Inhibition of histone methyltransferase EZH2 in Schistosoma mansoni *in vitro* by GSK343 reduces egg laying and decreases the expression of genes implicated in DNA replication and noncoding RNA metabolism. PLoS Negl Trop Dis 2018; 12(10): e0006873.
[http://dx.doi.org/10.1371/journal.pntd.0006873] [PMID: 30365505]

[75]   Anderson L, Gomes MR, daSilva LF, *et al*. Histone deacetylase inhibition modulates histone acetylation at gene promoter regions and affects genome-wide gene transcription in Schistosoma mansoni. PLoS Negl Trop Dis 2017; 11(4): e0005539.
[http://dx.doi.org/10.1371/journal.pntd.0005539] [PMID: 28406899]

[76]   Wang J, Paz C, Padalino G, *et al*. Large-scale RNAi screening uncovers therapeutic targets in the parasite *Schistosoma mansoni*. Science 2020; 369(6511): 1649-53.
[http://dx.doi.org/10.1126/science.abb7699] [PMID: 32973031]

[77]   Beckmann S, Long T, Scheld C, Geyer R, Caffrey CR, Grevelding CG. Serum albumin and α-1 acid glycoprotein impede the killing of Schistosoma mansoni by the tyrosine kinase inhibitor Imatinib. Int J Parasitol Drugs Drug Resist 2014; 4(3): 287-95.
[http://dx.doi.org/10.1016/j.ijpddr.2014.07.005] [PMID: 25516839]

[78]   Giuliani S, Silva AC, Borba JVVB, *et al*. Computationally-guided drug repurposing enables the discovery of kinase targets and inhibitors as new schistosomicidal agents. PLOS Comput Biol 2018; 14(10): e1006515.
[http://dx.doi.org/10.1371/journal.pcbi.1006515] [PMID: 30346968]

[79]   Avelar LGA, Gava SG, Neves RH, *et al*. Smp38 MAP kinase regulation in Schistosoma mansoni: roles in survival, oviposition, and protection against oxidative stress. Front Immunol 2019; 10: 21.
[http://dx.doi.org/10.3389/fimmu.2019.00021] [PMID: 30733716]

[80]   Long T, Neitz RJ, Beasley R, *et al*. Structure-bioactivity relationship for benzimidazole thiophene inhibitors of polo-like kinase 1 (PLK1), a potential drug target in Schistosoma mansoni. PLoS Negl Trop Dis 2016; 10(1): e0004356.
[http://dx.doi.org/10.1371/journal.pntd.0004356] [PMID: 26751972]

[81]   Wu K, Zhai X, Huang S, Jiang L, Yu Z, Huang J. Protein kinases: potential drug targets against Schistosoma japonicum. Front Cell Infect Microbiol 2021; 11: 691757.
[http://dx.doi.org/10.3389/fcimb.2021.691757] [PMID: 34277472]

[82]   Horn M, Fajtová P, Rojo Arreola L, *et al*. Trypsin- and Chymotrypsin-like serine proteases in schistosoma mansoni-- 'the undiscovered country'. PLoS Negl Trop Dis 2014; 8(3): e2766.
[http://dx.doi.org/10.1371/journal.pntd.0002766] [PMID: 24676141]

[83]   Cleenewerk L, Garssen J, Hogenkamp A. Clinical use of Schistosoma mansoni antigens as novel immunotherapies for autoimmune disorders. Front Immunol 2020; 11: 1821.
[http://dx.doi.org/10.3389/fimmu.2020.01821] [PMID: 32903582]

[84]   Yamamoto H, Fukui N, Adachi M, *et al.* Human molecular chaperone hsp60 and its apical domain suppress amyloid fibril formation of α-synuclein. Int J Mol Sci 2019; 21(1): 47.
[http://dx.doi.org/10.3390/ijms21010047] [PMID: 31861692]

[85]   López-Otín C, Bond JS. Proteases: multifunctional enzymes in life and disease. J Biol Chem 2008; 283(45): 30433-7.
[http://dx.doi.org/10.1074/jbc.R800035200] [PMID: 18650443]

[86]   Pakchotanon P, Molee P, Nuamtanong S, *et al.* Molecular characterization of serine protease inhibitor isoform 3, SmSPI, from Schistosoma mansoni. Parasitol Res 2016; 115(8): 2981-94.
[http://dx.doi.org/10.1007/s00436-016-5053-y] [PMID: 27083187]

[87]   Quezada LAL, McKerrow JH. Schistosome serine protease inhibitors: parasite defense or homeostasis? An Acad Bras Cienc 2011; 83(2): 663-72.
[http://dx.doi.org/10.1590/S0001-37652011000200025] [PMID: 21670886]

[88]   Nascimento I, Albino S, Menezes K, *et al.* Targeting SmCB1: Perspectives and insights to design antischistosomal drugs. Curr Med Chem 2023; 31.
[http://dx.doi.org/10.2174/0109298673255826231011114249]

[89]   Macedo Soares MF, Araújo C. Helminth products as a potential therapeutic strategy for inflammatory diseases. Inflamm Allergy Drug Targets 2008; 7(2): 113-8.
[http://dx.doi.org/10.2174/187152808785107606] [PMID: 18691141]

[90]   Quezada LAL, Sajid M, Lim KC, McKerrow JH. A blood fluke serine protease inhibitor regulates an endogenous larval elastase. J Biol Chem 2012; 287(10): 7074-83.
[http://dx.doi.org/10.1074/jbc.M111.313304] [PMID: 22174417]

[91]   Morais SB, Figueiredo BC, Assis NRG, *et al.* Schistosoma mansoni SmKI-1 serine protease inhibitor binds to elastase and impairs neutrophil function and inflammation. PLoS Pathog 2018; 14(2): e1006870.
[http://dx.doi.org/10.1371/journal.ppat.1006870] [PMID: 29425229]

[92]   Ranasinghe SL, Fischer K, Gobert GN, McManus DP. Functional expression of a novel Kunitz type protease inhibitor from the human blood fluke Schistosoma mansoni. Parasit Vectors 2015; 8(1): 408.
[http://dx.doi.org/10.1186/s13071-015-1022-z] [PMID: 26238343]

[93]   Abdulla MH, Lim KC, Sajid M, McKerrow JH, Caffrey CR. Schistosomiasis mansoni: novel chemotherapy using a cysteine protease inhibitor. PLoS Med 2007; 4(1): e14.
[http://dx.doi.org/10.1371/journal.pmed.0040014] [PMID: 17214506]

[94]   Sherif M. Abaza AAE-M, Ola A. Ismail, Maha M. Alabbassy. Cysteine proteases inhibitors (phenyl vinyl sulfone and valproic acid) in treatment of schistosomiasis mansoni-infected mice: An experimental study to evaluate their role in comparison to praziquantel. Parasitol United J 2013; 6(1): 99-108.

[95]   Molehin AJ, Gobert GN, Driguez P, McManus DP. Functional characterization of *SjB10*, an intracellular serpin from *Schistosoma japonicum*. Parasitology 2014; 141(13): 1746-60.
[http://dx.doi.org/10.1017/S0031182014001061] [PMID: 25137634]

[96]   Molehin AJ, Gobert GN, McMANUS DP. Serine protease inhibitors of parasitic helminths. Parasitology 2012; 139(6): 681-95.
[http://dx.doi.org/10.1017/S0031182011002435] [PMID: 22310379]

[97]   Huang W, Haas TA, Biesterfeldt J, Mankawsky L, Blanton RE, Lee X. Purification and crystallization of a novel membrane-anchored protein: the *Schistosoma haematobium* serpin. Acta Crystallogr D Biol Crystallogr 1999; 55(1): 350-2.
[http://dx.doi.org/10.1107/S0907444998008658] [PMID: 10089448]

[98] Ziniel PD, Karumudi B, Barnard AH, *et al.* The schistosoma mansoni cytochrome P450 (CYP3050A1) is essential for worm survival and egg development. PLoS Negl Trop Dis 2015; 9(12): e0004279.
[http://dx.doi.org/10.1371/journal.pntd.0004279] [PMID: 26713732]

[99] Elzoheiry MA, Elmehankar MS, Aboukamar WA, *et al.* Fluconazole as Schistosoma mansoni cytochrome P450 inhibitor: *in vivo* murine experimental study. Exp Parasitol 2022; 239: 108291.
[http://dx.doi.org/10.1016/j.exppara.2022.108291] [PMID: 35660528]

[100] Borst P, Elferink RO. Mammalian ABC transporters in health and disease. Annu Rev Biochem 2002; 71(1): 537-92.
[http://dx.doi.org/10.1146/annurev.biochem.71.102301.093055] [PMID: 12045106]

[101] Dassa E, Bouige P. The ABC of ABCs: a phylogenetic and functional classification of ABC systems in living organisms. Res Microbiol 2001; 152(3-4): 211-29.
[http://dx.doi.org/10.1016/S0923-2508(01)01194-9] [PMID: 11421270]

[102] Greenberg RM. ABC multidrug transporters in schistosomes and other parasitic flatworms. Parasitol Int 2013; 62(6): 647-53.
[http://dx.doi.org/10.1016/j.parint.2013.02.006] [PMID: 23474413]

[103] James CE, Hudson AL, Davey MW. Drug resistance mechanisms in helminths: is it survival of the fittest? Trends Parasitol 2009; 25(7): 328-35.
[http://dx.doi.org/10.1016/j.pt.2009.04.004] [PMID: 19541539]

[104] James CE, Hudson AL, Davey MW. An update on P-glycoprotein and drug resistance in Schistosoma mansoni. Trends Parasitol 2009; 25(12): 538-9.
[http://dx.doi.org/10.1016/j.pt.2009.09.007] [PMID: 19850522]

[105] Ardelli BF. Transport proteins of the ABC systems superfamily and their role in drug action and resistance in nematodes. Parasitol Int 2013; 62(6): 639-46.
[http://dx.doi.org/10.1016/j.parint.2013.02.008] [PMID: 23474412]

[106] Greenberg RM. New approaches for understanding mechanisms of drug resistance in schistosomes. Parasitology 2013; 140(12): 1534-46.
[http://dx.doi.org/10.1017/S0031182013000231] [PMID: 23552512]

[107] Lespine A, Ménez C, Bourguinat C, Prichard RK. P-glycoproteins and other multidrug resistance transporters in the pharmacology of anthelmintics: Prospects for reversing transport-dependent anthelmintic resistance. Int J Parasitol Drugs Drug Resist 2012; 2: 58-75.
[http://dx.doi.org/10.1016/j.ijpddr.2011.10.001] [PMID: 24533264]

[108] Walter M, Kuris A. Inventors; Institute for OneWorld Health, assignee. Methods for the inhibition of egg production in trematodes. United States 2003.

[109] Kasinathan RS, Greenberg RM. Pharmacology and potential physiological significance of schistosome multidrug resistance transporters. Exp Parasitol 2012; 132(1): 2-6.
[http://dx.doi.org/10.1016/j.exppara.2011.03.004] [PMID: 21420955]

[110] Kasinathan RS, Morgan WM, Greenberg RM. Genetic knockdown and pharmacological inhibition of parasite multidrug resistance transporters disrupts egg production in Schistosoma mansoni. PLoS Negl Trop Dis 2011; 5(12): e1425.
[http://dx.doi.org/10.1371/journal.pntd.0001425] [PMID: 22163059]

[111] Lago EM, Xavier RP, Teixeira TR, Silva LM, da Silva Filho AA, de Moraes J. Antischistosomal agents: state of art and perspectives. Future Med Chem 2018; 10(1): 89-120.
[http://dx.doi.org/10.4155/fmc-2017-0112] [PMID: 29235368]

[112] Han Q, Jia B, Hong Y, *et al.* Suppression of VAMP2 alters morphology of the tegument and affects glucose uptake, development and reproduction of schistosoma japonicum. Sci Rep 2017; 7(1): 5212.
[http://dx.doi.org/10.1038/s41598-017-05602-8] [PMID: 28701752]

[113] Han Q, Hong Y, Fu Z, *et al.* Characterization of VAMP2 in schistosoma japonicum and the evaluation

of protective efficacy induced by recombinant SjVAMP2 in mice. PLoS One 2015; 10(12): e0144584.
[http://dx.doi.org/10.1371/journal.pone.0144584] [PMID: 26641090]

[114] Tran MH, Freitas TC, Cooper L, *et al.* Suppression of mRNAs encoding tegument tetraspanins from Schistosoma mansoni results in impaired tegument turnover. PLoS Pathog 2010; 6(4): e1000840.
[http://dx.doi.org/10.1371/journal.ppat.1000840] [PMID: 20419145]

[115] Pearson MS, Pickering DA, McSorley HJ, *et al.* Enhanced protective efficacy of a chimeric form of the schistosomiasis vaccine antigen Sm-TSP-2. PLoS Negl Trop Dis 2012; 6(3): e1564.
[http://dx.doi.org/10.1371/journal.pntd.0001564] [PMID: 22428079]

[116] Zhang W, Li J, Duke M, *et al.* Inconsistent protective efficacy and marked polymorphism limits the value of Schistosoma japonicum tetraspanin-2 as a vaccine target. PLoS Negl Trop Dis 2011; 5(5): e1166.
[http://dx.doi.org/10.1371/journal.pntd.0001166] [PMID: 21655308]

[117] Mekonnen GG, Tedla BA, Pickering D, *et al. Schistosoma haematobium* extracellular vesicle proteins confer protection in a heterologous model of schistosomiasis. Vaccines (Basel) 2020; 8(3): 416.
[http://dx.doi.org/10.3390/vaccines8030416] [PMID: 32722279]

[118] Li XH, de Castro-Borges W, Parker-Manuel S, *et al.* The schistosome oesophageal gland: initiator of blood processing. PLoS Negl Trop Dis 2013; 7(7): e2337.
[http://dx.doi.org/10.1371/journal.pntd.0002337] [PMID: 23936568]

[119] DeMarco R, Mathieson W, Manuel SJ, *et al.* Protein variation in blood-dwelling schistosome worms generated by differential splicing of micro-exon gene transcripts. Genome Res 2010; 20(8): 1112-21.
[http://dx.doi.org/10.1101/gr.100099.109] [PMID: 20606017]

[120] Lee J, Chong T, Newmark PA. The esophageal gland mediates host immune evasion by the human parasite *Schistosoma mansoni.* Proc Natl Acad Sci USA 2020; 117(32): 19299-309.
[http://dx.doi.org/10.1073/pnas.2006553117] [PMID: 32737161]

[121] Romero AA, Cobb SA, Collins JNR, Kliewer SA, Mangelsdorf DJ, Collins JJ III. The Schistosoma mansoni nuclear receptor FTZ-F1 maintains esophageal gland function *via* transcriptional regulation of meg-8.3. PLoS Pathog 2021; 17(12): e1010140.
[http://dx.doi.org/10.1371/journal.ppat.1010140] [PMID: 34910770]

[122] van Wolfswinkel JC, Wagner DE, Reddien PW. Single-cell analysis reveals functionally distinct classes within the planarian stem cell compartment. Cell Stem Cell 2014; 15(3): 326-39.
[http://dx.doi.org/10.1016/j.stem.2014.06.007] [PMID: 25017721]

[123] Wendt G, Zhao L, Chen R, *et al.* A single-cell RNA-seq atlas of *Schistosoma mansoni* identifies a key regulator of blood feeding. Science 2020; 369(6511): 1644-9.
[http://dx.doi.org/10.1126/science.abb7709] [PMID: 32973030]

[124] Chen L, Luo S, Dupre A, *et al.* The nuclear receptor HNF4 drives a brush border gene program conserved across murine intestine, kidney, and embryonic yolk sac. Nat Commun 2021; 12(1): 2886.
[http://dx.doi.org/10.1038/s41467-021-22761-5] [PMID: 34001900]

[125] Chen L, Vasoya RP, Toke NH, *et al.* HNF4 regulates fatty acid oxidation and is required for renewal of intestinal stem cells in mice. Gastroenterology 2020; 158(4): 985-999.e9.
[http://dx.doi.org/10.1053/j.gastro.2019.11.031] [PMID: 31759926]

[126] Redman CA, Robertson A, Fallon PG, *et al.* Praziquantel: An urgent and exciting challenge. Parasitol Today 1996; 12(1): 14-20.
[http://dx.doi.org/10.1016/0169-4758(96)80640-5] [PMID: 15275303]

[127] Fallon PG, Mubarak JS, Fookes RE, *et al.* Schistosoma mansoni: maturation rate and drug susceptibility of different geographic isolates. Exp Parasitol 1997; 86(1): 29-36.
[http://dx.doi.org/10.1006/expr.1997.4149] [PMID: 9149238]

[128] Kasinathan RS, Goronga T, Messerli SM, Webb TR, Greenberg RM. Modulation of a *Schistosoma mansoni* multidrug transporter by the antischistosomal drug praziquantel. FASEB J 2010; 24(1): 128-

35.
[http://dx.doi.org/10.1096/fj.09-137091] [PMID: 19726755]

[129] Messerli SM, Kasinathan RS, Morgan W, Spranger S, Greenberg RM. Schistosoma mansoni P-glycoprotein levels increase in response to praziquantel exposure and correlate with reduced praziquantel susceptibility. Mol Biochem Parasitol 2009; 167(1): 54-9.
[http://dx.doi.org/10.1016/j.molbiopara.2009.04.007] [PMID: 19406169]

[130] Kasinathan RS, Morgan WM, Greenberg RM. Schistosoma mansoni express higher levels of multidrug resistance-associated protein 1 (SmMRP1) in juvenile worms and in response to praziquantel. Mol Biochem Parasitol 2010; 173(1): 25-31.
[http://dx.doi.org/10.1016/j.molbiopara.2010.05.003] [PMID: 20470831]

[131] Qokoyi NK, Masamba P, Kappo AP. Proteins as targets in anti-schistosomal drug discovery and vaccine development. Vaccines (Basel) 2021; 9(7): 762.
[http://dx.doi.org/10.3390/vaccines9070762] [PMID: 34358178]

[132] Molehin AJ, McManus DP, You H. Vaccines for human schistosomiasis: recent progress, new developments and future prospects. Int J Mol Sci 2022; 23(4): 2255.
[http://dx.doi.org/10.3390/ijms23042255] [PMID: 35216369]

[133] Furlong ST. Unique roles for lipids in Schistosoma mansoni. Parasitol Today 1991; 7(2): 59-62.
[http://dx.doi.org/10.1016/0169-4758(91)90192-Q] [PMID: 15463424]

[134] Tendler M, Simpson AJG. The biotechnology-value chain: Development of Sm14 as a schistosomiasis vaccine. Acta Trop 2008; 108(2-3): 263-6.
[http://dx.doi.org/10.1016/j.actatropica.2008.09.002] [PMID: 18834847]

[135] Tendler M, Brito CA, Vilar MM, et al. A Schistosoma mansoni fatty acid-binding protein, Sm14, is the potential basis of a dual-purpose anti-helminth vaccine. Proc Natl Acad Sci USA 1996; 93(1): 269-73.
[http://dx.doi.org/10.1073/pnas.93.1.269] [PMID: 8552619]

[136] Santini-Oliveira M, Coler RN, Parra J, et al. Schistosomiasis vaccine candidate Sm14/GLA-SE: Phase 1 safety and immunogenicity clinical trial in healthy, male adults. Vaccine 2016; 34(4): 586-94.
[http://dx.doi.org/10.1016/j.vaccine.2015.10.027] [PMID: 26571311]

[137] Tendler M, Almeida MS, Vilar MM, Pinto PM, Limaverde-Sousa G. Current status of the Sm14/GLA-SE schistosomiasis vaccine: Overcoming barriers and paradigms towards the first anti-parasitic human(itarian) vaccine. Trop Med Infect Dis 2018; 3(4): 121.
[http://dx.doi.org/10.3390/tropicalmed3040121] [PMID: 30469320]

[138] Cardoso FC, Macedo GC, Gava E, et al. Schistosoma mansoni tegument protein Sm29 is able to induce a Th1-type of immune response and protection against parasite infection. PLoS Negl Trop Dis 2008; 2(10): e308.
[http://dx.doi.org/10.1371/journal.pntd.0000308] [PMID: 18827884]

[139] Alves CC, Araujo N, Bernardes WPOS, Mendes MM, Oliveira SC, Fonseca CT. A strong humoral immune response induced by a vaccine formulation containing rSm29 adsorbed to alum is associated with protection against Schistosoma mansoni reinfection in mice. Front Immunol 2018; 9: 2488.
[http://dx.doi.org/10.3389/fimmu.2018.02488] [PMID: 30450095]

[140] Mossallam SF, Amer EI, Ewaisha RE, Khalil AM, Aboushleib HM, Bahey-El-Din M. Fusion protein comprised of the two schistosomal antigens, Sm14 and Sm29, provides significant protection against Schistosoma mansoni in murine infection model. BMC Infect Dis 2015; 15(1): 147.
[http://dx.doi.org/10.1186/s12879-015-0906-z] [PMID: 25887456]

CHAPTER 6

Progress in Medicinal Chemistry for Neglected Tropical Diseases: A Focus on Denv Drug Discovery (2014-2023)

Sheikh Murtuja[1], Shilpa Chatterjee[1], Gourav Rakshit[2], Rajendra Prasad Chatterjee[3] and Mohd Usman Mohd Siddique[4,*]

[1] *Department of Pharmaceutical Technology, School of Health and Medical Science, Adamas University, Kolkata, WB, India*

[2] *Department of Pharmaceutical Sciences & Technology, Birla Institute of Technology, Mesra, Ranchi, JH, India*

[3] *National Institute of Cholera and Enteric Diseases, Indian Council of Medical Research, Kolkata, WB, India*

[4] *Department of Pharmacy, SVKM's Institute of Pharmacy, Dhule, MH, India*

Abstract: Dengue is still a major concern as we are yet to identify a potent inhibitor, and unfortunately, there is loss of life associated with this disease; however, the fatalities are low, but every year, dengue is an added burden to the medical infrastructure. In a world hit by COVID-19 pandemic, dengue is yet another serious burden. To date, we do not have any approved medicine to combat this disease. Symptomatic treatment to reduce the fever and intensive care facilities for critical patients is the only treatment protocol adopted as of now. Earlier, it was a disease of tropical nations of the world, but now it has been observed that it has extended its reach beyond the tropical and subtropical nations. The WHO data suggest that the year 2023 saw a record over 5000 reported cases of death due to dengue in about 80 countries across the world. These data further call for the urgency in identifying inhibitors for dengue. In the book chapter, we have compiled the efforts made so far in the last decade to give a DENV inhibitor. Our extensive survey of the literature indicated that protease of DENV was the most explored target and besides these targets like NS5 methyltransferase, RdRp, and E proteins did report few molecules. The success of proteases for drug discovery in diseases like HIV and HCV has encouraged researchers to exploit the DENV proteases. In this book chapter, we identified varying scaffolds contributing to the inhibition of Dengue virus and by different mechanisms.

Keywords: DENV, Dengue virus, E protein, HTS, HTVS, Molecular docking, NS5 methyltransferase, RdRp.

* **Corresponding author Mohd Usman Mohd Siddique:** Department of Pharmacy, SVKM's Institute of Pharmacy, Dhule, MH, India; E-mail: palladiumsalt@gmail.com

Igor Jose dos Santos Nascimento & Ricardo Olimpio de Moura (Eds.)

INTRODUCTION

Dengue fever, a mosquito-borne disease caused by the dengue virus, is now considered a global public health problem that threatens half of the world's population. According to the World Health Organization (WHO), more than 3.9 billion people are at risk of infection and more than 20,000 die each year [1 - 3]. There are four closely related serotypes of the dengue virus (DENV 1–4), which is a single-stranded RNA virus belonging to the Flaviviridae family. Even though over 80% of cases of dengue are often mild, certain patients may experience severe infections that can result in coagulopathy and plasma leakage, which can be fatal and affect organ function as well as circulatory shock [4] Given that there is no clinically approved antiviral medication to treat dengue infection, treatment options for dengue infection are now restricted to supportive measures including careful fluid delivery and close observation during the critical phase, with the projected annual cost of dengue illness reaching US$8.9 billion worldwide, this has major economic repercussions [5].

The positive-sense, single-stranded genomic RNA of the dengue virus is 11 kb long and codes for a precursor polyprotein(5′-C-prME-NS1-NS2A-NS2B- NS3-NS4A-NS4BNS5-3′), which is cleaved into three structural proteins (capsid protein C, membrane protein prM and envelope protein E) and seven nonstructural proteins (NS1, NS2a, NS2b, NS3, NS4a, NS4b and NS5). Among these, the human mediator of IRF3 activation (MITA), a crucial adaptor protein, is cleaved by the NS2B/NS3 protease complex, which hence suppresses the host type I interferon (IFN) pathway. The E protein is important in the host cell-mediated viral attachment and its fusion with the membrane of the host cell [6, 7]. Once the viral replicase complex is assembled, the polyprotein precursor is processed by NS2B/NS3 proteins [6–9]. The N- and C-terminal sections of the NS5 contain RNA methyltransferase (MTase) and RNA-dependent RNA-polymerase (RdRp) respectively which are fused through a 9-amino acid linker [6 - 9]. E, NS5, and NS2B/NS3 proteins are thought to be viable candidates for the discovery of antiviral therapies based on their essential roles [10, 11].

A promising alternative is the design of small molecules directed to the allosteric site. The allosteric sites of DENV NS2B/NS3pro and other DENV proteins have been examined in several publications in the literature to find more powerful inhibitors [12 - 17]. In DENV NS2B/NS3pro, this binding site is located behind the active site and is formed mainly by the residues NS3-Asp71, NS3-Lys73, NS3-Lys74, NS3-Trp83, NS3-Leu85, NS3-Gly87, NS3-Glu88, NS3-Trp89, NS3-Glu91, NS3-Thr118, NS3-Thr120, NS3-Val147, NS3-Leu149, NS3-Asn152, NS3-Val155, NS3-Ala164, NS3-Ile165 and NS3-Asn167 [12] Furthermore, during replication, the DENV RdRp plays a pivotal role in synthesizing both positive- and negative-stranded RNA [18 - 20]. It presents an appealing possibility for the development of novel antiviral medications because it has no mammalian counterpart and its sequence is conserved across all four serotypes with approximately 65% homology [21, 22].

While coming across research in the field of dengue, the most putative target was found to be dengue protease. To some extent, very few research groups have targeted RdRp, while we also came across a few E protein inhibitors. This book chapter aims to accommodate the progress made in the last 10 years while encompassing chemical entities/scaffolds reported by various researchers across the globe. This chapter outlines our efforts in this area, offering insight into potential directions for the advancement of antiviral treatments in the future and assisting in the battle against the dengue virus.

TARGETS FOR DENGUE

Several potential drug targets for the Dengue virus include:

NS2B/NS3 Protease

Inhibiting the NS2B/NS3 protease can disrupt viral polyprotein processing, preventing viral replication.

NS5 Protein

Targeting the NS5 containing MTase and RdRp domain can hinder the viral replication process.

E protein

Blocking host cell receptors, such as dendritic cell-specific intercellular adhesion molecule-3-grabbing non-integrin (DC-SIGN), can prevent viral entry into host cells.

Other Non-structural Proteins

Various viral proteins involved in RNA synthesis, such as NS1,NS2B, NS4A, and NS4B are potential targets for antiviral intervention.

Protease

The dengue virus protease (Fig. **1**) is a crucial enzyme involved in the replication process of DENV. This enzyme is responsible for cleaving the viral polyproteins, a necessary step in the formation of mature and infectious virions. The DENV protease is a serine protease that relies on a serine residue in its active site for its catalytic function. The primary role of this protease is to process the viral polyprotein precursor, which is initially translated from the viral RNA genome, essential for viral replication and assembly. This cleavage process is crucial for the proper maturation of viral proteins, enabling them to fulfill their functions in the viral life cycle. Inhibition of the dengue virus protease has emerged as a potential therapeutic strategy to impede viral replication and curb the progression of dengue infections. Researchers are actively exploring the structural and functional aspects of the dengue virus protease to identify potential inhibitors. These inhibitors aim to disrupt the protease's role in polyprotein processing, thereby hindering the formation of infectious dengue virus particles. Efforts in drug discovery against dengue protease involve a combination of computational approaches, structural biology, and medicinal chemistry. Rational drug design and high-throughput screening are employed to identify small molecules or peptides that can serve as effective inhibitors. Successful development of dengue protease inhibitors holds promise for the development of antiviral therapeutics against dengue infections, addressing a significant global health concern.

Dengue virus protease covalently bound to a peptide [23].

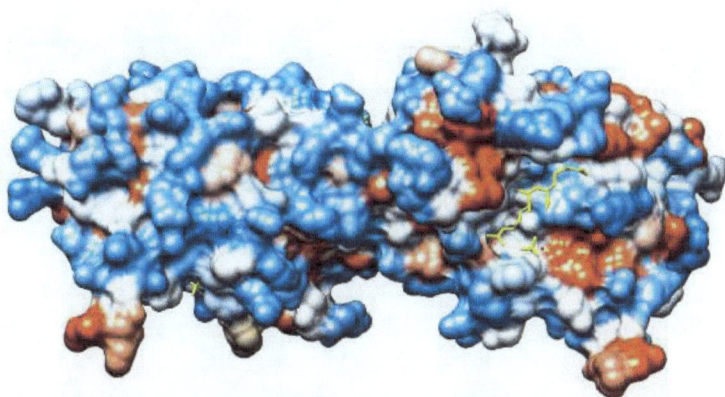

Fig. (1). Crystal structure of Dengue virus protease covalently bound to a peptide.

(hydrophobicity surface of protein & bound peptide inhibitor shown in yellow) [image generated using UCSF Chimera v17.3 [24]]

RdRp

The RDRP of DENV (Fig. **2**) is a multifunctional enzyme that plays a key role in the conversion of the viral RNA genome into replicative intermediates that serve as templates for the synthesis of new viral RNA strands. The enzyme achieves this by facilitating the complementary base pairing of nucleotides to the viral RNA template, resulting in the production of RNA strands that mirror the original genome. Given its crucial role in the viral life cycle, the DENV RdRp is a prime target for antiviral drug development. Inhibiting the activity of this enzyme is a strategy to disrupt viral replication and potentially curb the progression of dengue infections. Designing specific inhibitors that selectively bind to and interfere with the function of the RdRpis a focus of ongoing research in the field of antiviral drug discovery. Structural and functional studies of the Dengue virus RdRp are instrumental in understanding the enzyme's mechanisms and in designing effective inhibitors. Researchers employ various techniques, including X-ray crystallography, cryo-electron microscopy, and molecular modelling, to gain insights into the three-dimensional structure of the RdRp and to identify potential binding sites for inhibitors. Efforts to target the RdRp of Dengue virus represent a critical component of antiviral research, contributing to the development of therapeutics aimed at controlling Dengue infections. The goal is to discover and optimize compounds that can selectively inhibit the RDRP, offering a potential avenue for the treatment of Dengue viral infections.

PDB ID: 5F3Z

Dengue serotype 3 RNA-dependent RNA polymerase bound to PC-79-SH52 [25].

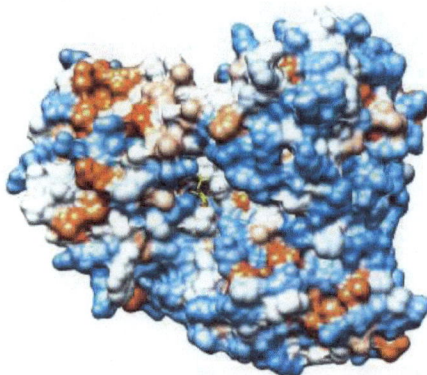

Fig. (2). Crystal structure of Dengue serotype 3 RNA-dependent RNA polymerase bound to PC-79-SH52 (hydrophobicity surface of protein & bound inhibitor shown in yellow) [image generated using UCSF Chimera v17.3 [24]].

Methyltransferase

Methyltransferases (Fig. **3**) play a crucial role in the replication and modification of the viral RNA. Methyltransferases are enzymes responsible for the transfer of methyl groups from a donor molecule to specific substrates, such as nucleic acids or proteins. In the context of the dengue virus, RNA methyltransferases are particularly important for the modification of the viral RNA genome. The dengue virus genome undergoes a series of modifications to ensure efficient replication and evasion of the host's immune response. One essential modification involves the addition of methyl groups to specific nucleotides within the viral RNA. This process is catalyzed by RNA methyltransferases, which facilitate the transfer of methyl groups from S-adenosylmethionine (SAM), a common methyl donor, to the RNA substrate. The methyltransferase activity is crucial for the stability of the viral RNA, modulation of host immune response evasion, and enhancement of viral replication. By methylating specific nucleotides, the virus can disguise its RNA from the host's immune surveillance, making it less recognizable to cellular sensors that typically detect foreign genetic material. Understanding the role of methyltransferases in dengue virus replication is important for the development of antiviral strategies. Targeting these enzymes could potentially disrupt the viral life cycle and limit the spread of the infection.

PDB ID: 3P8Z

Dengue Methyltransferase bound to a SAM-based inhibitor [26].

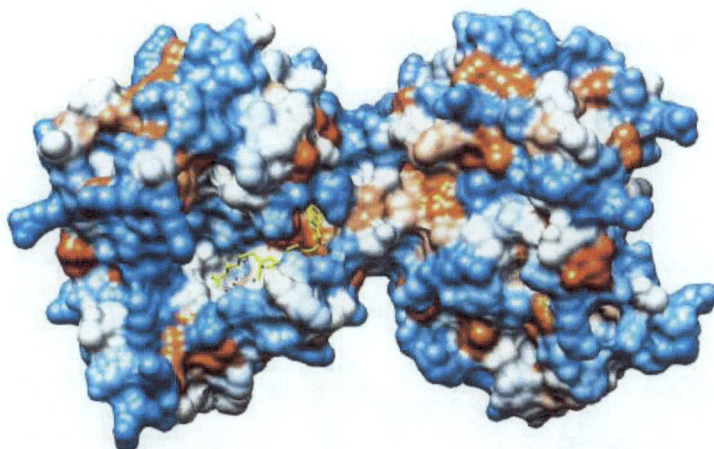

Fig. (3). Crystal structure of Dengue Methyltransferase bound to a SAM-based inhibitor.

(hydrophobicity surface of protein & bound inhibitor shown in yellow) [image generated using UCSF Chimera v17.3 [24]].

2.4E PROTEIN

The E protein of Dengue virus (Fig. **4**) is an attractive target for antiviral drug development due to its critical role in the viral life cycle, particularly in viral entry and fusion. Targeting the E protein offers a strategy to disrupt the infection process and inhibit viral replication. The following are key aspects of the E protein as a drug target:

Viral Entry Inhibition: The E protein is pivotal for mediating the fusion of the viral envelope with the host cell membrane during viral entry. Inhibiting this fusion process can prevent the release of the viral genome into the host cell, a crucial step in the establishment of infection [27].

Immunogenicity and Neutralization: The E protein is a major antigenic target, eliciting an immune response in the host. Antibodies generated against the E protein have the potential to neutralize the virus and protect against infection. This immunogenicity makes the E protein an attractive target for the development of vaccines to induce protective immunity.

Antibody-Dependent Enhancement (ADE): While the immune response against the E protein is critical for protection, it is important to note that ADE can occur. ADE is a phenomenon where non-neutralizing antibodies, instead of preventing infection, enhance viral entry into host cells [28].

PDB ID: 1OAN

Crystal structure of the dengue 2 virus envelope protein [29].

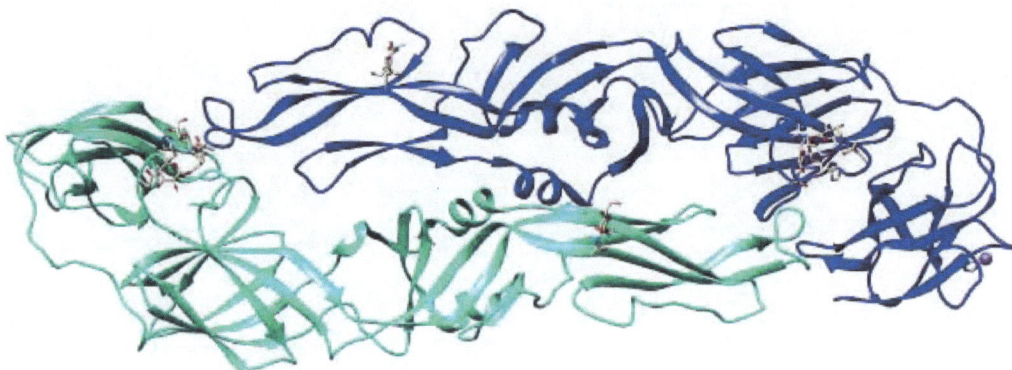

Fig. (4). Crystal structure of the dengue 2 virus envelope protein (chain representation) [image generated using UCSF Chimera v17.3 [24]].

This book chapter aims at providing the latest developments (in the last decade 2014-2023) pertaining to the targets of dengue. The main targets that were explored in the last decade were NS2B-NS3 protease, E protein, RNA-dependent-RNApolymerase and NS4B. All these targets have a significant role in the life cycle of the dengue virus.

INHIBITORS TARGETING PROTEASE

In the last two decades, this target, the protease, was the most explored one; DENV proteases have attracted researchers across the globe, and most of the work has been done on this target. The initial efforts were based upon the substrate mimics, which eventually led to the identification of tripeptide moieties, here we present the chronological progress of developing DENV protease inhibitors in the last decade (2014-2023).

In the year 2014, Behnam *et al.* reported substrate peptide conjugates, compound 1 (Fig. **5**) showed about 20 folds improvement (IC_{50}=0.6 µM) over the reference tripeptide (Bz-Arg-Lys-Nle-NH2, IC50=13.3 µM), their work involved the synthesis of thirty benzoyl capped tripeptides and application of fragment-based drug design approach through which eventually compound 1 was obtained [30].

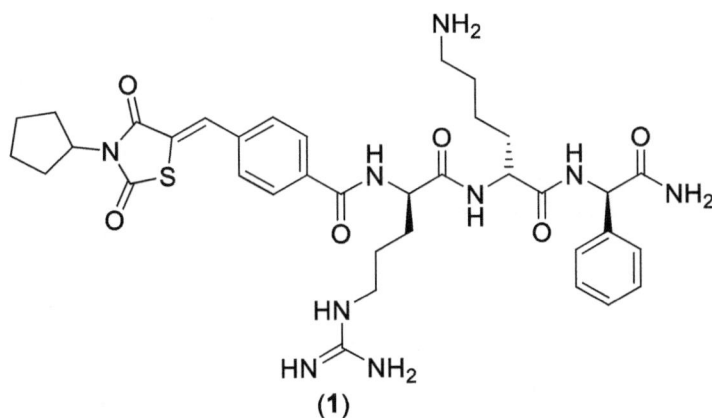

(1)

Fig. (5). Chemical structure of compound 1.

Further, Rothan *et al.*, in 2014, reported inhibitors from natural sources and screened nineteen traditional medicinal plant extracts which included, *Vernonia cinerea, Hemigraphisreptans, Hedyotis auricularia, Laurentia longiflora, Tridax procumbers* and *Senna angustifolia*. Their work identified Methanolic extract from *V. cinerea* leaves and ethanolic extract from *T. procumbers* stems showing good inhibitory activities with IC_{50} values of 23.7±4.1 and 25.6±3.8 µg/ml against DENV NS2B-NS3 protease, respectively. They believed that the activity was due to flavonoids [31].

Further, an HTS study performed by Liu *et al.* in 2014 (Fig. **6**) on a commercial library having approximately 7000 compounds identified a new lead, Thiadiazol pyrimidinone (compound **2)** (Fig. **6**). They attempted to synthesize this compound, however, in the process, a Transamidation product, thiadiazole acrylamide compound **3** (Fig. **6**) was formed and surprisingly the compound exhibited even better inhibitory activity than the cyclization product compound **2**. Amongst the synthesized analogues of thiadiazoloacrylamide, compound **4** (Fig. **6**) showed the best inhibitory activity against DENV2 NS2B-NS3 protease with an IC_{50} value of 2.24μM. Further modifications done to understand the significance of the linker enamide on the activity of the compound led to the synthesis of a dinitrile (compound **5**) and an olefin hydrogenation product (compound **6**) (Fig. **6**). Loss of activity indicated the significance of the enamide portion. Fig. (**6**), shows the schematic representation of the work. Docking studies were done for compound **4** and it was observed that one benzyl group attached to the thiadiazole group occupied the S3 pocket. The Benzyl group associated with the indole ring occupied the S2 pocket while the phenyl of the indole group occupied the S1 pocket [32].

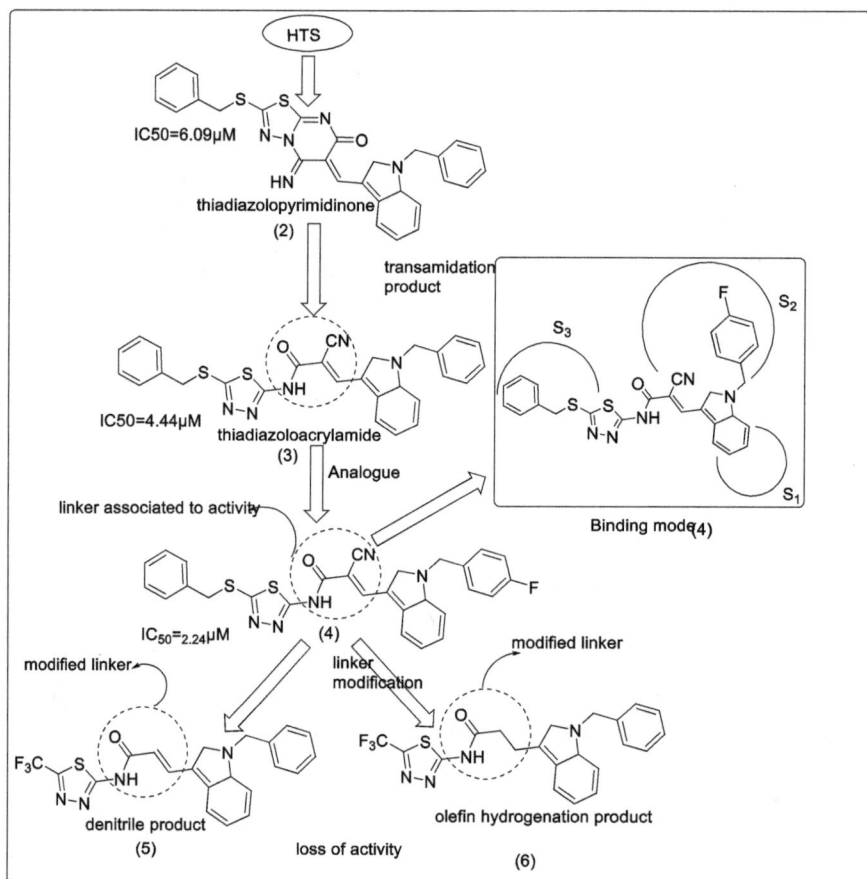

Fig. (6). Summary of Liu *et al.* work.

In 2014, Viswanathan *et al*. applied the HTVS approach and introduced their newly constructed and very efficient web-based drug discovery portal (DrugDiscovery@TACC) for structure-based drug discovery, The platform provided an option to screen multiple ligands for similar valid targets. Further, they independently screened two compiled virtual libraries against both, the inhibitor bound protease crystal structure (PDB 3U1I & 3U1J) and inhibitor devoid protease crystal structure (PDB 2FOM). The top-scoring Hits were further narrowed down to a few by applying suitable property filters and the resulting HITs were purchased from commercial sources and subjected to protease inhibition and protease kinetic assays. This exercise yielded a mixed non-competitive inhibitor, compound **7** (Fig. **7**) with a Ki value of 7µM.Drug-like properties of Compound **7** were calculated using the ORIS property calculator. Molecular modeling studies identified three hydrogen bonding interactions of the inhibitor with the amides of Gly133, Thr134, and Ser135. The hydrophobic interactions were shown by residues Val152, Val136, His51, Pro132, Asp129, Phe130, Tyr161, and Tyr150. The image was prepared using Ligplot+ [33].

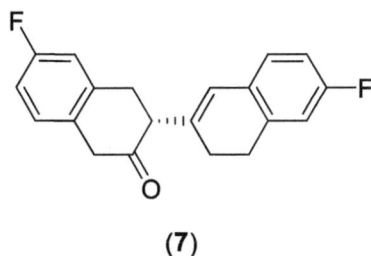

(7)

Fig. (7). Chemical structure of the compound 7.

In 2015, Weigel *et al*. designed substrate peptide analogues of the non-prime side, they observed a gap in the optimization of the S_2 pocket of the peptide hybrids and they found that previous modifications of peptide hybrids did not optimize the S_2 pocket, considering the target affinity [30, 34, 35]. In the process, arginine mimetic moieties were screened to eventually find a suitable replacement. For this, the already established tripeptide Bz-Arg-Lys-Phg-NH$_2$ (compound **8**) (Fig. **8**) was chosen [30] Further, several molecules were synthesized and in-vitrocharacterization was done and an arginine mimetic modification yielded a sub-micromolar range inhibitor against DENV2 NS2B NS3 protease. Following this, the cap was modified and, in the process, compound (**9**) Fig. (**8**) showing an IC$_{50}$ value of 0.21 µM and a K$_i$ value of 139 nM was obtained. A docking study of compound **9** was performed using protease crystal structure (PDB3U1I) wherein it was observed that arginine mimetic analog occupied the S_2 pocket the side chain of the lysine occupied the S_1 pocket, the N-terminal cap was positioned in the S_3 pocket, and the S_1'pocket was occupied by Phenylglycine [36].

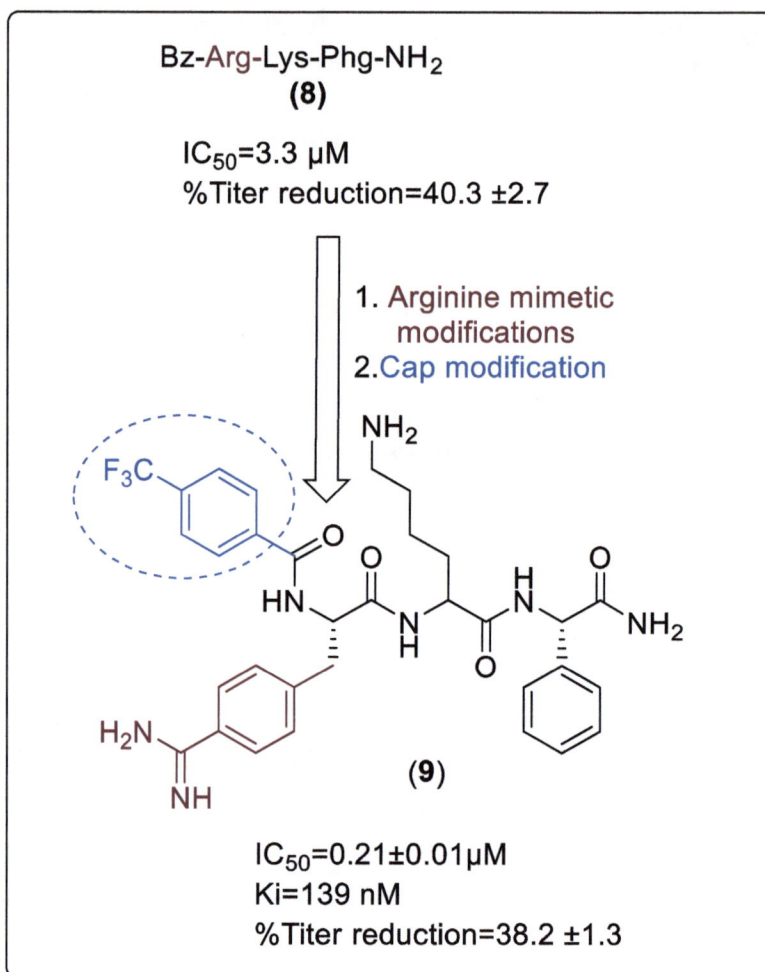

Fig. (8). Modification of Weigel *et al.*

Furthermore, Behnam *et al.* in 2015, explored their search for potential dual inhibitors of DENV and WNV protease and eventually went for the synthesis and biological evaluation of inhibitors housing benzyl ethers of 4-hydroxyphenylglycine in their structure as non-natural peptidic building blocks. For this purpose, a retro-peptide sequence (Bz-Arg-Lys-**Nle**-NH$_2$ **10**) (Fig. **9**), exhibiting good inhibitory activity against DENV2 protease was chosen as a template sequence [34]. Applying a small change in which Nle was substituted with Phg yielded compound **11** (Fig. **9**) having an IC$_{50}$ value of 3.32 μM [30]. Now this inhibitor witnessed a modification, yielding compound **12** (Fig. **9**), further, this compound was subjected to C-terminal and N-terminal modification, and followed by this, a fragment merging approach was applied, and eventually, two inhibitors (**13,14**) (Fig. **9**) having nano-molar affinity against DENV2 protease were identified. These inhibitors were also potent WNV protease inhibitors. Fig. (**9**). represents the schematic presentation of their work. Docking studies were performed using the crystal structure of DENV3 protease (PDB ID 3U1I) for compound **14** [37].

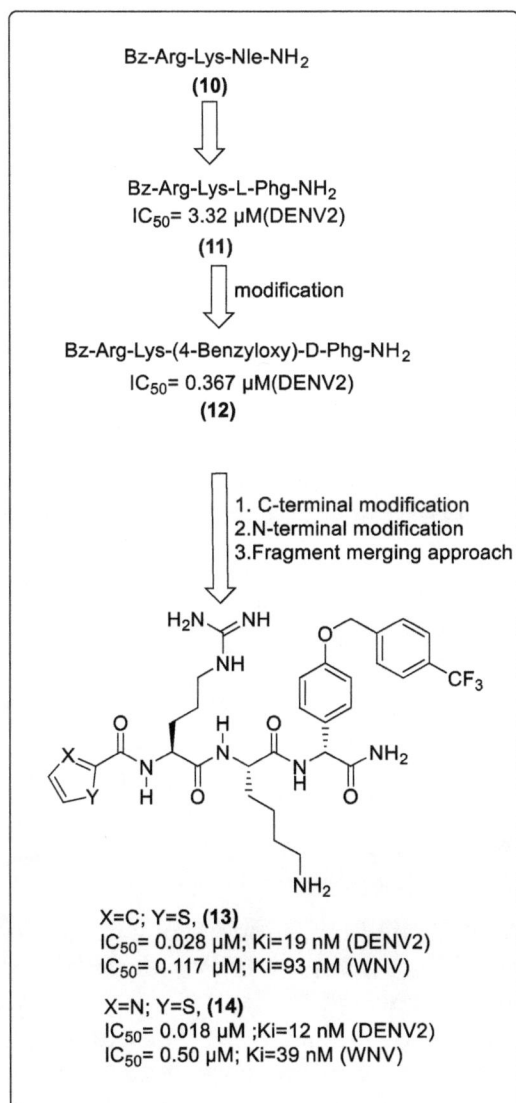

Bz-Arg-Lys-Nle-NH$_2$
(**10**)

Bz-Arg-Lys-L-Phg-NH$_2$
IC$_{50}$= 3.32 µM(DENV2)
(**11**)

modification

Bz-Arg-Lys-(4-Benzyloxy)-D-Phg-NH$_2$
IC$_{50}$= 0.367 µM(DENV2)
(**12**)

1. C-terminal modification
2. N-terminal modification
3. Fragment merging approach

X=C; Y=S, (**13**)
IC$_{50}$= 0.028 µM; Ki=19 nM (DENV2)
IC$_{50}$= 0.117 µM; Ki=93 nM (WNV)

X=N; Y=S, (**14**)
IC$_{50}$= 0.018 µM ;Ki=12 nM (DENV2)
IC$_{50}$= 0.50 µM; Ki=39 nM (WNV)

Fig. (9). Modifications of Behnam *et al*.

Further in 2015, Koh *et al*. in their effort at drug development, utilized the structure-guided optimization approach and modified a potent WNV protease inhibitor having an IC_{50} value of 0.105µM (compound **15**) (Fig. **10**), resulting in improved potency and selectivity for DENV protease. The selected WNV protease inhibitor was identified in an HTS exercise [38]. The resulting molecule, which was also a pyrazole ester derivative showed an IC_{50} value of 0.5± 0.1µM (compound **16**) (Fig. **10**), however, the ethereal modification (compound **17**) (Fig. **10**) showed a reduction in protease inhibition activity showing an IC_{50} value of 2.9 ± 0.5µM against DENV2 protease. Molecular docking studies were performed using DENV3 crystal structure (PDB ID 3U1I) with inhibitor **15**. The result of this drug development approach identified pyrazole ester derivatives as flaviviruses protease inhibitors and the takeaway point of this entire exercise (which included NMR validation of protein-inhibitor interaction) was that this inhibition was achieved using a targeted covalent modification of active site serine [39].

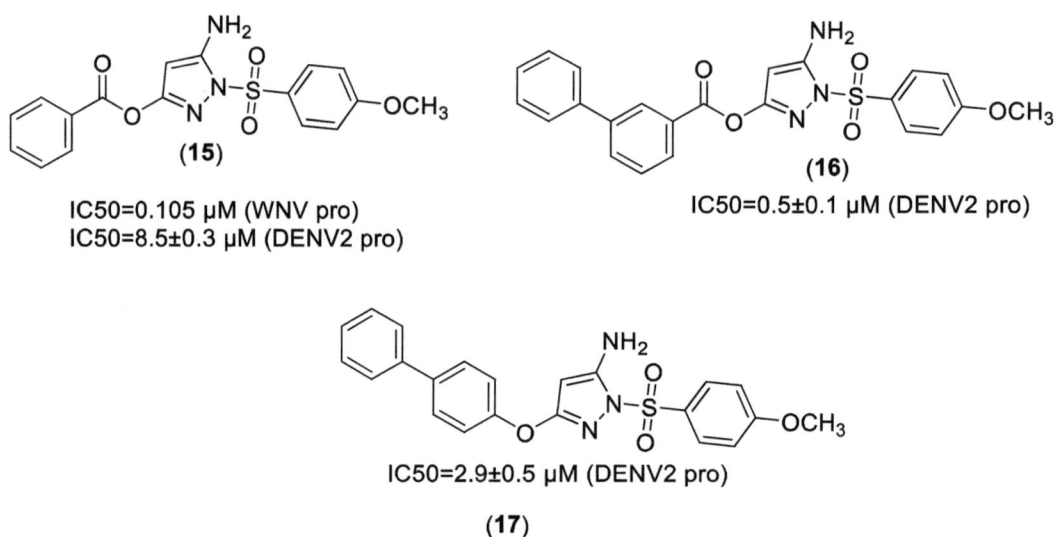

(15)

IC50=0.105 µM (WNV pro)
IC50=8.5±0.3 µM (DENV2 pro)

(16)

IC50=0.5±0.1 µM (DENV2 pro)

IC50=2.9±0.5 µM (DENV2 pro)

(17)

Fig. (10). Chemical structure of the compounds **15**, **16** and **17**.

In 2015, De Souse *et al.*, identified inhibitors from a natural source and evaluated six flavonoids for their DENV2 and DENV3NS2B-NS3 protease inhibition ability. Flavonoid, Agathisflavone (**18**, Fig. **11**) inhibited both the proteases of DENV2 and DENV3, and the IC_{50} values were found to be 15.1±2.2 and 17.5±1.4 µM, respectively. Docking studies of the same was done with DENV3 protease crystal structure, (PDB3U1I) [40].

(18)

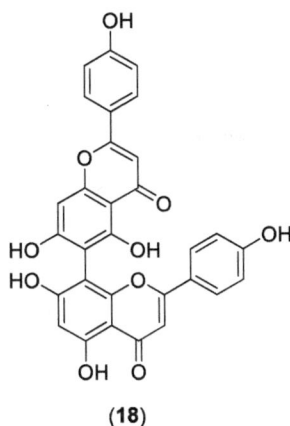

Fig. (11). Chemical structure of Agathisflavone **18**.

Further in 2015, Wu *et al.* performed an HTS exercise to identify compounds inhibiting DENV2-3 protease. This was done on their in-house library of about 250 compounds and a lead was eventually identified (compound **19**) (Fig. **12**). This compound was a diary this-ether derivative, several modifications were done on this lead in the anticipation of improved affinity against the DENV protease, as a result, seven analogues were synthesized, however, the best results were obtained for compound **20** (Fig. **12**) which showed IC_{50} value of 3.6±0.11 µM against DENV2 protease and displayed a non-competitive mode of inhibition [41].

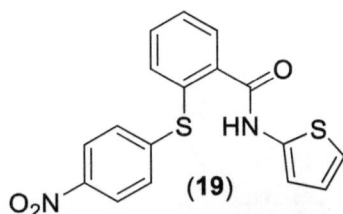

(19)

IC_{50}=31.8±4.5µM (DENV3 pro)
IC_{50}=98±4µM (DENV2 pro)
EC_{50}=3.5±0.3 µM (DENV2 pro)

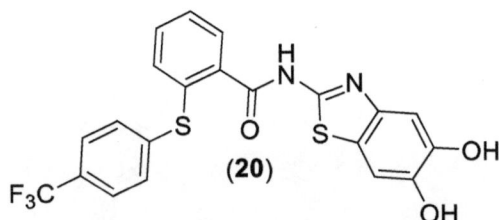

(20)

IC_{50}=9.1±1.02µM (DENV3 pro)
IC_{50}=3.6±0.11 µM (DENV2 pro)
EC_{50} >3µM (DENV2 pro)

Fig. (12). Chemical structure of the compounds **19** and **20**.

A very similar exercise was performed by Raut *et al.* in 2015, where they also screened their in-house library of approximately 1000 small molecules to identify DENV protease inhibitors. Compound **21** (Fig. **13**) which was a benzimidazole derivative displayed the best result as it inhibited all four serotypes in the cell-based assay and reduced the viral titer of DENV-1,2,3 and 4 by 50%, 83%, 75%, and 73% respectively. Further protease assay was also performed for this compound using cloned DENV-2 protease and the IC_{50} value was found to be 5.95 µM. The kinetic study suggested a mixed type of inhibition. Docking studies result indicated allosteric site binding [42].

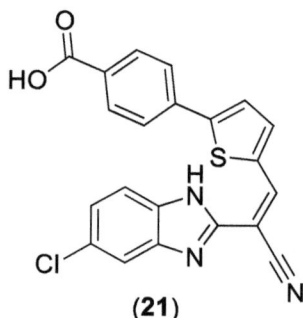

Fig. (13). Chemical structure of the compound **21**.

Furthermore, an HTVS approach to identify possible HIT against DENV 2 protease was attempted by Li *et al.* in 2015. They screened a library of 5 million compounds to identify small molecules of non-peptidic inhibitors. Based on the docking score, 14 compounds were evaluated and biological screening was performed. Compound **22** (Fig. **14**) displayed an EC_{50} value of 5.0µ. Mmolecular docking was performed for this compound using DENV3 crystal structure (PDB ID 3U1I) and the predicted binding affinity was found to be -10.65 Kcal/mole [43].

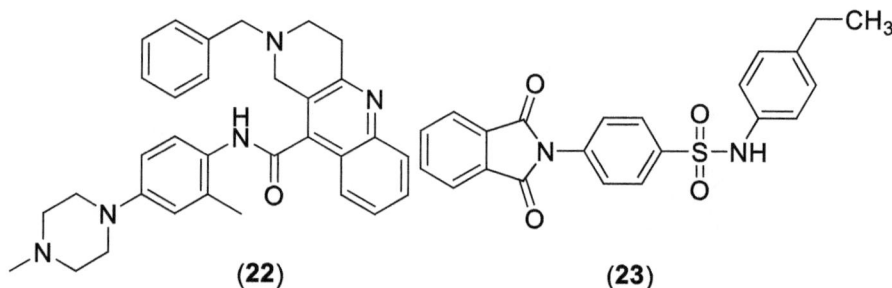

Fig. (14). Chemical structure of the compounds **22** and **23**.

Furthermore, another HTVS was performed by Timiri *et al.* in the year 2015 using the ZINC8 database. They performed the virtual screening and analyzed the top hundred compounds and eventually, decided to synthesize the phthalimide-sulphonamide derivatives of the 24 derivatives of 4-(1,3-dioxo-2,3-dihydo-1H-isoindol-2-yl) benzene- 1-sulphonamide. Compound **23** (Fig. **14**) showed considerable protease inhibition and the IC_{50} was found to be 48.2 μM. Further molecular docking was done and the predicted binding affinity was found to be - 5.12Kcal/mol [44].

Chu *et al.* in the year 2015 examined antiviral activities of 15 small molecules and peptide-based DENV2 S2B-NS3 protease inhibitors. Their work identified compound **24** (Fig. **15**), which was an anthraquinone derivative that showed promising results at 1 μM concentration. The compound reduced viral titer by more than 1 logPFU/ml. Also, it was not cytotoxic at this concentration [45].

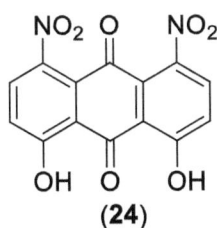

(24)

Fig. (15). Chemical structure of the compound **24**.

In an interesting work, Bhakta *et al.* in 2015 performed drug repurposing for identifying protease inhibitors of DENVNS2B-NS3, eventually nine peptidomimetics FDA-approved HIV/HCV inhibitors were analyzed through cell-based assay and *in silico* efforts. In the *in-silico* experiment , molecular docking and further MD were done. Docking was done using DENV3 protease crystal structure (PDB ID 3U1I) and the results revealed that these molecules bound the active site of the DENV NS2B NS3 protease inhibitors and Nelfinavir(compound **25**) (Fig. **16**) showed a binding affinity of (-8.9 kcal/mo. The *in silico* results corroborated with the cell-based antiviral assay results and the determined EC_{50} value for Nelfinavir was found to be 3.5 ± 0.4 μM, while the SI value was 4.6 this activity was the best among the nine selected inhibitors [46].

In a similar effort, Wu *et al.* in 2015 tested the potential of a topical hemostatic and antiseptic, pilocresulen for the DENV 2NS2B NS3 protease inhibition ability. This was chosen from their in-house library of approximately 1000 old drugs. Pilocresulen inhibited DENV2 protease competitively and the IC_{50} value was found to be 0.48 μg/mL. It also inhibited DENV 2 replication with an IC_{50} value of 4.99 μg/mL. Further docking studies were performed using NS2B NS3 protease model (PDB ID 2M9Q). Policresulen is not one entity but a mixture of various chemical entities and compound **26** (Fig. **16**) represents its main component [47].

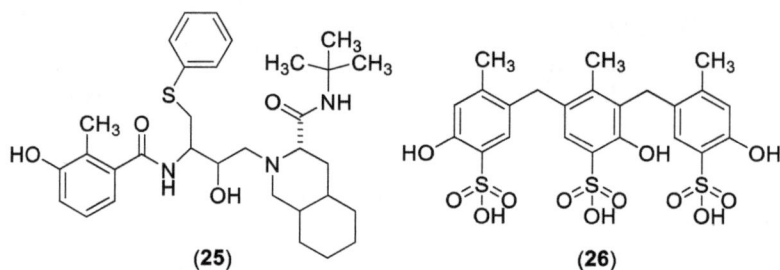

Fig. (16). Chemical structure of the compounds **25** and **26**.

In 2016 Dwivedi *et al.* showed the importance of triterpenoids as DENV NS2B NS3 protease inhibitors in their *in silico* study. They reported the binding affinity of Nimbin (-5.56 Kcal/mol), desacetylnimbin (−5.24 Kcal/mol), and desacetylsalannin (−3.43 Kcal/mol) from the docking studies done on the DENV crystal structure, PDB ID 2VBC. Nimbin's (compound **27**) (Fig. **17**) high binding affinity accounted for its interaction with the residues of the catalytic triad through hydrogen bonds besides other interactions such as hydrophobic interactions with the other residues of the protease [48].

In yet another effort, in 2016, Lee *et al.* reported dengue inhibitors from natural origin. They identified predinin (compound **28**) (Fig. **17**), which shares similarities with carotene. It inhibited DENV2 replication with an EC_{50} of 4.5±0.46 μM, and the EC_{50} for DENV 1,3, and 4 was found to be in the range of 5.84-7.62 μM. Further it showed DENV2 protease inhibition and the obtained EC_{50} was 8.5±0.41 μM [49].

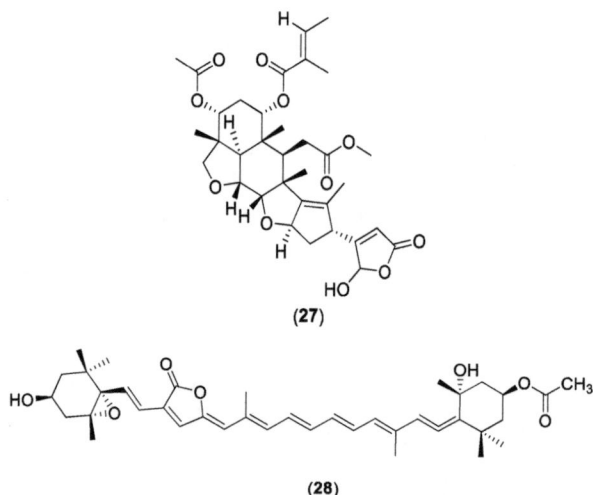

Fig. (17). Chemical structure of the compounds **27** and **28**.

An HTS exercise was performed by Balasubramanian *et al.* in 2016 to identify potent DENV protease inhibitors. About 1,20,000 compounds were screened and compounds **29** and **30** (Fig. **18**) were found to inhibit DENV1-4 protease with an IC_{50} ranging between 0.64–1.15μM and 0.13–0.77μM respectively. While for compound **29,** the EC_{50} value for DENV2 replication inhibition was found to be 2.29±0.3 μM. These compounds were competitive inhibitors of DENV2 protease and the docking studies predicted their binding to the active site. The identified compound belonged to the polyphenolic and catechol class [50].

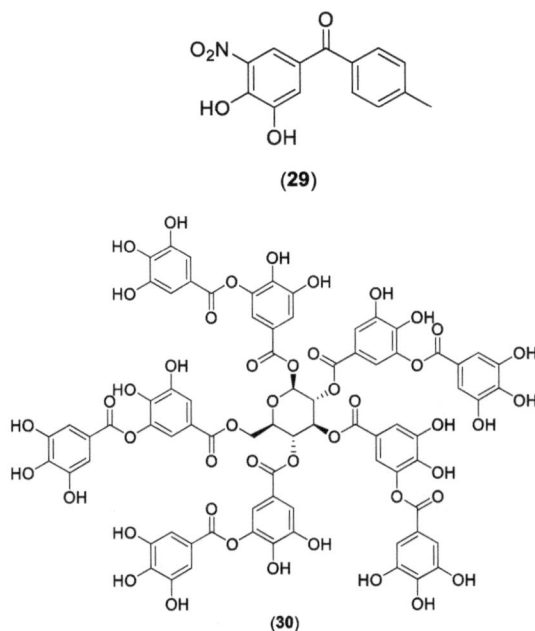

(29)

(30)

Fig. (18). Chemical structure of the compounds **29** and **30**.

Lin *et al.* in 2017 reported a cyclic peptide based on the structure of aprotinin. Aprotinin showed a high affinity for DENV2 protease, which is well reflected by its K_i value (26.9nM). In their study, they exploited the significance of the prime side in affecting DENV protease binding affinity [51] and designed cyclic peptides showing binding interactions with both the sides of the active site of the protease. Their design was based on the structure of aprotinin having two loops linked with a glycine linker. They designed various cyclic peptides based on this and ultimately the best activity was obtained for a cyclic peptide (compound **31**) (Table **1**) which had P3-P3'residues. PCRARI in their binding loop while the second loop residues included YGGCA (from residue 35-39), the structure was devoid of glycine linker and the K_i value reported against wild-type DENV3 protease was 2.9 μM [52].

Table 1. Cyclic peptide designed by Lin *et al.*

Binding loop (loop1) residues							No glycine linker	Loop 2 residues					K_i
Cyclic peptide (Compound 31)	P	C*	R	A	R	I#		Y#	G	G	C*	A	2.9±0.8 µM
Cyclic structure attained due to peptide bond(#) and disulphide bond(*)between the residues													

In the year 2017, Takaji *et al.* reported a cyclic peptide for DENV2 NS2B NS3 protease inhibition. Molecular docking was performed for this structure and it was found that the inhibitor (compound **32**) (Fig. **19**) acquired a β turn-like conformation inside the protease. The IC_{50} value for this inhibitor was 0.95µM. However, the molecule showed poor antiviral activity, possibly due to the high hydrophilicity of the cyclic peptide. The side chain hydrophilicity prevented the permeability of the inhibitor in the antiviral assay [53].

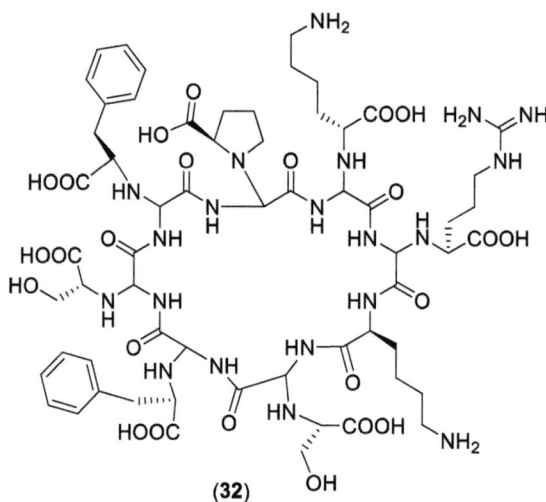

(32)

Fig. (19). Chemical structure of compound **32**.

In the same year, Pelliccia *et al.* using the HTVS approach identified allosteric inhibitors against DENV NS2B-NS3 protease. Their work led to the designing and synthesis of various compounds amongst which compound **33** (Fig. **20**) showed considerable EC_{50} values in the cell-based (6.7 ± 0.78µM) and enzyme-based assay (4.7 ± 0.3µM) [54].

Further in the year 2017, Gan *et al.* applied a rational approach and identified two inhibitors showing good antiviral activity against DENV2. The EC_{50} value of these piperidinyl derivatives was found in the low micromolar range. For compound **34** (Fig. **21**), the value was 3.2 µM while for compound **35** (Fig. **21**), it was 2.4 µM. However, these molecules failed as potent DENV protease inhibitors as the IC_{50} values were on the higher side [55].

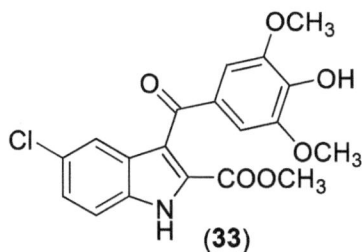

Fig. (20). Chemical structure of compound **33**.

A similar rational approach was applied by Osman *et al.* in 2017 wherein they exploited the benefits of α, β-unsaturated ketones for the DENV protease inhibition. Piperidone moiety was incorporated into the α, β-unsaturated ketone system. Further DENV protease inhibition assay was performed and the IC_{50} value for the best compound (**36**) (Fig. **21**) among the ten synthesized compounds was found to be 15.2µmol/L. Molecular docking was done using DENV2 crystal structure (PDB ID 2FOM) and the inhibitor was predicted to occupy the active site [56].

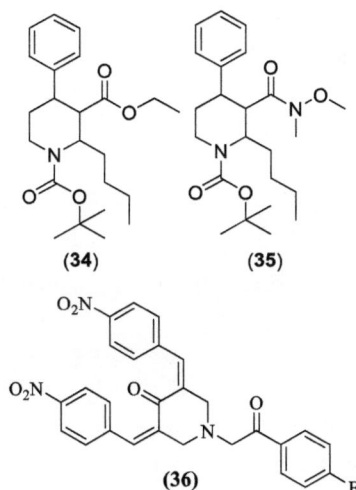

Fig. (21). Chemical structure of compounds **34**, **35**, and **36**.

Weng *et al.* took the opportunity of modifying a previously reported DENV2NS2B NS3 protease inhibitor [57], a linear dipeptide that showed an IC_{50}

value of 1.2 ± 0.4 µM (compound **37**) (Fig. **22**). Eventually, a new series of fused bicyclic compounds of pyrrolidino [1,2-c] imidazolidinone derivatives were synthesized and these were evaluated for DENV NS2B NS3 protease inhibition and wild-type DENV2 virus. Compound **38** (Fig. **22**) showed a very similar IC_{50} against the DENV2 protease (1.2 ± 0.4 µM) as that of the linear dipeptide, also the EC_{50} was found to be 39.4 ± 6.2 µM and this value too was quite close to the value of EC_{50} obtained for compound **37** (38.7 ± 5.4 µM). This study provided a new non-peptidic scaffold that could be explored for future DENV drug discovery. Further, a molecular docking study was done using DENV2 protease crystal structure (PDB ID 2FOM) to understand the binding interactions [58].

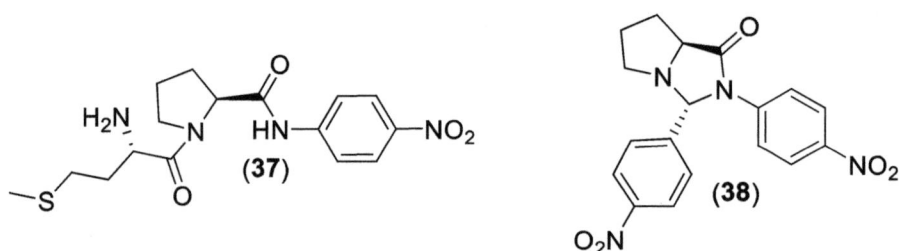

Fig. (22). Chemical structure of the compounds **37** and **38**.

In the year, 2018 a rational approach was applied by Padampriya *et al.* to identify inhibitors for DENVas they were encouraged by the antiviral role of thiosemicarbazones. Eventually, they synthesized thiosemicarbazone derived phenyl-acetyl derivatives, compound **39** (Fig. **23**) showed antiviral activity against the DENV2 serotype. Using DENV2 protease crystal structure (PDB ID 2FOM), an effort was made to understand the binding interaction and the study revealed the occupancy of the inhibitor near the active site [59].

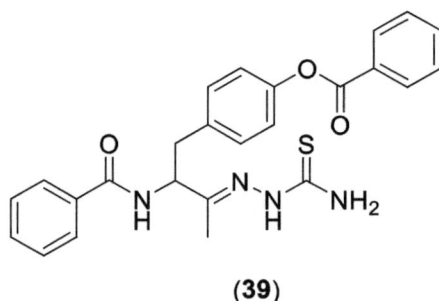

(39)

Fig. (23). Chemical structure of compound **39**.

Further, Li *et al.* in 2018 adopted a drug repurposing approach to identify DENV protease inhibitors. They reported Erythrocin B (compound **40**) (Fig. **24**), which is an FDA-approved food additive as a DENV protease inhibitor. IC_{50} value reported for this compound was found to be15μM and it was found to be a non-competitive inhibitor inhibiting the interaction of DENV2 NS2B & NS3. Further viral plaque reduction assay experiment gave an EC_{50} value of 1.2 μM against DENV2 [60].

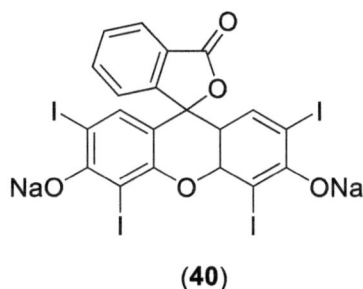

(40)

Fig. (24). Chemical structure of compound **40**.

In the year 2019, Hariono *et al.*, performed HTVS and identified a HIT against DENV2 NS2B-NS3 protease, which showed an IC_{50} value of 62 μM experimentally against DENV2 NS2B-NS3 protease. Further, this compound was modified and the resulting thioguanine scaffold (compound **41**) (Fig. **25**) gave much better results as the determined IC_{50} for this compound was found to be 0.38 μM [61].

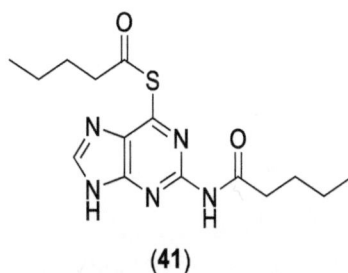

(41)

Fig. (25). Chemical structure of compound **41**.

Balasubramanian *et al.* in 2019 synthesized four analogues of curcumin and evaluated the *in vitro* DENV protease efficiency, the analogues displayed a very moderate IC_{50} ranging between 36.23μM –60.98μM. However, the results of the DENV replication inhibition were quite encouraging and compound **42** (Fig. **26**) showed an EC_{50} value of 8.07±1.52μM and EC_{50}value for plaque assay was found to be 2.34±0.21μM. Further compound **43** (Fig. **26**), a cyclopentanone analog of curcumin displayed a better selectivity index (16.27) and was found to be less toxic [62].

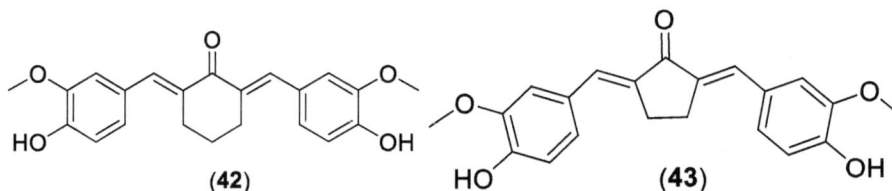

Fig. (26). Chemical structure of the compounds **42** and **43**.

In 2019, Sunderman *et al.* explored a previously reported structure [63]. compound **44 (a** dibasic 4-guanidinobenzoate) (Fig. **27**), which exhibited DENV2 protease inhibition in a low micro-molar range. They applied modifications rationally [64] and therefore introduced modifications like replacing the ester group with amide and introducing carbamates between two aromatic rings. Eventually, they synthesized 19 analogues but none of the modifications produced good results when they were evaluated against both the DENV and WNV protease [65].

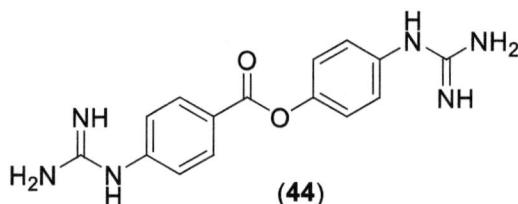

Fig. (27). Chemical structure of the compounds **44**.

In 2020, Dwivedi *et al.*, explored the anti-dengue properties of *Azadirachtaindica* and performed virtual screening on 49 previously reported bioflavonoids. The top four compounds identified as potent DENV NS2B NS3 protease inhibitors based on docking score were kaempferol-3-O-rutinoside (compound **45**,-9.55Kcal/mol), rutin (-9.32Kcal/mol), hyperoside (-7.87Kcal/mol) and epicatechenin (compound **46**,-7.62 Kcal/mol) (Fig. **28**). Further cell viability and *in vitro* antiviral studies were done for the reference compound quercetin, kaempferol-3-O-rutinoside, and epicatechin and it was found that kaempferol-3-O-rutinoside proved to be strong DENV infection inhibitor (77.7% at 100 µM conc.) while epicatechenin (66.2% at 1000 µM conc.) was a moderate inhibitor when compared to the reference quercetin [66].

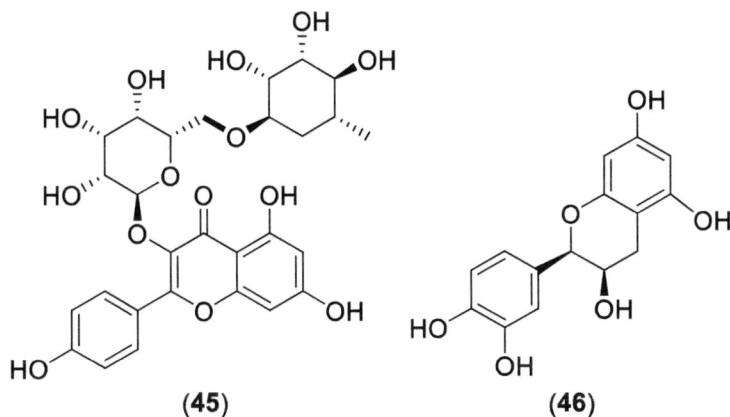

Fig. (28). Chemical structure of the compounds **45** and **46**.

In 2020, Kuhl *et al.* approached rationally towards identifying non-peptidic small-molecule inhibitors of DENV2 protease. Eventually, they synthesized fifty-five derivatives of 4-benzyloxyphenylglycine. In their designed molecule, different variants were produced by a fragment merging approach supported with biochemical assays to put appropriate residues at appropriate places. Finally, compound **47** (Fig. 29) showed an EC_{50} value of 0.49±0.08µM in the DENV2 protease HeLa activity. Compound **47** appeared to be L-isomer while its D-isomer was 20-fold less potent. Further molecular docking studies were done to understand the binding mode using DENV 3 NS2B NS3 crystal structure (PDB ID 3U1I) [67].

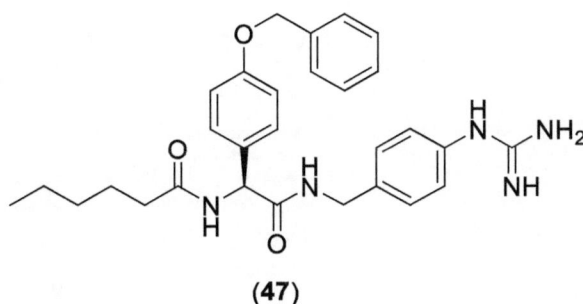

(47)

Fig. (29). Chemical structure of the compounds **47**.

Very recently in 2023 Behrouz *et al.* reported potent peptidic inhibitors of DENV2 protease housing a sulfonyl moiety as the N-terminal cap,thissulfonamide-peptide hybrid showed nanomolar affinity against DENV-2 protease and their *Ki* reported for compound **48** (Fig. **30**) was 78 nM against DENV-2 protease while the IC_{50} was found to be 0.12±0.4µM [68].

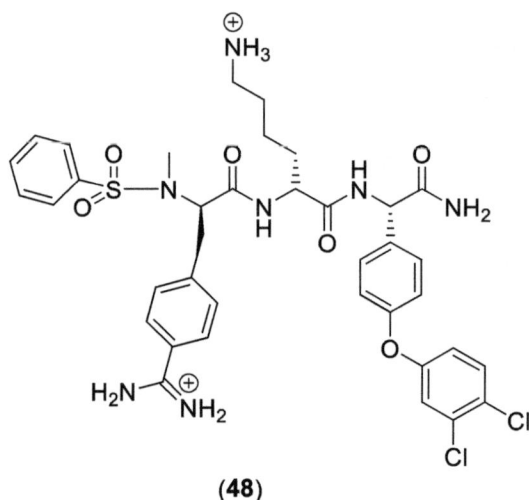

(48)

Fig. (30). Chemical structure of the compounds **48**.

INHIBITORS TARGETING RdRp

Over the past decade, there has been an increase in interest in DENV NS5 protein, and mainly several RNA-dependent RNA polymerase (RdRp) inhibitors have been identified.A study performed by Xu *et al*. identified an active-site metal ion chelator (compound **49**) (Fig. **31**) that acts against DENV NS5 polymerase by inhibiting viral RdRp activity of DENV serotypes 1 to 4 with EC_{50} of <3 µM and IC_{50} of 5-6.7 µM [69] Another study performed by Yokokawa *et al*. in 2016, identified one promising allosteric inhibitor of DENV RdRp (compound **50**) (Fig. **31**), which demonstrated substantial activity against all clinically relevant dengue virus serotypes with IC_{50} value of 0.172 µM and EC_{50} of 1.8-2.3 µM [70].

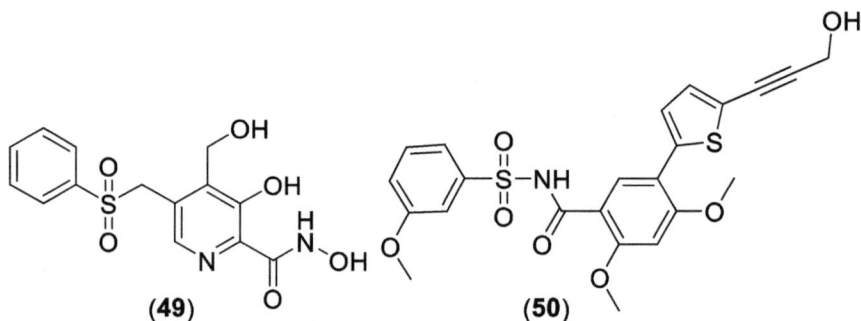

(49)   (50)

Fig. (31). Chemical structure of the compounds **49** and **50**.

Lim *et al*. performed a fragment-based screening on DENV NS5 polymerase and designed a few potent allosteric DENV NS5 inhibitors targeting the RdRp N pocket (allosteric binding pocket), which showed EC_{50} values in the range of 1–2 µM against all four DENV serotypes in cell culture assays. This range of EC_{50} was achieved by adopting a design strategy where the acyl sulphonamide replaced the charged acidic groups. Compound **51** (Fig. **32**) was the most active compound of the series, with an 8-quinolinol scaffold, and displayed IC_{50} values ranging between 0.013-0.038µM across DENV1-4 polymerase, while theEC$_{50}$ value for this compound was 1.9±0.2 µM in the DENV2 replicon cell-based assay [71].

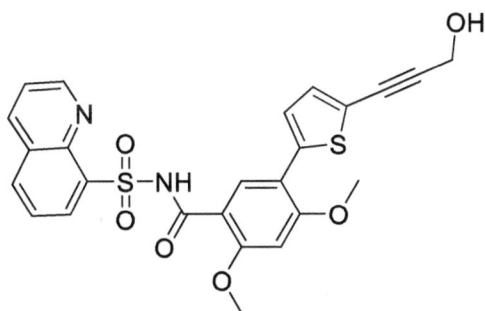

(51)

Fig. (32). Chemical structure of the compounds **51**.

In the year 2016, Manvar *et al*. reported thiazolidinone-thiadiazole derivative (Compound **52**) (Fig. **33**) as another DENV2 NS5 RdRp inhibitor with IC_{50} of 2.1 ± 0.4 µM [72].

Cannalire *et al*. in 2018, further carried out a virtual screening study against DENV RdRp and identified a new potent pyridobenzothiazole derivative (compound **53**) (Fig. **33**) inhibitor against DENV3 with an IC50 value of 0.6 µM [73].

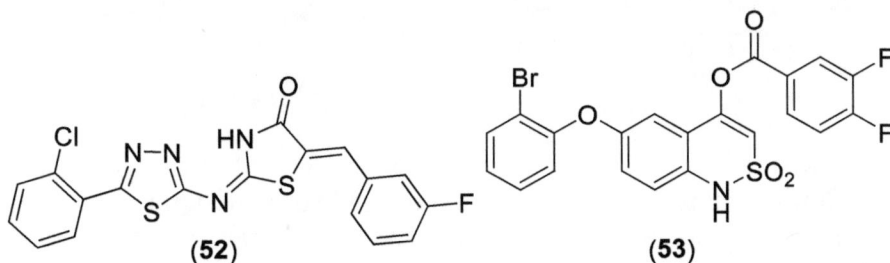

(52)   **(53)**

Fig. (33). Chemical structure of the compounds **52** and **53**.

In the year 2019, Shimizu *et al.*, screened 16240 small molecule inhibitors for their ability to inhibit DENV 2 NS 5 RdRp, this *in vitro* exercise identified compound **54** (Fig. **34**) which showed an EC_{50} value of 6.0μM. Further studies identified that this molecule bound two sites in DENV RdRp, the first site was the thumb domain while the second site was located within the active site [74].

(54)

Fig. (34). Chemical structure of the compounds **54**.

Zong *et al.* in 2023 identified a few small molecules as NS5RdRp inhibitors. Among these molecules, compound **55** and compound **56** (Fig. **35**) showed similar or superior activity against DENV2, with IC_{50} values of 3.58 ± 0.29 μM and 23.94 ± 1.00 μM, respectively [75].

(55)   **(56)**

Fig. (35). Chemical structure of the compounds **55** and **56**.

INHIBITORS TARGETING NS5 METHYL TRANSFERASE

Aouadi *et al.* in the year 2017 performed a screening of Prestwick Chemical Library® of 2000 compounds, which included 1280 FDA-approved drugs to identify methyltransferase inhibitors against some important viruses which also included DENV. They screened 20 compounds using dengue NS5 methyltransferase and human RNA *N*7-methyltransferase (hRNMT) and the screening results showed 98.9% and 97.8% inhibition for compound **57** and compound **58** (Fig. **36**) at 50 μM concentration for DENV NS5 methyltransferase, respectively. A limitation demanded an optimization in the structure for these two compounds as it inhibited hRNMT too [76].

Fig. (36). Chemical structure of the compounds **57** and **58**.

In 2017, Benmansour *et al.* identified a NS5 methyltransferase inhibitor of DENV in a rational way composed of a systematic approach. They applied fragment-based screening on a library of 500 fragments followed by fragment-based X-ray crystallographic screening resulting in the identification of a few fragments, these fragments were subjected to an enzyme assay, and then the approach of merging these fragments computationally was followed in the anticipation of forming a compound with increased affinity against Methyltransferase. Eventually, a new structure of non-nucleoside inhibitors of flavivirus Methyltransferase was designed and 41 analogues of it were synthesized. Compound **59** (Fig. **37**) displayed the best activity with an IC50 value of 91μM against NS5 methyltransferase. Further, this compound showed no toxicity at 100 mM concentration [77].

Fig. (37). Chemical structure of the compounds **59**.

Further in 2018, Yao *et al.* identified compound **60** (Diasarone I) (Fig. **38**) showing an antiviral effect against dengue. This compound was obtained from the ethanolic extract of rhizomes of *Acorus tatarinowii Schott* (*A. tatarinowii*). Compound **60** showed ant dengue activity for DENV 1,2 and 4 with an EC_{50} value of 4.27, 4.5, and 4.54 μM respectively. The docking studies indicated good affinity of this compound with 2' -*O* methyltransferase of NS5 (docking score- 7.2 kcal/mol), after analyzing the binding interaction they established that the anti-DENV activity was due to the inhibition of NS5 methyltransferase [78].

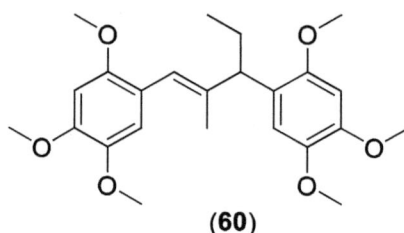

(60)

Fig. (38). Chemical structure of the compounds **60**.

In the year 2019, Hernandez *et al.* modified compound **59** (see Fig. **37**) reported by Benmansour *et al.* and eventually synthesized nitro-sulfonamide ester derivative (compound **61**) and aniline-sulfone ester derivative (compound **62**) (Fig. **39**). Further these compounds were evaluated by *in vitro* DenV-3 2' -*O*-Methyltransferase assays. The IC_{50} values reported for these compounds were found to be 24 and 26μM, which was better than compound **59** [79].

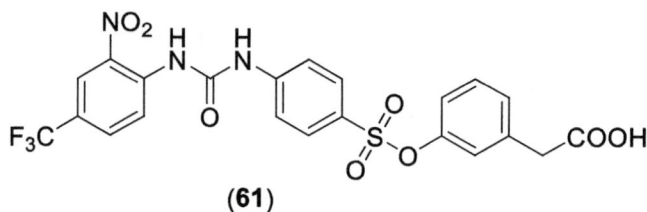

(61)

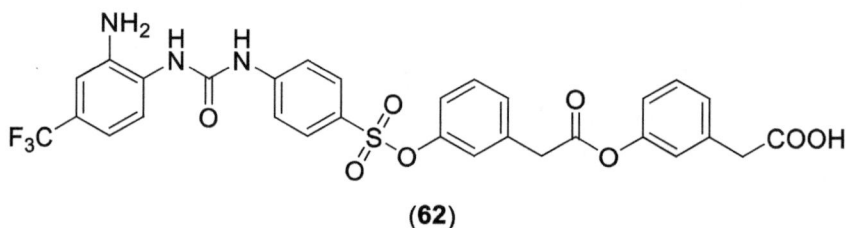

(62)

Fig. (39). Chemical structure of the compounds **61** and **62**.

Furthermore, Spizzichino *et al.* in 2020 performed structure-based virtual screening and identified carbazoyl-aryl-urea compounds as new DENV NS5 Methyltransferase inhibitors. The HIT, compound **63** (Fig. **40**) was subjected to *in vitro* against DENV NS5 MTase, assay and showed an IC50 value of 38 μM. Further this structure was optimized and eventually, many analogues were synthesized and subjected to the same assay and displayed IC_{50} values ranging between (38-267 μM). Amongst the derivatives, only the best IC_{50} value was shown by compound **64** (Fig. **40**) and thus provided a scaffold around which future modifications could be done to obtain a potent NS5 methyltransferase inhibitor [80].

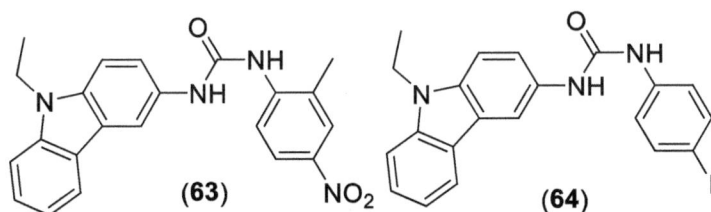

Fig. (40). Chemical structure of the compounds 63 and 64.

INHIBITORS TARGETING E PROTEIN

In the year 2014, Panya *et al.* reported that n-octyl-β-D-glycoside (BOG) or hydrophobic pocket of DENV Envelop (E) protein is important for the protein-ligand interaction. In this study, the researchers designed a few small peptides that specifically bind to the hydrophobic pocket of the E protein. Among them, Lys-Glu-Asn (compound **65**) and Glu-Phe (compound **66**) showed promising effects against DENV with IC_{50} of 331.9 μM and 96.50 μM respectively [81] Further, in 2015, Jadav *et al.* in their work designed a few pyrazoline and thiazolyl hydrazine analogues targeting DENV E protein and identified a potent inhibitor, compound **67** (Fig. **41**) with an EC_{50} value of 1.32 ± 0.41μM in the virus yield reduction assay done for DENV-2 [82].

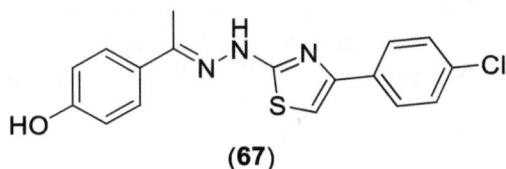

Fig. (41). Chemical structure of the compounds 67.

Further, Budigi *et al.* 2018 tested the ability of VIS513, an engineered cross-neutralizing humanized antibody targeting the DENV E protein domain III, to overcome antibody-enhanced infections and high but brief viremia, which are commonly encountered in dengue patients, in various *in vitro* and *in vivo* models. They observed that VIS513 efficiently neutralizes DENV at clinically relevant viral loads or in the presence of enhancing levels of DENV immune sera [83].

Further in the year 2020, Yamamoto *et al.* reported an *in vitro* quantitative mosquito-cell-based membrane-fusion assay for the E protein using dual split proteins (DSPs). DSP assay is a useful means of studying the mechanism of membrane fusion in Flaviviruses. In their assay, it was seen that the antimalarial drug atovaquone (compound **68**) (Fig. **42**) blocked the *in vitro* infection of mammalian cellsby Zika viruses as well as by the four DENV serotypes. The IC_{90} for DENV1-4 inhibition was in the range of 1.6–2.5 µM [84].

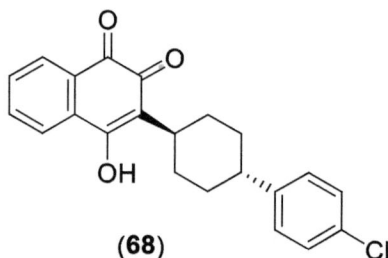

Fig. (42). Chemical structure of the compounds **68**.

In the year 2022, Hour *et al.* synthesized a library of the known and novel Glycyrrhizic acid (GL) derivatives bearing amino acid residues or their methyl/ethyl esters in the carbohydrate part and studied their DENV inhibition ability *in vitro* using the cytopathic effect (CPE), viral infectivity and virus yield assays with DENV-2 in Vero E6 and A549 cells. Two GL derivatives, compounds**69** and **70** (Fig. **43**) showed good antiviral activity with IC_{50} values of 0.5±0.0.17 µM and 0.18±0.01in Vero E6 cells and 0.12±0.028 µM and µM1.56±0.49 µM in A549 cells, respectively. Docking results showed that Compounds **69** and **70** showed hydrophobic interactions in the hydrophobic pocket lying at the interfaces of Domains I, II, and the stem region of the DENV2 envelope (E) protein. Further these two molecules open avenues for developing DENV E protein inhibitors with this approach [85].

MISCELLANEOUS

Given that NS4B is an indispensable element of the viral replication complex, an inhibitor may work by preventing protein-protein interactions from occurring when the virus is making RNA, and that makes NS4B a potent antiviral target. A study by Wang *et al.* in 2015 identified a number of spiropyrazolopyridone scaffolds as an effective inhibitor of NS4B of DENV-2 and -3 and among them, compound **71** (Fig. **44**) showed potent antiviral activity against DENV withEC$_{50}$ value of 0.042 ± 0.016 µM [86].

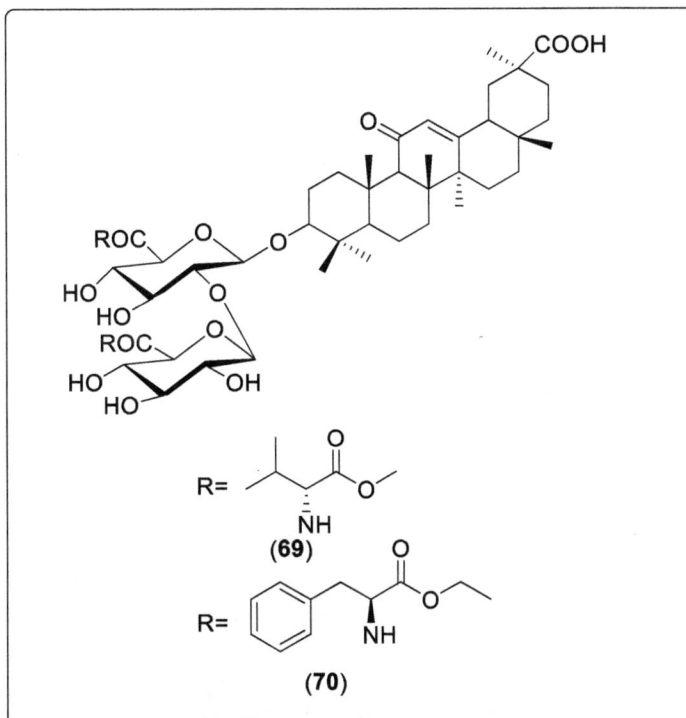

Fig. (43). Chemical structure of the compounds **69** and **70**.

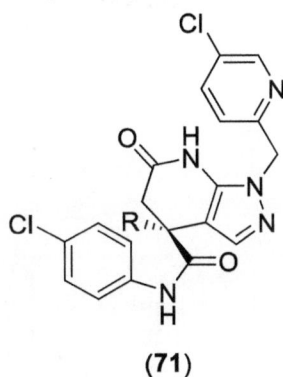

(71)

Fig. (44). Chemical structure of the compounds **71**.

In 2021, Kaptein *et al.* described a highly potent dengue virus inhibitor compound **72** (Fig. **45**) that exerts nanomolar to picomolar activity against a panel of 21 clinical isolates that represent the natural genetic diversity of known genotypes and serotypes. The molecule has a high barrier to resistance and prevents the formation of the viral replication complex by blocking the interaction between two viral proteins (NS3 and NS4B), thus revealing a previously undescribed mechanism of antiviral action [87].

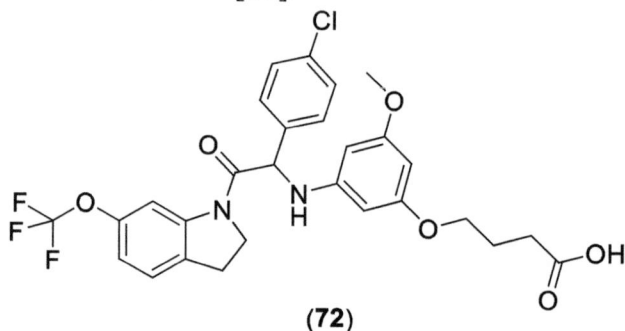

(72)

Fig. (45). Chemical structure of the compounds **72**.

Good *et al.*in 2021 showed that compound **73** (Fig. **46**), the free base of AT-752 (a sulphate salt), an orally available double prodrug of a guanosine nucleotide analogue, inhibits viral replication of DENV serotypes 2 and 3 *in vitro* with EC$_{50}$ values of 0.48 and 0.77 µM respectively in Huh-7 cells [88].

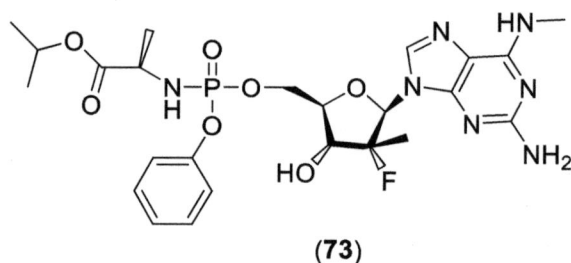

(73)

Fig. (46). Chemical structure of the compounds **73**.

CONCLUSION

Based upon our extensive search for designing inhibitors against the dengue virus, it was observed that the most explored target was DENV NS2B-NS3 protease for which, there were numerous inhibitors belonging to various chemical classes, the best efficiency was obtained for the peptide inhibitors which showed sub-micromolar to nanomolar affinities, however, there were few limitations as the protease inhibitors did not excel well in the cell-based assays, besides this many small molecule inhibitors of the varying scaffold were identified and they showed lower micromolar affinities. Inhibitors of natural origin were also reported, and further HTS, HTVS, and drug-repurposing approaches were also employed to explore and identify inhibitors of protease. While searching for inhibitors for other targets of dengue viruses, we found that very a small number of inhibitors were reported, which indicates that there is a lot to be explored for targets like E-protein, NS4B, and NS5 polymerase including RdRp.

One major limitation in containing dengue is that there is still a search for a widely accepted tetravalent vaccine as the previously reported vaccines were not able to show the desired protection, also antibody-dependent enhancement effect remains a major concern in the path of vaccine development. Despite all these limitations, various research groups are still working towards identifying inhibitors against the dengue virus, however, currently, only palliative treatment remains an option.

REFERENCES

[1]   Organization WH. Global strategy for dengue prevention and control 2012; 2012.

[2]   Stanaway JD, Shepard DS, Undurraga EA, *et al*. The global burden of dengue: an analysis from the Global Burden of Disease Study 2013. Lancet Infect Dis 2016; 16(6): 712-23.
        [http://dx.doi.org/10.1016/S1473-3099(16)00026-8] [PMID: 26874619]

[3]   Messina JP, Brady OJ, Golding N, *et al*. The current and future global distribution and population at risk of dengue. Nat Microbiol 2019; 4(9): 1508-15.
        [http://dx.doi.org/10.1038/s41564-019-0476-8] [PMID: 31182801]

[4]   Guzman MG, Gubler DJ, Izquierdo A, Martinez E, Halstead SB. Dengue infection. Nat Rev Dis Primers 2016; 2(1): 16055.
        [http://dx.doi.org/10.1038/nrdp.2016.55] [PMID: 27534439]

[5]   Shepard DS, Undurraga EA, Halasa YA, Stanaway JD. The global economic burden of dengue: a systematic analysis. Lancet Infect Dis 2016; 16(8): 935-41.
        [http://dx.doi.org/10.1016/S1473-3099(16)00146-8] [PMID: 27091092]

[6]   Kuhn RJ, Zhang W, Rossmann MG, *et al*. Structure of dengue virus: implications for flavivirus organization, maturation, and fusion. Cell 2002; 108(5): 717-25.
        [http://dx.doi.org/10.1016/S0092-8674(02)00660-8] [PMID: 11893341]

[7]   Yu CY, Chang TH, Liang JJ, *et al*. Dengue virus targets the adaptor protein MITA to subvert host innate immunity. PLoS Pathog 2012; 8(6): e1002780.
        [http://dx.doi.org/10.1371/journal.ppat.1002780] [PMID: 22761576]

[8]   Green AM, Beatty PR, Hadjilaou A, Harris E. Innate immunity to dengue virus infection and subversion of antiviral responses. J Mol Biol 2014; 426(6): 1148-60.
        [http://dx.doi.org/10.1016/j.jmb.2013.11.023] [PMID: 24316047]

[9]   Su YC, Huang YF, Wu YW, *et al*. MicroRNA-155 inhibits dengue virus replication by inducing heme oxygenase-1-mediated antiviral interferon responses. FASEB J 2020; 34(6): 7283-94.
        [http://dx.doi.org/10.1096/fj.201902878R] [PMID: 32277848]

[10]   Brecher M, Zhang J, Li H. The flavivirus protease as a target for drug discovery. Virol Sin 2013; 28(6): 326-36.
        [http://dx.doi.org/10.1007/s12250-013-3390-x] [PMID: 24242363]

[11]   Luo D, Vasudevan SG, Lescar J. The flavivirus NS2B–NS3 protease–helicase as a target for antiviral drug development. Antiviral Res 2015; 118: 148-58.
        [http://dx.doi.org/10.1016/j.antiviral.2015.03.014] [PMID: 25842996]

[12]   Merdanovic M, Mönig T, Ehrmann M, Kaiser M. Diversity of allosteric regulation in proteases. ACS Chem Biol 2013; 8(1): 19-26.
       [http://dx.doi.org/10.1021/cb3005935] [PMID: 23181429]

[13]   Hauske P, Ottmann C, Meltzer M, Ehrmann M, Kaiser M. Allosteric regulation of proteases. ChemBioChem 2008; 9(18): 2920-8.
       [http://dx.doi.org/10.1002/cbic.200800528] [PMID: 19021141]

[14]   Mukhametov A, Newhouse EI, Aziz NA, Saito JA, Alam M. Allosteric pocket of the dengue virus (serotype 2) NS2B/NS3 protease: *In silico* ligand screening and molecular dynamics studies of inhibition. J Mol Graph Model 2014; 52: 103-13.
       [http://dx.doi.org/10.1016/j.jmgm.2014.06.008] [PMID: 25023665]

[15]   Millies B, von Hammerstein F, Gellert A, *et al.* Proline-based allosteric inhibitors of zika and dengue virus NS2B/NS3 proteases. J Med Chem 2019; 62(24): 11359-82.
       [http://dx.doi.org/10.1021/acs.jmedchem.9b01697] [PMID: 31769670]

[16]   Lim L, Dang M, Roy A, Kang J, Song J. Curcumin allosterically inhibits the dengue NS2B-NS3 protease by disrupting its active conformation. ACS Omega 2020; 5(40): 25677-86.
       [http://dx.doi.org/10.1021/acsomega.0c00039] [PMID: 33073093]

[17]   Yildiz M, Ghosh S, Bell JA, Sherman W, Hardy JA. Allosteric inhibition of the NS2B-NS3 protease from dengue virus. ACS Chem Biol 2013; 8(12): 2744-52.
       [http://dx.doi.org/10.1021/cb400612h] [PMID: 24164286]

[18]   Acosta eg, Kumar A, Bartenschlager R. Revisiting dengue virus-host cell interaction: new insights into molecular and cellular virology. Adv Virus Res 2014; 88: 1-109.
       [http://dx.doi.org/10.1016/B978-0-12-800098-4.00001-5] [PMID: 24373310]

[19]   Selisko B, Wang C, Harris E, Canard B. Regulation of Flavivirus RNA synthesis and replication. Curr Opin Virol 2014; 9: 74-83.
       [http://dx.doi.org/10.1016/j.coviro.2014.09.011] [PMID: 25462437]

[20]   Bollati M, Milani M, Mastrangelo E, *et al.* Recognition of RNA cap in the Wesselsbron virus NS5 methyltransferase domain: implications for RNA-capping mechanisms in Flavivirus. J Mol Biol 2009; 385(1): 140-52.
       [http://dx.doi.org/10.1016/j.jmb.2008.10.028] [PMID: 18976670]

[21]   Lim SP, Noble CG, Shi PY. The dengue virus NS5 protein as a target for drug discovery. Antiviral Res 2015; 119: 57-67.
       [http://dx.doi.org/10.1016/j.antiviral.2015.04.010] [PMID: 25912817]

[22]   Koonin EV. Computer-assisted identification of a putative methyltransferase domain in NS5 protein of flaviviruses and 2 protein of reovirus. J Gen Virol 1993; 74(4): 733-40.
       [http://dx.doi.org/10.1099/0022-1317-74-4-733] [PMID: 8385698]

[23]   Noble CG, Seh CC, Chao AT, Shi PY. Ligand-bound structures of the dengue virus protease reveal the active conformation. J Virol 2012; 86(1): 438-46.
       [http://dx.doi.org/10.1128/JVI.06225-11] [PMID: 22031935]

[24]   Pettersen EF, Goddard TD, Huang CC, *et al.* UCSF Chimera—A visualization system for exploratory research and analysis. J Comput Chem 2004; 25(13): 1605-12.
       [http://dx.doi.org/10.1002/jcc.20084] [PMID: 15264254]

[25]   Noble CG, Lim SP, Arora R, *et al.* A conserved pocket in the dengue virus polymerase identified through fragment-based screening. J Biol Chem 2016; 291(16): 8541-8.
       [http://dx.doi.org/10.1074/jbc.M115.710731] [PMID: 26872970]

[26]   Lim SP, Sonntag LS, Noble C, *et al.* Small molecule inhibitors that selectively block dengue virus methyltransferase. J Biol Chem 2011; 286(8): 6233-40.
       [http://dx.doi.org/10.1074/jbc.M110.179184] [PMID: 21147775]

[27]   De La Guardia C, Lleonart R. Progress in the identification of dengue virus entry/fusion inhibitors. Biomed Res Int 2014; 2014

[28]   Halstead SB. Dengue antibody-dependent enhancement: knowns and unknowns. Antibodies for Infectious Diseases 2015; pp. 249-71.

[29]   Modis Y, Ogata S, Clements D, Harrison SC. A ligand-binding pocket in the dengue virus envelope glycoprotein. Proc Natl Acad Sci USA 2003; 100(12): 6986-91.
[http://dx.doi.org/10.1073/pnas.0832193100] [PMID: 12759475]

[30]   Behnam MAM, Nitsche C, Vechi SM, Klein CD. C-terminal residue optimization and fragment merging: discovery of a potent Peptide-hybrid inhibitor of dengue protease. ACS Med Chem Lett 2014; 5(9): 1037-42.
[http://dx.doi.org/10.1021/ml500245v] [PMID: 25221663]

[31]   Rothan HA, Zulqarnain M, Ammar YA, Tan EC, Rahman NA, Yusof R. Screening of antiviral activities in medicinal plants extracts against dengue virus using dengue NS2B-NS3 protease assay. Trop Biomed 2014; 31(2): 286-96.
[PMID: 25134897]

[32]   Liu H, Wu R, Sun Y, *et al.* Identification of novel thiadiazoloacrylamide analogues as inhibitors of dengue-2 virus NS2B/NS3 protease. Bioorg Med Chem 2014; 22(22): 6344-52.
[http://dx.doi.org/10.1016/j.bmc.2014.09.057] [PMID: 25438757]

[33]   Viswanathan U, Tomlinson SM, Fonner JM, Mock SA, Watowich SJ. Identification of a novel inhibitor of dengue virus protease through use of a virtual screening drug discovery Web portal. J Chem Inf Model 2014; 54(10): 2816-25.
[http://dx.doi.org/10.1021/ci500531r] [PMID: 25263519]

[34]   Nitsche C, Behnam MAM, Steuer C, Klein CD. Retro peptide-hybrids as selective inhibitors of the Dengue virus NS2B-NS3 protease. Antiviral Res 2012; 94(1): 72-9.
[http://dx.doi.org/10.1016/j.antiviral.2012.02.008] [PMID: 22391061]

[35]   Nitsche C, Schreier VN, Behnam MAM, Kumar A, Bartenschlager R, Klein CD. Thiazolidinone-peptide hybrids as dengue virus protease inhibitors with antiviral activity in cell culture. J Med Chem 2013; 56(21): 8389-403.
[http://dx.doi.org/10.1021/jm400828u] [PMID: 24083834]

[36]   Weigel LF, Nitsche C, Graf D, Bartenschlager R, Klein CD. Phenylalanine and phenylglycine analogues as arginine mimetics in dengue protease inhibitors. J Med Chem 2015; 58(19): 7719-33.
[http://dx.doi.org/10.1021/acs.jmedchem.5b00612] [PMID: 26367391]

[37]   Behnam MAM, Graf D, Bartenschlager R, Zlotos DP, Klein CD. Discovery of nanomolar dengue and west nile virus protease inhibitors containing a 4-benzyloxyphenylglycine residue. J Med Chem 2015; 58(23): 9354-70.
[http://dx.doi.org/10.1021/acs.jmedchem.5b01441] [PMID: 26562070]

[38]   Johnston PA, Phillips J, Shun TY, *et al.* HTS identifies novel and specific uncompetitive inhibitors of the two-component NS2B-NS3 proteinase of West Nile virus. Assay Drug Dev Technol 2007; 5(6): 737-50.
[http://dx.doi.org/10.1089/adt.2007.101] [PMID: 18181690]

[39]   Koh-Stenta X, Joy J, Wang SF, *et al.* Identification of covalent active site inhibitors of dengue virus protease. Drug Des Devel Ther 2015; 9(December): 6389-99.
[http://dx.doi.org/10.2147/DDDT.S94207] [PMID: 26677315]

[40]   de Sousa LRF, Wu H, Nebo L, *et al.* Flavonoids as noncompetitive inhibitors of Dengue virus NS2B-NS3 protease: Inhibition kinetics and docking studies. Bioorg Med Chem 2015; 23(3): 466-70.
[http://dx.doi.org/10.1016/j.bmc.2014.12.015] [PMID: 25564380]

[41]   Wu H, Bock S, Snitko M, *et al.* Novel dengue virus NS2B/NS3 protease inhibitors. Antimicrob Agents Chemother 2015; 59(2): 1100-9.

[http://dx.doi.org/10.1128/AAC.03543-14] [PMID: 25487800]

[42]   Raut R, Beesetti H, Tyagi P, *et al*. A small molecule inhibitor of dengue virus type 2 protease inhibits the replication of all four dengue virus serotypes in cell culture. Virol J 2015; 12(1): 16.
[http://dx.doi.org/10.1186/s12985-015-0248-x] [PMID: 25886260]

[43]   Li L, Basavannacharya C, Chan KWK, Shang L, Vasudevan SG, Yin Z. Structure-guided discovery of a novel non-peptide inhibitor of dengue virus NS2B-NS3 protease. Chem Biol Drug Des 2015; 86(3): 255-64.
[http://dx.doi.org/10.1111/cbdd.12500] [PMID: 25533891]

[44]   Timiri AK, Selvarasu S, Kesherwani M, *et al*. Synthesis and molecular modelling studies of novel sulphonamide derivatives as dengue virus 2 protease inhibitors. Bioorg Chem 2015; 62: 74-82.
[http://dx.doi.org/10.1016/j.bioorg.2015.07.005] [PMID: 26247308]

[45]   Chu JJH, Lee RCH, Ang MJY, *et al*. Antiviral activities of 15 dengue NS2B-NS3 protease inhibitors using a human cell-based viral quantification assay. Antiviral Res 2015; 118: 68-74.
[http://dx.doi.org/10.1016/j.antiviral.2015.03.010] [PMID: 25823617]

[46]   Bhakat S, Delang L, Kaptein S, Neyts J, Leyssen P, Jayaprakash V. Reaching beyond HIV/HCV: nelfinavir as a potential starting point for broad-spectrum protease inhibitors against dengue and chikungunya virus. RSC Advances 2015; 5(104): 85938-49.
[http://dx.doi.org/10.1039/C5RA14469H]

[47]   Wu D, Mao F, Ye Y, *et al*. Policresulen, a novel NS2B/NS3 protease inhibitor, effectively inhibits the replication of DENV2 virus in BHK-21 cells. Acta Pharmacol Sin 2015; 36(9): 1126-36.
[http://dx.doi.org/10.1038/aps.2015.56] [PMID: 26279156]

[48]   Mishra SK, Dwivedi VD, Tripathi IP. *In silico* evaluation of inhibitory potential of triterpenoids from Azadirachta indica against therapeutic target of dengue virus, NS2B-NS3 protease. J Vector Borne Dis 2016; 53(2): 156-61.
[http://dx.doi.org/10.4103/0972-9062.184848] [PMID: 27353586]

[49]   Lee JC, Chang FR, Chen SR, *et al*. Anti-dengue virus constituents from Formosan zoanthid Palythoa mutuki. Mar Drugs 2016; 14(8): 151.
[http://dx.doi.org/10.3390/md14080151] [PMID: 27517937]

[50]   Balasubramanian A, Manzano M, Teramoto T, Pilankatta R, Padmanabhan R. High-throughput screening for the identification of small-molecule inhibitors of the flaviviral protease. Antiviral Res 2016; 134: 6-16.
[http://dx.doi.org/10.1016/j.antiviral.2016.08.014] [PMID: 27539384]

[51]   Lin KH, Nalivaika EA, Prachanronarong KL, Yilmaz NK, Schiffer CA. Dengue protease substrate recognition: binding of the prime side. ACS Infect Dis 2016; 2(10): 734-43.
[http://dx.doi.org/10.1021/acsinfecdis.6b00131] [PMID: 27657335]

[52]   Lin KH, Ali A, Rusere L, Soumana DI, Kurt Yilmaz N, Schiffer CA. Dengue virus NS2B/NS3 protease inhibitors exploiting the prime side. J Virol 2017; 91(10): e00045-17.
[http://dx.doi.org/10.1128/JVI.00045-17] [PMID: 28298600]

[53]   Takagi Y, Matsui K, Nobori H, *et al*. Discovery of novel cyclic peptide inhibitors of dengue virus NS2B-NS3 protease with antiviral activity. Bioorg Med Chem Lett 2017; 27(15): 3586-90.
[http://dx.doi.org/10.1016/j.bmcl.2017.05.027] [PMID: 28539222]

[54]   Pelliccia S, Wu YH, Coluccia A, *et al*. Inhibition of dengue virus replication by novel inhibitors of RNA-dependent RNA polymerase and protease activities. J Enzyme Inhib Med Chem 2017; 32(1): 1091-101.
[http://dx.doi.org/10.1080/14756366.2017.1355791] [PMID: 28776445]

[55]   Gan CS, Lee YK, Heh CH, Rahman NA, Yusof R, Othman S. The synthetic molecules YK51 and YK73 attenuate replication of dengue virus serotype 2. Trop Biomed 2017; 34(2): 270-83.
[PMID: 33593007]

[56]   Osman H, Idris NH, Kamarulzaman EE, Wahab HA, Hassan MZ. 3,5-Bis(arylidene)-4-piperidones as potential dengue protease inhibitors. Acta Pharm Sin B 2017; 7(4): 479-84.
[http://dx.doi.org/10.1016/j.apsb.2017.04.009] [PMID: 28752033]

[57]   Zhou GC, Weng Z, Shao X, *et al.* Discovery and SAR studies of methionine–proline anilides as dengue virus NS2B-NS3 protease inhibitors. Bioorg Med Chem Lett 2013; 23(24): 6549-54.
[http://dx.doi.org/10.1016/j.bmcl.2013.10.071] [PMID: 24268549]

[58]   Weng Z, Shao X, Graf D, *et al.* Identification of fused bicyclic derivatives of pyrrolidine and imidazolidinone as dengue virus-2 NS2B-NS3 protease inhibitors. Eur J Med Chem 2017; 125(125): 751-9.
[http://dx.doi.org/10.1016/j.ejmech.2016.09.063] [PMID: 27721158]

[59]   Padmapriya P, Gracy Fathima S, Ramanathan G, *et al.* Development of antiviral inhibitor against dengue 2 targeting Ns3 protein: *in vitro* and in silico significant studies. Acta Trop 2018; 188: 1-8.
[http://dx.doi.org/10.1016/j.actatropica.2018.08.022] [PMID: 30145258]

[60]   Li Z, Sakamuru S, Huang R, *et al.* Erythrosin B is a potent and broad-spectrum orthosteric inhibitor of the flavivirus NS2B-NS3 protease. Antiviral Res 2018; 150(150): 217-25.
[http://dx.doi.org/10.1016/j.antiviral.2017.12.018] [PMID: 29288700]

[61]   Hariono M, Choi SB, Roslim RF, *et al.* Thioguanine-based DENV-2 NS2B/NS3 protease inhibitors: Virtual screening, synthesis, biological evaluation and molecular modelling. PLoS One 2019; 14(1): e0210869.
[http://dx.doi.org/10.1371/journal.pone.0210869] [PMID: 30677071]

[62]   Balasubramanian A, Pilankatta R, Teramoto T, *et al.* Inhibition of dengue virus by curcuminoids. Antiviral Res 2019; 162(162): 71-8.
[http://dx.doi.org/10.1016/j.antiviral.2018.12.002] [PMID: 30529358]

[63]   Knehans T, Schüller A, Doan DN, *et al.* Structure-guided fragment-based *in silico* drug design of dengue protease inhibitors. J Comput Aided Mol Des 2011; 25(3): 263-74.
[http://dx.doi.org/10.1007/s10822-011-9418-0] [PMID: 21344277]

[64]   Bartolini M, Cavrini V, Andrisano V. Characterization of reversible and pseudo-irreversible acetylcholinesterase inhibitors by means of an immobilized enzyme reactor. J Chromatogr A 2007; 1144(1): 102-10.
[http://dx.doi.org/10.1016/j.chroma.2006.11.029] [PMID: 17134713]

[65]   Sundermann TR, Benzin CV, Dražić T, Klein CD. Synthesis and structure-activity relationships of small-molecular di-basic esters, amides and carbamates as flaviviral protease inhibitors. Eur J Med Chem 2019; 176: 187-94.
[http://dx.doi.org/10.1016/j.ejmech.2019.05.025] [PMID: 31103899]

[66]   Dwivedi VD, Bharadwaj S, Afroz S, Khan N, Ansari MA, Yadava U, *et al.* Anti-dengue infectivity evaluation of bioflavonoid from Azadirachta indica by dengue virus serine protease inhibition. J Biomol Struct Dyn 2020; 1102.
[PMID: 32107969]

[67]   Kühl N, Graf D, Bock J, Behnam MAM, Leuthold MM, Klein CD. A new class of dengue and west nile virus protease inhibitors with submicromolar activity in reporter gene DENV-2 protease and viral replication assays. J Med Chem 2020; 63(15): 8179-97.
[http://dx.doi.org/10.1021/acs.jmedchem.0c00413] [PMID: 32605372]

[68]   Behrouz S, Kühl N, Klein CD. N-sulfonyl peptide-hybrids as a new class of dengue virus protease inhibitors. Eur J Med Chem 2023; 251: 115227.
[http://dx.doi.org/10.1016/j.ejmech.2023.115227] [PMID: 36893626]

[69]   Xu HT, Colby-Germinario SP, Hassounah S, *et al.* Identification of a pyridoxine-derived small-molecule inhibitor targeting dengue virus RNA-dependent RNA polymerase. Antimicrob Agents Chemother 2016; 60(1): 600-8.

[http://dx.doi.org/10.1128/AAC.02203-15] [PMID: 26574011]

[70]   Yokokawa F, Nilar S, Noble CG, *et al.* Discovery of potent non-nucleoside inhibitors of dengue viral RNA-dependent RNA polymerase from a fragment hit using structure-based drug design. J Med Chem 2016; 59(8): 3935-52.
[http://dx.doi.org/10.1021/acs.jmedchem.6b00143] [PMID: 26984786]

[71]   Lim SP, Noble CG, Seh CC, *et al.* Potent allosteric dengue virus NS5 polymerase inhibitors: mechanism of action and resistance profiling. PLoS Pathog 2016; 12(8): e1005737.
[http://dx.doi.org/10.1371/journal.ppat.1005737] [PMID: 27500641]

[72]   Manvar D, Küçükgüzel İ, Erensoy G, *et al.* Discovery of conjugated thiazolidinone-thiadiazole scaffold as anti-dengue virus polymerase inhibitors. Biochem Biophys Res Commun 2016; 469(3): 743-7.
[http://dx.doi.org/10.1016/j.bbrc.2015.12.042] [PMID: 26697747]

[73]   Cannalire R, Tarantino D, Astolfi A, *et al.* Functionalized 2,1-benzothiazine 2,2-dioxides as new inhibitors of Dengue NS5 RNA-dependent RNA polymerase. Eur J Med Chem 2018; 143: 1667-76.
[http://dx.doi.org/10.1016/j.ejmech.2017.10.064] [PMID: 29137867]

[74]   Shimizu H, Saito A, Mikuni J, *et al.* Discovery of a small molecule inhibitor targeting dengue virus NS5 RNA-dependent RNA polymerase. PLoS Negl Trop Dis 2019; 13(11): e0007894.
[http://dx.doi.org/10.1371/journal.pntd.0007894] [PMID: 31738758]

[75]   Zong K, Li W, Xu Y, *et al.* Design, synthesis, evaluation and molecular dynamics simulation of dengue virus NS5-RdRp inhibitors. Pharmaceuticals (Basel) 2023; 16(11): 1625.
[http://dx.doi.org/10.3390/ph16111625] [PMID: 38004490]

[76]   Aouadi W, Eydoux C, Coutard B, *et al.* Toward the identification of viral cap-methyltransferase inhibitors by fluorescence screening assay. Antiviral Res 2017; 144: 330-9.
[http://dx.doi.org/10.1016/j.antiviral.2017.06.021] [PMID: 28676301]

[77]   Benmansour F, Trist I, Coutard B, *et al.* Discovery of novel dengue virus NS5 methyltransferase non-nucleoside inhibitors by fragment-based drug design. Eur J Med Chem 2017; 125: 865-80.
[http://dx.doi.org/10.1016/j.ejmech.2016.10.007] [PMID: 27750202]

[78]   Yao X, Ling Y, Guo S, *et al.* Inhibition of dengue viral infection by diasarone-I is associated with 2'O methyltransferase of NS5. Eur J Pharmacol 2018; 821: 11-20.
[http://dx.doi.org/10.1016/j.ejphar.2017.12.029] [PMID: 29246851]

[79]   Hernandez J, Hoffer L, Coutard B, *et al.* Optimization of a fragment linking hit toward Dengue and Zika virus NS5 methyltransferases inhibitors. Eur J Med Chem 2019; 161: 323-33.
[http://dx.doi.org/10.1016/j.ejmech.2018.09.056] [PMID: 30368131]

[80]   Spizzichino S, Mattedi G, Lauder K, *et al.* Design, synthesis and discovery of *N,N'* -Carbazoyl-ar-l-urea inhibitors of zika NS5 methyltransferase and virus replication. ChemMedChem 2020; 15(4): 385-90.
[http://dx.doi.org/10.1002/cmdc.201900533] [PMID: 31805205]

[81]   Panya A, Bangphoomi K, Choowongkomon K, Yenchitsomanus P. Peptide inhibitors against dengue virus infection. Chem Biol Drug Des 2014; 84(2): 148-57.
[http://dx.doi.org/10.1111/cbdd.12309] [PMID: 24612829]

[82]   Jadav SS, Kaptein S, Timiri A, *et al.* Design, synthesis, optimization and antiviral activity of a class of hybrid dengue virus E protein inhibitors. Bioorg Med Chem Lett 2015; 25(8): 1747-52.
[http://dx.doi.org/10.1016/j.bmcl.2015.02.059] [PMID: 25791449]

[83]   Budigi Y, Ong EZ, Robinson LN, *et al.* Neutralization of antibody-enhanced dengue infection by VIS513, a pan serotype reactive monoclonal antibody targeting domain III of the dengue E protein. de Silva AM, editor. PLoS Negl Trop Dis. 2018; 12: p. (2)e0006209.

[84]   Yamamoto M, Ichinohe T, Watanabe A, *et al.* The antimalarial compound atovaquone inhibits Zika and dengue virus infection by blocking E protein-mediated membrane fusion. Viruses 2020; 12(12):

1475.
[http://dx.doi.org/10.3390/v12121475] [PMID: 33371476]

[85]   Hour MJ, Chen Y, Lin CS, *et al.* Glycyrrhizic acid derivatives bearing amino acid residues in the carbohydrate part as dengue virus E protein inhibitors: Synthesis and antiviral activity. Int J Mol Sci 2022; 23(18): 10309.
[http://dx.doi.org/10.3390/ijms231810309] [PMID: 36142222]

[86]   Wang QY, Dong H, Zou B, *et al.* Discovery of dengue virus NS4B inhibitors. J Virol 2015; 89(16): 8233-44.
[http://dx.doi.org/10.1128/JVI.00855-15] [PMID: 26018165]

[87]   Kaptein SJF, Goethals O, Kiemel D, *et al.* A pan-serotype dengue virus inhibitor targeting the NS3–NS4B interaction. Nature 2021; 598(7881): 504-9.
[http://dx.doi.org/10.1038/s41586-021-03990-6] [PMID: 34616043]

[88]   Good SS, Shannon A, Lin K, *et al.* Evaluation of AT-752, a double prodrug of a guanosine nucleotide analog with *in vitro* and *in vivo* activity against dengue and other flaviviruses. Antimicrob Agents Chemother 2021; 65(11): e00988-21.
[http://dx.doi.org/10.1128/AAC.00988-21] [PMID: 34424050]

CHAPTER 7

Malaria: State of the Art and New Perspectives

Samyak Bajaj[1,#], **Akankcha Gupta**[1,#], **Priyanshu Nema**[1], **Mitali Mishra**[1] and **Sushil Kumar Kashaw**[1,*]

[1] *Integrated Drug Discovery Research Laboratory, Department of Pharmaceutical Sciences, Dr. Harisingh Gour University (A Central University), Sagar (MP), India*

Abstract: Malaria continues to endanger over half of the world's population, claiming 1-2 million lives each year. The main causative agents are *Plasmodium falciparum* (Pf) and *Plasmodium vivax* (Pv). Both cause widespread mortality and morbidity, and they impose a significant socioeconomic burden, particularly in poor nations. The emergence and dissemination of resistance to currently available antimalarial medications have generated a crisis scenario among experts. Unfortunately, artemisinin-resistant parasitic strains have been observed in Southeast Asia. Several approaches that include, combination therapy, exploitation of natural products, drug resistance reversers, covalent bitherapy, identification of novel targets, and development of vaccines, have been explored to surmount the issue of drug resistance. In the absence of effective vaccinations, the disease has been mostly managed with chemotherapy and chemoprophylaxis. Over the past year, breakthroughs in technology such as molecular evolutionary and population genetic techniques have exposed the malaria parasite genome, considerably contributing to the understanding of the targets and dissemination of parasite treatment resistance. The rapid discovery and molecular characterization of novel targets have paved the path for the development of new antimalarial medicines. To find chemically varied, efficacious medications, new pharmacophores, and validated targets are necessary. Functional genomics and structure-based drug design can help in the search for novel potential targets and therapeutic candidates. Once the putative targets are validated, which are capable of providing effective and safe drugs, they can be used for screening compounds to discover new leads, which, successively, can be utilized in the lead optimization process. Combinatorial chemistry, along with as well as high throughput screening technologies, is used to generate huge numbers of structurally diverse compounds. This chapter discusses possible chemotherapeutic targets for antimalarial therapy and their locations inside the malaria parasite, as well as new lead compounds for rationally designing new antimalarial medicines.

Keywords: Apicoplast, Aquaporins, CDKs, Medicinal chemistry, NPPs, Plasmodium vivax, Plasmodium falciparum.

---
* **Corresponding author Sushil Kumar Kashaw:** Integrated Drug Discovery Research Laboratory, Department of Pharmaceutical Sciences, Dr. Harisingh Gour University (A Central University), Sagar (MP), India; Tel: +91-9425655720; E-mail: sushilkashaw@gmail.com
# These authors contributed equally to this work.

Igor Jose dos Santos Nascimento & Ricardo Olimpio de Moura (Eds.)

INTRODUCTION

Malaria still poses a threat to about half of the world's population, which claims 1-2 million lives annually. Among the four species of malaria parasite, two strains, *Plasmodium falciparum* (Pf) and Plasmodium vivax, are the predominant causal agents. They have developed resistance to nearly all existing antimalarial drugs [1, 2]. Both are major socioeconomic burdens, particularly for emerging nations, and are to blame for the high rates of death and morbidity. Researchers are now facing a serious predicament as a result of the formation and spread of resistance to currently available antimalarial medications. Unfortunately, in recent reports, artemisinins-resistant parasitic strains have been observed in Southeast Asia [3 - 5]. Moreover, no viable therapeutic candidate for malaria has been made available for clinical usage in the pipeline.

To overcome the problem of drug resistance, several strategies have been investigated, including combination therapy, natural products, drug resistance reversers, covalent biotherapy, identification of novel targets, and vaccine development [6]. All these strategies need to be specifically focused on lowering the price of the drug discovery process so that developing nations can benefit to the fullest.

Chemotherapy and chemoprophylaxis have been the mainstays of illness management in the absence of viable vaccinations. Over the past year, advancements in technology such as molecular evolutionary and population genetic techniques have exposed the malaria parasite genome, which has considerably contributed to understanding the targets and dissemination of parasite treatment resistance [7].

The rapid identification and molecular characterisation of novel targets have offered a new path for developing new antimalarial medicines. Additionally, the advent of high throughput screening and combinatorial chemistry coupled with bioinformatics has revolutionized the drug discovery process [8]. To design new antimalarial medications, this book chapter focuses on prospective chemotherapeutic targets for antimalarial therapy and their locations inside the malaria parasite. It also emphasizes the ongoing development of the targets and particular inhibitors.

Chemotherapeutic Targets for Antimalarial Therapy

The primary metabolic distinctions between the malaria parasite and its host form the basis of the current arsenal of antimalarial medications. Antimalarial drug design has identified key processes of *P. falciparum* as targets, including heme detoxification, fatty acid biosynthesis, nucleic acid metabolism, and oxidative stress. Although most of them have been used for decades, their usage is currently limited due to the advent of resistance [9]. The literature claims that no antimalarial medication is now in use that was created to inhibit a recognized therapeutic target in a completely logical manner. Rather, anti-malarial potency has always been found by investigations using *in vitro* or animal models. As a result, the target of action for most current medicines within the malaria parasite is unknown [10]. Furthermore, for most medications, the processes behind the establishment of resistance are poorly known. Genetic, molecular, and pharmacological approaches have shown that several targets of older treatments are resistant due to changes in their key transporters or enzymes [11]. Also, the list of drug resistance does not exclude artemisinin and its derivatives, which are the most effective anti-malarial drugs. Artemisinins are potent inhibitors of phosphatidylinositol-3-kinase (PfPI3K). *P. falciparum* Kelch13 (PfKelch13) contains a significant marker of artemisinin resistance, the C580Y mutation, which has been linked to elevated PfPI3K in clinically resistant strains [12]. Thus, medication resistance resulting from mutations is a significant concern and the identification of new targets is mandatory to design new drugs against resistant malarial parasites.

The Need for New Target for Anti-malarial Drugs

The emergence and dissemination of resistance to conventional antimalarial medications due to genetic changes have resulted in the development of novel antimalarial compounds with distinct mechanisms of action. However, malaria elimination necessitates a comprehensive strategy that includes new and old medications, vaccines, vector control, and public health control issues [13]. The most innovative technique is most likely to identify novel targets and then produce compounds that act on these targets. This can be accomplished in two ways: by focusing on validated targets to find novel chemical entities, or by investigating the malaria parasite's vital metabolic pathways to find new possible targets. The search for new potential targets becomes crucial because, the dearth of structural diversity in the armory of antimalarial drugs, except artemisinin-type compounds, led to considerable cross-resistance between drugs with existing targets.

Consequently, the hunt for new potential targets has become imperative. Furthermore, to find safe and effective compounds, new targets need to be carefully verified [14, 15]. To combat the problem of resistance, new target discovery and the search for inhibitors tailored to these targets are currently widely employed strategies. Therefore, screening of inhibitors specific for new target proteins of the malaria parasite has been utilized to identify therapeutic targets and is now being studied [16].

Targets for Malaria Parasite

To ensure that the drug has little to no effect on the host, the identified pharmacological target must have distinct metabolic pathways or processes that are particular to the parasite and differ greatly from those of the host. Although the genomic host and proteomic information are in the exploratory stage, the mapping of the *P. falciparum* genome has provided a significant boost to this discovery process. Several recently found metabolic pathways are now being targeted for the development of innovative anti-malarial medications to better understand the parasites' life cycle, growth, and survival [17].

TARGETING THE PROCESSES IN THE PARASITE MEMBRANE

Targeting Channels/Transporters

To survive, the parasite's intraerythrocytic stage creates new permeability pathways (NPPs) in the host membrane of infected red blood cells (RBCs) 10-15 hours after invasion [18]. NPPs are produced to produce ionic and pH gradients, as well as to aid in the diffusion of certain purines and vitamins, nutrients (such as pantothenic acid, glucose, and glycerol), and biosynthetic precursors (such as hypoxanthine, cysteine, tyrosine, glutamine, and proline). They can also be used to remove harmful metabolic waste products (such as lactic acid and amino acids) from parasite cells and transport medications to them. These channels provide a sequential diffusive conduit for nutrients to reach the intracellular pathogen through: i) A "metabolic window," defined as a specific area where the membranes of the parasite, erythrocyte, and parasitophorous vacuole unite to allow for the uptake of substances across a single membrane [19]. A "tubovesicular network" fuses the erythrocyte membrane with the parasitophorous vacuole membrane extensions, allowing solutes to be taken up directly into the parasitophorous vacuole space [20]. iii) A "parasitophorous duct" that, by keeping the extensions of the parasitophorous vacuole open to the extracellular fluid, permits the parasite plasma membrane to be exposed to the outside world [21, 22]. By preventing the parasite from using its energy source, producing a build-up of cytotoxic metabolites, or producing cytotoxic drugs that can only enter through these induced transporters, blocking these channels would only have a limited impact on the parasite's growth. Here are some descriptions of some of the special channels/transporters.

Aquaporin Channel

The membrane proteins known as aquaporins (AQP) are essential for membrane function and can be categorised into two main groups: i) Orthodox aquaporins are limited to water channels [23, 24], and ii) Aquaglyceroporins are permeable to minor solutes such as glycerol, urea, nitrate, hydrogen peroxide, and gases like ammonia, carbon dioxide, and nitric oxide [25, 26].

Aquaporins and apicomplexes are engaged in numerous biological processes.

1) They protect the parasite from osmotic stress during kidney passages or transmembrane fluid transport by accumulating or releasing compatible solutes;

2) They promote glycerol uptake, a precursor for membrane lipid biosynthesis;

3) They also reduce oxidative stress by increasing the NADH/NAD+ ratio; and

4) release toxic metabolites such as ammonia or arsenite [27 - 29].

As a result, inhibition might negatively impact parasite growth. According to Martins *et al.* [30], auphen just slightly inhibits water permeability but selectively inhibits glycerol transport in AQP3. Due to its excellent water solubility and low toxicity, it is a good option for the next *in vivo* research. According to recent reports, pentamidine, an aromatic diamidine, inhibits aquaglyceroporin in Trypanosoma brucei at the nanomolar level [31, 32]. As a result, using these inhibitors could offer helpful pharmacological tools for researching the potential target of parasite AQPs.

Plasmodial Surface Anion Channel

An intriguing novel therapeutic target has surfaced: the plasmodial surface anion channel (PSAC), a peculiar small-conductance ion channel produced on the membrane of Plasmodium-infected erythrocytes. It appears to be a new ion channel based on the number of functional features. Unlike almost all human chloride channels, it is permeable to selective anions (SCN− > I− > Br− > Cl−). The capacity of PSAC to retain low Na+ permeability in spite of Cl's high permeability is another distinctive property. Additionally, PSAC has emerged as a major marker. It exhibits voltage-dependent gating, with opening events happening far more frequently at negative membrane potentials than positive ones. As a result, these PSAC features may be a target for the development of specific inhibitors and potent antimalarial medicines [33].

Phloridzin [34], furosemide, NPPB [nitro-2-(3-phenyl-propylamino) benzoic acid] [35], glybenclamide [36], and dantrolene [37] are a few high-affinity inhibitors that have been found. They all have quantitatively similar effects on PSAC. Two PSAC inhibitors that are presently undergoing Phase I clinical trials—E912-0081 (MBX 2366) and C791-0105—showed efficient inhibition of plasmodial proliferation and demonstrated inhibitory activity in the nanomolar range [38]. Recent high-throughput screening has revealed a novel family of PSAC inhibitors: furoquinoline [39] and benzamide derivatives (PRT-1 & PRT1-20) [40]. These inhibitors are distinct from current blockers and have different effects on channel-mediated transport.

Hexose Transporter

P. falciparum encodes the facilitative sodium-independent hexose transporter (PfHT), which is crucial for glucose uptake and has been studied extensively as a possible therapeutic target. Since parasites lack energy reserves, their intra-erythrocytic stages are solely dependent on the glucose produced by their hosts for energy synthesis. Throughout the parasite's life cycle, a hexose transporter localizes to the plasma membrane [41]. 3-O-((undec-10-en)-1-yl)-D-glucose (CM3361) is an O-3 hexose derivative that inhibits PfHT's glucose and fructose absorption while having no effect on the major mammalian glucose and fructose transporters (GLUT1 and 5) [42]. It also eliminates parasites in culture and an infected animal model [43].

The finding that a single amino acid alteration (Q196N) renders PfHT1 incapable of transporting fructose while maintaining glucose transport at wild-type levels is a noteworthy finding [44]. This suggests that this residue is specifically crucial for substrate specificity. PFI0785c and PFI0955w, two more putative sugar transporters found in the genomic sequence of *P. falciparum*, differ from known glucose transporters more than PfHT1 does [45]. All three of these transporters are expressed during the intra-erythrocyte life cycle, according to an analysis of their transcripts. PfHT1 expresses itself relatively early after infection, whilst the other two express themselves considerably later [46]. Since hexose transporters have been demonstrated to be crucial to the survival of parasites in their infectious stage, they may serve as targets for the creation of novel anti-parasitic medications [47].

Choline Transporter

In the search for novel antimalarial medicines, parasite transporters are of great interest as therapeutic targets and as potential pathways for selective drug administration in blood-stage parasites. Given that the parasite is known to produce phosphatidylcholine (PC) *de novo* by absorbing choline from the external media, the parasite's choline carrier became the emerging focal point for the investigations. In this system, choline transport—which controls the precursor supply—is a rate-limiting step, while choline phosphate cytidylyl transferase is a regulatory step [48].

The crucial necessity of phospholipid metabolism to the parasite makes it an ideal target for novel treatment. When a person has malaria, their erythrocyte phospholipid concentration can rise by 500%. Normally, mature human erythrocytes do not undergo phospholipid metabolism. PC and PE, which together account for around 85% of the entire phospholipid pool, are the principal phospholipids found in infected erythrocytes. Complete descriptions of *de novo* processes in plasmodium-infected erythrocytes have been published for PC and PE production from choline and ethanolamine, respectively [49].

Many compounds that were intended to resemble the structure of choline have been synthesised in recent years. Lead compounds having a bis-quaternary ammonium or diamidine structure have been shown to exhibit good *in vivo* efficacy against P cynomolgi in rhesus and Aotus monkeys, and strong *in vitro* activity against *Plasmodium vivax* and P falciparum, respectively [50].

In the search for new antimalarial medications, parasite transporters are of great interest as therapeutic targets and as potential selective drug delivery channels in blood-stage parasites [51]. Since the parasite is known to absorb choline from the external medium for the *de novo* production of phosphatidylcholine (PC), we have concentrated on the parasite choline carrier in this investigation. The rate-limiting stage in this system is choline transport, which regulates the precursor supply, while choline phosphate cytidylyltransferase is a regulatory step [52].

Given the critical role that phospholipid metabolism plays for the parasite, it is a prime candidate for novel chemotherapeutic targets. Mature human erythrocytes do not undergo phospholipid metabolism. However, during malarial infection, the phospholipid content of erythrocytes can increase by up to 500%. The two main phospholipids in the infected erythrocyte, accounting for around 85% of the total phospholipid pool, are [53, 54] PC and phosphatidylethanolamine (PE). In Plasmodium-infected erythrocytes, *de novo* mechanisms for PC and PE production from choline and ethanolamine have been comprehensively documented, respectively [55].

Many compounds that were intended to resemble the structure of choline have been synthesised in recent years. Lead compounds with bis-quaternary ammonium or diamidine structure have shown strong *in vitro* activity against *Plasmodium vivax* and *P. falciparum* [56] and good *in vivo* action against *P. falciparum* and P. cynomolgi in Aotus and rhesus monkeys, respectively [57].

TARGETING THE APICOPLAST

It was discovered through molecular and cell biology investigation that apicomplexan parasites, such as *P. falciparum*, contain an organelle known as the apicoplast that resembles a plastid.

One of the main functions of the apicoplast is the production of fatty acids. These apicoplasts feature unique metabolic pathways, such as the synthesis of fatty acids, isoprenoid compounds, and heme, that are not found in the human host. As a result, these particular metabolic pathways seen in parasites are a fantastic supply of possible treatment targets [58].

The synthesis of fatty acids is essential for cell division, proliferation, and homeostasis. Fatty acids are produced by all living things, with the exception of mycoplasmas. One of the main roles of the apicoplast is fatty acid production (FAS).

FAS is caused by the following enzymes: betaketoacyl-ACP synthase (Fab H, B/F), enoyl-ACP reductase (Fab I), beta-ketoacyl-ACP reductase (Fab G), beta-hydroxyacyl-ACP dehydrase (Fab A/Z), and acetyl-CoA carboxylase (ACC). Because the human host (type I) and the parasite (type II) have fundamentally different fatty acid synthesis pathways, they are good targets for the development of antimalarial medications.

Thiolactomycin has been demonstrated to decrease *P. falciparum* growth *in vitro* and to inhibit FabH [59]. This implies that the synthesis of type II fatty acids in apicoplasts depends on _-ketoacyl-ACP synthase III (Fab H). Recent studies on enoyl-ACP reductase (Fab I) activity have shown that triclosan inhibits Fab I, which is how it exerts its antiparasitic effects [59].

FOCUSING ON CYCLIN-DEPENDENT PROTEIN KINASES (CDKs) FOUND IN PARASITES

The class of protein kinases known as cyclin-dependent kinases (CDK) was originally linked to the control of the cell cycle. Furthermore, transcription and mRNA processing are regulated by CDKs. Proteins with serine and threonine amino acid residues are phosphorylated by serine/threonine kinases or CDKs. A cyclin-dependent kinase is activated and a cyclin-dependent kinase complex is created when it combines forces with a cyclin. It has been determined that many *P. falciparum* kinases are homologs of the mammalian CDKs. It is anticipated that plasmodial CDKs will be essential for parasite proliferation since CDKs are conserved among species [60].

The cell cycle of a parasite differs greatly from that of a eukaryotic organism. Every cell cycle in eukaryotes results in the production of two identical daughter cells through a single round of DNA replication. The parasite goes through several rounds of nuclear division and DNA replication during schizogony before cytokinesis. A single multinucleate syncytium emerges as a result. Eight to thirty-two merozoites are produced by a single parasite. The regulation of parasitic cell division differs from that of mammals. It has been revealed that several *P. falciparum* CDKs resemble their mammalian homologs in terms of both sequence and structure [61]. Consequently, CDKs are becoming desirable targets for cutting-edge antimalarial medications.

Human CDK7 has the most sequence identity (46%) and similarity (64%), when compared to Pfmrk. CDK7 is a transcription factor that regulates transcription and DNA repair; it is also a kinase that activates cyclin-dependent kinase. Similar to Pfmrk, the parasite kinase, has a dual function, making it a prime candidate for CDK inhibitor development. To rationally design effective and selective Pfmrk inhibitors as antimalarial treatments, structural investigations would be beneficial.

TARGETING NUCLEIC ACID METABOLISM

The starting point for the production of DNA and RNA is nucleotides. The human host and *P. falciparum* have different metabolic routes for nucleic acids. Mammalian cells synthesise pyrimidines *via* a *de novo* pathway and purines by either *de novo* or salvage pathways, whereas plasmodia synthesise purines through salvage and/or *de novo* pathways. Numerous vital enzymes are involved in the two routes, and therapeutic intervention might be directed toward them.

The Purine Pathway

This pathway is used to create novel antimalarial drugs that specifically target PNP enzymes and the parasite HGPRT. The main structures of the parasite and human HGPRT differ in substrate preference (xanthine for plasmodia) and have a partial sequence similarity of 46%. Purine nucleotide phosphorylase (PNP) catalyses the phosphorolysis of inosine to hypoxanthine, which is the mechanism by which hypoxanthine is produced in humans and parasites. It has been demonstrated that the transition state analogue immucillin-H kills the parasite by inhibiting PNP [62].

The Pyrimidine Pathway

Pyrimidine nucleotides are derived from scratch by malaria parasites. Pre-made pyrimidine nucleosides are not something they can use. Both *de novo* and salvage mechanisms are possible in mammalian cells. The salvage enzymes, uridine kinase, and thymidine kinase, are absent from the parasite. The enzymes that are generated from scratch include orotate phosphoribosyl transferase, aspartate transcarbamylase, dihydroorotase, dihydroorotate dehydrogenase (DHODase), and orotidine 5-phosphate decarboxylase. Thymidylate synthase (TS) and dihydrofolate reductase are related. It is a recognized target of antimalarial chemotherapy as well. Because TS is a highly conserved protein, designing specific inhibitors may be difficult. Combining a nucleoside that the host can use with an efficient TS inhibitor could be a different tactic. Since N5–N10-methylene tetrahydrofolate analogs suppress TS without entering the nucleotide pool through metabolism, they are viewed as attractive alternatives [63]. It is necessary to investigate these analogs further.

TARGETING PARASITE TRANSPORTERS

Malaria-infected erythrocytes show a marked increase in the host membrane's permeability to a wide range of solutes. Significant changes occur in molecular trafficking of the kind and strength of the molecules that cross the host erythrocyte membrane. Numerous charged, low-molecular-weight solutes have improved permeability thanks to the induced permeability pathways, also known as novel permeability pathways (NPPs). They are polyspecific and anion-selective. It is believed that these NPPs are the main source of pantothenate, one of the vital nutrients needed by the parasites. Additionally, they facilitate the release of different waste products from metabolism, including lactic acid, from the contaminated cell [64].

TARGETING THE MITOCHONDRIAL SYSTEM

The mitochondrial DNA sequence of *P. falciparum* has been determined. The synthesis of proteins and the movement of electrons are the two main functions of mitochondria. These appear to be essential for survival and might be the focus of chemotherapy in the treatment of malaria. The 6 kb genome of the mitochondrial DNA of the malaria parasite encodes three proteins: cytochrome b and subunits I and III of cytochrome c oxidase, a respiratory chain terminal oxidase [65]. Transcripts of the 6 kb segment are most common in the later phases of the asexual life cycle. The cytochrome b gene of the ubiquinol–cytochrome c reductase (complex III) does not originate primarily from gametocytes; rather, asexual life stages are. It is expected that chemotherapy would focus on the structural differences in mitochondria between malaria parasites and their host, as evidenced by the discrepancies between the plasmodial and mammalian forms of cytochrome b [66].

TARGETING THE REDOX SYSTEM

Oxidative stress has a role in the destruction of intracellular parasites, such as malaria. The production of reactive oxygen is out of balance with the ability of a biological system to rapidly detoxify the reactive intermediates or reverse the damage they cause. This imbalance leads to oxidative stress. The cellular environment of all living organisms is constantly decreasing. Enzymes retain the reduced state by continuously supplying metabolic energy. This keeps the reducing environment intact. Reactive oxygen species are created by the parasites themselves, the erythrocyte, or the host immune cells during the intraerythrocytic stage of malaria. The parasite makes its own antioxidant enzymes to guard against oxidative damage. Therefore, antimalarial chemotherapy drugs may be able to attack the parasite's antioxidant defense. The primary *P. falciparum* enzymes involved in redox metabolism are glutathione reductase, glutathione peroxidase, thioredoxin reductase, and thioredoxin peroxiredoxin [67].

TARGETING THE SHIKIMATE PATHWAY

Apicomplexan parasites, such as *P. falciparum*, have a shikimate pathway that offers multiple targets for the synthesis of novel antiparasitic drugs. Mammals do not have this route [68]. Nevertheless, it is exclusive to the chloroplast in plants and can be found in the cytoplasm of bacteria and fungus. Seven enzymes are involved in the shikimate pathway, which catalyzes the sequential conversion of erythrose 4-phosphate and phosphoenolpyruvate to chorismate. It has been demonstrated that chorismate synthase is necessary for both normal growth and the RNA interference-induced interruption of expression, which inhibits parasite growth [69]. As a result, *P. falciparum* chorismate synthase is a verified target for medication development.

TARGETING ISOPRENOID BIOSYNTHESIS

As a potential therapeutic target, inhibition of the Plasmodium protein farnesyltransferase (PfPFT) is being investigated. PFT inhibitors work by obstructing posttranslational modification pathways, and they are used to treat cancer in humans. Medicinal chemistry and pharmacokinetics are investigating a related idea to create PFT inhibitors that combat parasites [70]. 1-deoxy-d-xylulose-5-phosphate (1-DOXP) is used as a precursor molecule by bacteria and *Plasmodium falciparum* through the mevalonate-independent mechanism. One possible target for antimalarial treatment has been suggested to be the plastid-encoded mevalonate-independent route of isoprenoid production [71].

TARGETING PARASITE PROTEASES

Plasmodium are parasites that feed on blood. Proteases hydrolyze a large amount of the proteins in the host erythrocyte, which is crucial for the survival of the parasite. A portion of the individual amino acids that are produced by the breakdown of 80% of the hemoglobin in host cells is utilized to synthesise parasite proteins [72]. It appears that many Plasmodium proteases are in charge of the essential cleavage of host proteins. Two functional groups can be distinguished from the malarial parasite's spectrum of proteolytic activity:

i. Proteases implicated in hemoglobin degradation; (ii) an erythrocyte's invasion and rupture [73].

The host-parasite interactions are still unclear at the molecular level during the invasion phase. It is clear that a great deal of surface proteins are modified by proteases, and the success of merozoite invasion is dependent upon these mechanisms [74]. The merozoite surface protein MSP-1 is involved in the invasion process. *P. falciparum*, the malaria parasite, invades human red blood cells. To infect new erythrocytes, the merozoites need to escape their host cell and enter the blood plasma. At this point, proteases are thought to have a significant role. Cysteine protease inhibitors are used to study the merozoite release mechanism in combination with immunoelectron microscopy and fluorescence microscopy. The inhibitors stop the host cell membrane from rupturing, which leads to clustered merozoite formations. Leupeptin, chymostatin, and E64 are examples of cysteine protease inhibitors that may be used as a model to create new inhibitors specific to plasmodial proteases [75].

TARGETING PARASITE MEMBRANE BIOSYNTHESIS

Various membranes, such as the parasitophorous vacuole membrane, the feeding vacuolar membrane, and the parasite plasma membrane (PPM), are present in intraerythrocytic parasites. Hence, compared to normal erythrocytes, infected erythrocytes have a much larger amount of lipid. Plasmid fatty acids are converted into phospholipids, which are needed in high quantities by malaria parasites for growth and division. The main phospholipid found in parasites is phosphatidylcholine (PC). Using choline, seventy to eighty percent of PCs are created from scratch. Choline mobility in infected red blood cells (RBCs) is significantly boosted with the use of a constitutive choline carrier. Either overactivity of a constitutive host cell transporter or carrier synthesis driven by parasites for this occurs. Targeting the parasite's PC supply, molecules are being developed. G25, a lead chemical, significantly reduced the development of *Plasmodium vivax* and *P. falciparumin vitro* [76].

TARGETING THE pfTBP–pfTFIIB INTERFACE

As of right now, there are no antimalarial medications that specifically target nuclear transcription, an essential step in every stage of *P. falciparum* reproduction. Owing to its crucial role in the start of transcription, novel antimalarial chemotherapeutic drugs are being investigated as potential targets for the pfTBP–pfTFIIB interaction. TATA box binding protein (TBP) and transcription factor IIB (TFIIB) have to work together for transcription to start [77]. Many transcriptional regulators include TFIIB and TBP as their primary targets [78]. The same TFIIB regions appear to be interacting with both activators and inhibitors. The amino- and carboxy-terminal domains of natural TFIIB (TFIIBn and TFIIBc, respectively) are shown to interact intramolecularly in certain investigations [79]. Acidic activators cause this intramolecular connection to break down, revealing TFIIB binding sites that engage with other transcription factors and promote the start of transcription. TFIIBn connects with the RNA polymerase II dock domain [80], while TFIIBc attaches to TBP and DNA following the loss of the TFIIB intramolecular connection. Despite experimental evidence supporting both positive and negative transcriptional regulation functions for Negative Cofactor 2 (NC2) [81], crystallographic data, on the other hand, indicate that NC2's inhibitory activity is mediated by the direct interaction between its beta sub-unit and TBP, which sterically inhibits TBP's association with TFIIB. One plausible mechanism for novel antimalarial types is the natural action of NC2 in transcription inhibition [82].

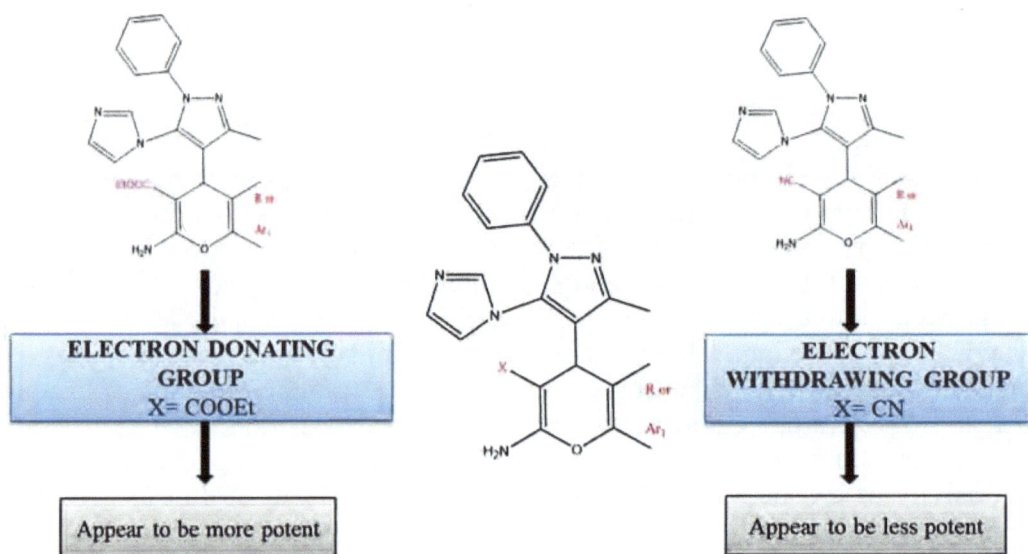

Fig. (1). Structure activity relationship of 5-imidazopyrazole incorporated fused Pyran.

Malaria-related morbidity and mortality have decreased over the past 15 years, but the durability of these gains is endangered by the emergence of resistance to first-line artemisinin-based antimalarials, the scarcity of efficient vaccines, and the limited availability of chemotherapeutic options. Recently, a detailed proposal for the best candidate compounds and pharmaceuticals likely to successfully advance into the final stages of clinical development was accepted by the malaria drug discovery community, which will serve as a template to guide future designs of novel treatments. This book chapter serves as an audit of current advancements in malaria chemotherapy especially during the past five years, depicts a landscape of varied compounds at different phases of drug development, and talks about their advancement. For the purpose of developing antimalarial drugs, researchers are searching for chemicals with target profiles in order to prevent or treat single-exposure radicals. This effort is motivated by worries regarding the rise of resistance to existing antimalarial drugs. These are creative molecular skeletons for future creative treatment concepts [83-85].

NOVEL 5-IMIDAZOPYRAZOLE INCORPORATED FUSED PYRANS

Analogs of pyrazole constitute a significant class of heterocycles. A wide range of pharmacological actions, including anticancer [86], antibacterial [87], antiviral [88], analgesic [89], and anti-inflammatory [90], are exhibited by pyrazole derivatives. Imidazole compounds, on the other hand, have been linked to several biological characteristics, including analgesic, anti-inflammatory, anti-convulsant, anti-antitubercular, antibacterial, anticancer, and anti-Parkinson's effects [91 - 95]. The fused pyran ring, a prominent structural motif, and important heterocyclic core composition, is present in many pharmaceutically active drugs. Due to its significant pharmacophore role in both antimicrobial and antituberculosis activity, the fused pyran scaffold is still considered a viable lead structure for the synthesis of more effective and broad-spectrum antibacterial and antituberculosis medicines. A significant class of substances with a high activity profile are fused pyran derivatives. The antimalarial activity of all newly fused pyran derivatives was assessed against the *P. falciparum* strain [96-98].

According to the structure-activity relationship analysis, pyran was found to have a wide variety of antimalarial activities due to several heteromeric motifs attached at positions 5 and 6 (Fig. 1). Compound 6 [IC_{50}=0.049] having N-methyl barbituric acid substitution exhibited better antimalarial efficacy against P. falciparum. *P. falciparum* was effectively inhibited by compounds 4 [IC_{50}=0.062] and 3 [IC_{50}=0.034] that contained 3-methyl-1-phenyl pyrazol-5-one. The ester group in Compound 6 [IC_{50}=0.049] enhanced its antimalarial efficacy against P. falciparum. Compound 5 [IC_{50}=0.082], which has a carbonitrile group, exhibited weak defense against P. falciparum. Three-methyl-1-phenyl pyrazol-5-one is present in compounds 3 [IC_{50}=0.034] and 4 [IC_{50}=0.062]. Of these, compound 4 [IC_{50}=0.062], which has an ester group, exhibited superior antimalarial activity (Fig. 2) [98-100].

2-AMIDOBENZIMIDAZOLE DERIVATIVES

The benzimidazole skeleton (BZ) is a key component in medicinal chemistry. Substitutions in various places of the molecule provide compounds with a wide range of applications, including antihypertensive [101], antidiabetic [102], antitumoral [103], antibacterial [104], and anti-inflammatory [105]. For the past five years, a number of research teams have been focusing on the synthesis of BZ compounds that may have antimalarial effects. 2-phenyl-1H-benzimidazole derivatives demonstrated good activity against *P. falciparum in vitro*; the IC50 values of the most potent compounds ranged from 18 nM to 1.30 µM. Many BZ compounds were investigated for *in vitro* anti-Pf activity in this work. This paper examined the *in vitro* anti-Pf activity of many BZ drugs. These compounds contain an amide spacer between the BZ nucleus and the heterocyclic fragment (ring B). The molecules' capacity for exocyclic tautomerization, which could facilitate deeper bonding with their target and potentially increase activity, is provided by the amide region. It is possible to enhance or impede the production of the exocyclic tautomer by including electron donor or acceptor groups into ring A. As an alternative, one may make a new connection—a hydrogen bond could form with the methoxy group, increasing the level of activity—or enlarge the BZ to better match the target. With relation to ring B, the viability of larger (quinoline, isoquinoline) or medium-sized (pyridine) heterocycles has been studied. (Fig. **3**). Even the kind and location of certain substituents on the pyridine ring along with the majority of active chemicals' cytotoxicity toward the Vero cell line are explained, and the associated selectivity index (SI) is also computed. A number of mechanistic investigations were included for some compounds that had good activity but insufficient selectivity in order to obtain insight into potential variations between the lead compounds BZ 1 and 5 in terms of how they affect parasites [106].

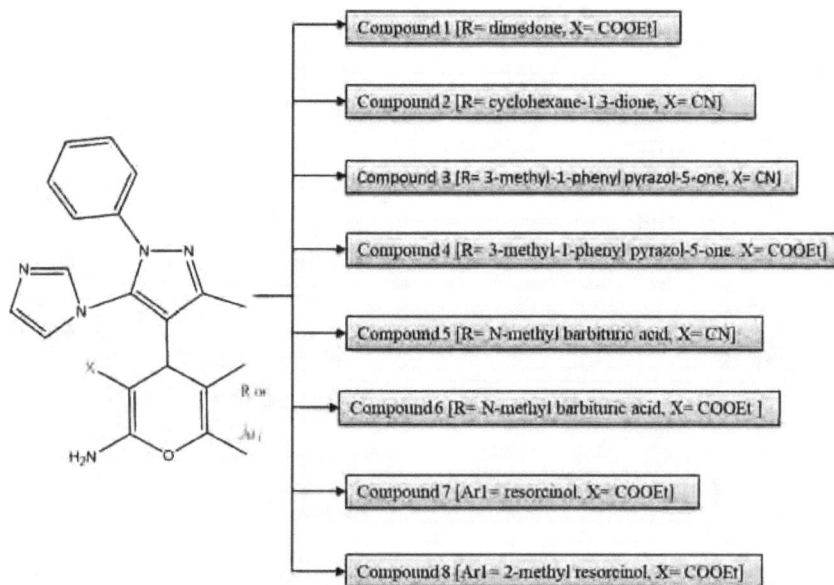

Fig. (2). Substitution of 5-imidazopyrazole incorporated fused Pyran.

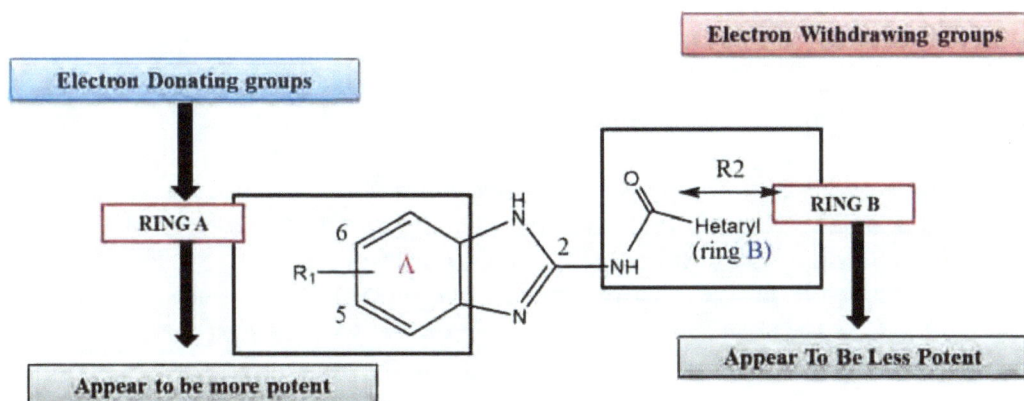

Fig. (3). Structural Activity relationship of 2-amido benzimidazole derivative.

Derivatives of benzimidazole were evaluated at 10 μM against the Pf HB3 strain, and the IC50 values were calculated for those compounds that showed a percentage of growth inhibition (% GI) greater than 50%. To determine their selectivity indexes (SI), their cytotoxicity on epithelial Vero cell cultures was also assessed. A lead compound is predicted to have an index of 10 or higher. Compounds are arranged first by complexity of ring B, then by substituent on ring A. In the BZ system, ring A exhibits electron-withdrawing groups (EWG; 5-Cl, 5-NO2, 5-NHCOR, or 5,6-diCH3) or electron-donating groups (EDG; 5-CH3, 5-OCH3, 5-NH2, 5-NHCOR, or 5,6-diCH3). Ring B heterocycles can be pyridines with nitrogen in ortho, meta, or para position, quinolines, or isoquinolines.

Therefore, it appears that Compounds 1 and 4 are more effective (Fig. **4**), since they showed methyl as an electron donor group in ring A.

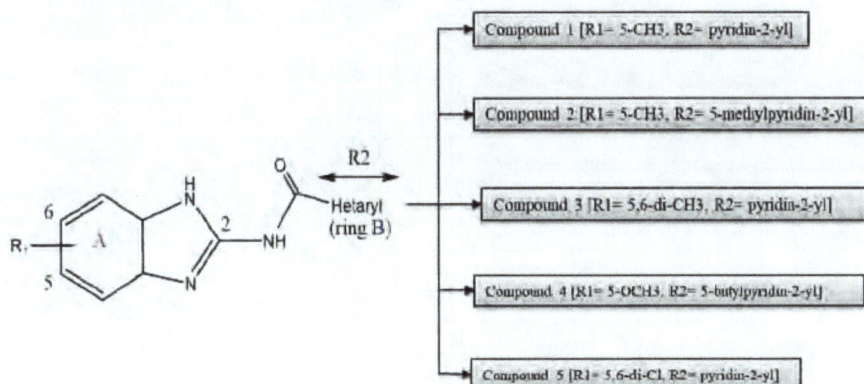

Fig. (4). Substitution of 2-amidobenzimidazole derivative.

PHENOXYARYL-4(1H)-PYRIDONES

They mainly concentrate on a class of 4(1H)-pyridones associated with clopidol, an anticoccidial medication. Studies conducted in the late 1960s under the auspices of the Walter Reed Army Institute of Research showed that clopidol was active against many animal models of Plasmodium sp., including those resistant to chloroquine [107]. Human clinical studies verified efficacy against chloroquine-resistant *P. falciparum*; nonetheless, the results were insufficient to justify additional research and development. At the time, there were unsuccessful attempts to increase activity by using a variety of basic compounds. Later, data showed that clopidol inhibited mitochondrial respiration as part of its mechanism of action [108]. Additionally, it has been demonstrated that clopidol retains its antimalarial efficacy against an atovaquone-resistant strain while enhancing the antimalarial activity of hydroxynaphthoquinones both *in vitro* and *in vivo* [109]. This suggested that clopidol was working through a different mechanism, and its straightforward structure provided some room for modification to enhance antimalarial efficacy (Fig. **5**). The purpose of this study, which we present here, was to find compounds with significantly better activity than clopidol against *P. falciparumin vitro* and murine *P. yoelii in vivo*, with the potential for the treatment of malaria [110]. We also looked into the relationship between the structure and antimalarial activity of 4-pyridones.

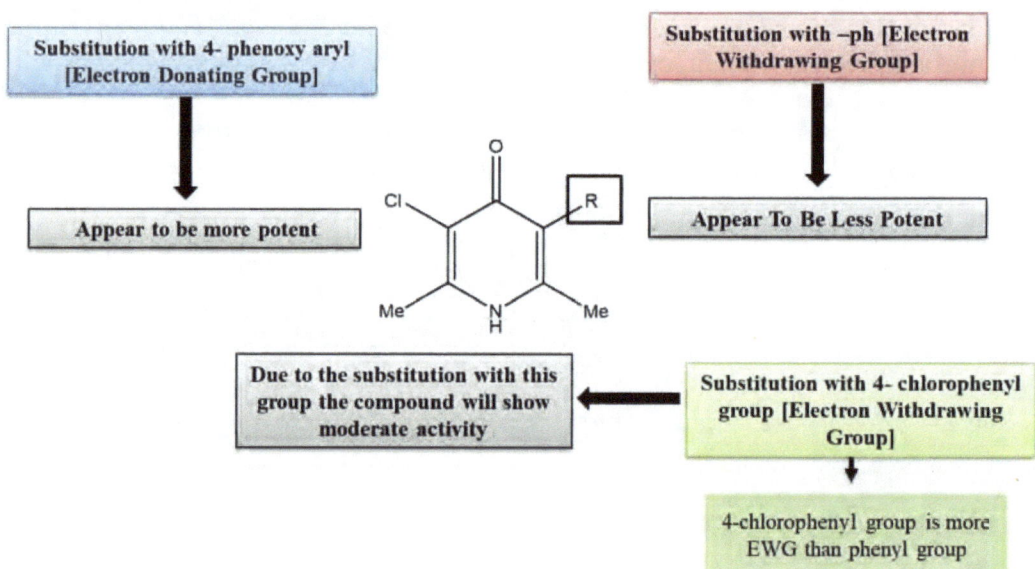

Fig. (5). Structure activity relationship of 4(1H)-pyridones derivatives.

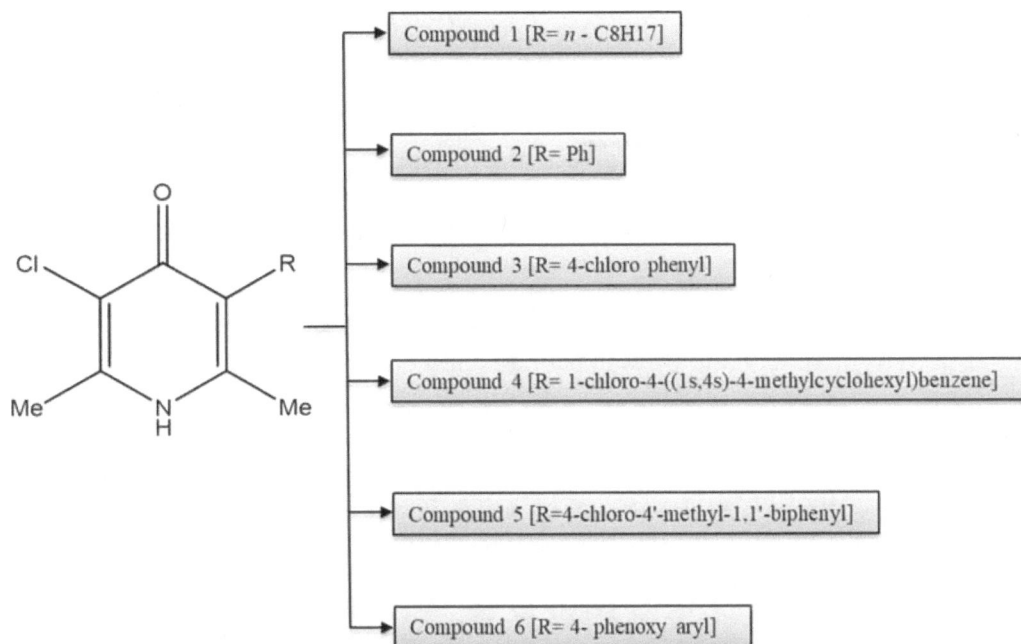

Fig. (6). Substitution of 4(1H)-pyridones derivatives.

Fig. (**6**) summarizes the antimalarial activity of a cross-section of the first series of 4-pyridones produced. The activity of the 3-octyl derivative 1 was increased. The replacement of R= 1-chloro-4-((1s,4s)-4-methylcyclohexyl)benzene resulted in compound 4, which had the most powerful action of all the compounds with an IC50 value of 0.05.

SAR OF HYDROXYFERROQUINE DERIVATIVES

It has been demonstrated that ferroquine works astonishingly well against *P. falciparum*, which is resistant to CQ [111]. It is thought that FQ and CQ have similar modes of action, most likely involving hematin as the pharmacological target and suppression of hemozoin formation [112]. Similarities to CQ's metabolism were found in a recent study on FQ metabolism in hepatic models from animals and humans [113]. One important distinction is that FQ metabolites showed considerable effectiveness despite the fact that the two primary CQ metabolites are inactive against *P. falciparum* which is resistant to CQ. It is also crucial to remember that hydroxychloroquine (HCQ), the near relative of CQ, was discovered to be inert against *P. falciparum*, a CQ-resistant strain while being believed to be less hazardous than CQ [113].

in vitro testing of metallocenes against *P. falciparum's* CQ-sensitive HB3 strain and CQ-resistant W2 strain was conducted. Against the resistant strain, the three hydroxy compounds showed more efficacy than CQ. The unsubstituted 1 [IC_{50}= 15.4± 5.5&133.2 ± 7.4] and the N-ethyl-substituted 3 [IC_{50}=.11.7 ± 5.7&20.4 ± 1.1] of these amino-alcohol derivatives had the highest activity. It should be noted that, against both *P. falciparum* strains, the most active product 3, which was 3, was even more effective than mefloquine and just marginally less effective than FQ [110].

Derivative 3 of hydroxyferroquine (IC50 = 11.7 ± 5.7 & 20.4 ± 1.1) had much higher activity than CQ and only marginally lower activity than FQ and MF. With MF, there was no cross-resistance, but with CQ, there was a little cross-reaction. Nearly the same amount of activity was seen in Metallocene 3 as in FQ. Anticipatedly, among the isolates examined, a strong association was seen between the IC50 of FQ and 3 [IC_{50}= 11.7 ± 5.7&20.4 ± 1.1]. This implies that the two substances function similarly and/or are absorbed by the parasite. When it comes to *P. falciparum* strains that are resistant to HCQ, the toxicity and antimalarial properties of HCQ seem to be absent [114]. Our objective was to create a possibly less toxic compound with strong antimalarial activity based on the high activity of FQ (Fig. 7). Compound 3 [IC_{50}= 11.7 ± 5.7&20.4 ± 1.1] (Fig. 8) among the three hydroxyferroquine-type derivatives synthesized showed strong antimalarial activity against all strains and isolates of *P. falciparum* tested, being only 1.5 times less active than FQ, and much more active than CQ (6-fold). Of the three compounds produced, this product is the most lipophilic and has high FQ action against strains of *P. falciparum* that are resistant to CQ [112]. 3 [IC_{50}= 11.7 ± 5.7&20.4 ± 1.1] is more active than 1 [IC_{50}= 15.4± 5.5&133.2 ± 7.4] and 2 [IC 50= 21.5 ± 14.5&30 ± 8.8].

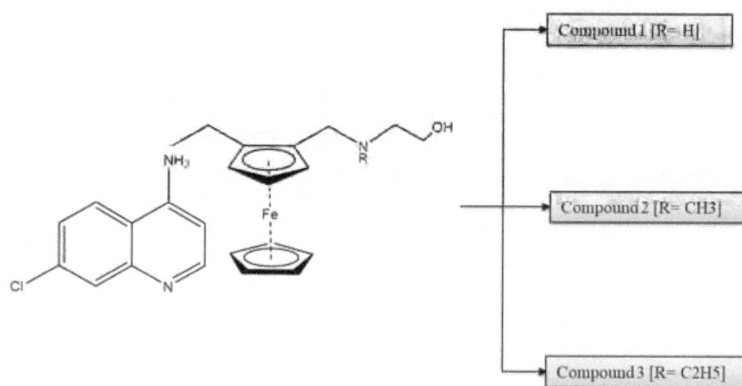

Fig. (7). Substitution of hydroxyferroquine derivatives.

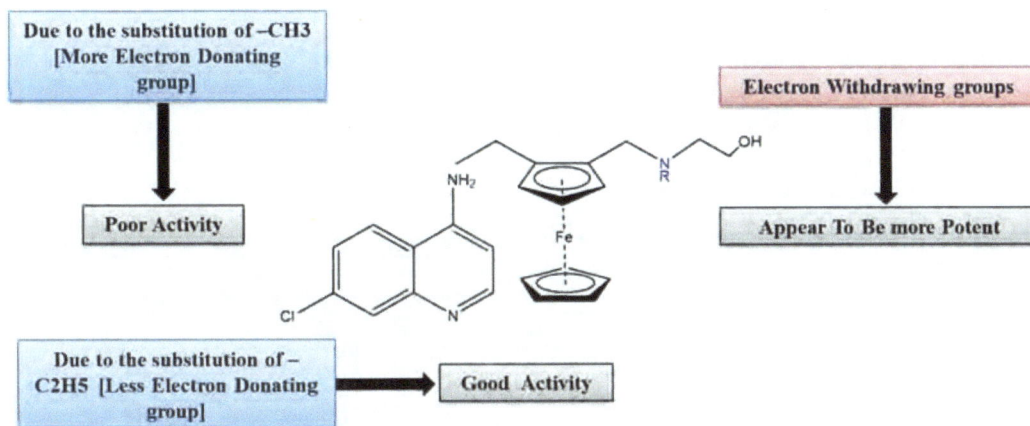

Fig. (8). Structure-activity Relationship of Hydroxyferroquine Derivatives.

NOVEL INDOLEAMIDE DERIVATIVES

Reports on the antimalarial properties of compounds based on indole are few. Currently undergoing a phase-I clinical study, a spiroindolone class antimalarial drug has demonstrated strong antimalarial efficacy against all isolates of *P. vivax* and *P. falciparum in vitro*, with an IC50 of less than 10nM [116]. In addition, a large number of additional compounds based on indole show antimalarial activity in the 39–0.65 µM range [117, 118]. With an IC50 of 0.65 µM, vitexin, a violet pigment derived from indole and isolated from Chromobacterium violaceum, had shown strong antimalarial properties [118]. Novel indole-based compounds with antiplasmodial action that have an IC50 range of 19 to 2.9 µM have recently been described by the Garcia C.R.S group [119].

Using chloroquine as a reference medication, these compounds' *in vitro* antiplasmodial efficacy against *P. falciparum* strains that were CQ sensitive (3D7) and CQ resistant (K1) was assessed. Compounds 1 and 2 of adamantyl sulfonamides had moderate to excellent efficacy; compound 1 displayed IC50 values of 1.87 and 1.69 µM against strains that were sensitive and resistant, respectively, while compound 2 displayed IC50 values of 1.93 and 2.12 µM. Cycloheptyl sulfonamides 3 and 4 likewise showed moderate to excellent efficacy; compound 3 demonstrated an IC 50 of 2.00 and 1.60 µM against strains that were sensitive and resistant, respectively, while compound 4 demonstrated an IC 50 of 2.17 and 2.19 µM. It is interesting to note that compounds 1 and 3 have more effectiveness against resistant strains than sensitive strains when combined with the bulky terbutylphenyl sulfonamide at the N1 position of indole (Fig. **9**). Compounds 2 and 4, which include bulky 4-chloro-2,5-dimethylphenyl sulfonamides, have likewise demonstrated good action. Their respective IC50 values are 1.93 and 2.17 µM for sensitive strain and 2.12 and 2.19 µM for resistant strain (Fig. **10**), [115].

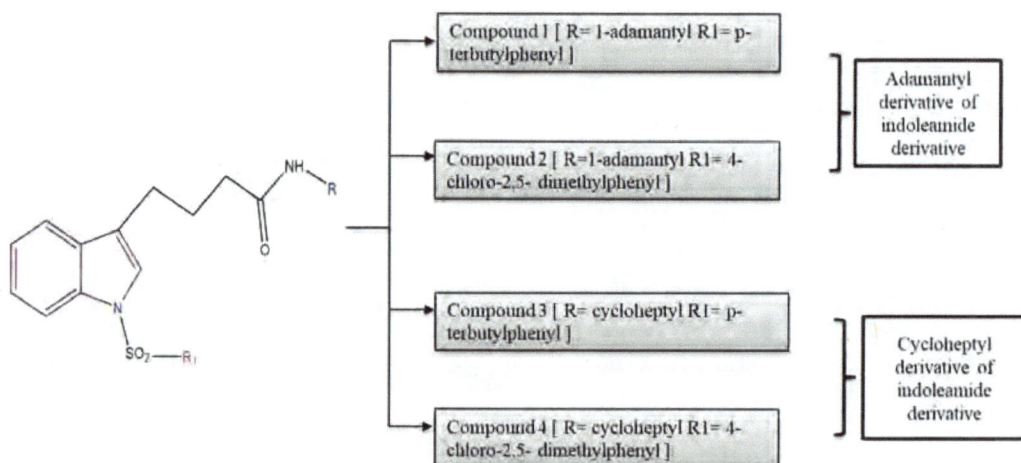

Fig. (9). Substitution of indoleamide derivatives.

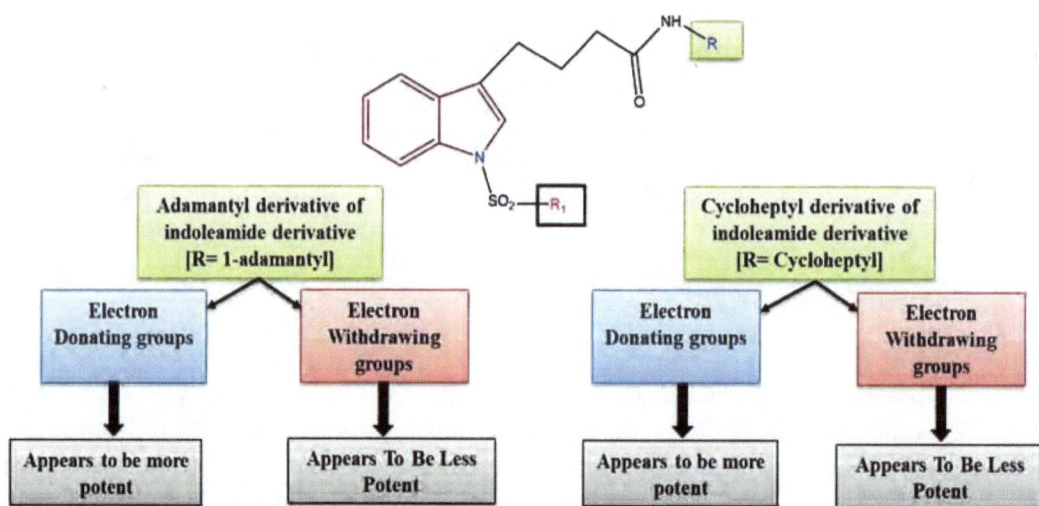

Fig. (10). Structure-activity Relationship of Indoleamide Derivatives.

CHROMANO-CHALCONES AND CHROMENO-CHALCONES DERIVATIVES

Chalcone with oxygen to date, the most promising antimalarial compound found in Chinese licorice roots has been identified as licochalcone A (I). Natural chalcone has been shown to inhibit the development of both chloroquine-susceptible (CQ S) 3D7 and chloroquine-resistant (CQ R) Dd2 strains of

Plasmodium falciparum.

Structural Activity Relationship of Chromano-chalcones Derivatives

In the structural activity relation, halogen groups on ring-A, electron-withdrawing groups (EWGs), and electron-donating groups (EDGs) appear to be less powerful (MIC >25 μM) compared to the synthesis of prenylated chalcone derivatives by Tadigoppula N. *et al.* The activity of chalcones 1f (MIC = 126.90 μM) and 1g (MIC = 122.54 μM), which have an additional alkyl chain on the benzopyran core, was equally low (**6**) (Fig. **11b**). When chromanochalcones (Fig. **11a**) were compared to C-prenylated chalcones, their antimalarial activity was shown to be less effective due to the cyclization of a prenyl/geranyl group.

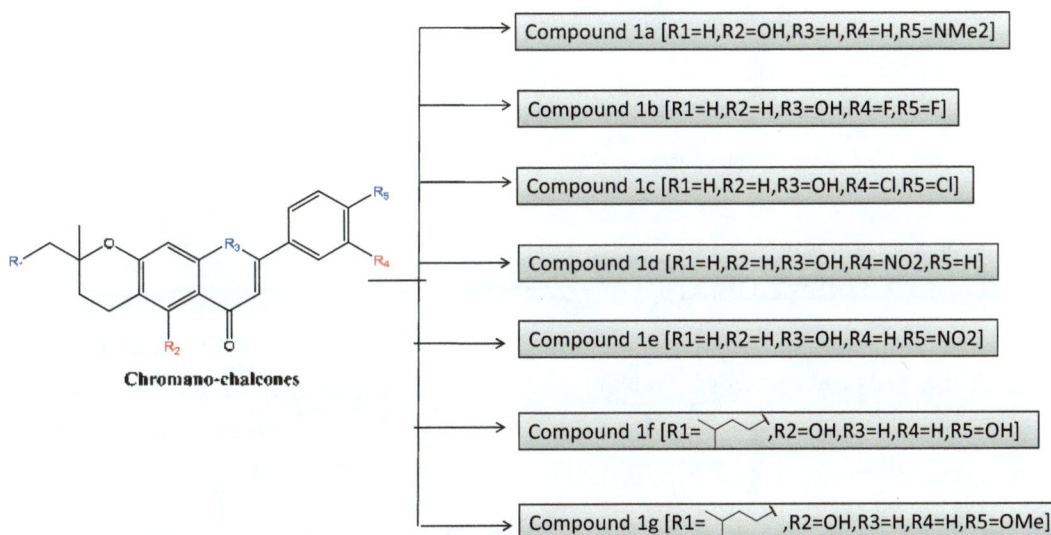

Compound 1a [R1=H,R2=OH,R3=H,R4=H,R5=NMe2]

Compound 1b [R1=H,R2=H,R3=OH,R4=F,R5=F]

Compound 1c [R1=H,R2=H,R3=OH,R4=Cl,R5=Cl]

Compound 1d [R1=H,R2=H,R3=OH,R4=NO2,R5=H]

Compound 1e [R1=H,R2=H,R3=OH,R4=H,R5=NO2]

Compound 1f [R1= ,R2=OH,R3=H,R4=H,R5=OH]

Compound 1g [R1= ,R2=OH,R3=H,R4=H,R5=OMe]

Chromano-chalcones

Fig. (11a). Substitution of chromano-chalcones derivatives.

SAR of Chromeno-chalcone's Antimalarial Activity

Instead of chroman, we discover the activity profile of the chromene (benzopyran) moiety in structural relations. The EDGs on ring-A are located on chromenochalcones 30–36. Of them, the antimalarial activity of compounds 1-4 and 6 was low (MIC = 126–155 μM range), while that of compounds 5 (MIC = 27.47 μM) and 7 (MIC = 25.25 μM) was moderate. With the exception of chromenochalcone 13 (MIC = 5.34 μM), the activity of the other chalcones (8–12) with mono- or 3,4-dihalogen substituents on ring-A is low (MIC = 105–155 μM). The combination of EDGs and halogen substituents on ring-A in chromenochalcone 14 (MIC = 135.86 μM) (Fig. **12b**) and its regioisomer 15 (>135.86 μM) showed unsatisfactory action.

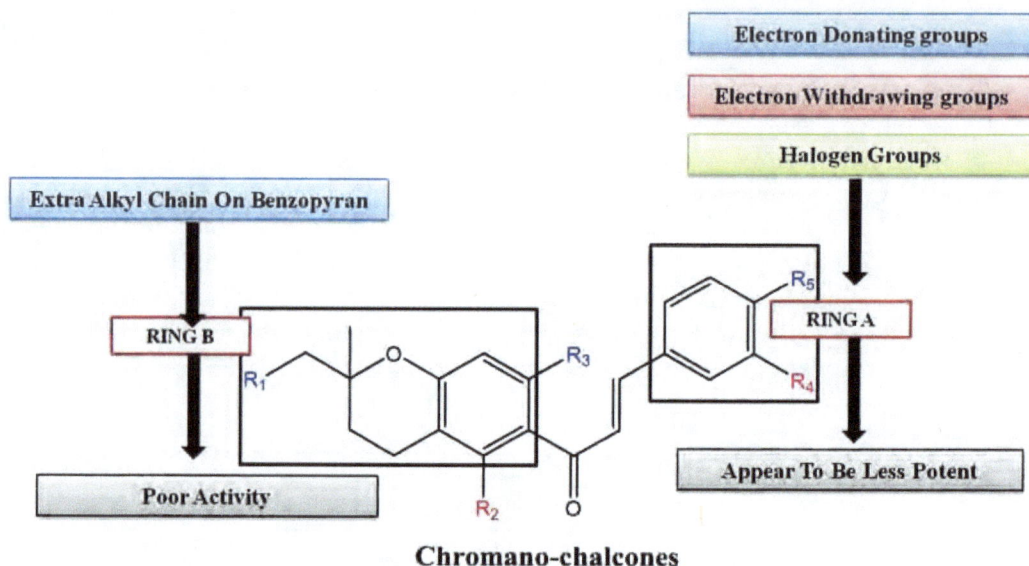

Chromano-chalcones

Fig. (11b). Structural Activity Relationship of Chromano-chalcones Derivatives.

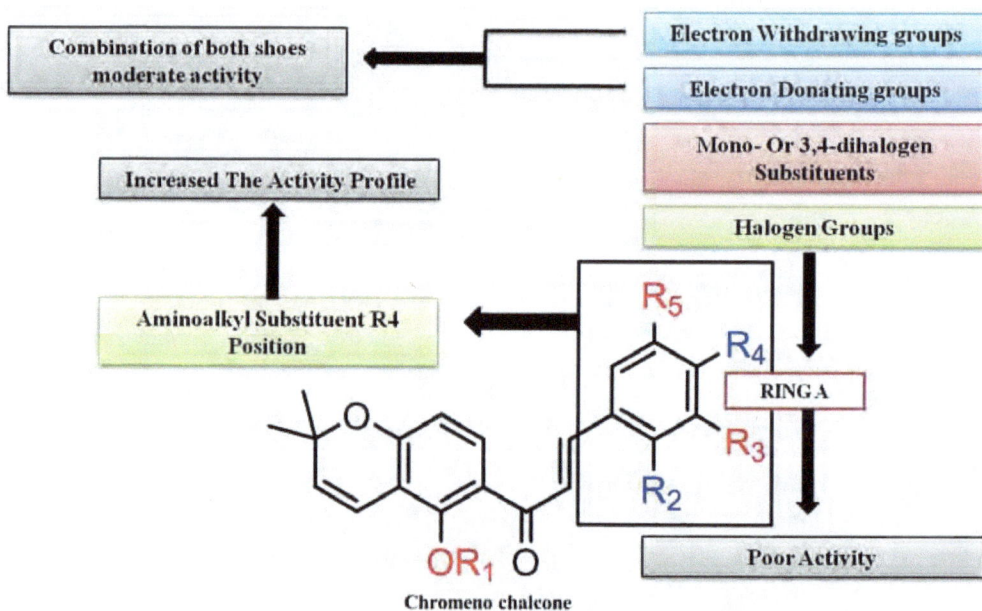

Chromeno chalcone

Fig. (12a). Structural Activity relationship of Chromano-chalcones Derivatives.

Compounds 16 and 17, which comprise EWGs, likewise exhibited little activity. Conversely, compound 18, which substitutes a mix of EDGs and EWGs for ring-A, showed moderate activity (MIC = 28.57 μM). The activity profile **6** [123] was greatly enhanced by the addition of an aminoalkyl substituent, such as in 19 (MIC = 3.67 μM), on the hydroxyl group of 33 (MIC = 155.27 μM) [123] (Fig. **12a**).

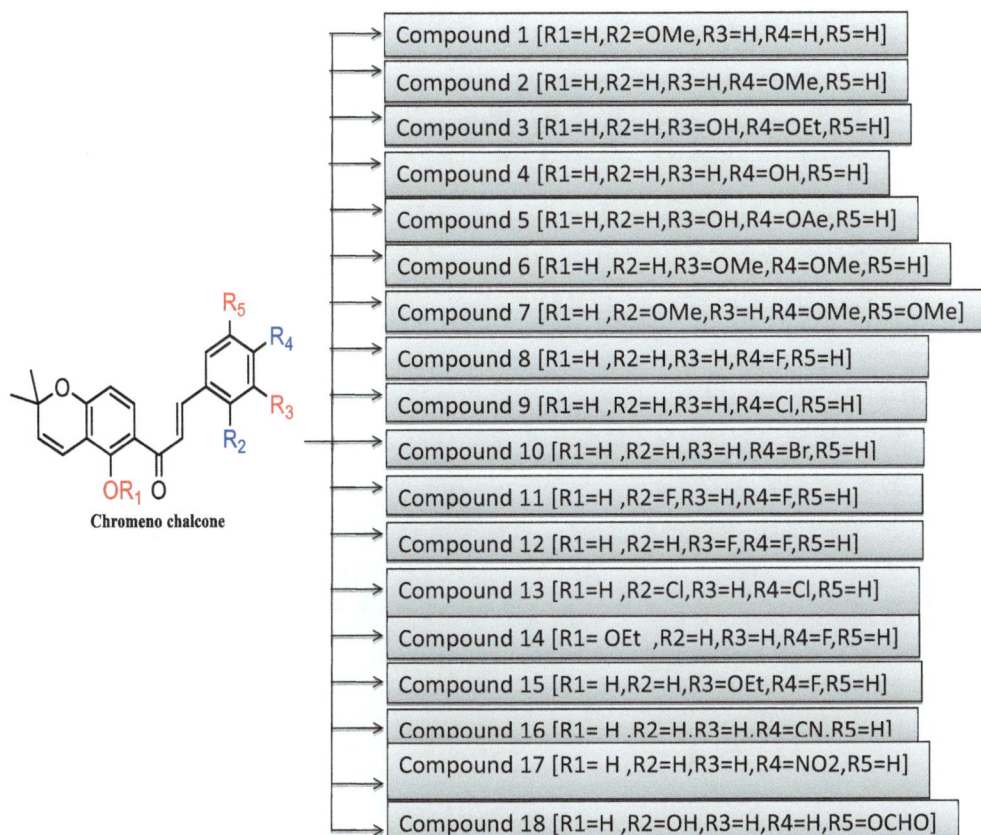

Compound 1 [R1=H,R2=OMe,R3=H,R4=H,R5=H]

Compound 2 [R1=H,R2=H,R3=H,R4=OMe,R5=H]

Compound 3 [R1=H,R2=H,R3=OH,R4=OEt,R5=H]

Compound 4 [R1=H,R2=H,R3=H,R4=OH,R5=H]

Compound 5 [R1=H,R2=H,R3=OH,R4=OAe,R5=H]

Compound 6 [R1=H ,R2=H,R3=OMe,R4=OMe,R5=H]

Compound 7 [R1=H ,R2=OMe,R3=H,R4=OMe,R5=OMe]

Compound 8 [R1=H ,R2=H,R3=H,R4=F,R5=H]

Compound 9 [R1=H ,R2=H,R3=H,R4=Cl,R5=H]

Compound 10 [R1=H ,R2=H,R3=H,R4=Br,R5=H]

Compound 11 [R1=H ,R2=F,R3=H,R4=F,R5=H]

Compound 12 [R1=H ,R2=H,R3=F,R4=F,R5=H]

Compound 13 [R1=H ,R2=Cl,R3=H,R4=Cl,R5=H]

Compound 14 [R1= OEt ,R2=H,R3=H,R4=F,R5=H]

Compound 15 [R1= H,R2=H,R3=OEt,R4=F,R5=H]

Compound 16 [R1= H ,R2=H,R3=H,R4=CN,R5=H]

Compound 17 [R1= H ,R2=H,R3=H,R4=NO2,R5=H]

Compound 18 [R1=H ,R2=OH,R3=H,R4=H,R5=OCHO]

R_5
R_4
R_3
R_2
OR_1 O
Chromeno chalcone

Fig. (12b). Substitution of chromeno-chalcone derivatives.

NOVEL BENZOXABOROLES DERIVATIVES

Compounds 1 through 20 were evaluated for their *in vitro* inhibitory activity against *P. falciparum*, the malaria parasite, and their IC 50 values are compiled in Fig. (**13**). The purpose of designing and synthesizing Compounds 1-3 was to examine the impact of side-chain length. Compound 1 was 24 times more effective than compound 2 with C3 space because it had two carbon spaces (C 2) between the benzene ring and the carboxylic acid group. Increasing the gap to compound 3's C4 resulted in an additional loss of potency of three times. Compounds 1-6 exhibit the impact of variation in side-chain atoms. The IC50 values are 0.46, 0.95, and >5 lM, respectively, when the side-chain next-t--benzene CH2 of 1 is replaced by an O-atom of 4, an NH of 5, and an NMe of 6.

The potency was sensitive to the side-chain electron change from CH2 to O to NH, and the steric variation of the chain from NH to NMe.

To investigate the impact of side-chain terminal functional group change, compounds 7–14 were synthesized. With 2.72 lM IC50, ketone compound 7 exhibited modest action, whereas methyl ester 8 had 0.32 lM IC50. A molecule 10 with an IC 50 >5 lM was produced by adding dimethyl to the amide nitrogen, but the main amide 9 with an IC 50 of 1.30 lM was 50 times less powerful than the acid 1. The efficacy was improved thrice by adding a cyclopropyl sulfonyl group to the amide nitrogen, from 1.30 lM of 9 to 0.46 lM of 11, which contains the acidic C(O)NHSO2 group. An IC50 of 1.02 lM was obtained by substituting the cyano group in 12 for the carboxylic group in 1, with a 39-fold reduction in potency. The potency increased by two and six times, respectively, when the cyano group was transformed to the aminomethyl of 13 and the tetrazole of 14. Based on side chain terminal alteration, tetrazole compound 14 was the most powerful among compounds 7–14 (Fig. **14**).

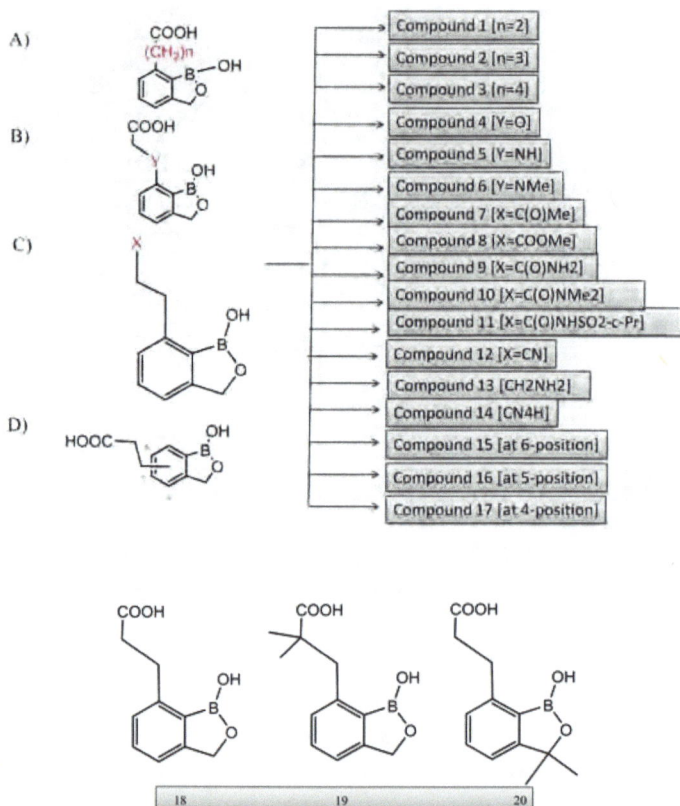

Fig. (13). Substitution of novel benzoxaboroles derivatives.

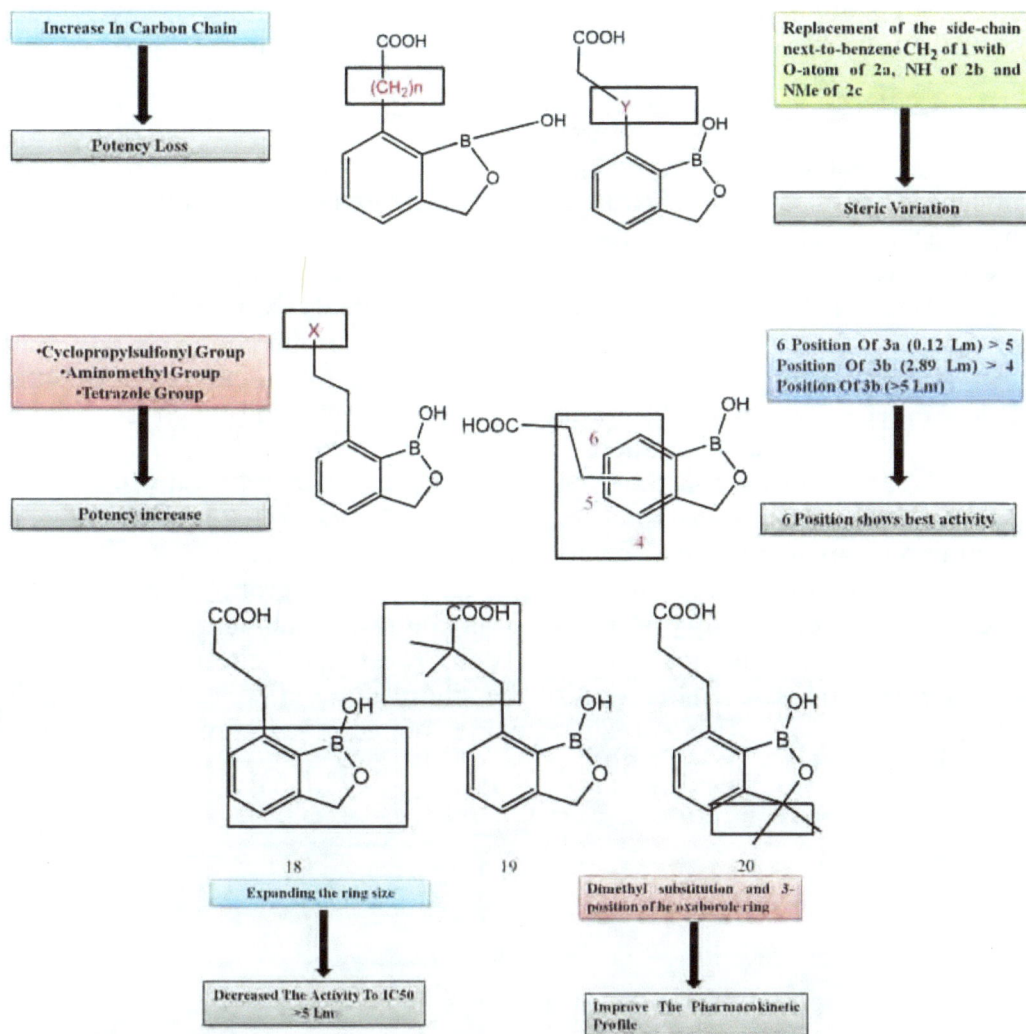

Fig. (14). Structural Activity Relationship of Benzoxaboroles Derivatives.

Among compounds 1 through 17, the impact of side-chain substitution position modification on antimalarial activity is distinctly shown in a potency sequence: 7-position of compound 1 (26 nM) > 6-position of compound 15 (0.12 lM) > 5-position of compound 16 (2.89 lM) > 4-position of compound 17 (>5 lM). When the ring size was increased to six members instead of eighteen, the activity was reduced to IC50 >5 lM. Dimethyl substitution is expected to improve the pharmacokinetic profile of 1 by reducing the possibility of carboxylic acid glucuronidation or by minimizing boron oxidative metabolism through the steric hindrance of the dimethyl groups on the side chain carbon next to COOH in 19 or on the 3-position of the oxaborole ring in 20. However, these substitutions resulted in the loss of antimalarial activity (>5 lM) [124].

CURCUMINS

Numerous therapeutic benefits of curcumin have been shown, including anticancer, antibacterial, antifungal, anti-inflammatory, anti-plasmodial, and antioxidant properties [125 - 129]. Its two methoxy phenolic groups are the main locations responsible for its bioactivity, and their study of its chemical structure has allowed for their identification. Since the electrons from the hydroxy group are delocalized into the aromatic ring, the hydroxy group connected at the para position of the aromatic phenyl group aids in the stability of curcumin. Dohutia *et al.* looked at how curcumin's antimalarial activity changed when O-acetyl and methoxy groups were substituted for the hydroxy group (Fig. **15**). The *in vitro* study's IC50 results demonstrated that replacing an O-acetyl group (IC50 = 2.34 µM) had potency comparable to curcumin (IC50 = 3.25 µM); however, substituting a methoxy group resulted in a significant drop in potency (IC50 = 7.86 µM). This was believed to be caused by the acetyl group's biodegradability by ester bond breakage by esters, which, in contrast to the bond connected to an alkyl group, which is not easily cleaved, regenerates the parent curcumin structure. Given that the alteration of the site resulted in the loss of curcumin's antimalarial action, these results demonstrated the significance of the unsubstituted phenol group [130].

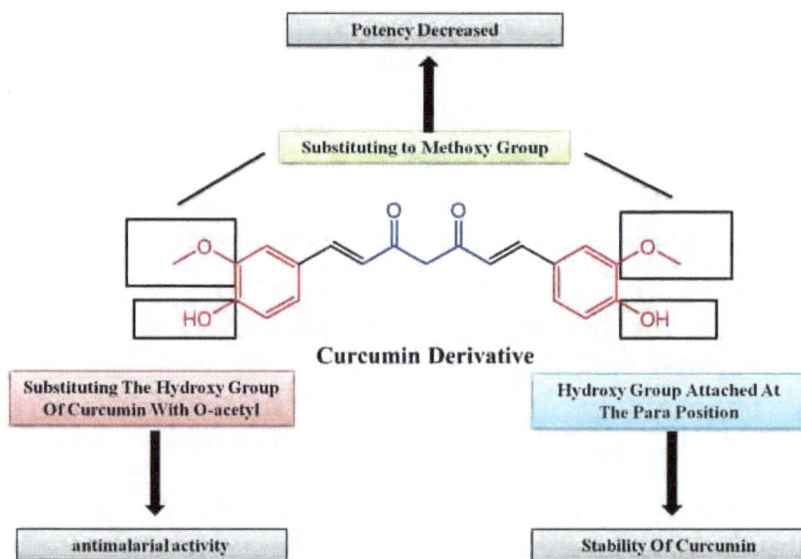

Fig. (15). Structural activity relationship of curcumin derivatives.

4-OXO-3-CARBOXYL QUINOLONES

7-methoxy quinolones' antimalarial efficacy ranged widely in terms of EC50 values. The most effective antimalarial efficacy was exhibited by carboxyl ester 7 (EC50 0.25 lM against K1 and 3D7 strains). Its efficacy against both bacteria was eliminated when the 3-carboxyl ester group was substituted with 3-carboxylic acid or 3-carboxylic amide (Fig. **17**). The potency decreased by over 90% when an acetyl group was added at position 3 (Fig. **16**). We also noticed that the drug was ineffective against both strains in the absence of a carboxylic ester group. More than 100 lM of compounds containing 3-carboxylate, 3-acid, and 3-amide groups were soluble in phosphate-buffered saline (PBS) containing DMSO at a pH of 7.4. The solubility of compounds without three substituents was lower (3 and 1 lM, respectively). Additionally, we found that all of the compounds in series had acceptable permeability. Hydrophilic compound groups were unable to pierce the lipid layer. We concentrated our attention on compounds having the 7-methoxy and 3-carboxyl ester substituents [131] due to the constraints of 5-methoxy and 7-methoxy quinolones bearing carboxylate at the 3-position.

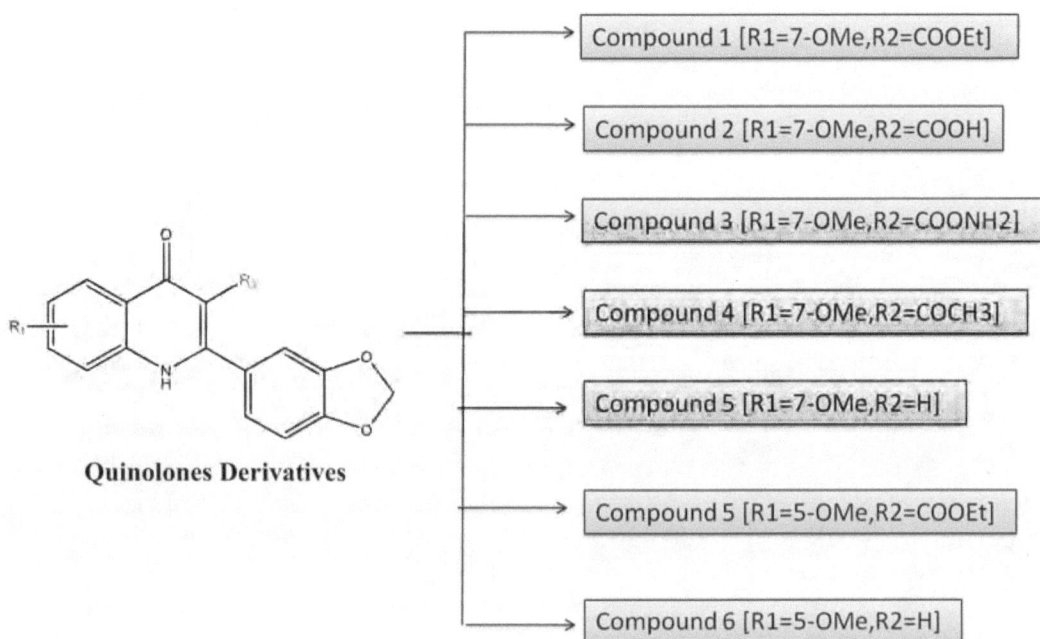

Fig. (16). Substitution of novel 4-oxo-3-carboxyl quinolones Derivatives.

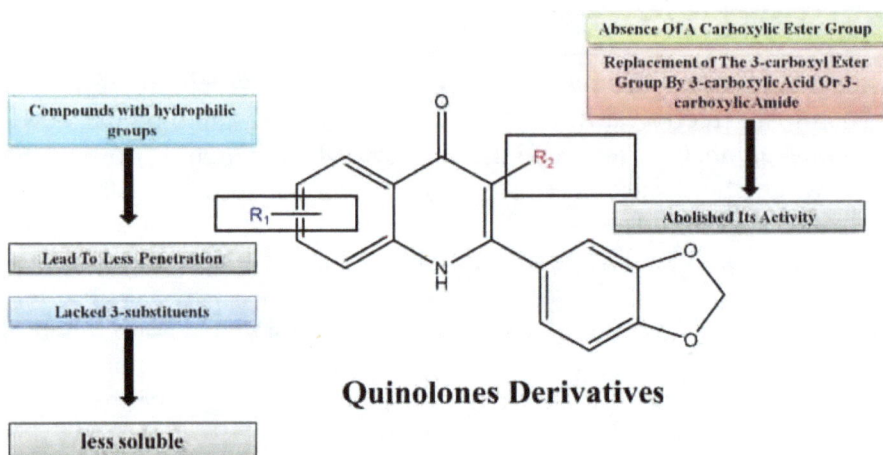

Fig. (17). Structural Activity relationship of 4-oxo-3-carboxyl quinolones Derivatives.

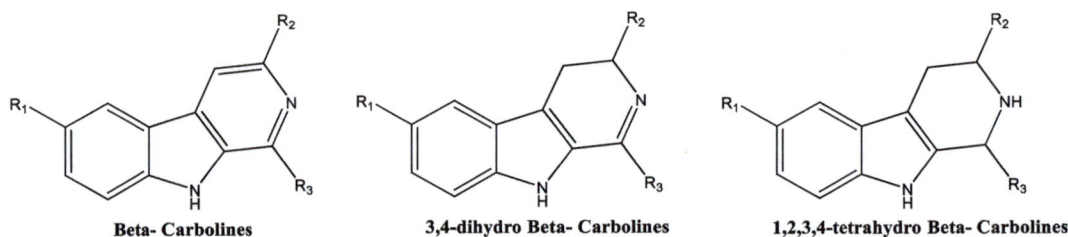

Fig. (18). Structure of Beta-carbolines Derivatives.

β-CARBOLINE DERIVATIVE

A pyrido [3,4-b]indole ring surrounds the tricyclic nucleus of β-carboline. It may be separated into three scaffolds based on how unsaturated the pyridine ring is. As shown in Fig. **(18)**, β-carbolines are completely unsaturated aromatic pyridine ring compounds, while 3,4-dihydro β-carbolines are partially saturated compounds [120]. Conversely, the compounds with completely saturated pyridine rings are referred to as 1,2,3,4-tetrahydro β-carbolines [121]. The antiplasmodial properties of β-carbolines and tetrahydroβ-carbolines N-methyl quaternary salts are also investigated.

In order to leverage the therapeutic properties of β-carboline and create drugs that might offer robust protection against malaria, a thorough comprehension of the compound's structure-activity relationship (SAR) is required (Fig. **19**). As a result, the next sections include a comprehensive SAR study spanning a variety of artificial and natural β-carboxylates.

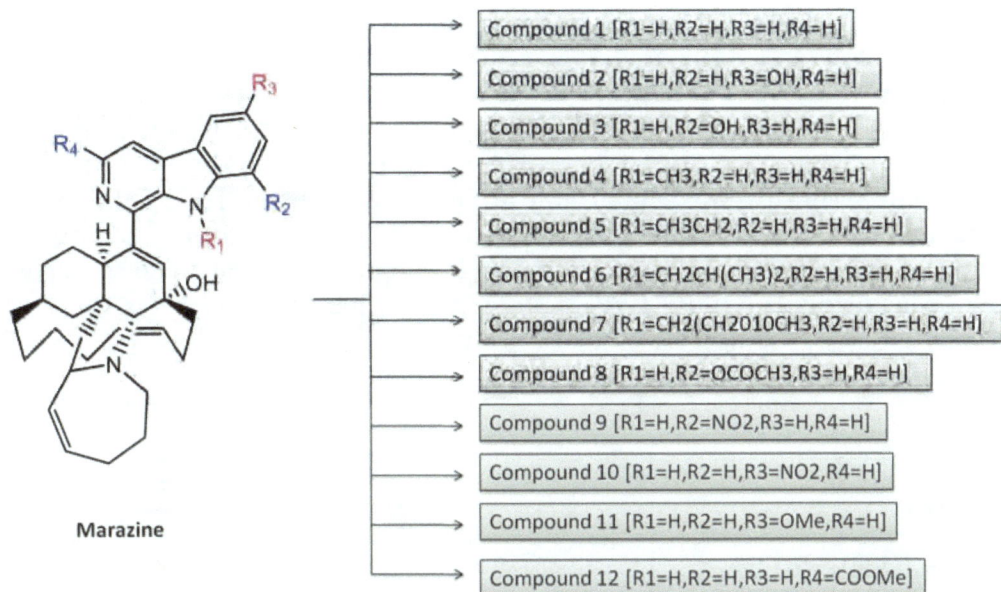

Fig. (19). Substitution of β-Carboline Derivatives.

Several alkaloids that are found in nature and have skeletons made of β-carboline or tetrahydroβ-carboline have been demonstrated to be effective antimalarial medications. Manzamine is a naturally occurring alkaloid that possesses a β-carboline moiety and a pentacyclic diamine ring structure. More research is being done to determine its ability to fight malaria. Sakai *et al.* [122] brought attention to this beneficial alkaloid in 1986 when they announced the discovery of a novel anticancer alkaloid called manzamine from Okinawa sea sponges (Haliclona). Consequently, some marine sponge species generated Manzamine-like alkaloids that demonstrated potent inhibitory effects on both drug-sensitive and drug-resistant strains of the malaria-causing *Plasmodium* parasite. A number of manzamine alkaloids and their derivatives with antiparasitic properties and modifications at the C6, C8, and N1 locations of the β-carboline moiety are shown in Figure. The following significant SAR analysis features become clear upon close inspection of the figure (Fig. **20**). The hydrochloride salt of hydroxymanzamine A demonstrated a considerable increase in activity (IC50 = 6.1 ± 2.4 ng/mL), but the C8 position hydroxy group of manzamine A produced a single overlap reduction in activity. Additionally, manzamine Y's activity against the D6 and W2 clones of *P. falciparum* was lower than that of 8-hydroxy manzamine A (IC50 420 and 850 ng/mL, respectively), indicating that the change in hydroxyl shifting the positioning of the β-carboxy line moiety from its C8 to

C6 position decreases the antimalarial activity. Additionally, the addition of alkyl and lipophilic groups at the N9 position of the β-carboline ring resulted in a notable reduction in antimalarial activity when compared to the parent medication manzamine A, indicating that the antimalarial action requires the retention of 9-NH. Similarly, compared to manzamine A, the activity was lowered by 70 times upon the insertion of a nitro group at position C8. Moreover, manzamine A's antiparasitic efficacy was about four times lower than that of the original molecule due to the C6 nitro substitution. On the other hand, the analogues of manzamine A were still less active than their parent compound, even if they have shown considerable activity (IC50 = 28 ng/mL for the ester and 11 ng/mL for the methoxy group at position C6 at the C3 position).

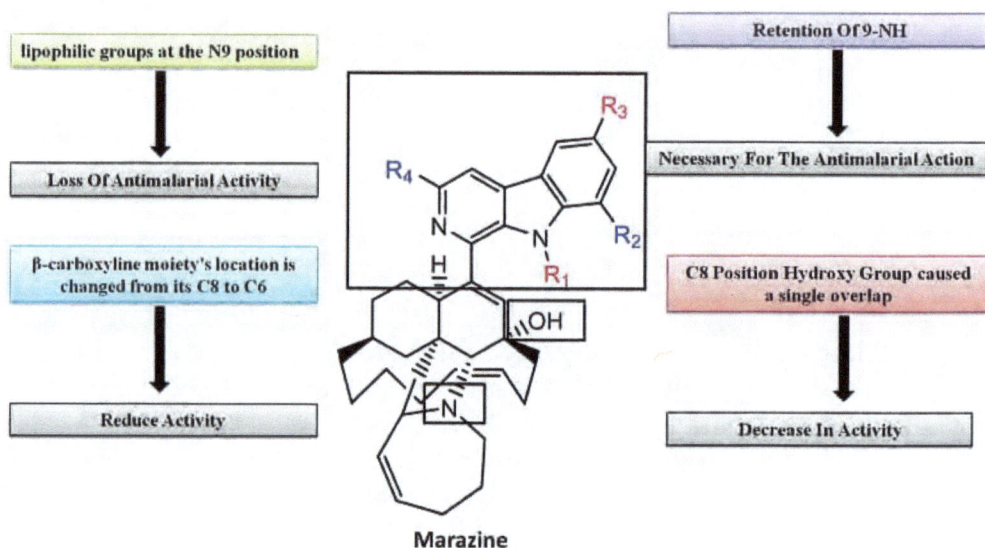

Marazine

Fig. (20). Structural Activity Relationship of Beta-carbolines Derivatives.

QUINAZOLINE-CHALCONE HYBRIDS

The cost-effective Claisen-Schmidt condensation reaction was used to synthesize quinazoline-chalcone hybrids covalently linked by amine linkage. The hybrids were then tested for their *in vitro* antimalarial activity against chloroquine-sensitive (MRC-2) and chloroquine-resistant (RKL-9) *P. falciparum* strains, with chloroquine serving as a positive control. A total of five compounds were found to be more or equipotent to chloroquine (IC50 = 0.40 μM), with values between IC50 = 0.217-0.453 μM. (Fig. **21**) [132].

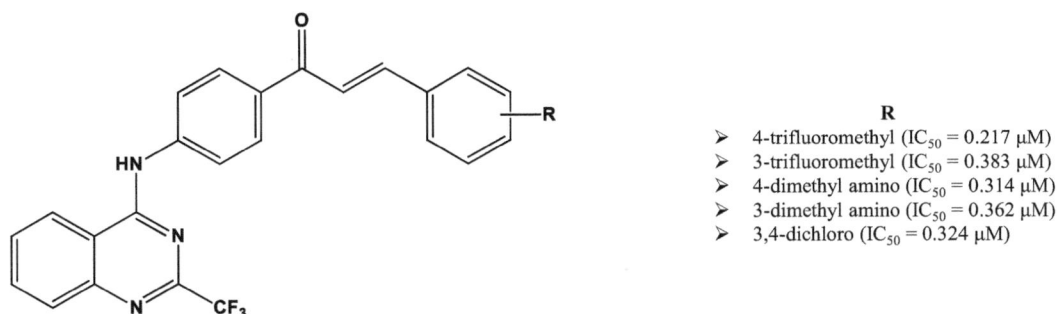

Fig. (21). Quinazoline chalcone hybrid molecule.

R
- 4-trifluoromethyl (IC_{50} = 0.217 μM)
- 3-trifluoromethyl (IC_{50} = 0.383 μM)
- 4-dimethyl amino (IC_{50} = 0.314 μM)
- 3-dimethyl amino (IC_{50} = 0.362 μM)
- 3,4-dichloro (IC_{50} = 0.324 μM)

CONCLUSION

The resistance of malaria parasites to existing drugs carries on growing and progressively limiting our ability to manage this severe disease and finally leading to a massive global health burden. Till now, malaria control has relied upon the traditional quinoline, antifolate, and artemisinin compounds. Very few new antimalarials were developed in the past 50 years. Among recent approaches, the identification of novel chemotherapeutic targets, exploration of natural products with medicinal significance, covalent biotherapy having a dual mode of action into a single hybrid molecule and malaria vaccine development are explored heavily. The proper execution of these approaches and proper investment from international agencies will accelerate the discovery of drugs that provide new hope for the control or eventual eradication of this global infectious disease. In this review, various strategies for the evaluation and development of new antimalarial drugs were discussed. New approaches should be introduced by systematically reviewing the status and scientific value of previous approaches and providing pragmatic forecasts for future developments. So that new powerful anti-malaria medicines can be explored.

REFERENCES

[1]   Cui L, Mharakurwa S, Ndiaye D, Rathod PK, Rosenthal PJ. Antimalarial drug resistance: Literature review and activities and findings of the ICEMR network. Am J Trop Med Hyg 2015; 93(3_Suppl) (Suppl.): 57-68.
      [http://dx.doi.org/10.4269/ajtmh.15-0007] [PMID: 26259943]

[2]   Hastings IM, Watkins WM, White NJ. The evolution of drug–resistant malaria: the role of drug elimination half–life. Philos Trans R Soc Lond B Biol Sci 2002; 357(1420): 505-19.
      [http://dx.doi.org/10.1098/rstb.2001.1036] [PMID: 12028788]

[3]   Woodrow CJ, White NJ. The clinical impact of artemisinin resistance in Southeast Asia and the potential for future spread. FEMS Microbiol Rev 2017; 41(1): 34-48.
      [http://dx.doi.org/10.1093/femsre/fuw037] [PMID: 27613271]

[4]   Brandyce St. Laurent, Becky Miller, Timothy A. Burton, *et al.* Fairhurs Artemisinin-resistant *Plasmodium falciparum* clinical isolates can infect diverse mosquito vectors of Southeast Asia and Africa. Nat Commun 2015; 6: 8614.

[http://dx.doi.org/10.1038/ncomms9614]

[5]   Elizabeth A, Ashley . Spread of artemisinin resistance in *plasmodium falciparum* malaria N Engl J Med 2014; 371(9): 411-23.
         [http://dx.doi.org/10.1056/NEJMoa1314981]

[6]   Mishra M, Mishra VK, Kashaw V, Iyer AK, Kashaw SK. Comprehensive review on various strategies for antimalarial drug discovery. Eur J Med Chem 2017; 125: 1300-20.
         [http://dx.doi.org/10.1016/j.ejmech.2016.11.025] [PMID: 27886547]

[7]   Horn D, Duraisingh MT. Antiparasitic chemotherapy: from genomes to mechanisms. Annu Rev Pharmacol Toxicol 2014; 54(1): 71-94.
         [http://dx.doi.org/10.1146/annurev-pharmtox-011613-135915] [PMID: 24050701]

[8]   Muregi FW, Wamakima HN, Kimani FT. Novel drug targets in malaria parasite with potential to yield antimalarial drugs with long useful therapeutic lives. Curr Pharm Des 2012; 18(24): 3505-21.
         [PMID: 22607143]

[9]   De Azevedo Teotônio Cavalcanti M, Da Silva Menezes KJ, De Oliveira Viana J, *et al.* Current trends to design antimalarial drugs targeting N -myristoyltransferase. Future Microbiol 2024; 19: 1601-8.
         [http://dx.doi.org/10.1080/17460913.2024.2412397]

[10]   Belete TM. Recent progress in the development of new antimalarial drugs with novel targets. Drug Des Devel Ther 2020; 14: 3875-89.
         [http://dx.doi.org/10.2147/DDDT.S265602] [PMID: 33061294]

[11]   Ramos-Martín F, D'Amelio N. Drug resistance: an incessant fight against evolutionary strategies of survival. Microbiol Res (Pavia) 2023; 14(2): 507-42.
         [http://dx.doi.org/10.3390/microbiolres14020037]

[12]   Noreen N, Ullah A, Salman SM, Mabkhot Y, Alsayari A, Badshah SL. New insights into the spread of resistance to artemisinin and its analogues. J Glob Antimicrob Resist 2021; 27: 142-9.
         [http://dx.doi.org/10.1016/j.jgar.2021.09.001] [PMID: 34517141]

[13]   Santos-Júnior PFS, Nascimento IJS, Neto GJS, *et al.* Design of antimalarial compounds on quinoline scaffold: From plant to drug. Alkaloids Other Nitrogen-Containing Deriv 2023; 189-237.
         [http://dx.doi.org/10.2174/9789815123678123030010]

[14]   Prabhu P, Patravale V. Novel targets for malaria therapy. Curr Drug Targets 2011; 12(14): 2129-43.
         [http://dx.doi.org/10.2174/138945011798829384] [PMID: 21756223]

[15]   Oladele TO, Bewaji CO, Sadiku JS. Drug target selection for malaria: Molecular basis for the drug discovery process. Centrepoint Journal 2012; 18(2): 111-24.

[16]   de Azevedo Teotônio Cavalcanti M, Da Silva Menezes KJ, De Oliveira Viana J, *et al.* Current trends to design antimalarial drugs targeting N -myristoyltransferase. Future Microbiol 2024; 19: 1601-8.
         [http://dx.doi.org/10.1080/17460913.2024.2412397]

[17]   Miller LH, Ackerman HC, Su X, Wellems TE. Malaria biology and disease pathogenesis: insights for new treatments. Nat Med 2013; 19(2): 156-67.
         [http://dx.doi.org/10.1038/nm.3073] [PMID: 23389616]

[18]   Staines Henry M, Ellory J C, Chibale Kelly. The new permeability pathways: Targets and selective routes for the development of new antimalarial agents Combinatorial Chemistry & High Throughput Screening 2005; 8(1): 81-8.
         [http://dx.doi.org/10.2174/1386207053328138]

[19]   Bodammer JE, Bahr GF. The initiation of a "metabolic window" in the surface of host erythrocytes by Plasmodium berghei NYU-2. Lab Invest 1973; 28(6): 708-18.
         [PMID: 4351644]

[20]   Lauer SA, Rathod PK, Ghori N, Haldar K. A membrane network for nutrient import in red cells infected with the malaria parasite. Science 1997; 276(5315): 1122-5.

[http://dx.doi.org/10.1126/science.276.5315.1122] [PMID: 9148808]

[21] Pouvelle B, Spiegel R, Hsiao L, *et al.* Direct access to serum macromolecules by intraerythrocytic malaria parasites. Nature 1991; 353(6339): 73-5.
[http://dx.doi.org/10.1038/353073a0] [PMID: 1715521]

[22] Kirk K. Membrane transport in the malaria-infected erythrocyte. Physiol Rev 2001; 81(2): 495-537.
[http://dx.doi.org/10.1152/physrev.2001.81.2.495] [PMID: 11274338]

[23] Verkman AS, Anderson MO, Papadopoulos MC. Aquaporins: important but elusive drug targets. Nat Rev Drug Discov 2014; 13(4): 259-77.
[http://dx.doi.org/10.1038/nrd4226] [PMID: 24625825]

[24] Song J. Mak E, Wu B, Beitz E. Parasite aquaporins: Current developments in drug facilitation and resistance. Biochim Biophys Acta 2013.
[http://dx.doi.org/10.1016/j.bbagen.2013.10.014] [PMID: 24140393]

[25] Mukhopadhyay R, Bhattacharjee H, Rosen BP. Aquaglyceroporins: Generalized metalloid channels. Biochim Biophys Acta, Gen Subj 2014; 1840(5): 1583-91.
[http://dx.doi.org/10.1016/j.bbagen.2013.11.021] [PMID: 24291688]

[26] Almasalmeh A, Krenc D, Wu B, Beitz E. Structural determinants of the hydrogen peroxide permeability of aquaporins. FEBS J 2014; 281(3): 647-56.
[http://dx.doi.org/10.1111/febs.12653] [PMID: 24286224]

[27] Fadiel A, Isokpehi RD, Stambouli N, Hamza A, Benammar-Elgaaied A, Scalise TJ. Protozoan parasite aquaporins. Expert Rev Proteomics 2009; 6(2): 199-211.
[http://dx.doi.org/10.1586/epr.09.10] [PMID: 19385945]

[28] Zeuthen T, Wu B, Pavlovic-Djuranovic S, *et al.* Ammonia permeability of the aquaglyceroporins from *Plasmodium falciparum*, *Toxoplasma gondii* and *Trypansoma brucei*. Mol Microbiol 2006; 61(6): 1598-608.
[http://dx.doi.org/10.1111/j.1365-2958.2006.05325.x] [PMID: 16889642]

[29] Wu B, Song J, Beitz E. Novel channel enzyme fusion proteins confer arsenate resistance. J Biol Chem 2010; 285(51): 40081-7.
[http://dx.doi.org/10.1074/jbc.M110.184457] [PMID: 20947511]

[30] Martins AP, Ciancetta A, de Almeida A, *et al.* Aquaporin inhibition by gold(III) compounds: new insights. ChemMedChem 2013; 8(7): 1086-92.
[http://dx.doi.org/10.1002/cmdc.201300107] [PMID: 23653381]

[31] Munday JC, Eze AA, Baker N, *et al.* Trypanosoma brucei aquaglyceroporin 2 is a high-affinity transporter for pentamidine and melaminophenyl arsenic drugs and the main genetic determinant of resistance to these drugs. J Antimicrob Chemother 2014; 69(3): 651-63.
[http://dx.doi.org/10.1093/jac/dkt442] [PMID: 24235095]

[32] Song J, Baker N, Rothert M, *et al.* Pentamidine is not a permeant but a nanomolar inhibitor of the trypanosoma brucei aquaglyceroporin-2. PLoS Pathog 2016; 12(2): e1005436.
[http://dx.doi.org/10.1371/journal.ppat.1005436] [PMID: 26828608]

[33] Lisk G, Desai SA. The plasmodial surface anion channel is functionally conserved in divergent malaria parasites. Eukaryot Cell 2005; 4(12): 2153-9.
[http://dx.doi.org/10.1128/EC.4.12.2153-2159.2005] [PMID: 16339732]

[34] Kutner S, Breuer WV, Ginsburg H, Cabantchik ZI. On the mode of action of phlorizin as an antimalarial agent in *in vitro* cultures of plasmodium falciparum. Biochem Pharmacol 1987; 36(1): 123-9.
[http://dx.doi.org/10.1016/0006-2952(87)90389-3] [PMID: 3099799]

[35] Kirk K, Horner HA, Elford BC, Ellory JC, Newbold CI. Transport of diverse substrates into malaria-infected erythrocytes *via* a pathway showing functional characteristics of a chloride channel. J Biol Chem 1994; 269(5): 3339-47.

[http://dx.doi.org/10.1016/S0021-9258(17)41868-0] [PMID: 8106373]

[36]   Kirk K, Horner HA, Spillett DJ, Elford BC. Glibenclamide and meglitinide block the transport of low molecular weight solutes into malaria-infected erythrocytes. FEBS Lett 1993; 323(1-2): 123-8.
[http://dx.doi.org/10.1016/0014-5793(93)81462-9] [PMID: 8495724]

[37]   Lisk G, Kang M, Cohn JV, Desai SA. Specific inhibition of the plasmodial surface anion channel by dantrolene. Eukaryot Cell 2006; 5(11): 1882-93.
[http://dx.doi.org/10.1128/EC.00212-06] [PMID: 16950925]

[38]   Available from: https://www.sbir.gov/sbirsearch/detail/399750

[39]   Pillai AD, Pain M, Solomon T, Bokhari AAB, Desai SA. A cell-based high-throughput screen validates the plasmodial surface anion channel as an antimalarial target. Mol Pharmacol 2010; 77(5): 724-33.
[http://dx.doi.org/10.1124/mol.109.062711] [PMID: 20101003]

[40]   Pain M, Fuller AW, Basore K, *et al.* Synergistic malaria parasite killing by two types of plasmodial surface anion channel inhibitors. PLoS One 2016; 11(2): e0149214.
[http://dx.doi.org/10.1371/journal.pone.0149214] [PMID: 26866812]

[41]   Blume M, Hliscs M, Rodriguez-Contreras D, *et al.* A constitutive pan-hexose permease for the *Plasmodium* life cycle and transgenic models for screening of antimalarial sugar analogs. FASEB J 2011; 25(4): 1218-29.
[http://dx.doi.org/10.1096/fj.10-173278] [PMID: 21169382]

[42]   Slavic K, Krishna S, Derbyshire ET, Staines HM. Plasmodial sugar transporters as anti-malarial drug targets and comparisons with other protozoa. Malar J 2011; 10(1): 165.
[http://dx.doi.org/10.1186/1475-2875-10-165] [PMID: 21676209]

[43]   Nigussie D, Beyene T, Shah NA, Belew S. New targets in malaria parasite chemotherapy: A review. Malar Control Elimin 2015; s1: 1.
[http://dx.doi.org/10.4172/2470-6965.1000S1-007]

[44]   Woodrow CJ, Burchmore RJ, Krishna S. Hexose permeation pathways in *Plasmodium falciparum* - infected erythrocytes. Proc Natl Acad Sci USA 2000; 97(18): 9931-6.
[http://dx.doi.org/10.1073/pnas.170153097] [PMID: 10954735]

[45]   Martin RE, Henry RI, Abbey JL, Clements JD, Kirk K. The 'permeome' of the malaria parasite: an overview of the membrane transport proteins of Plasmodium falciparum. Genome Biol 2005; 6(3): R26.
[http://dx.doi.org/10.1186/gb-2005-6-3-r26] [PMID: 15774027]

[46]   Dean P, Major P, Nakjang S, Hirt RP, Embley TM. Transport proteins of parasitic protists and their role in nutrient salvage. Front Plant Sci 2014; 5: 153.
[http://dx.doi.org/10.3389/fpls.2014.00153] [PMID: 24808897]

[47]   Landfear SM. Glucose transporters in parasitic protozoa. Methods Mol Biol 2010; 637: 245-62.
[http://dx.doi.org/10.1007/978-1-60761-700-6_13] [PMID: 20419439]

[48]   Krishna S, Eckstein-Ludwig U, Joët T, *et al.* Transport processes in Plasmodium falciparum-infected erythrocytes: potential as new drug targets. Int J Parasitol 2002; 32(13): 1567-73.
[http://dx.doi.org/10.1016/S0020-7519(02)00185-6] [PMID: 12435441]

[49]   Biagini GA, O'Neill PM, Nzila A, Ward SA, Bray PG. Antimalarial chemotherapy: young guns or back to the future? Trends Parasitol 2003; 19(11): 479-87.
[http://dx.doi.org/10.1016/j.pt.2003.09.011] [PMID: 14580958]

[50]   Stead AMW, Bray PG, Edwards IG, *et al.* Diamidine compounds: selective uptake and targeting in Plasmodium falciparum. Mol Pharmacol 2001; 59(5): 1298-306.
[http://dx.doi.org/10.1016/S0026-895X(24)12591-6] [PMID: 11306715]

[51]   Gero A, Dunn C, Brown D, *et al.* New malaria chemotherapy developed by utilization of a unique

parasite transport system. Curr Pharm Des 2003; 9(11): 867-77.
[http://dx.doi.org/10.2174/1381612033455233] [PMID: 12678871]

[52]   Ancelin ML, Vial HJ. Regulation of phosphatidylcholine biosynthesis in Plasmodium-infected erythrocytes. Biochim Biophys Acta Lipids Lipid Metab 1989; 1001(1): 82-9.
[http://dx.doi.org/10.1016/0005-2760(89)90310-X] [PMID: 2536284]

[53]   Holz GG Jr. Lipids and the malarial parasite. Bull World Health Organ 1977; 55(2-3): 237-48.
[PMID: 412602]

[54]   Vial HJ, Ancelin ML. Malarial Lipids. Subcell Biochem 1992; 18: 259-306.
[http://dx.doi.org/10.1007/978-1-4899-1651-8_8] [PMID: 1485354]

[55]   Vial HJ, Eldin P, Martin D, Gannoun L, Calas M, Ancelin ML. Transport of phospholipid synthesis precursors and lipid trafficking into malaria-infected erythrocytes. Novartis Found Symp 1999; 226: 74-83.
[http://dx.doi.org/10.1002/9780470515730.ch6] [PMID: 10645539]

[56]   Ancelin ML, Calas M, Bompart J, *et al.* Antimalarial activity of 77 phospholipid polar head analogs: close correlation between inhibition of phospholipid metabolism and *in vitroPlasmodium falciparum* growth. Blood 1998; 91(4): 1426-37.
[http://dx.doi.org/10.1182/blood.V91.4.1426] [PMID: 9454774]

[57]   Wengelnik K, Vidal V, Ancelin ML, *et al.* A class of potent antimalarials and their specific accumulation in infected erythrocytes. Science 2002; 295(5558): 1311-4.
[http://dx.doi.org/10.1126/science.1067236] [PMID: 11847346]

[58]   Pala ZR, Saxena V, Saggu GS, Garg S. Recent advances in the [Fe–S] cluster biogenesis (SUF) pathway functional in the apicoplast of plasmodium. Trends Parasitol 2018; 34(9): 800-9.
[http://dx.doi.org/10.1016/j.pt.2018.05.010] [PMID: 30064903]

[59]   Ben Mamoun C, Prigge ST, Vial H. Targeting the lipid metabolic pathways for the treatment of malaria. Drug Dev Res 2010; 71(1): 44-55.
[http://dx.doi.org/10.1002/ddr.20347] [PMID: 20559451]

[60]   Halbert J, Ayong L, Equinet L, *et al.* A *Plasmodium falciparum* transcriptional cyclin-dependent kinase-related kinase with a crucial role in parasite proliferation associates with histone deacetylase activity. Eukaryot Cell 2010; 9(6): 952-9.
[http://dx.doi.org/10.1128/EC.00005-10] [PMID: 20305001]

[61]   Hammarton TC, Mottram JC, Doerig C. The cell cycle of parasitic protozoa: potential for chemotherapeutic exploitation. Prog Cell Cycle Res 2003; 5: 91-101.
[PMID: 14593704]

[62]   Kicska GA, Tyler PC, Evans GB, Furneaux RH, Kim K, Schramm VL. Transition state analogue inhibitors of purine nucleoside phosphorylase from Plasmodium falciparum. J Biol Chem 2002; 277(5): 3219-25.
[http://dx.doi.org/10.1074/jbc.M105905200] [PMID: 11707439]

[63]   Sahu NK, Sahu S, Kohli DV. Novel molecular targets for antimalarial drug development. Chem Biol Drug Des 2008; 71(4): 287-97.
[http://dx.doi.org/10.1111/j.1747-0285.2008.00640.x] [PMID: 18298458]

[64]   Desai SA. Why do malaria parasites increase host erythrocyte permeability? Trends Parasitol 2014; 30: 151-9.
[http://dx.doi.org/10.1016/j.pt.2014.01.003]

[65]   Fisher N, Antoine T, Ward SA, Biagini GA. Mitochondrial electron transport chain of *Plasmodium falciparum*. In: Hommel M, Kremsner P, Eds. Encyclopedia of Malaria. New York, NY: Springer 2014.
[http://dx.doi.org/10.1007/978-1-4614-8757-9_12-1]

[66]   Ross LS, Fidock DA. Elucidating mechanisms of drug-resistant plasmodium falciparum. Cell Host

Microbe 2019; 26(1): 35-47.
[http://dx.doi.org/10.1016/j.chom.2019.06.001] [PMID: 31295423]

[67]   Jortzik E, Becker K. Thioredoxin and glutathione systems in Plasmodium falciparum. Int J Med Microbiol 2012; 302(4-5): 187-94.
[http://dx.doi.org/10.1016/j.ijmm.2012.07.007] [PMID: 22939033]

[68]   Roberts F, Roberts CW, Johnson JJ, *et al.* Evidence for the shikimate pathway in apicomplexan parasites. Nature 1998; 393(6687): 801-5.
[http://dx.doi.org/10.1038/31723] [PMID: 9655396]

[69]   Valenciano AL, Fernández-Murga ML, Merino EF, *et al.* Metabolic dependency of chorismate in *Plasmodium falciparum* suggests an alternative source for the ubiquinone biosynthesis precursor. Sci Rep 2019; 9(1): 13936.
[http://dx.doi.org/10.1038/s41598-019-50319-5] [PMID: 31558748]

[70]   Sharma K. A review on plasmodium falciparum-protein farnesyltransferase inhibitors as antimalarial drug targets. Curr Drug Targets 2017; 18(14): 1676-86.
[http://dx.doi.org/10.2174/1389450117666160823165004] [PMID: 27557819]

[71]   Saggu Gagandeep S, Pala Zarna R, Garg Shilpi, Saxena Vishal. New insight into isoprenoids biosynthesis process and future prospects for drug designing in plasmodium Front Microbiol 2016; 7.
[http://dx.doi.org/10.3389/fmicb.2016.01421]

[72]   Mishra M, Singh V, Singh S. Structural insights into key *Plasmodium* proteases as therapeutic drug targets. Front Microbiol 2019; 10: 394.
[http://dx.doi.org/10.3389/fmicb.2019.00394] [PMID: 30891019]

[73]   Pandey KC, Singh N, Arastu-Kapur S, Bogyo M, Rosenthal PJ. Falstatin, a cysteine protease inhibitor of Plasmodium falciparum, facilitates erythrocyte invasion. PLoS Pathog 2006; 2(11): e117.
[http://dx.doi.org/10.1371/journal.ppat.0020117] [PMID: 17083274]

[74]   Boyle MJ, Langer C, Chan JA, *et al.* Sequential processing of merozoite surface proteins during and after erythrocyte invasion by Plasmodium falciparum. Infect Immun 2014; 82(3): 924-36.
[http://dx.doi.org/10.1128/IAI.00866-13] [PMID: 24218484]

[75]   Patrick G L. Falcipains as drug targets in antimalarial therapy Antimalarial Agents 2019; 271-317.
[http://dx.doi.org/10.1016/B978-0-08-101210-9.00008-1]

[76]   Kumar S, Bhardwaj TR, Prasad DN, Singh RK. Drug targets for resistant malaria: Historic to future perspectives. Biomed Pharmacother 2018; 104: 8-27.
[http://dx.doi.org/10.1016/j.biopha.2018.05.009] [PMID: 29758416]

[77]   Lima WR, Moraes M, Alves E, Azevedo MF, Passos DO, Garcia CRS. The PfNF-YB transcription factor is a downstream target of melatonin and cAMP signalling in the human malaria parasite *Plasmodium falciparum.* J Pineal Res 2013; 54(2): 145-53.
[http://dx.doi.org/10.1111/j.1600-079X.2012.01021.x] [PMID: 22804732]

[78]   Butt TR, Karathanasis SK. Transcription factors as drug targets: opportunities for therapeutic selectivity. Gene Expr 1995; 4(6): 319-36.
[PMID: 7549464]

[79]   Bratkowski M, Unarta IC, Zhu L, Shubbar M, Huang X, Liu X. Structural dissection of an interaction between transcription initiation and termination factors implicated in promoter-terminator cross-talk. J Biol Chem 2018; 293(5): 1651-65.
[http://dx.doi.org/10.1074/jbc.M117.811521] [PMID: 29158257]

[80]   Zhang DY, Carson DJ, Ma J. The role of TFIIB-RNA polymerase II interaction in start site selection in yeast cells. Nucleic Acids Res 2002; 30(14): 3078-85.
[http://dx.doi.org/10.1093/nar/gkf422] [PMID: 12136090]

[81]   Cang Y, Prelich G. Direct stimulation of transcription by negative cofactor 2 (NC2) through TATA-binding protein (TBP). Proc Natl Acad Sci USA 2002; 99(20): 12727-32.

[http://dx.doi.org/10.1073/pnas.202236699] [PMID: 12237409]

[82]   Shibeshi MA, Kifle ZD, Atnafie SA. Antimalarial drug resistance and novel targets for antimalarial drug discovery. Infect Drug Resist 2020; 13: 4047-60.
[http://dx.doi.org/10.2147/IDR.S279433] [PMID: 33204122]

[83]   Kalaria PN, Satasia SP, Raval DK. Synthesis, characterization and biological screening of novel 5-imidazopyrazole incorporated fused pyran motifs under microwave irradiation. New J Chem 2014; 38(4): 1512-21.
[http://dx.doi.org/10.1039/c3nj01327h]

[84]   World Malaria Report 2011 summary (Report). World Health Organization

[85]   Nadjm B, Behrens RH. Malaria. Infect Dis Clin North Am 2012; 26(2): 243-59.
[http://dx.doi.org/10.1016/j.idc.2012.03.010] [PMID: 22632637]

[86]   Fletcher S, Keaney EP, Cummings CG, *et al.* Structure-based design and synthesis of potent, ethylenediamine-based, mammalian farnesyltransferase inhibitors as anticancer agents. J Med Chem 2010; 53(19): 6867-88.
[http://dx.doi.org/10.1021/jm1001748] [PMID: 20822181]

[87]   Tanitame A, Oyamada Y, Ofuji K, *et al.* Synthesis and antibacterial activity of a novel series of potent DNA gyrase inhibitors. Pyrazole derivatives. J Med Chem 2004; 47(14): 3693-6.
[http://dx.doi.org/10.1021/jm030394f] [PMID: 15214796]

[88]   Ouyang G, Cai XJ, Chen Z, *et al.* Synthesis and antiviral activities of pyrazole derivatives containing an oxime moiety. J Agric Food Chem 2008; 56(21): 10160-7.
[http://dx.doi.org/10.1021/jf802489e] [PMID: 18939848]

[89]   Hall A, Billinton A, Brown SH, *et al.* Non-acidic pyrazole EP1 receptor antagonists with *in vivo* analgesic efficacy. Bioorg Med Chem Lett 2008; 18(11): 3392-9.
[http://dx.doi.org/10.1016/j.bmcl.2008.04.018] [PMID: 18462938]

[90]   Bandgar BP, Gawande SS, Bodade RG, Gawande NM, Khobragade CN. Synthesis and biological evaluation of a novel series of pyrazole chalcones as anti-inflammatory, antioxidant and antimicrobial agents. Bioorg Med Chem 2009; 17(24): 8168-73.
[http://dx.doi.org/10.1016/j.bmc.2009.10.035] [PMID: 19896853]

[91]   Suzuki F, Kuroda T, Tamura T, Sato S, Ohmori K, Ichikawa S. New antiinflammatory agents. 2. 5-Phenyl-3H-imidazo[4,5-c][1,8]naphthyridin-4(5H)-ones: a new class of nonsteroidal antiinflammatory agents with potent activity like glucocorticoids. J Med Chem 1992; 35(15): 2863-70.
[http://dx.doi.org/10.1021/jm00093a020] [PMID: 1495017]

[92]   Pinza M, Farina C, Cerri A, *et al.* Synthesis and pharmacological activity of a series of dihydro-1--pyrrolo[1,2-a]imidazole-2,5(3H,6H)-diones, a novel class of potent cognition enhancers. J Med Chem 1993; 36(26): 4214-20.
[http://dx.doi.org/10.1021/jm00078a011] [PMID: 8277504]

[93]   Pandey J, Tiwari VK, Verma SS, *et al.* Synthesis and antitubercular screening of imidazole derivatives. Eur J Med Chem 2009; 44(8): 3350-5.
[http://dx.doi.org/10.1016/j.ejmech.2009.02.013] [PMID: 19272678]

[94]   Takeuchi I, Sugiura M, Yamamoto K, Ito T, Hamada Y. Syntheses and Antimicrobial Activities of cis-1-[2-Phenyl-4-(phenoxy or Phenylthio) methyl-1, 3-dioxolan-2-ylmethyl]-1H-imidazole Derivatives. Yakugaku Zasshi 1985; 105(6): 554-61.
[http://dx.doi.org/10.1248/yakushi1947.105.6_554] [PMID: 4067820]

[95]   Miyachi H, Kiyota H, Segawa M. Novel imidazole derivatives with subtype-selective antimuscarinic activity (1). Bioorg Med Chem Lett 1998; 8(14): 1807-12.
[http://dx.doi.org/10.1016/S0960-894X(98)00312-6] [PMID: 9873438]

[96]   Bonsignore L, Loy G, Secci D, Calignano A. Synthesis and pharmacological activity of 2-oxo-(2H) 1-benzopyran-3-carboxamide derivatives. Eur J Med Chem 1993; 28(6): 517-20.

[http://dx.doi.org/10.1016/0223-5234(93)90020-F]

[97]   Thumar NJ, Patel MP. ARKIVOC 2009; 13: 363.

[98]   Shamroukh AH, Zaki MEA, Morsy EMH, Abdel-Motti FM, Abdel-Megeid FME. Synthesis of Pyrazolo[4',3':5,6]pyrano[2,3- *d*]pyrimidine Derivatives for Antiviral Evaluation. Arch Pharm (Weinheim) 2007; 340(5): 236-43.
[http://dx.doi.org/10.1002/ardp.200700005]

[99]   Ough M, Lewis A, Bey EA, *et al.* Efficacy of beta-lapachone in pancreatic cancer treatment: Exploiting the novel, therapeutic target NQO1. Cancer Biol Ther 2005; 4(1): 102-9.
[http://dx.doi.org/10.4161/cbt.4.1.1382] [PMID: 15662131]

[100]   Escala N, Pineda LM, Ng MG, Coronado LM, Spadafora C, del Olmo E. Antiplasmodial activity, structure–activity relationship and studies on the action of novel benzimidazole derivatives. Sci Rep 2023; 13(1): 285.
[http://dx.doi.org/10.1038/s41598-022-27351-z] [PMID: 36609676]

[101]   Vyas VK, Ghate M. Substituted benzimidazole derivatives as angiotensin II-AT1 receptor antagonist: a review. Mini Rev Med Chem 2010; 10(14): 1366-84.
[http://dx.doi.org/10.2174/138955710793564151] [PMID: 20937029]

[102]   Gaba M, Singh S, Mohan C. Benzimidazole: An emerging scaffold for analgesic and anti-inflammatory agents. Eur J Med Chem 2014; 76: 494-505.
[http://dx.doi.org/10.1016/j.ejmech.2014.01.030] [PMID: 24602792]

[103]   Shrivastava N, Naim MJ, Alam MJ, Nawaz F, Ahmed S, Alam O. Benzimidazole scafold as anticancer agent: Synthetic approaches and structure-activity relationship. Arch. Pharm. (Weinheim). 2017 Jun;350(6).
[http://dx.doi.org/10.1002/ardp.201700040] [PMID: 28544162]

[104]   Bansal Y, Kaur M, Bansal G. Antimicrobial potential of benzimidazole derived molecules. Mini Rev Med Chem 2019; 19(8): 624-46.
[http://dx.doi.org/10.2174/1389557517666171101104024] [PMID: 29090668]

[105]   Veerasamy R, Roy A, Karanakaran R, Rajak H. Structure-activity relationship analysis of benzimidazoles as emerging antiinfammatory agents: An overview. Pharmaceuticals 14(7): 633.

[106]   Yeates CL, Batchelor JF, Capon EC, *et al.* Synthesis and structure-activity relationships of 4-pyridones as potential antimalarials. J Med Chem 2008; 51(9): 2845-52.
[http://dx.doi.org/10.1021/jm0705760] [PMID: 18396855]

[107]   Markley LD, Van Heertum JC, Doorenbos HE. Antimalarial activity of clopidol, 3,5-dichloro-2-6-dimethyl-4-pyridinol, and its esters, carbonates, and sulfonates. J Med Chem 1972; 15(11): 1188-9.
[http://dx.doi.org/10.1021/jm00281a029] [PMID: 4569924]

[108]   Fry M, Williams RB. Effects of decoquinate and clopidol on electron transport in mitochondria of Eimeria tenella (Apicomplexa: coccidia). Biochem Pharmacol 1984; 33(2): 229-40.
[http://dx.doi.org/10.1016/0006-2952(84)90480-5] [PMID: 6704148]

[109]   Latter VS, Hudson AT, Richards WHG, Randall AW. Antiprotozoal Agents. U.S. Patent 5,053,418, 1991.

[110]   Biot C, Daher W, Chavain N, *et al.* Design and synthesis of hydroxyferroquine derivatives with antimalarial and antiviral activities. J Med Chem 2006; 49(9): 2845-9.
[http://dx.doi.org/10.1021/jm0601856] [PMID: 16640347]

[111]   Biot C. Ferroquine: a new weapon in the fight against malaria. Curr. Med. Chem. Antiinfect Agents 2004; 3: 135-47.

[112]   Biot C, Taramelli D, Forfar-Bares I, *et al.* Insights into the mechanism of action of ferroquine. Relationship between physicochemical properties and antiplasmodial activity. Mol Pharm 2005; 2(3): 185-93.

[http://dx.doi.org/10.1021/mp0500061] [PMID: 15934779]

[113]   Daher W, Pelinski L, Klieber S, *et al. in vitro* metabolism of ferroquine (SSR97193) in animal and human hepatic models and antimalarial activity of major metabolites on Plasmodium falciparum. Drug Metab Dispos 2006; 34(4): 667-82.
[http://dx.doi.org/10.1124/dmd.104.003202] [PMID: 16415117]

[114]   Warhurst DC, Steele JC, Adagu IS, Craig JC, Cullander C. Hydroxychloroquine is much less active than chloroquine against chloroquine-resistant Plasmodium falciparum, in agreement with its physicochemical properties. J Antimicrob Chemother 2003; 52(2): 188-93.
[http://dx.doi.org/10.1093/jac/dkg319] [PMID: 12837731]

[115]   Devender N, Gunjan S, Tripathi R, Tripathi RP. Synthesis and antiplasmodial activity of novel indoleamide derivatives bearing sulfonamide and triazole pharmacophores. Eur J Med Chem 2017; 131: 171-84.
[http://dx.doi.org/10.1016/j.ejmech.2017.03.010] [PMID: 28319782]

[116]   Rottmann M, McNamara C, Yeung BKS, *et al.* Spiroindolones, a potent compound class for the treatment of malaria. Science 2010; 329(5996): 1175-80.
[http://dx.doi.org/10.1126/science.1193225] [PMID: 20813948]

[117]   Zhu J, Chen T, Chen L, *et al.* 2-amido-3-(1H-indol-3-yl)-N-substituted-propanamides as a new class of falcipain-2 inhibitors. 1. Design, synthesis, biological evaluation and binding model studies. Molecules 2009; 14(1): 494-508.
[http://dx.doi.org/10.3390/molecules14010494] [PMID: 19158658]

[118]   Lopes SCP, Blanco YC, Justo GZ, *et al.* Violacein extracted from Chromobacterium violaceum inhibits Plasmodium growth *in vitro* and *in vivo*. Antimicrob Agents Chemother 2009; 53(5): 2149-52.
[http://dx.doi.org/10.1128/AAC.00693-08] [PMID: 19273690]

[119]   Schuck DC, Jordão AK, Nakabashi M, Cunha AC, Ferreira VF, Garcia CRS. Synthetic indole and melatonin derivatives exhibit antimalarial activity on the cell cycle of the human malaria parasite Plasmodium falciparum. Eur J Med Chem 2014; 78: 375-82.
[http://dx.doi.org/10.1016/j.ejmech.2014.03.055] [PMID: 24699367]

[120]   Flannery EL, Chatterjee AK, Winzeler EA. Antimalarial drug discovery — approaches and progress towards new medicines. Nat Rev Microbiol 2013; 11(12): 849-62.
[http://dx.doi.org/10.1038/nrmicro3138] [PMID: 24217412]

[121]   Price RN, Douglas NM. Expanding the use of primaquine for the radical cure of plasmodium vivax. Clin Infect Dis 2018; 67(7): 1008-9.
[http://dx.doi.org/10.1093/cid/ciy236] [PMID: 29590343]

[122]   Sakai R, Higa T, Jefford CW, Bernardinelli G, Manzamine A. Manzamine A, a novel antitumor alkaloid from a sponge. J Am Chem Soc 1986; 108(20): 6404-5.
[http://dx.doi.org/10.1021/ja00280a055]

[123]   Tadigoppula N, Korthikunta V, Gupta S, *et al.* Synthesis and insight into the structure-activity relationships of chalcones as antimalarial agents. J Med Chem 2013; 56(1): 31-45.
[http://dx.doi.org/10.1021/jm300588j] [PMID: 23270565]

[124]   Zhang YK, Plattner JJ, Freund YR, *et al.* Synthesis and structure–activity relationships of novel benzoxaboroles as a new class of antimalarial agents. Bioorg Med Chem Lett 2011; 21(2): 644-51.
[http://dx.doi.org/10.1016/j.bmcl.2010.12.034] [PMID: 21195617]

[125]   Lee KH, Ab Aziz FH, Syahida A, *et al.* Synthesis and biological evaluation of curcumin-like diarylpentanoid analogues for anti-inflammatory, antioxidant and anti-tyrosinase activities. Eur J Med Chem 2009; 44(8): 3195-200.
[http://dx.doi.org/10.1016/j.ejmech.2009.03.020] [PMID: 19359068]

[126]   Hatcher H, Planalp R, Cho J, Torti FM, Torti SV. Curcumin: From ancient medicine to current clinical trials. Cell Mol Life Sci 2008; 65(11): 1631-52.

[http://dx.doi.org/10.1007/s00018-008-7452-4] [PMID: 18324353]

[127] Dovigo LN, Pavarina AC, Ribeiro APD, *et al.* Investigation of the photodynamic effects of curcumin against Candida albicans. Photochem Photobiol 2011; 87(4): 895-903.
[http://dx.doi.org/10.1111/j.1751-1097.2011.00937.x] [PMID: 21517888]

[128] Tong SYC, Davis JS, Eichenberger E, Holland TL, Fowler VG Jr. Staphylococcus aureus infections: epidemiology, pathophysiology, clinical manifestations, and management. Clin Microbiol Rev 2015; 28(3): 603-61.
[http://dx.doi.org/10.1128/CMR.00134-14] [PMID: 26016486]

[129] Jagetia G, Rajanikant G. Curcumin stimulates the antioxidant mechanisms in mouse skin exposed to fractionated γ irradiation. Antioxidants 2015; 4(1): 25-41.
[http://dx.doi.org/10.3390/antiox4010025] [PMID: 26785336]

[130] Jamil SNH, Ali AH, Feroz SR, *et al.* Curcumin and its derivatives as potential antimalarial and anti-inflammatory agents: A review on structure–activity relationship and mechanism of action. Pharmaceuticals (Basel) 2023; 16(4): 609.
[http://dx.doi.org/10.3390/ph16040609] [PMID: 37111366]

[131] Zhang Y, Guiguemde WA, Sigal M, *et al.* Synthesis and structure–activity relationships of antimalarial 4-oxo-3-carboxyl quinolones. Bioorg Med Chem 2010; 18(7): 2756-66.
[http://dx.doi.org/10.1016/j.bmc.2010.02.013] [PMID: 20206533]

[132] Mishra M, Mishra VK, Kashaw V, Agrawal RK, Kashaw SK. Novel quinazoline-chalcone hybrids as antiplasmodium agents: synthesis, biological evaluation and molecular docking. Int J Adv Sci Res 2020; 11: 85-99.

CHAPTER 8

On the Trail of Zika Virus: Understanding its Druggable Targets

Leandro Rocha Silva[1] and **Edeildo Ferreira da Silva-Júnior**[1,*]

[1] *Research Group on Biological and Molecular Chemistry, Institute of Chemistry and Biotechnology, Federal University of Alagoas, Lourival Melo Mota Avenue, 57072-970, Maceió, Brazil*

Abstract: The Zika virus (ZIKV) is responsible for the infection of millions of people, causing mild flu-like symptoms and even severe symptoms, which are related to the nervous system, including Guillain-Barré syndrome and microcephaly. Nonetheless, it still remains with no antiviral treatments or effective vaccine to prevent it. Thus, several efforts have been addressed to discover a medicinal alternative to disrupt the ZIKV infection worldwide. Notwithstanding these facts, this chapter will focus on the main antiviral targets associated with ZIKV and their inhibitors identified so far. In principle, viral and host factors related to the ZIKV life cycle could be targeted for the development of novel drugs. In fact, there are some macromolecular targets that could be further investigated aiming to develop anti-ZIKV drugs, some of which remain still a few explored. In summary, this chapter encourages the exploration of new opportunities for medicinal chemists to design novel anti-ZIKV agents, providing a solid hope for future treatments against this disease.

Keywords: Flavivirus, Non-structural proteins, Structural proteins, ZIKV.

INTRODUCTION

ZIKV belongs to the *Flaviviridae* family, which also includes other pathogens with a significant impact on human health, such as Yellow Fever virus (YFV), Dengue virus (DENV), and West Nile virus (WNV), which are transmitted by infected mosquitoes (arthropod-borne viruses). ZIKV genome is composed of a single -strand positive-sense RNA (ssRNA(+)) that encodes a single open-reading frame (ORF). It is flanked by 5'-untranslate region (UTR) and 3'-structural proteins (named capsid (C), pre-membrane (prM), end envelope (E)), which are involved in the assembly of new viral particles; whereas seven non-structural proteins (named NS1, NS2A, NSB, NS3, NS4A, NS4B, and NS5) responsible for

---

* **Corresponding author Edeildo Ferreira da Silva-Júnior:** Research Group on Biological and Molecular Chemistry, Institute of Chemistry and Biotechnology, Federal University of Alagoas, Lourival Melo Mota Avenue, 57072-970, Maceió, Brazil; E-mail: edeildo.junior@iqb.ufal.br

Igor Jose dos Santos Nascimento & Ricardo Olimpio de Moura (Eds.)

viral genome replication by processing the polyprotein; particle assembly; and evasion of innate antiviral response [1]. Seven G-rich sequences have been found in the coding regions for prM, E, NS1 (two G-rich sequences, NS1A and NS1B), NS3, and NS5 (two G-rich sequences, NS5A and NS5B) proteins, and one G-rich sequence has been also found at the 3'-end of the ZIKV genome.

These G-rich sequences may fold to form the RNA G-quadruplex structures of two G-tetrads under physiological conditions. ZIKV RNA G-quadruplex sequences have been found to play important biological roles in virus entry, transcription, translation, and genome stability [2 - 6]. Regarding the ZIKV-related epidemiologic aspects, it was first reported in 1947 as a mild and obscure human pathogen, which was isolated from febrile sentinel rhesus monkeys in Uganda. ZIKV has emerged as a major threat to public health, being an arthropod-borne virus with rapid dissemination in regions with tropical and subtropical climates [7, 8]. Still, it is genotypically classified into three strains, being East African, West African, and Asian lineages. Still, the Asian lineage is further classified by geographical origin, named Micronesian, Cambodian, and Malaysian [2, 9]. Generally, the ZIKV infection is asymptomatic, otherwise, it causes symptoms similar to the common flu, or mild symptoms (known as Zika fever). On the other hand, some cases can evolve into neurological complications due to ZIKV tropism, manifesting Guillain-Barré syndrome in adults, whereas microcephaly in fetuses and/or newborns [7, 10, 11]. Currently, there are no drugs or vaccines to treat or even prevent ZIKV infection, respectively. However, research works have described several drug-like compounds targeting ZIKV, such as chelerythrine chloride [12], chalcones [13], lycorine [14], gemcitabine, saliphenylhamide, and obatoclax [15]. Throughout this chapter, the reader will be guided into discussions involving the main ZIKV targets associated with the development of antiviral drugs within the last five years. Furthermore, advances in the discovery of new classes of active molecules against ZIKV will be covered, as well.

NON-STRUCTURAL PROTEINS OF ZIKA VIRUS AND THEIR INHIBITORS

Non-Structural Protein 1

Non-Structural Protein 1 (NS1). The NS1 is a highly conserved glycoprotein that presents several functions in Flaviviruses and is found in elevated concentrations during acute infection by ZIKV. It is also related to ZIKV tropism, pro-inflammatory and immunogenic processes, as well as, it exerts pathogenic effects on vascular permeability tissues [16]. The NS1 similarity index among flaviviruses is very high and among ZIKV strains the similarity is greater than

90% [17]. Its general role includes immune invasion, interactions with ribosomal subunits during the viral replication complex, RNA replication, and when produced extracellularly, it interacts with host immunological factors to improve immune evasion and pathogenesis [18]. In the extracellular environment, NS1 forms multimeric structures that can dimerize, in which trimers of dimers (hexamers) can be formed *via* hydrophobic interactions; being potential biomarkers in diagnosis [19, 20].

The mature form of NS1 presents a dimer of identical monomeric subunits. The structurally conserved monomer has three domains, being a small *N*-terminal *β*-hairpin (residues 1–29), a *"wing"* domain (residues 30–180), and, the largest, *C*-terminal *"β-ladder"* domain (residues 181–352) [21, 22] (Fig. 1). A three-stranded β-sheet is formed by segments comprising the wing and β-ladder domains, involving residues 30–37 and 152– 180 [16, 21]. As aforementioned, the intracellular dimer form of NS1 plays a role in genome replication, while the secreted hexamer one plays a role in immune evasion [17]. The dimerized form of NS1 is constituted by a β-hairpin (swapped domain), which is composed of the N-terminus of each monomer, consisting of two β-strands, from which extends a wing-ladder domain and the β-ladder [19]. Extracellularly, NS1 dimers are secreted as a proteolipid particle forming a putative barrel-shaped hexameric coat [16]. Within the hexamer, the main dimerization characteristic is attributed to the β-ladder domain, which presents a significant number of contact regions at the dimeric interface. Then, the virulence can be reduced by eliminating dimer formation, which can be done through point mutations in the β-ladder domain. Comparing the crystal structures of Flavivirus β-ladder dimers with the internal domain of the NS1 dimer, both maintain highly-conversed structural aspects. DNA synthesis depends on the dimeric form of NS1, which binds to the endoplasmic reticulum membrane after being formed. Structurally, this domain consists of 10 β-strands arranged like a ladder rung and connected through short loops or turns, except a 53-long residue (composed of 219–272 residues), called as "spaghetti loop", located between β13 and β14 strands. The presence of the spaghetti loop gives rise to two different surfaces: the membrane side of the continuous β-sheet and the luminal side of the irregular loop surface [19].

A recent study demonstrated that there is an association between secreted NS1 and High-Density Lipoprotein (HDL). HDL binds to SR-B1 (scavenger receptor class B type 1), which functions as a receptor and can trigger proinflammatory responses in cultured cells. Evidence have shown that sNS1 probably does not exist as hexamers, either in the blood of infected patients or supernatants, but rather is found mainly in the dimeric form complexed with HDL. This fact is justified due to the initial evidence of sNS1 as hexameric structures, which were found in less than 3.5% of the particles, with the tetrameric form being the main form observed in a sample. The altered metabolism observed in lipoproteins in patients with DENV could be explained by the fact that sNS1 interacts indirectly as a complex with HDL, or indirectly with SRB1 for subsequent internalization, contributing to the rupture of the endothelial glycocalyx and viral replication. The way sNS1–SRB1 interactions may influence flaviviral tropism is still unclear, it was identified that β-ladder is involved in inducing endothelial hyperpermeability and NS1 wing domain as the primary determinant for cell- binding specificity [16].

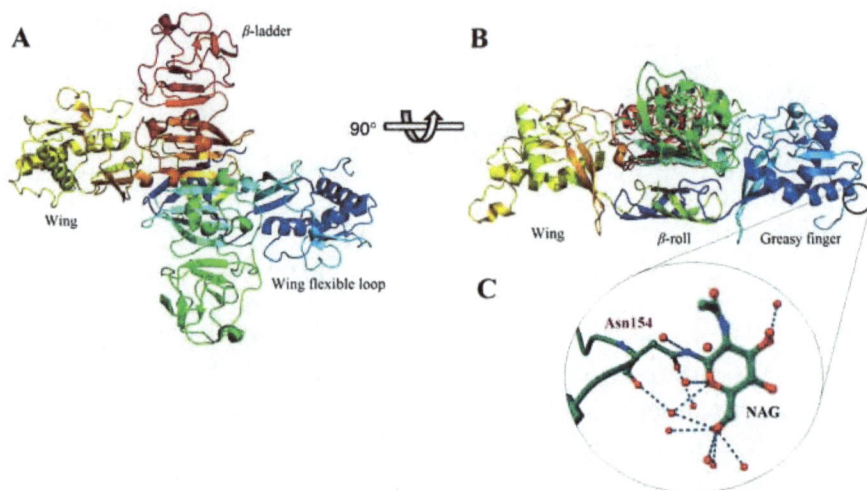

Fig. (1). Structure of Zika NS1 protein (PDB: 5K6K). (**A**) Representation of the dimeric form of ZIKV NS1, showing the wing domain (residues 30–180), β-ladder domain (residues 181–352), and wing flexible loop (residues 108–129). (**B**) NS1 dimer rotated 90° about the horizontal axis, showing the greasy finger (residues 159–163), wing domain (residues 30–180), and β-roll (residues 1–29). (**C**) NAG cocrystallized on the ZIKV NS1, showing its interaction with Asn[154] residue and water solvation (red spheres).

In the NS1 monomer, there are six disulfides, two of which are located in the β-ladder domain. These disulfides are of great importance in the stability and folding of proteins, since after their translation, there is an increase in the conformational barrier for unfolding as a consequence of the decrease in entropy, which leads to structurally more stable and functional polypeptide chains. ZIKV dimerization cannot be readily inhibited by Cys-Ala mutations on the wing and swapping domain, however, mutations of the disulfide-related Cys residues of the β-ladder domain lead to significant inhibition in ZIKV assembly and dimerization. Also, it has been seen that the ZIKV dimerization cysteine in NS1 demonstrates the great influence of β-ladder disulfides on the oligomerization and maturation of the protein [23].

NS1 Inhibitors

A series of glycyrrhetinic acid (GA) derivatives were synthetized targeting ZIKV inhibition. Four active compounds were found among the GA derivatives tested, **1** (IC$_{50}$: 0.13 µM), **2** (IC$_{50}$: 0.55 µM), **3** (IC$_{50}$: 0.29 µM), and **4** (IC$_{50}$: 0.56 µM) (Fig. **2**). All four effective GA derivatives meaningfully inhibited the entry and post-entry stages of ZIKV infection in a concentration-dependent manner. The entry mode assay demonstrated that compound **4** (IC$_{50}$: 0.50 µM) was a more potent inhibitor on the entry-stage than compounds **1** (IC$_{50}$: 0.68 µM), **2** (IC$_{50}$: 1.09 µM), and **3** (IC$_{50}$: 0.52 µM). In the post-entry assay, compound **4** also had the highest inhibitory effect on ZIKV replication (IC$_{50}$: 0.43 µM) than compounds **1** (IC$_{50}$: 1.00 µM), **2** (IC$_{50}$: 0.81 µM), and **3** (IC$_{50}$: 1.94 µM). Four hit-compounds **1**, **2**, **3**, and **4** with high inhibitory activity were found to inhibit the cytopathogenic effect (CPE), NS1 production, and infectivity of ZIKV. Furthermore, molecular docking studies showed that compounds **1** and **4** also can be bound in the binding pocket of NS2B-NS3 ZIKV protease and form hydrogen-bonding interactions with the catalytic triad (His[51], Asp[75], and Ser[135]) [24].

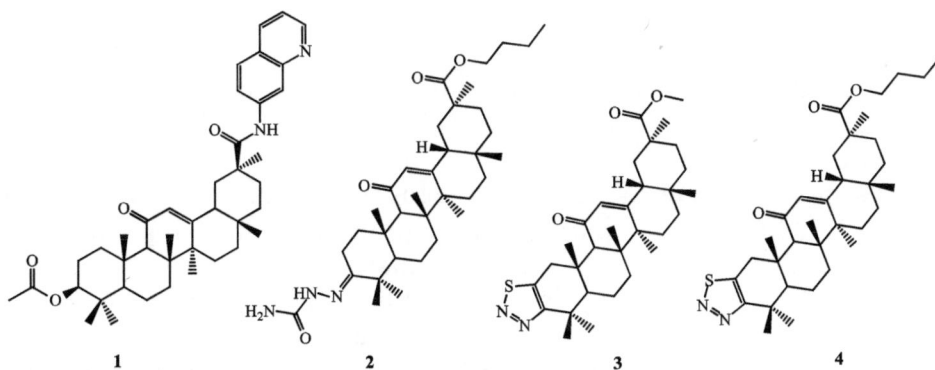

Fig. (2). Glycyrrhetinic acid derivatives as Zika NS1 inhibitors.

Non-Structural Protein 2A (NS2A)

Non-Structural Protein 2A (NS2A). The NS2A is composed of 226 amino acids, being the first NS protein to have multiple transmembrane helixes. It contains seven transmembrane segments (pTMS), with the N-terminal region (pTMS1–pTMS2) near the endoplasmic reticulum lumen, pTMS3 across the endoplasmic reticulum membrane, and the C-terminal region (pTMS4–pTMS7) near the cytoplasm. Still, it antagonizes MDA5/RIG-I-mediated interferon-β (IFβ) and NF-κB production, promotes the degradation of STAT1 and STAT2 to suppress interferon pathway, and induces the degradation of karyopherin subunit α-2 *via* chaperone-mediated autophagy, which is the primary nucleocytoplasmic transporter for some transcription factors to activate cellular proliferation and differentiation [16, 25].

Still, NS2A plays an important role in virion assembly and RNA synthesis. In addition, it acts by recruiting structural proteins and viral RNA to the viral particle assembly site, and as an antagonist of the immune response of the infected individual [16]. So far, there are no specific inhibitors targeting NS2A.

Non-Structural Protein 2B (NS2B)

NS2B is composed of a transmembrane region, anchoring the protease to the endoplasmic reticulum, and its C-terminal cofactor region (NS2Bcf), essential for proper folding of the NS3 serine protease (NS3pro) catalytic domain [26 - 29]. Due to its role as a cofactor for NS3pro, NS2B is considered an important protein for the diagnosis of ZIKV. The complex formed, NS2B-NS3, plays a pivotal role in the viral cycle, whether in the maturation of viral proteins or participating in the hydrolysis process [30]. Finally, there are no selective inhibitors against NS2Bcf so far.

Non-Structural Protein 3 (NS3)

NS3 has the N-terminal performing proteolytic activity, while the C-terminal region contains NTPase (NS3NTPase) and helicase (NS3hel) domains [31]. The N-terminal domain (aa 1–170) of NS3 codes for the trypsin-like serine protease followed by a flexible linker of ~20 amino acids, which has conserved domains found in RNA helicases [32]. NS3pro is a protease with a high degree of conservation among flaviviruses, having more than 50% similarity. It belongs to the S7 subfamily of the chymotrypsin family, it has a catalytic site that presents the residues His^{51}, Asp^{75}, and Ser^{135}. The viral protease is formed from a hetero-dimeric complex, NS2B-containing four transmembrane (TM) helices linked to the $NS3^{pro}$ domain, which is then self-cleaved at the NS2B-NS3 junction site [32]. NS3pro requires NS2B as a cofactor to perform its full proteolytic activity. NS2B plays a crucial role in anchoring the enzyme in addition to contributing to maintaining protein activity. The most important features of the complex formed include, in addition to the catalytic triad, the chymotrypsin-like fold and S2 pocket [31].

Non-Structural NS2B/NS3 Serino Protease

The NS3 protease domain is located at the N-terminus, whereas a helicase domain is found at the C-terminus. However, without the cofactor NS2B to stabilize the structure of NS3, it is practically inactive [27, 33 - 35]. The NS2B- NS3 protease (Fig. **3**) is responsible for all cytoplasmic cleavages and plays a crucial role in the viral replicative cycle. Since it is responsible for the cleavage of the junctions between S2B/NS3NS2A/NS2B, NS4B/NS5 and NS3/NS4A, the NS2B-NS3 protease is an important target for the development of new antivirals [36].

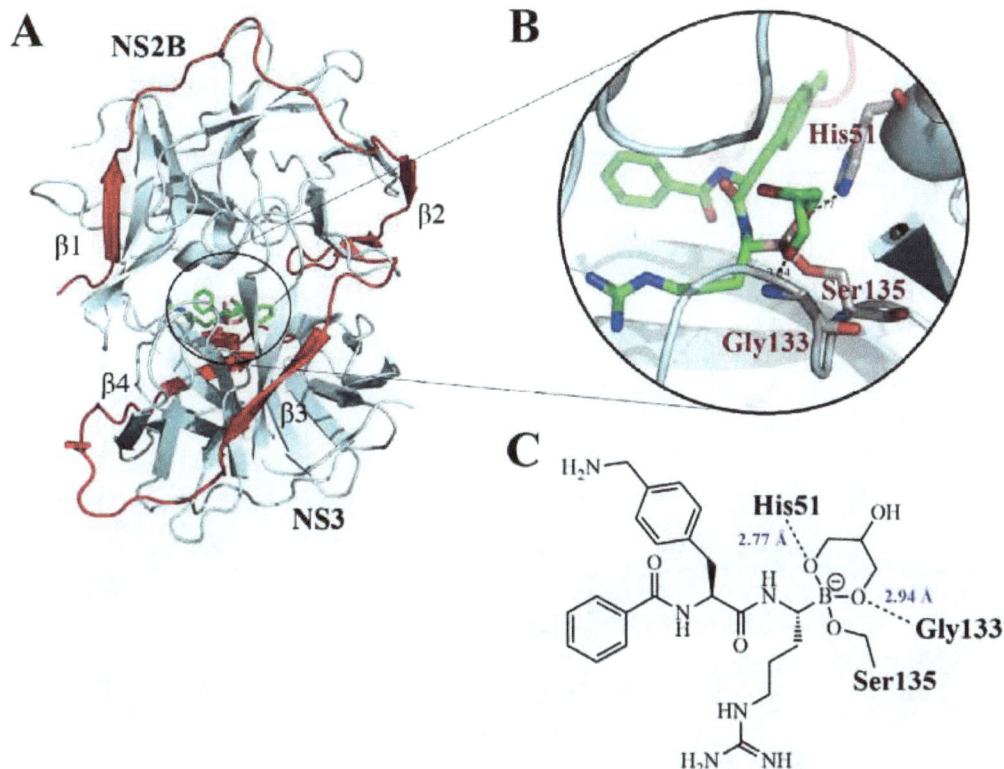

Fig. (3). Structure of Zika NS2B/NS3 protease in complex with a boronic acid derivative. (**A**) Ribbon representation of NS2B/NS3 complex, showing NS2B cofactor (red) and NS3 protease (pale cyan). (**B**) Covalent complex involving a boronate analog with Ser[135] residue. (**C**) The structure of the boronate analog is covalently connected with Ser[135], also showing the stabilization by H-bonding interactions with His[51] and Gly[133] at 2.77 and 2.94 Å, respectively.

The substrate-binding pocket of the ZIKV NS2B/NS3 protease has two crucial catalytic sites, S1 and S2. S1 contains the signature catalytic triad composed of His[51], Asp[75], and Ser[135], whereas S2 is located in NS2B [37]. The NS2B/NS3 can exist in two distinct conformations, in which the catalytically active conformation is known as the closed conformation, presenting NS2B wraps around NS3 and forms a β-turn with its C-terminus contributing to the formation of the S2- and S3-binding pockets [26, 38]. By contrast, in the open conformation, the β-turn segment of NS2B is disordered and does not interact with NS3. The open conformation of the protease is inactive since the S2 pocket is incomplete and lacks key residues from NS2B that interact with the P2 residue of the substrates.

An allosteric binding pocket around Ala[125] was first identified with surface cysteine mutagenesis and cysteine reactive probes. It was proposed that binding of the compound into this site may rearrange the 120s loop, thus locking the protein in its open conformation [26, 33].

Still, NS2B/NS3 is responsible for processing at least four sites on the polyprotein cleaving after Arg-Arg or Lys-Arg (at P2 and P1 positions), and complementing this the protease active site is highly negatively charged and relatively flat [33]. A highly negatively charged active site significantly reduces important characteristics, such as permeability and stability, impairing its druggability, and since there are similarities with other enzymes, such as furin, thrombin, and trypsin, nonspecific cleavages may occur [31].

NS2B/NS3 Inhibitors

Most of the reported competitive inhibitors targeting NS2B/NS3 are peptidomimetic, which have poor cellular activity and pharmacokinetic properties, limiting their potential for preclinical development. Considering the characteristics of the active site of the NS2B-NS3 protease and its importance in the viral cycle, efforts have been directed towards the development of non-basic inhibitors [31, 39].

Non-competitive inhibitors of NS2B/NS3 protease containing a common quinoxaline core with a proline or cyclic amine moiety at 2-position and diverse substituents at 3- and 7-positions, competing with NS2B cofactor for binding to NS3. Among them, compound **5** showed good inhibitory activity (IC$_{50}$: 30 mM) upon this target [33].

Compound **6** was discovered as a non-competitive inhibitor (IC$_{50}$: 6.85 mM), significantly reducing protease activity, symptoms, and damage in a mouse model. The efficacy of this compound was better and presented lower cytotoxicity than temoporfin (IC$_{50}$: 18.77 μM), which is a clinical drug capable of inhibiting the viral replication of several flaviviruses, *e.g.* DENV, impairing the protease performance. Furthermore, the treatment with compound 6 (Fig. **4**) can reduce the risks of neurodegeneration by partially blocking the entry of monocytes into the brain in tests carried out on mice infected with ZIKV [40].

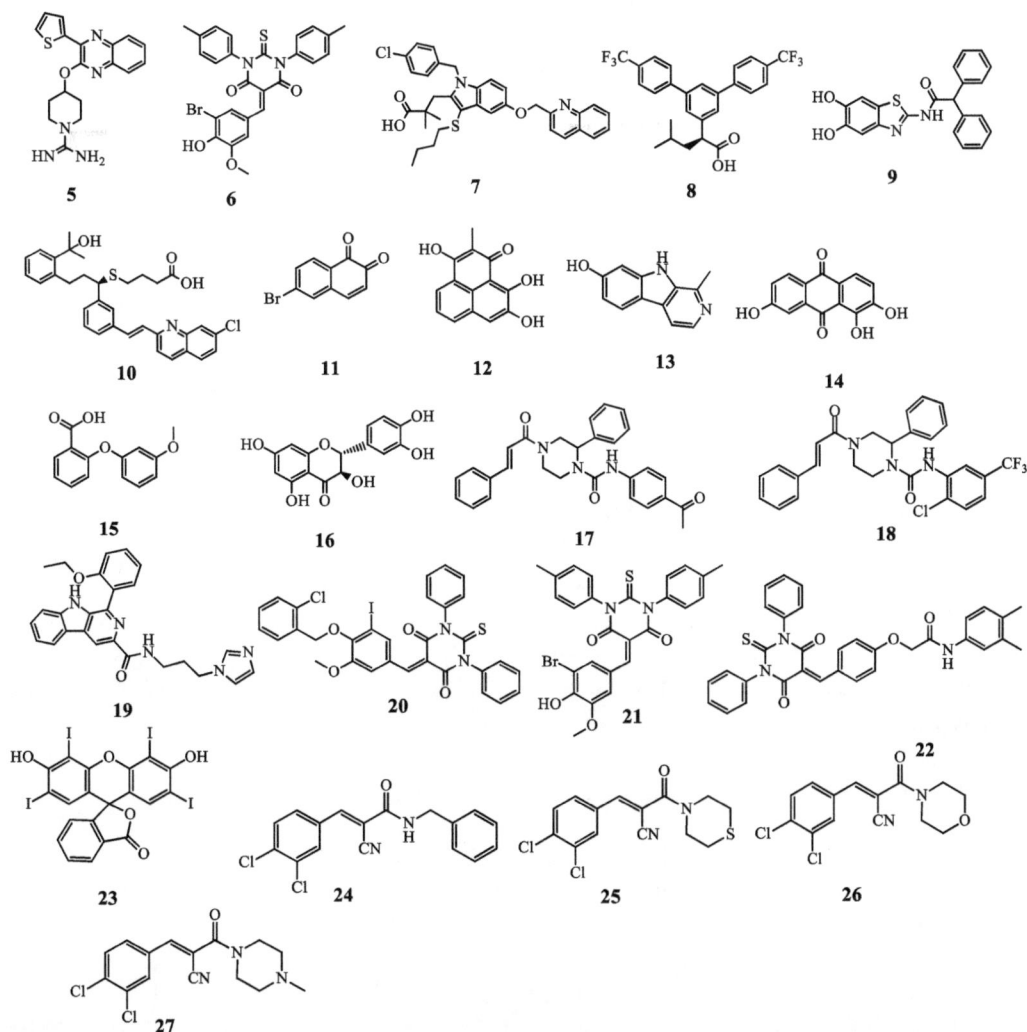

Fig. (4). Inhibitors of Zika virus NS2B/NS3 protease.

By performing a high-throughput screening (HTS), Teramoto *et al.* identified 11 active compounds toward ZIKV protease, with IC_{50} values ranging from 1.0 to 9.3 μM, whereas EC_{50} values for viral replication in neural stem cell (NSC) varying from 1.2 to 10.8 μM. Compounds MK-591 (**7**) and JNJ-40418677 (**8**) (Fig. **4**) were the most active ones, with similar IC_{50} and EC_{50} values for protease inhibition and NSC-based assays, respectively; being 3.0 and 3.1 μM for MK-591 (**7**) and 3.9 and 3.2 μM for JNJ-40418677(**8**). These results suggest that both of these compounds inhibit viral replication by blocking viral protease activity [32].

A series of benzothiazoles targeting an allosteric pocket of ZIKV NS2B/NS3 protease was developed, having a larger hydrophobic contact surface, binding to previously unaddressed regions of the allosteric NS2B/NS3 pocket. These efforts resulted in the identification of compounds that inhibited ZIKV protease in a low micromolar range (IC_{50}: 0.09- 6.48 µM). Then, compound **9** (Fig. **4**), a Y-shaped inhibitor, was found to be the most promising molecule, with a sub- micromolar IC_{50} value of 0 .09 µM [26].

in silico studies showed the potential mechanism of action for Montelukast (**10**) (Fig. **4**) against the ZIKV-replicon infected cells, which was further validated through *in vitro* protease assay. Thus, *in vitro* protease inhibition assay, enzymatic kinetics, thrombin, and trypsin assays were carried out on Montelukast (**10**), proving that it could bind to NS2B-NS3 proteases of ZIKV as a competitive inhibitor without any off-target effects [6].

in vivo and *in vitro* assays revealed that compound (**11**) (Fig. **4**) performs a specific inhibitory effect since it was able to inhibit the cytopathogenic effects induced by viruses at up to 20 µM, in a concentration-dependent inhibition manner. Also, the inhibition of protease activity was dependent on compound concentration, in which its IC_{50} value was found to be 67.47 µM. It was also observed that even during increased viral load, viral proteins and RNA were significantly reduced when the cells were treated after infection, which continued to present normal morphology. These results suggest that the inhibitory effect is related to its action in the phase initial stage of virus replication [41].

To identify new active compounds against ZIKV, Andrade *et al.* performed a screening involving 2,320 compounds from the chemical library of the National Natural History Museum of Paris [42]. From 2,320 compounds screened, five of them were analyzed for their inhibitory mechanisms by kinetics assays and computational approaches. Compounds **12-14** (uncompetitive inhibitors), **15** (a competitive inhibitor), and **16** (a noncompetitive inhibitor) exhibited IC_{50} values of 1.05, 1.62, 1.68, 1.34, and 2.10 µM, respectively (Fig. **4**); having K_i values of 0.49, 10.72, 2.47, 0.49, and 4.63 µM, respectively. *in silico* results obtained using ZIKV NS2B-NS3pro 3D-structure in closed conformation suggested that the competitive inhibitor (**15**) presented a score of −6.6 kcal/mol, interacting by hydrogen bonds with Thr[134] and Ser[135] residues. In addition, this inhibitor interacts by π-π stacking with His[51] and Tyr[161], whereas hydrophobic contacts were observed with Leu[76] and Val[155] residues in the NS3. The uncompetitive inhibitors (**12-14**) perform hydrogen-bonding interactions with Trp[89], while hydrophobic interactions with Ala[88]. In general, these compounds presented similar docking score values, ranging from −6.1 to −5.7 kcal/mol. Compounds **12** and **14** have in common the interaction with Gln[167] through hydrogen bonds and hydrophobic interaction with Ile[123]. These findings suggest a probable uncompetitive mode of inhibition [42].

García-Lozano *et al.* synthetized a series of piperazine-derived small molecules as potent NS3 protease inhibitors. Compounds **17** (IC$_{50}$: 6.6 µM) and **18** (IC$_{50}$: 1.9 µM) (Fig. **4**) were the most promising, with high SI values (60.5 and 33.5, respectively), whereas very similar docking scores values (−5.78 and −5.79, respectively), respectively. Both compounds interact with NS2B-NS3 protease active site, interacting His[77], Ser[161], Tyr[176], and Tyr[187] residues [43].

A computer-aided structure-based approach was used by Mirza *et al.* to screen a diverse library of compounds against ZIKV NS2B-NS3 protease. After selection and biological investigations, eight compounds showed promising activity against ZIKV protease, with inhibitions greater than 25%, in which three of them displayed ~50% inhibition at 10 µM concentration. Of these, only one compound (**19**) (Fig. **4**) produced whole-cell anti-ZIKV activity, and the binding mode was extensively analyzed through long-run molecular dynamics (MD) simulations. Finally, this compound showed anti-ZIKV activity in the cell-based assay with EC$_{50}$ and IC$_{50}$ values of 9.79 ± 1.20 and 7.8 µM, respectively; while lacking mammalian cytotoxicity (CC$_{50}$ > 100 µM) [37].

Using fluorescence-based enzymatic assay of peptide cleavage, Lin *et al.* were able to identify 11 compounds (**20-22**) (Fig. **4**) with inhibitory potential for the ZIKV NS2B-NS3 protease. The IC$_{50}$ values observed for compounds **20** (14.01 µM), **21** (6.85 µM), and **22** (14.2 µM) showed their high activity. In addition to the activity values found, non-bonding interactions and even hydrogen bonds were observed with important amino acid residues of the allosteric site, including (Gln[139], Trp[148], Leu[150], and Val[220]) [40].

Some FDA-approved compounds for other uses, such as Erythrosin B (**23**) (Fig. **4**), which is originally a food additive, have been evaluated as ZIKV NS2B-NS3 protease inhibitors. Erythrosin B (**23**) prevents the docking of NS2B to NS3, directly interfering with the stability of the complex (IC$_{50}$: 0.42 µM), and at the same time acts directly on the protease (IC$_{50}$: 7.9 µM). It was also observed that treatment with Erythrosin B (**23**) does not cause morphological changes in 3D-mini-forebrain organoids and has preventive potential against ZIKV in human cortical tissue [44].

Cyanoacrylamide and cyanoacrylate analogs were developed by our research team, in the study of Vilela *et al.* (2022), through pharmacology-based drug design, starting from an in-house virtual library composed of 340 small molecules, which were then screened through molecular docking, using NS2B-NS3pro as a target, after fragments with FitScore values higher were combined to lead to 27 new compounds. Among them, LQM467 (**24**) ($K_i = 15.1 \pm 0.9$ μM), LQM471 (**25**) ($K_i = 13.2 \pm 0.43$ μM), LQM472 (**26**) ($K_i = 15.8 \pm 2.0$ μM) and LQM474 (**27**) ($K_i = 20.3 \pm 2.1$ μM) (Fig. **4**) were found to be active. Compound **25** was the most promising compound exhibiting an EC_{50} value of 35.07 μM on infected cells. Results of qPCR showed that the most active derivative, compound **25** is able to reduce the viral RNA copies. The stability of the NS2B-NS3pr--ligand complexes was proven by means of dynamic simulations at 200 ns. The binding mode and interactions observed between the compounds and NS2B-NS3pro were similar and included interactions with amino acid residues His[51], Asp[75], as well as, Leu[128] for all inhibitors [45].

Non-Structural Protein 4B (NS4B)

The NS4B contains 274 amino acid residues and is an integral membrane protein whose N-terminal region contains the signal peptide that generates the mature form of NS4B after being cleaved. In its mature form, NS4B has five transmembrane helices domains called pTM1, pTM2, TM3, TM4, and TM5, both probably present in the lumen of the endoplasmic reticulum [12, 46]. NS4B is a protein that plays an important role in viral pathogenesis, as it interacts with viral and host proteins, and is involved, together with NS4A, in the induction of autophagy and inhibition of neurogenesis [46]. NS4B can suppress STAT1 phosphorylation by inhibiting IFN-I signaling, which can have its response modulated by the protein. NS4B also blocks the phosphorylation of TANK-binding kinase 1 (TBK1) through inhibition of RIG-I-mediated signaling, in addition to reducing the activation of interferon regulatory factor in the TLR4 and DNA sensing pathways [46]. ZIKV NS4B also interacted with 7-dehydrocholesterol reductase (DHCR7) and enhanced DHCR7 expression to block TBK1 and IRF3 activation and results in reduced IFN-β and ISGs productions, facilitating the ZIKV infection in glial cells [47].

NS4B inhibitor

To identify new inhibitors against ZIKV, Loe *et al.* performed a virtual screening of a library comprising 502 natural products. Chelerythrine (**28**) (Fig. **5**) chloride showed the most promising results. During the experimental investigation, chelerythrine chloride (**28**) was observed to be effective against ZIKV-infected BHK-21 (IC_{50}: 0.43 mM), Huh7 (IC_{50}: 0.42 mM), HEK293T (IC_{50}: 0.61 mM), HUVEC (IC_{50}: 0.46 mM), and JEG-3 (IC_{50}: 0.25 mM) cell lines. Studies aiming to elucidate its mechanism of action revealed that chelerythrine chlorine (**28**) treatment resulted in both delayed ZIKV replication kinetics and reduced peak viral titer. Also, chelerythrine chloride (**28**) mediates the inhibition of ZIKV protein synthesis by interfering with NS4B [12].

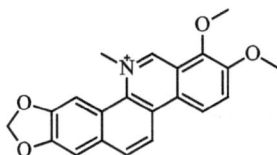

28

Fig. (5). Chelerythrine chloride as an inhibitor of Zika virus NS4B protein.

Non-Structural Protein 5 (NS5)

One of the most studied viral targets is the NS5, the largest one (~100 kDa) and, the most conserved non-structural protein among flaviviruses. NS5 carries essential enzymatic activities hosted in two domains, an N-terminal methyltransferase (MTase) domain and an RNA-dependent RNA polymerase (RdRp) domain at the C-terminal end [48, 49]. Its N-terminal domain has guanine N-7 and ribose 2'-O-methylation activities that can methylate GpppA- capped and m(7)GpppA-capped RNAs sequentially, yielding m(7)GpppA and m(7)GpppAm RNA products in the presence of S-adenosyl methionine methyl donor. The conserved motif, Lys^{61}–Asp^{146}–Lys^{182}–Glu^{218} is important for guanine N-7 and ribose 2-O-methylation reactions N-7-methylation requires only Asp^{146} residue, although other amino acids of the motif facilitate the reaction [8, 32]. NS5 is a multifunctional protein with central roles in the antagonism of host IFN responses [50]. The MTase domain uses S-adenosyl-L- methionine, which is necessary for the translation of viral mRNA to catalyze the formation of N-7-methyl-guanosine and 2-O-methyl-adenosine and add the RNA cap [3, 51, 52]. Thus, the ZIKV NS5 protein plays an important role in several phases of the viral cycle, including viral replication, activation of NOD-, LRR-, and pyrin domain-containing protein 3 (NLRP3), in the formation of the inflammasome and evasion of the immune system [53]. As it remains highly conserved among flaviviruses, NS5 is a target of great importance for the development of new drugs against viruses of this genus [3]. The last step in maintaining viral pathogenesis is carried out by the MTase domain, through post-transcriptional changes to the newly synthesized mRNA. The stability and translation of mRNA depend on the capping and methylation of the new mRNA, which are carried out after its synthesis by RdRp, which prevents the host's immune response. The host can detect uncapped RNA molecules and trigger responses to degrade them in the cytoplasm [36]. Through a *De novo* mechanism, the NS5 RdRp domain acts in viral replication and viral RNA synthesis, generating copies of the RNA genome, both positive and negative sense. During this process, RdRp uses a different RNA template than host RNA biosynthesis, not requiring a primer to elongate the nascent RNA [8, 36, 54].

The crystal structure of ZIKV NS5 RdRp has been reported, which adopts a classic "right-hand" structure consisting of the "palm", "finger", and "thumb" sub-domains [55] (Fig. **6**). Due to the fact that NS5 RdRp generates double-stranded RNA, it is an important target for the planning and development of effective and safe antivirals and, based on it, several compounds have been identified with potential anti-RdRp activity [13, 49, 52, 56]. Indeed, both nucleotide inhibitors (NIs) and non-nucleoside inhibitors (NNIs) have been reported targeting ZIKV NS5 RdRp for the development of direct-acting antiviral (DAA) agents. NIs integrate into the nascent RNA as a substrate analog and result in strand termination or lethal replication, such as Favipiravir [57], Ribavirin [58], Sofosbuvir [59], NITD008 [60], 7-Deaza-7-fluoro-2'-*C*-methyladenosine [61].

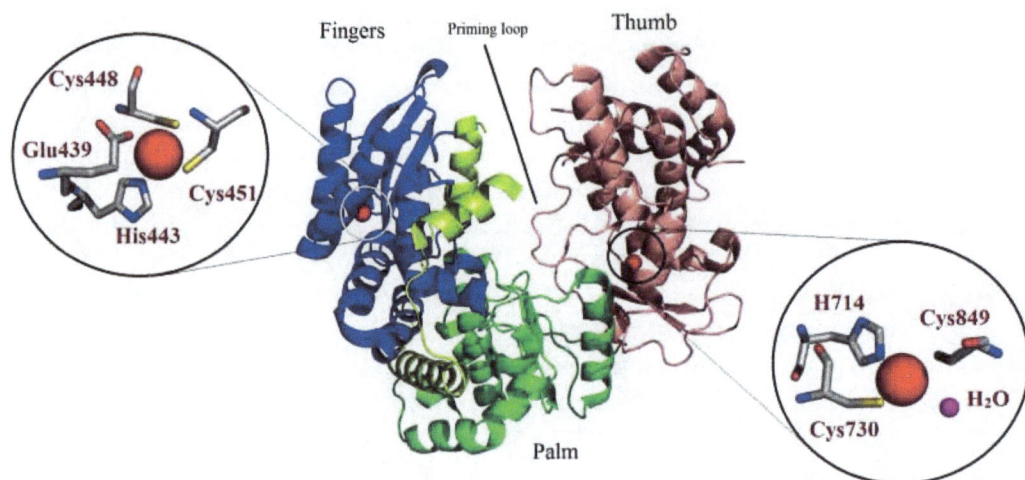

Fig. (6). Structure of Zika NS5-RNA-dependent RNA polymerase (RdRp). Ribbon representation of the overall fold with the three subdomains: fingers (blue), palm (green), thumb (light red), and the putative NLS region (yellow). The priming loop is highlighted by a black line. The catalytic residues are indicated by stick representation. The two zinc-binding sites are highlighted by circles, and detailed interactions are shown as sticks. The zinc ions are displayed as red spheres, and the water interacting with the zinc ions is displayed as pink spheres.

FDA has approved some RdRp inhibitors, most of which are nucleoside analogs, these compounds are acted upon by host kinases that convert them into triphosphate forms, which function as terminators of the nascent viral nucleic acid chain, preventing the continuation of replication of the viral genome. In this context, ribavirin is an FDA-approved drug active against several viruses, acting by inhibition of RdRp protein since it competes with its GTP substrate [3]. To exert their inhibitory activity efficiently, nucleoside analogs undergo modifications in 5'-triphosphate after entering the cell. Additionally, the process of synthesizing nucleotide triphosphates is an obstacle to be overcome, as it is a time-consuming process, which requires attention to the development of other RdRp inhibitors, which are more effective and easier to obtain [3].

NS5 Inhibitors

NNIs, such as Fidaxomicin and Cinnamic Acid, significantly inhibited ZIKV replication and improved the survival rate of mice ZIKV infected by inhibiting NS5 RdRp activity [49, 62]. Zhou *et al.* explored derivatives of fused tricyclic compounds of imidazolidinone and indole in an attempt to discover new and potent inhibitors of the NS5 RdRp. In this way, compounds **29-31** (Fig. **7**) showed the best activity, which directly inhibits RdRp activity in a dose-dependent manner, exhibiting IC_{50} values of 8.52, 9.89, and 10.67 μM, respectively [8]. The compound ZFD-10 (**32**) (Fig. **7**) is an indole derivative with activity against RdRp. It protects NS5 from thermally induced aggregation by binding directly to the target in a dose-dependent manner, with an IC_{50} value of 6.89 μM being observed [54].

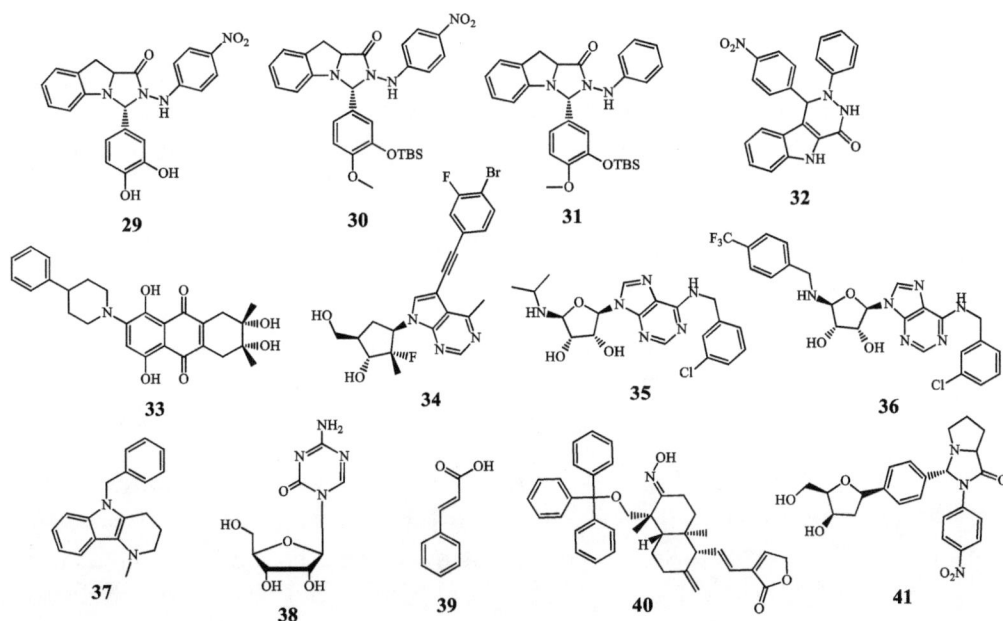

Fig. (7). Inhibitors targeting Zika NS5-RNA-dependent RNA polymerase (RdRp).

Anthraquinones have been discovered to have a wide range of applications, including anti-virus activity. Zhu *et al.* developed anthraquinone analogs as anti-ZIKV agents. Compound **33** (Fig. **7**) has a piperidine moiety as a linker, which is a rigid structure and can keep a more stable binding conformation with the protein with no meaningful cytotoxic effects. The results suggest that compound **33** inhibits the replication of ZIKV by binding to and suppressing ZIKV non-structural protein NS5 RdRp [55].

Studies performed by Yao *et al.* demonstrated that compound **34** (Fig. **7**), a nucleoside analog, directly bounds to the ZIKV RdRp domain with anti-ZIKV activity (K_D: 1.87 μM) [63]. Several nucleotide-like inhibitors of the ZIKV RdRp have been identified such as 2'-*C*-methylated nucleoside triphosphates [64], 10-undecenoic acid zinc salt [65], and Sofosbuvir triphosphate [66]. Only one non-nucleotide inhibitor, thienylcarbonyl-piperazinyl-benzothiophene (TBP) compound, has been described for the ZIKV RdRp with an IC_{50} value of 94 nM [67].

Based on previous studies that showed compound TZY12-9 (**35**) (Fig. **7**) as a promising analog, Chen *et al.* used this molecule as a starting point for designing novel potential inhibitors, providing a series of new NI analogs, in which compound XSJ2-46 (**36**) (Fig. **7**) was discovered with the high potential for *in vitro* inhibition of ZIKV (IC_{50}: 2.15 μM), with also excellent *in vivo* activity, and reasonable RdRp inhibition. XSJ2-46 (**36**) showed potential for inhibiting RNA replication, viral protein, and the spread of infectious particles, in a dose-dependent manner with the significant suppression of viral RNA at 1.25 μM. Data obtained suggest that XSJ2-46 (**36**) exerts its activity mainly in the stages after the virus enters the cell so that it could inhibit RNA production at some stages. XSJ2-46 (**36**) was able to inhibit NS5 RdRp activity by 17.52% (12.5 μM) and 62.37% (50 μM) in a dose-dependent manner, effectively inhibiting ZIKV RNA replication with an IC_{50} value of 8.78 μM [68].

The repurposing of clinically approved drugs is a strategy that has been pursued for ZIKV drug discovery. Zhou *et al.* identified mebhydolin napadisylate (MHL) (**37**) (Fig. **7**) as an effective antiviral agent against ZIKV, which suppresses viral RNA synthesis by interfering with ZIKV RdRp *in vitro*. The results of the surface plasmon resonance (SPR) assay showed that MHL could directly bind with ZIKV NS5 RdRp (K_D: 49.2 μM). Similarly, the results of the MST assay also revealed that MHL binds to ZIKV NS5 RdRp with a K_D value of 22.62 ± 2.91 μM. The binding pocket of MHL is located in the central channel of ZIKV NS5 RdRp. MHL interacts with the active site of RdRp *via* charge interactions with Asp[665] and Asp[666], which are reported to be involved in the binding of two magnesium ions at the catalytic center, therefore, the binding of MHL may block the active sites of the ZIKV [69].

Seeking to overcome the challenge associated with the conversion of nucleoside analogs into triphosphate forms, Wang *et al.* used secretory Gaussia-luciferase (Gluc) to develop cellular assays with the purpose of evaluating the activity of nucleotide compounds targeting ZIKV RdRp, avoiding conversion into active nucleotide triphosphates. From cellular assays, it was observed that 5- Azacitidine (**38**) (Fig. **7**) was able to inhibit ZIKV replication (EC_{50}: 12.5 µM) and NS5-dependent Gluc expression (EC_{50}: 4.9 µM), suppressing viral RNA synthesis and reducing the activity of the ZIKV RdRp [3].

The study by Chen *et al.* identified that unsubstituted cinnamic acid (**39**) (Fig. **7**) interferes with protein synthesis and viral RNA replication, blocking viral replication in multiple cell types. Through immunofluorescence detection, Cinnamic Acid (**39**) was able to inhibit infection or reduce viral load, at 100 µM concentration. The formed RdRp-cinnamic acid complex showed hydrogen bonds and other interactions with the residues Ser[56], Lys[105], His[110], Asp[131], Val[132], Asp[146], and Arg[354] of RdRp [49].

Qian *et al.* reported the first MTase inhibitor (**40**) (Fig. **7**) of andrographolide derivatives. Compound **40** showed a CC_{50} value greater than 200 µM and good activity on ZIKV-infected Vero, Huh7, and A549 cells, during the plaque formation screening. On Vero cells, its inhibition was observed with a CC_{50} value of 0.76 µM. Compound **40** was also capable of inhibiting the activity of ZIKV MTase, and is even more potent than the drug Sinefungin, used as a positive control for MTase. Studies carried out using molecular docking showed the interaction of compound **40** with the MTase domain of ZIKV NS5. In addition, it exerts inhibitory activity against MTase through two interactions with two phenyl groups from C19-large bulky ether, which favor binding, contributing to the inhibition of infection and viral replication [36].

ZDL-116 (**41**), a hexylhydropyrrol[1,2-*e*]imidazo-1-one derivative (Fig. **7**), showed 100% inhibition of ZIKV at all the tested concentrations without any morphological alteration of the ZDL-116-treated cell monolayers and not cytotoxicity for cells, showing CC_{50} values > 500 µM and great SI values. Studies of molecular docking showed that compound **41** can tightly bind the NS5 MTase and construct multiply interactions, including key amino acids such as Asp[146], Glu[149], and Arg[160], showing a significant docking score value of −6.38 kcal/mol [20].

STRUCTURAL PROTEINS OF ZIKA VIRUS AND THEIR INHIBITORS

Envelop (E) Protein

E protein is related to viral tropism, assists in virulence by mediating viral entry, membrane fusion, and receptor binding, is closely linked to immunogenicity, and is a good target for obtaining neutralizing antibodies [70]. E protein consists of an ectodomain (ED) and a stem/transmembrane domain. The ED can be further divided into three subdomains (EDI, EDII, and EDIII) [70] (Fig. **8**). Although neutralizing anti-bodies can bind to the ED epitopes in all three subdomains, the EDI (35% similarity) and EDII (51%similarity) subdomains are more likely to cross-react with ZIKV and DENV, as compared with ED III (29% similarity) [71]. This protein plays an important role in the production of neutralizing antibodies, which are likely to neutralize viral infection, and plays key roles in host cell binding, attachment, and membrane fusion [71, 72].

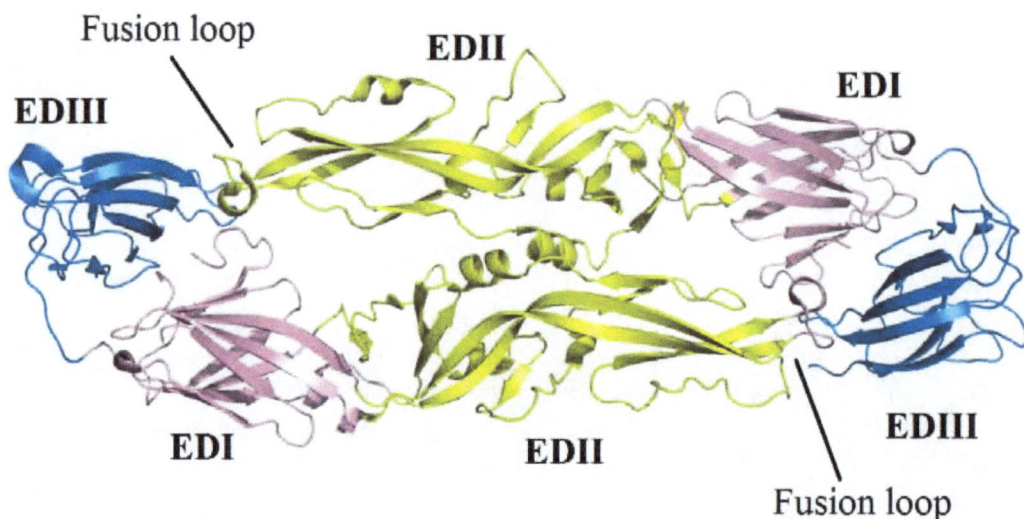

Fig. (8). ZIKV Envelope Protein (E) Structure in its dimeric form. The dimeric structure is composed of three distinct domains (EDI, EDII, and EDIII). Domain one is β-barrel-shaped, domain two is finger-like and is responsible for the dimerization of ZIKV E protein, and domain three is immunoglobulin-like. The fusion loop is between EDI and EDII of the second monomer of the protein.

The entry stage of ZIKV infection can be divided into adsorption and subsequent internalization, which is predominantly mediated by ZIKV E protein. First, the ZIKV E protein is adsorbed to the cell surface through recognizing viral entry receptors, of which AXL is the key receptor. Then, ZIKV internalizes host cells *via* clathrin-mediated endocytosis. Finally, the virus membrane fuses with the endosome releases its genome, and begins to replicate [73, 74].

ZIKV has several receptors that facilitate its entry into macrophages, monocytes, fetal cells, and neural progenitor cells (NPCs), these include the TIM-1, TAM (Tyro3, Axl, Mer), and DC-SIGN receptors. The AXL receptor plays an important role in cellular autophagy and acts as an entry receptor, however, its inhibition did not affect ZIKV entry and it seems [75, 76].

E Protein Inhibitors

Atranorin (**42**) (Fig. **9**) was confirmed to inhibit ZIKV envelope protein (4G2) expression in SNB-19 cells [23]. The results of the time-of-addition assay indicated that atranorin acted primarily by disturbing the viral entry process directly targeting the viral envelope protein and lowered ZIKV infectivity by blocking ZIKV internalization without affecting adsorption. The docking results showed the optimal conformation of the atranorin molecule and E protein located between EDI and EDIII. Atranorin showed little toxicity and could protect SNB-19 cells from cytopathic effects with an EC_{50} value of 11.90 μM [23].

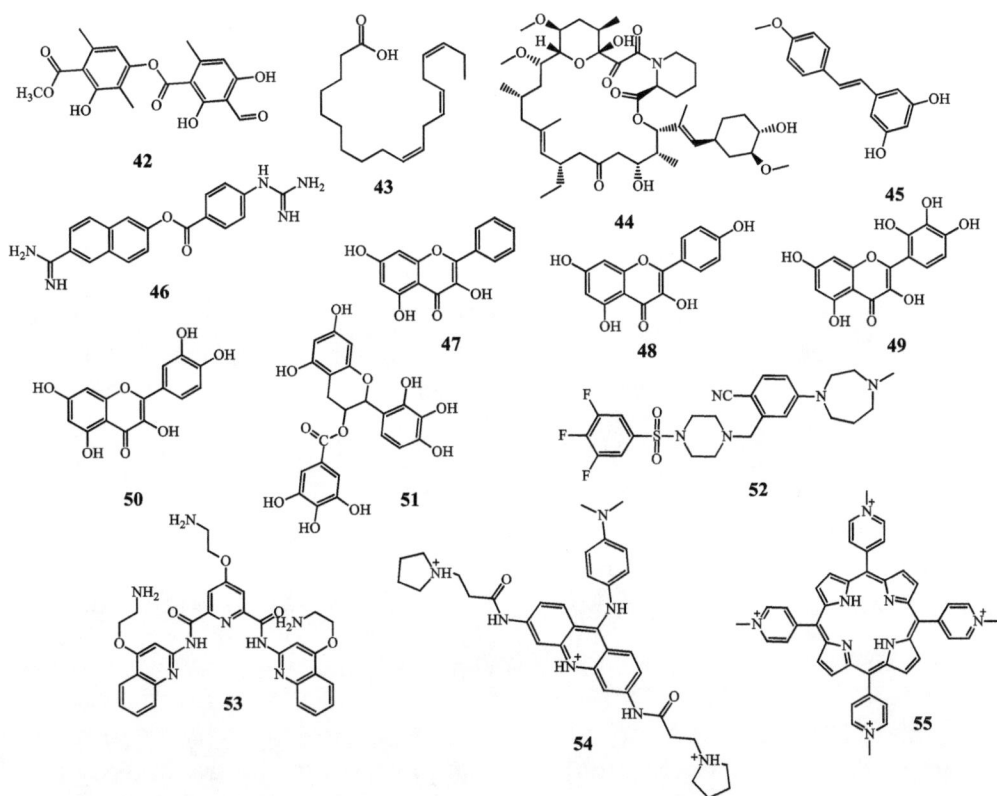

Fig. (9). Inhibitors targeting Zika Envelope (E) protein.

Monoclonal antibodies (mAbs) are synthetic antibodies that can be used to treat viral infections. To date, there have been at least 400 reported types of mice or humans' mAbs against the Zika E protein of which over 70 exhibit neutralizing activity (antiviral activity). Ten mAbs were generated using conventional hybridoma technology, one of them (8B6) exhibited neutralization ability, while the remaining 9 mAbs showed only substantial capacity to bid to the ZIKV EDIII protein [71]. The mAB 8B6, showed a high affinity towards ZIKV EDIII with a K_D value of 1.05 ± 0.22 µM. Also, it could neutralize ZIKV and recognize the ZIKV EDIII epitope (GRLITANPVITESTE), which was located at sites 646 to 660 within the polyprotein [71].

Recently, it was reported that the USP38 gene (ubiquitin-specific peptidase 38), when binding to the E protein through its C-terminal domain, can repress ZIKV infection, attenuating its K63-linked and K48-linked polyubiquitylation and subsequently can be used to generate mRNA display set, which can inhibit the virus [77].

Zou *et al.* showed that IFN-induced transmembrane protein 3 containing extracellular vesicles (IFITM-3-Exos)-treated cells exhibited strong suppression of ZIKV E protein production. To restrict entry, IFITM3 on the surface of lysosomes and late endosomes directly blocks the fusion mediated by the E protein of flavivirus. IFITM3 is also highly expressed in the placenta, and its expression is elevated during pregnancy, suggesting that IFITM3 plays a role in the fetus's defense against pathogens [78].

Alpha-linoleic acid (ALA) (**43**) (Fig. **9**) inhibited ZIKV E protein expression significantly at concentrations above 25 µM and the plaque assay and indirect immunofluorescence assay also suggested that ALA inhibited ZIKV progeny virus and cytoplasmatic expression of ZIKV E protein. Treatment of Vero cells with ALA (**43**) caused a 99% reduction rate of E mRNA level and ZIKV E protein expression, suggesting that ALA (**43**) inhibits ZIKV replication. ALA (**43**) at 5-50 mM prevented ZIKV infection by inhibiting ZIKV adsorption to Vero cells and at 15-50 mM, it inhibited ZIKV entry into Vero cells. In addition, ALA (**43**) substantially suppressed ZIKV mRNA loads, indicating a dose-dependent destruction of viral membrane integrity. Thus, ALA (**43**) interrupts the early stages of ZIKV replication, including virus binding, adsorption, and entry [72].

Ascomycin (**44**) (Fig. **9**), a macrolide obtained from *Streptomyces hygroscopicus*, was discovered such as a ZIKV inhibitor, demonstrating antiviral activity against both *in vitro* and *in vivo* ZIKV infection. Ascomycin (**44**) also inhibited ZIKV infection in human glioblastoma SNB-19 cells and hepatoma Huh7 cells. Upon SNB-19 cells, it demonstrated the best result (IC$_{50}$: 0.06 µM), which suggested that the selective index (SI) was more than 700, thus showing the safety of Ascomycin (**44**) on SNB-19 cells. The levels of ZIKV E protein and RNA were decreased along with an increasing concentration of Ascomycin (**44**). From a time-addiction experiment, it was observed that the main step affected by

Ascomicyn (**44**) is the virus replication step independent of IFN-related pathways [79].

Desoxyrhapontigenin (DES) (**45**) (Fig. **9**) was identified such a potent antiviral against ZIKV infection by blocking virus entry, downregulating receptors, and interacting with envelope protein (E). Yu *et al.* also demonstrated that DES can reduce the level of maternal-fetal transmission of ZIKV in mice (IC_{50}: 2.25 mM and SI: 62.6), reducing harm to the fetus. *in silico* molecular docking analysis showed that DES has a higher binding affinity to ZIKV E protein, specifically domain III (PDB: 5JHM (ZIKV E protein)). The consequences associated with damage to the brain and testes are related to the activation of caspase-3, and it has been observed that treatment with DES restricts this activation and protects these organs from suffering damage [80].

Nafamostat (**46**) (Fig. **9**) exhibits anti-ZIKV activity in the early stages of infection, targeting DIII and the viral internalization and adsorption phases. In Vero and BHK cell lines, IC_{50} values equal to 11.78 ± 5.67 and 6.83 ± 0.39 µM, respectively, were observed for protection from the cytopathogenic effect. The interaction between Nafamostat (**46**) and E protein DIII was confirmed using SPR assay technology, showing a dose-dependent activity, and the results indicated that Nafamostat (**46**) interacts directly with the E protein [81].

It is known that flavonoids are potential inhibitors of ZIKV infections and many methods have been used for the validation of these compounds, such as Galangin (**47**), Kaempferide (**48**), Myricetin (**49**), Quercetin (**50**), and Epigallocatechin Gallate (EGCG) (**51**) (Fig. **9**). These are examples of flavonoids with inhibitory activity on ZIKV RNA production, acting mainly in the early stages of infection on Vero cells in a dose-dependent manner, and time-of-addition assay suggests that E protein could be involved with their activities [82].

Quan *et al.* identified a series of *N*-phenylsulfonyl-2-(piperazin-1-yl)methyl-benzonitrile derivatives as ZIKV entry inhibitors, of which compound (**52**) (Fig. **9**) with lower cytotoxicity ($CC_{50} > 20$ mM) acts on the early entry stage of ZIKV cycle, dependently inhibiting protein synthesis and ZIKV RNA replication in ZIKV-infected HUVECs (EC_{50}: 5.34 µM) and Vero cells (EC_{50}: 3.27 µM) [83].

Zou *et al.* showed that Pyridostatin (PDS) (**53**) (Fig. **9**) is an excellent binder towards ZIKV RNA G-quadruplexes and exerted antiviral activity (EC_{50}: 4.2 µM) at the post-entry process of ZIKV infection, which could lead to the inhibition of the ZIKV mRNA replication and protein synthesis, preventing the release of progeny virus. PDS can also cause a dose-dependent reduction in both E and NS1 protein synthesis and interfere with the activity of NS2B/NS3 protease by covalent and non-covalent binding. PDS binds and stabilizes the G- quadruplexes

(GQs) of ZIKV positive-stranded RNA and double-stranded RNA, thus inhibiting viral mRNA replication and protein synthesis. Thus, PDS is a potential multi-target inhibitor of ZIKV infection [5].

Majee *et al.* identified four new ZIKV GQs conserved in the NS2, NS4B, and NS5 genes of ZIKV genome, which can be stabilized through the binding of Braco-19 (**54**) and TMPyP4 (**55**) (Fig. **9**). Both compounds inhibited virus growth significantly, at 100 µM of Braco-19 (**54**), cell viability was greater than 85%, inhibition of virus growth was most significant (> 80-fold) at 96 hpi compared to the untreated control. At a concentration of 10 µM of TMPyP4, at which cell viability was over 80%, the infectious virus yields in the supernatants at 72 hpi and 96 hpi were reduced nearly120-fold and 170-fold, respectively; when compared to the untreated control. The increasing concentrations of Braco-19 (**54**) caused a marked reduction in E protein expression while increasing the dose of TMPyP4 (**55**) resulted in increased molecular mass of the E protein. The results suggest that GQ-binding compounds Braco-19 (**54**) and TMPyP4 (**55**) inhibit ZIKV growth infectious progeny production. *in vitro* studies also suggest that Braco-19 (**54**) and TMPyP4 (**55**) inhibit the activities of the RNA template and that binding of these compounds to the GQ structures inhibits the movement of the viral RNA polymerase, resulting in an overall reduction of viral RNA copy numbers [84].

Precursor of Membrane (prM) Protein

The ZIKV prM protein is involved in ZIKV-mediated neuro-pathogenicity. In fact, it has been demonstrated that the higher neurovirulence/tropism of African strains could be linked to differences in ten amino acid residues in prM proteins of the two ZIKV strains, African and Asian [85]. African strains also display higher transmissibility and fetal pathogenicity than Asian strains. The antiviral response elicited against the two strains upon infection of human neural progenitors and astrocytes could also contribute to the higher neurovirulence of the African strains [85]. The prM of flaviviruses facilitates the folding and trafficking of the E protein at the time of virus particle biogenesis [86]. The cellular protease furin cleaves prM during particle egress, releasing an *N*-terminal fragment (pr)-containing the single *N*-linked glycan of prM. This cleavage is required for infectivity in flaviviruses [87].

The main mechanism by which ZIKV infiltrates host cells is receptor-mediated viral recognition, and clathrin-mediated endocytosis, followed by fusion with endosome membrane and release of the genetic material. AXL, a TAM family kinase receptor that was highly expressed in astrocytes, microglia, and radial glia cells, has been described as the main entry receptor for ZIKV recognition.

Clathrin-mediated endocytosis, which is a vesicular trafficking process and is mostly involved in physiological processes, has been shown to be used by ZIKV to enter cells. After clathrin-mediated uptake, the endocytic vesicle carrying the virus is delivered to the initial endosomes, which mature into late endosomes, and then the viral membrane fuses with the endosome membrane, and viral RNA is released into the cytoplasm. Since membrane fusion is an essential step in the infection of enveloped viruses, inhibitors of membrane fusion are expected to exhibit potent antiviral effects [88].

Xu *et al.* revealed that hemin, an iron-binding porphyrin, demonstrates anti-ZIKV activity by acting on the process of virus-endosome fusion restricting ZIKV infection-elicited inflammatory responses in SNB-19 cells and in Heme Oxygenase-1-independent pathway, which is a stress-inducible, anti-inflammatory, and cytoprotective enzyme expressed in most cell types in the organism. Also, it has been reported that hemin can exert significant antiviral activity against a wide variety of viruses. Also, hemin decreased ZIKV NS1, NS2B, and NS3 protein expressions, including ZIKV NS1 gene expression, as well [88, 89]. Although, there are no specific inhibitors targeting ZIKV prM protein so far.

Capsid (C) Protein

C protein (122 amino acids length) forms the icosahedral capsid of the virion, supplemented with RNA and surrounded by the globular lipid bilayer and has been identified as one of the main targets of CD4$^+$ and CD8$^+$ T-cells [72, 90, 91]. Along with encapsidation of the genomic RNA, capsid protein has been shown to interact with host intracellular biomolecules, such as viral RNA to perform important processes for the viral cycle [92]. It includes host immune response suppression, RNA chaperone activity, cellular metabolism, apoptosis, and viral replication [93].

C protein is 104 amino acids long and remains bound to the endoplasmic reticulum (ER), even after its translation by ORF. To remain linked to the ER it uses a capsid anchor at its C-terminal end, the N-terminal region is oriented towards the cytosol. The C protein anchor is found as the fifth α-helix, therefore named α-5. It is anchored to the ER through a region a-5, or capsid anchor, which is a transmembrane region. This transmembrane is responsible for separating the capsid from the prM protein (Fig. **10**). The mature C protein is released into the cytoplasm during polyprotein maturation and after NS2B-NS3 leaves the ER region [92, 94]. The host signal peptidase recognizes the CA-prM junction in the ER lumen as a cleavage site, then the CA is incorporated into the membrane of the two proteins and separated [95]. The C protein facilitates the ZIKV genome packaging into the virus particles [86, 96], and acts in the protection of the RNA genome and viral assembly [18]. Lastly, the flaviviral C protein offers an attractive target for a potential therapeutic strategy since it performs multiple functions regulating the viral life cycle and virulence [93], although there are no specific inhibitors against ZIKV C protein so far.

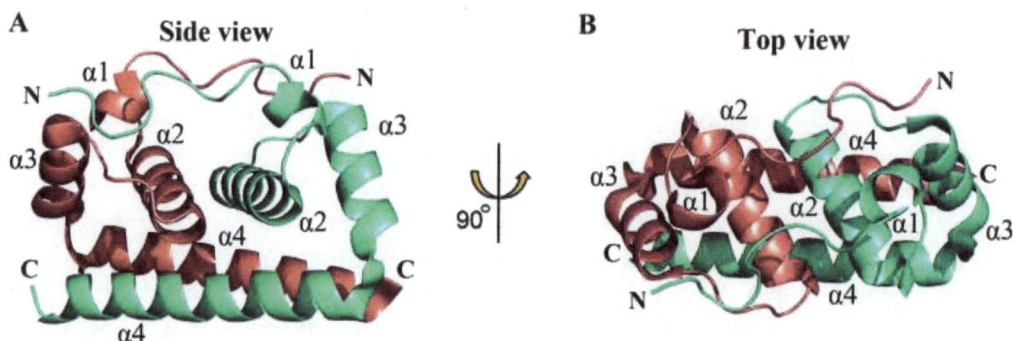

Fig. (10). Ribbon representation of ZIKV Capsid (C) structure, showing its dimeric form. (**A**) One monomer is colored in salmon, and the other is colored in pale green. (**B**) Rotation of dimer along Y-axis by 90°.

Alternative Pathways of Inhibition of ZIKV

According to Lai *et al.*, viral replication and even maturation can be delayed if defined viral-induced inflammatory pathways are blocked. During ZIKV infection occurs a statistically significant increase in *N*-Acylethanolamine acid amidase (NAAA) expression, suggesting that NAAA plays a role in viral replication [72]. The authors showed that NAAA inhibition with ARN736 was able to slow viral replication, inhibit viral maturation, and reduce inflammation, consequently, the virion release dropped ~5-fold. Furthermore, NAAA inhibition hinders prM maturation and reduces furin activity [97, 98]. Inhibiting NAAA through gene-editing or drugs moderately reduces ZIKV replication by approximately one $\log_{10}$ in Human Neural Stem Cells, while also releasing immature virions that have lost their infectivity. This inhibition impairs furin-mediated prM cleavage, ultimately blocking ZIKV maturation [97].

ML-SA1 (**56**) (Fig. **11**), a selective TRPML agonist, acting as an activator of TRPMLs has potent antiviral activity against ZIKV RNA (IC$_{50}$: 52.99 µM) and protein levels. ML-SA1 has no significant antiviral activity against ZIKV at the attachment stage, the effect of ML-SA1 on viruses mainly occurs at the entry stage of the viral life cycle, which includes receptor-mediated endocytosis of viral particles, acidification of the endosomes, and unravelling of the nucleocapsid resulting in the degradation of viral pathogens [99].

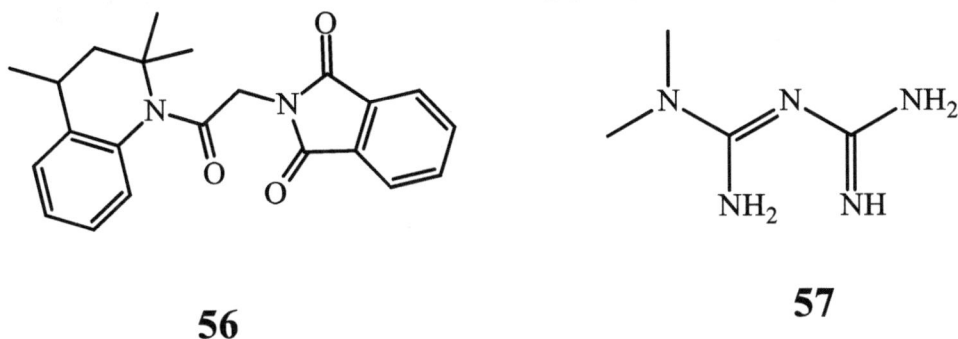

Fig. (11). Compounds capable of inducing anti-Zika virus *via* multiple targets' pathways.

Metformin (**57**) (Fig. **11**), an established drug used in the treatment of diabetes *mellitus*, can diminish ZIKV replication without the alteration of viral entry and phagocytosis. Data showed Metformin (**57**) reduced ZIKV-induced inflammatory responses but upregulated type I and III IFNs, such as IFNα2, IFNβ1 and IFNλ3, in microglia and that the antiviral function of Metformin (**57**) might be associated with multiple signaling pathways, including cell proliferation, apoptosis, AMPK, NF-κB, mTOR, MAPK, and PI3K-Akt signaling pathways, viral infection pathways, protein processing in endoplasmic reticulum, regulation of actin cytoskeleton and EGFR tyrosine kinase inhibitor resistance. ZIKV mainly infects fetal microglia and induces elevated levels of pro-inflammatory mediators including TNFα, IL1β, IL6, CCL2, and CXCL10. The Metformin (**57**) treatment downregulates these markers accompanied by the downregulation of ISG transcript levels, including IRF9, GBP4, MDA5, OAS1, MX1, and ISG15, demonstrating that the administration of Metformin (**57**) decreases ZIKV-induced inflammatory responses in microglia and that the upregulated type I and III may contribute to the suppression of ZIKV replication and further decrease the ZIKV-induced ISG levels in microglia. Finally, Metformin (**57**) does not alter ZIKV entry into microglia, instead might inhibit ZIKV replication after viral entry [100].

CONCLUSION

A comprehensive understanding of pathogenic organisms such as the ZIKV virus is a great necessity for drug development. Thus, understanding all structural and non-structural components, including amino acid sequence and protein conformation is important to medicinal chemistry to discover useful new therapies against this threatening pathogen. Although factors related to the viral cycle and the host can be considered as possible targets for the development of new anti-ZIKV agents, there is a greater effort for certain targets, while others are less addressed but could allow the development of new and diversified scaffolds. Developing new assays and exploring targets that are currently underexplored in more depth is the first step towards the efficient identification of new anti-ZIKV drugs that could generate promising treatments. Finally, we hope that this chapter can inspire researchers around the world and that the knowledge compiled here can be used in their research. This enables the discovery of new anti-ZIKV drugs that can provide new hope against this disease, which has caused serious damage to the world's population.

ACKNOWLEDGEMENTS

The authors express their gratitude to the National Council for Scientific and Technological Development – CNPq (grant number: 306323/2022-2) and the Coordination for the Improvement of Higher Education Personnel – CAPES (finance code: 001).

REFERENCES

[1]   Rodrigues ÉE da S. Maus H, Hammerschmidt SJ, *et al*. The medicinal chemistry of zika virus. In: Ahmad SI, Ed. Hum Viruses Dis Treat Vaccines new insights. 1st ed. Cham: Springer International Publishing 2021; pp. 233-95.
[http://dx.doi.org/10.1007/978-3-030-71165-8_13]

[2]   Hernández-Sarmiento LJ, Valdés-López JF, Urcuqui-Inchima S. American-Asian- and African lineages of Zika virus induce differential pro-inflammatory and Interleukin 27-dependent antiviral responses in human monocytes. Virus Res 2023; 325: 199040.
[http://dx.doi.org/10.1016/j.virusres.2023.199040] [PMID: 36610657]

[3]   Wang L, Zhou R, Liu Y, *et al*. A cell-based assay to discover inhibitors of Zika virus RNA-dependent RNA polymerase. Virology 2024; 589: 109939.
[http://dx.doi.org/10.1016/j.virol.2023.109939] [PMID: 37979208]

[4]   de Sales-Neto JM, Madruga Carvalho DC, Arruda Magalhães DW, Araujo Medeiros AB, Soares MM, Rodrigues-Mascarenhas S. Zika virus: Antiviral immune response, inflammation, and cardiotonic steroids as antiviral agents. Int Immunopharmacol 2024; 127: 111368.
[http://dx.doi.org/10.1016/j.intimp.2023.111368] [PMID: 38103408]

[5]   Zou M, Li JY, Zhang MJ, *et al*. G-quadruplex binder pyridostatin as an effective multi-target ZIKV inhibitor. Int J Biol Macromol 2021; 190: 178-88.
[http://dx.doi.org/10.1016/j.ijbiomac.2021.08.121] [PMID: 34461156]

[6]   Jiang H, Zhang Y, Wu Y, *et al*. Identification of Montelukast as flavivirus NS2B-NS3 protease inhibitor by inverse virtual screening and experimental validation. Biochem Biophys Res Commun 2022; 606: 87-93.
[http://dx.doi.org/10.1016/j.bbrc.2022.03.064] [PMID: 35339757]

[7]   Song G, Lee EM, Pan J, *et al*. An integrated systems biology approach identifies the proteasome as a critical host machinery for ZIKV and DENV replication. Genomics Proteomics Bioinformatics 2021; 19(1): 108-22.
[http://dx.doi.org/10.1016/j.gpb.2020.06.016] [PMID: 33610792]

[8]   Zhou GF, Li F, Xue JX, *et al*. Antiviral effects of the fused tricyclic derivatives of indoline and imidazolidinone on ZIKV infection and RdRp activities of ZIKV and DENV. Virus Res 2023; 326: 199062.
[http://dx.doi.org/10.1016/j.virusres.2023.199062] [PMID: 36746341]

[9]   Kasprzykowski JI, Fukutani KF, Fabio H, *et al.* A recursive sub-typing screening surveillance system detects the appearance of the ZIKV African lineage in Brazil: Is there a risk of a new epidemic? Int J Infect Dis 2020; 96: 579-81.
[http://dx.doi.org/10.1016/j.ijid.2020.05.090] [PMID: 32497802]

[10]   Fowler A, Ye C, Clarke EC, *et al.* A method for mapping the linear epitopes targeted by the natural antibody response to Zika virus infection using a VLP platform technology. Virology 2023; 579: 101-10.
[http://dx.doi.org/10.1016/j.virol.2023.01.001] [PMID: 36623351]

[11]   Lee CYP, Carissimo G, Teo TH, *et al.* CD8+ T cells trigger auricular dermatitis and blepharitis in mice after zika virus infection in the absence of CD4+ T cells. J Invest Dermatol 2023; 143(6): 1031-1041.e8.
[http://dx.doi.org/10.1016/j.jid.2022.11.020] [PMID: 36566875]

[12]   Loe MWC, Lee RCH, Chin WX, *et al.* Chelerythrine chloride inhibits Zika virus infection by targeting the viral NS4B protein. Antiviral Res 2023; 219: 105732.
[http://dx.doi.org/10.1016/j.antiviral.2023.105732] [PMID: 37832876]

[13]   Mottin M, Caesar LK, Brodsky D, *et al.* Chalcones from Angelica keiskei (ashitaba) inhibit key Zika virus replication proteins. Bioorg Chem 2022; 120: 105649.
[http://dx.doi.org/10.1016/j.bioorg.2022.105649] [PMID: 35124513]

[14]   Chen H, Lao Z, Xu J, *et al.* Antiviral activity of lycorine against Zika virus *in vivo* and *in vitro*. Virology 2020; 546: 88-97.
[http://dx.doi.org/10.1016/j.virol.2020.04.009] [PMID: 32452420]

[15]   Kuivanen S, Bespalov MM, Nandania J, *et al.* Obatoclax, saliphenylhalamide and gemcitabine inhibit Zika virus infection *in vitro* and differentially affect cellular signaling, transcription and metabolism. Antiviral Res 2017; 139: 117-28.
[http://dx.doi.org/10.1016/j.antiviral.2016.12.022] [PMID: 28049006]

[16]   van den Elsen K, Chew BLA, Ho JS, Luo D. Flavivirus nonstructural proteins and replication complexes as antiviral drug targets. Curr Opin Virol 2023; 59: 101305.
[http://dx.doi.org/10.1016/j.coviro.2023.101305] [PMID: 36870091]

[17]   Zhan Y, Pang Z, Du Y, *et al.* NS1-based DNA vaccination confers mouse protective immunity against ZIKV challenge. Infect Genet Evol 2020; 85: 104521.
[http://dx.doi.org/10.1016/j.meegid.2020.104521] [PMID: 32882433]

[18]   Bhat EA, Ali T, Sajjad N, kumar R, Bron P. Insights into the structure, functional perspective, and pathogenesis of ZIKV: an updated review. Biomed Pharmacother 2023; 165: 115175.
[http://dx.doi.org/10.1016/j.biopha.2023.115175] [PMID: 37473686]

[19]   Roy P, Roy S, Sengupta N. Disulfide reduction allosterically destabilizes the β-ladder subdomain assembly within the NS1 dimer of ZIKV. Biophys J 2020; 119(8): 1525-37.
[http://dx.doi.org/10.1016/j.bpj.2020.08.036] [PMID: 32946768]

[20]   Chen R, Francese R, Wang N, *et al.* Exploration of novel hexahydropyrrolo[1,2-e]imidazol-1-one derivatives as antiviral agents against ZIKV and USUV. Eur J Med Chem 2023; 248: 115081.
[http://dx.doi.org/10.1016/j.ejmech.2022.115081] [PMID: 36623328]

[21]   Zeng Q, Liu J, Hao C, Zhang B, Zhang H. Making sense of flavivirus non-strctural protein 1 in innate immune evasion and inducing tissue-specific damage. Virus Res 2023; 336: 199222.
[http://dx.doi.org/10.1016/j.virusres.2023.199222] [PMID: 37716670]

[22]   Brown WC, Akey DL, Konwerski JR, *et al.* Extended surface for membrane association in Zika virus NS1 structure. Nat Struct Mol Biol 2016; 23(9): 865-7.
[http://dx.doi.org/10.1038/nsmb.3268] [PMID: 27455458]

[23]   Huang G, Wang H, Wang X, *et al.* Atranorin inhibits Zika virus infection in human glioblastoma cell line SNB-19 *via* targeting Zika virus envelope protein. Phytomedicine 2024; 125: 155343.

[http://dx.doi.org/10.1016/j.phymed.2024.155343] [PMID: 38290230]

[24]   Baltina LA, Lai HC, Liu YC, *et al.* Glycyrrhetinic acid derivatives as Zika virus inhibitors: Synthesis and antiviral activity *in vitro*. Bioorg Med Chem 2021; 41: 116204.
[http://dx.doi.org/10.1016/j.bmc.2021.116204] [PMID: 34022526]

[25]   Yu Y, Chen Y, Wang J, *et al.* A peptide derived from the N-terminal of NS2A for the preparation of ZIKV NS2A recognition polyclonal antibody. J Immunol Methods 2023; 512: 113396.
[http://dx.doi.org/10.1016/j.jim.2022.113396] [PMID: 36463933]

[26]   Maus H, Barthels F, Hammerschmidt SJ, *et al.* SAR of novel benzothiazoles targeting an allosteric pocket of DENV and ZIKV NS2B/NS3 proteases. Bioorg Med Chem 2021; 47: 116392.
[http://dx.doi.org/10.1016/j.bmc.2021.116392] [PMID: 34509861]

[27]   Nitsche C. Proteases from dengue, West Nile and Zika viruses as drug targets. Biophys Rev 2019; 11(2): 157-65.
[http://dx.doi.org/10.1007/s12551-019-00508-3] [PMID: 30806881]

[28]   Voss S, Nitsche C. Inhibitors of the Zika virus protease NS2B-NS3. Bioorg Med Chem Lett 2020; 30(5): 126965.
[http://dx.doi.org/10.1016/j.bmcl.2020.126965] [PMID: 31980339]

[29]   Nitsche C, Holloway S, Schirmeister T, Klein CD. Biochemistry and medicinal chemistry of the dengue virus protease. Chem Rev 2014; 114(22): 11348-81.
[http://dx.doi.org/10.1021/cr500233q] [PMID: 25268322]

[30]   Cláudia Marinho da Silva A, Lima Amaral CM, Maestre Herazo MA, *et al.* Production and characterization of egg yolk antibodies against the ZIKV NS2B expressed in Nicotiana benthamiana. Int Immunopharmacol 2023; 125(Pt A): 111088.
[http://dx.doi.org/10.1016/j.intimp.2023.111088] [PMID: 37925945]

[31]   Manzato VM, Di Santo C, Torquato RJS, *et al.* Boophilin D1, a Kunitz type protease inhibitor, as a source of inhibitors for the ZIKA virus NS2B-NS3 protease. Biochimie 2023; 214(Pt B): 96-101.
[http://dx.doi.org/10.1016/j.biochi.2023.06.010] [PMID: 37364769]

[32]   Teramoto T, Choi KH, Padmanabhan R. Flavivirus proteases: The viral Achilles heel to prevent future pandemics. Antiviral Res 2023; 210: 105516.
[http://dx.doi.org/10.1016/j.antiviral.2022.105516] [PMID: 36586467]

[33]   Zephyr J, Rao DN, Johnson C, *et al.* Allosteric quinoxaline-based inhibitors of the flavivirus NS2B/NS3 protease. Bioorg Chem 2023; 131: 106269.
[http://dx.doi.org/10.1016/j.bioorg.2022.106269] [PMID: 36446201]

[34]   Kang C, Keller TH, Luo D. Zika virus protease: An antiviral drug target. Trends Microbiol 2017; 25(10): 797-808.
[http://dx.doi.org/10.1016/j.tim.2017.07.001] [PMID: 28789826]

[35]   Lei J, Hansen G, Nitsche C, Klein CD, Zhang L, Hilgenfeld R. Crystal structure of zika virus NS2B-NS3 protease in complex with a boronate inhibitor Science (80-) 2016; 353: 503-5.
[http://dx.doi.org/10.1126/science.aag2419]

[36]   Qian W, Zhou GF, Ge X, *et al.* Discovery of dehydroandrographolide derivatives with C19 hindered ether as potent anti-ZIKV agents with inhibitory activities to MTase of ZIKV NS5. Eur J Med Chem 2022; 243: 114710.
[http://dx.doi.org/10.1016/j.ejmech.2022.114710] [PMID: 36055002]

[37]   Mirza MU, Alanko I, Vanmeert M, *et al.* The discovery of Zika virus NS2B-NS3 inhibitors with antiviral activity *via* an integrated virtual screening approach. Eur J Pharm Sci 2022; 175: 106220.
[http://dx.doi.org/10.1016/j.ejps.2022.106220] [PMID: 35618201]

[38]   Maus H, Hammerschmidt SJ, Hinze G, *et al.* The effects of allosteric and competitive inhibitors on ZIKV protease conformational dynamics explored through smFRET, nanoDSF, DSF, and ^{19}F NMR. Eur J Med Chem 2023; 258: 115573.

[http://dx.doi.org/10.1016/j.ejmech.2023.115573] [PMID: 37379675]

[39] da Silva-Júnior EF, de Araújo-Júnior JX. Peptide derivatives as inhibitors of NS2B-NS3 protease from Dengue, West Nile, and Zika flaviviruses. Bioorg Med Chem 2019; 27(18): 3963-78.
[http://dx.doi.org/10.1016/j.bmc.2019.07.038] [PMID: 31351847]

[40] Lin WW, Huang YJ, Wang YT, *et al.* Development of NS2B-NS3 protease inhibitor that impairs Zika virus replication. Virus Res 2023; 329: 199092.
[http://dx.doi.org/10.1016/j.virusres.2023.199092] [PMID: 36965673]

[41] Miao J, Yuan H, Rao J, *et al.* Identification of a small compound that specifically inhibits Zika virus *in vitro* and *in vivo* by targeting the NS2B-NS3 protease. Antiviral Res 2022; 199: 105255.
[http://dx.doi.org/10.1016/j.antiviral.2022.105255] [PMID: 35143853]

[42] Andrade MA, Mottin M, Sousa BKP, *et al.* Identification of novel Zika virus NS3 protease inhibitors with different inhibition modes by integrative experimental and computational approaches. Biochimie 2023; 212: 143-52.
[http://dx.doi.org/10.1016/j.biochi.2023.04.004] [PMID: 37088408]

[43] del Rosario García-Lozano M, Dragoni F, Gallego P, *et al.* Piperazine-derived small molecules as potential Flaviviridae NS3 protease inhibitors. *in vitro* antiviral activity evaluation against Zika and Dengue viruses. Bioorg Chem 2023; 133: 106408.
[http://dx.doi.org/10.1016/j.bioorg.2023.106408] [PMID: 36801791]

[44] Li Z, Xu J, Lang Y, *et al. in vitro* and *in vivo* characterization of erythrosin B and derivatives against Zika virus. Acta Pharm Sin B 2022; 12(4): 1662-70.
[http://dx.doi.org/10.1016/j.apsb.2021.10.017] [PMID: 35847519]

[45] Vilela GG, Silva WFS, Batista VM, *et al.* Fragment-based design of α-cyanoacrylates and α-cyanoacrylamides targeting Dengue and Zika NS2B/NS3 proteases. New J Chem 2022; 46(42): 20322-46.
[http://dx.doi.org/10.1039/D2NJ01983C]

[46] Sarratea MB, Alberti AS, Redolfi DM, *et al.* Zika virus NS4B protein targets TANK-binding kinase 1 and inhibits type I interferon production. Biochim Biophys Acta, Gen Subj 2023; 1867(12): 130483.
[http://dx.doi.org/10.1016/j.bbagen.2023.130483] [PMID: 37802371]

[47] Chen W, Li Y, Yu X, *et al.* Zika virus non-structural protein 4B interacts with DHCR7 to facilitate viral infection. Virol Sin 2023; 38(1): 23-33.
[http://dx.doi.org/10.1016/j.virs.2022.09.009] [PMID: 36182074]

[48] Baltina LA, Hour MJ, Liu YC, *et al.* Antiviral activity of glycyrrhizic acid conjugates with amino acid esters against Zika virus. Virus Res 2021; 294: 198290.
[http://dx.doi.org/10.1016/j.virusres.2020.198290] [PMID: 33388394]

[49] Chen Y, Li Z, Pan P, *et al.* Cinnamic acid inhibits Zika virus by inhibiting RdRp activity. Antiviral Res 2021; 192: 105117.
[http://dx.doi.org/10.1016/j.antiviral.2021.105117] [PMID: 34174248]

[50] Ponia SS, Robertson SJ, McNally KL, *et al.* Mitophagy antagonism by ZIKV reveals Ajuba as a regulator of PINK1 signaling, PKR-dependent inflammation, and viral invasion of tissues. Cell Rep 2021; 37(4): 109888.
[http://dx.doi.org/10.1016/j.celrep.2021.109888] [PMID: 34706234]

[51] Quintana VM, Selisko B, Brunetti JE, *et al.* Antiviral activity of the natural alkaloid anisomycin against dengue and Zika viruses. Antiviral Res 2020; 176: 104749.
[http://dx.doi.org/10.1016/j.antiviral.2020.104749] [PMID: 32081740]

[52] Nascimento IJS, Santos-Júnior PFS, Aquino TM, Araújo-Júnior JX, Silva-Júnior EF. Insights on Dengue and Zika NS5 RNA-dependent RNA polymerase (RdRp) inhibitors. Eur J Med Chem 2021; 224: 113698.
[http://dx.doi.org/10.1016/j.ejmech.2021.113698] [PMID: 34274831]

[53]   Shrivastava G, Valenzuela-Leon PC, Botello K, Calvo E. *Aedes aegypti* saliva modulates inflammasome activation and facilitates flavivirus infection *in vitro*. iScience 2024; 27(1): 108620.
[http://dx.doi.org/10.1016/j.isci.2023.108620] [PMID: 38188518]

[54]   Zhou GF, Qian W, Li F, *et al*. Discovery of ZFD-10 of a pyridazino[4,5-b]indol-4(5H)-one derivative as an anti-ZIKV agent and a ZIKV NS5 RdRp inhibitor. Antiviral Res 2023; 214: 105607.
[http://dx.doi.org/10.1016/j.antiviral.2023.105607] [PMID: 37088168]

[55]   Zhu Y, Yu J, Chen T, *et al*. Design, synthesis, and biological evaluation of a series of new anthraquinone derivatives as anti-ZIKV agents. Eur J Med Chem 2023; 258: 115620.
[http://dx.doi.org/10.1016/j.ejmech.2023.115620] [PMID: 37421888]

[56]   Gharbi-Ayachi A, Santhanakrishnan S, Wong YH, *et al*. Non-nucleoside inhibitors of zika virus RNA-dependent RNA polymerase. J Virol 2020; 94(21): e00794-20.
[http://dx.doi.org/10.1128/JVI.00794-20] [PMID: 32796069]

[57]   Kim JA, Seong RK, Kumar M, Shin O. Favipiravir and ribavirin inhibit replication of asian and african strains of zika virus in different cell models. Viruses 2018; 10(2): 72.
[http://dx.doi.org/10.3390/v10020072] [PMID: 29425176]

[58]   Kamiyama N, Soma R, Hidano S, *et al*. Ribavirin inhibits Zika virus (ZIKV) replication *in vitro* and suppresses viremia in ZIKV-infected STAT1-deficient mice. Antiviral Res 2017; 146: 1-11.
[http://dx.doi.org/10.1016/j.antiviral.2017.08.007] [PMID: 28818572]

[59]   Mumtaz N, Jimmerson LC, Bushman LR, *et al*. Cell-line dependent antiviral activity of sofosbuvir against Zika virus. Antiviral Res 2017; 146: 161-3.
[http://dx.doi.org/10.1016/j.antiviral.2017.09.004] [PMID: 28912011]

[60]   Deng YQ, Zhang NN, Li CF, *et al*. Adenosine analog NITD008 is a potent inhibitor of zika virus. Open Forum Infect Dis 2016; 3(4): ofw175.
[http://dx.doi.org/10.1093/ofid/ofw175] [PMID: 27747251]

[61]   Olsen DB, Eldrup AB, Bartholomew L, *et al*. A 7-deaza-adenosine analog is a potent and selective inhibitor of hepatitis C virus replication with excellent pharmacokinetic properties. Antimicrob Agents Chemother 2004; 48(10): 3944-53.
[http://dx.doi.org/10.1128/AAC.48.10.3944-3953.2004] [PMID: 15388457]

[62]   Yuan J, Yu J, Huang Y, *et al*. Antibiotic fidaxomicin is an RdRp inhibitor as a potential new therapeutic agent against Zika virus. BMC Med 2020; 18(1): 204.
[http://dx.doi.org/10.1186/s12916-020-01663-1] [PMID: 32731873]

[63]   Yao G, Yu J, Lin C, *et al*. Design, synthesis, and biological evaluation of novel 2′-methyl-2′-fluoo-6-methyl-7-alkynyl-7-deazapurine nucleoside analogs as anti-Zika virus agents. Eur J Med Chem 2022; 234: 114275.
[http://dx.doi.org/10.1016/j.ejmech.2022.114275] [PMID: 35306290]

[64]   Hercík K, Kozak J, Šála M, *et al*. Adenosine triphosphate analogs can efficiently inhibit the Zika virus RNA-dependent RNA polymerase. Antiviral Res 2017; 137: 131-3.
[http://dx.doi.org/10.1016/j.antiviral.2016.11.020] [PMID: 27902932]

[65]   Lin Y, Zhang H, Song W, Si S, Han Y, Jiang J. Identification and characterization of Zika virus NS5 RNA-dependent RNA polymerase inhibitors. Int J Antimicrob Agents 2019; 54(4): 502-6.
[http://dx.doi.org/10.1016/j.ijantimicag.2019.07.010] [PMID: 31310806]

[66]   Sacramento CQ, de Melo GR, de Freitas CS, *et al*. The clinically approved antiviral drug sofosbuvir inhibits Zika virus replication. Sci Rep 2017; 7(1): 40920.
[http://dx.doi.org/10.1038/srep40920] [PMID: 28098253]

[67]   Pattnaik A, Palermo N, Sahoo BR, *et al*. Discovery of a non-nucleoside RNA polymerase inhibitor for blocking Zika virus replication through *in silico* screening. Antiviral Res 2018; 151: 78-86.
[http://dx.doi.org/10.1016/j.antiviral.2017.12.016] [PMID: 29274845]

[68] Chen X, Yan Y, Song H, *et al.* Investigation of novel 5'-amino adenosine derivatives with potential anti-Zika virus activity. Eur J Med Chem 2023; 261: 115852.
[http://dx.doi.org/10.1016/j.ejmech.2023.115852] [PMID: 37801825]

[69] Zhou R, Li Q, Yang B, *et al.* Repurposing of the antihistamine mebhydrolin napadisylate for treatment of Zika virus infection. Bioorg Chem 2022; 128: 106024.
[http://dx.doi.org/10.1016/j.bioorg.2022.106024] [PMID: 35901544]

[70] Dai L, Song J, Lu X, *et al.* Structures of the zika virus envelope protein and its complex with a flavivirus broadly protective antibody. Cell Host Microbe 2016; 19(5): 696-704.
[http://dx.doi.org/10.1016/j.chom.2016.04.013] [PMID: 27158114]

[71] Hu H, Liu R, Li Q, *et al.* Development of a neutralizing antibody targeting linear epitope of the envelope protein domain III of ZIKV. Virus Res 2021; 306: 198601.
[http://dx.doi.org/10.1016/j.virusres.2021.198601] [PMID: 34678322]

[72] Feng Y, Yang Y, Zou S, *et al.* Identification of alpha-linolenic acid as a broad-spectrum antiviral against zika, dengue, herpes simplex, influenza virus and SARS-CoV-2 infection. Antiviral Res 2023; 216: 105666.
[http://dx.doi.org/10.1016/j.antiviral.2023.105666] [PMID: 37429528]

[73] Sirohi D, Kuhn RJ. Zika Virus Structure, Maturation, and Receptors. J Infect Dis 2017; 216 (Suppl. 10): S935-44.
[http://dx.doi.org/10.1093/infdis/jix515] [PMID: 29267925]

[74] Lunardelli VAS, de Souza Apostolico J, Souza HFS, *et al.* ZIKV-envelope proteins induce specific humoral and cellular immunity in distinct mice strains. Sci Rep 2022; 12(1): 15733.
[http://dx.doi.org/10.1038/s41598-022-20183-x] [PMID: 36131132]

[75] Mwaliko C, Nyaruaba R, Zhao L, *et al.* Zika virus pathogenesis and current therapeutic advances. Pathog Glob Health 2021; 115(1): 21-39.
[http://dx.doi.org/10.1080/20477724.2020.1845005] [PMID: 33191867]

[76] Brango-Vanegas J, Leite ML, de Oliveira KBS, da Cunha NB, Franco OL. From exploring cancer and virus targets to discovering active peptides through mRNA display. Pharmacol Ther 2023; 252: 108559.
[http://dx.doi.org/10.1016/j.pharmthera.2023.108559] [PMID: 37952905]

[77] Wang Y, Li Q, Hu D, *et al.* USP38 inhibits zika virus infection by removing envelope protein ubiquitination. Viruses 2021; 13(10): 2029.
[http://dx.doi.org/10.3390/v13102029] [PMID: 34696459]

[78] Zou X, Yuan M, Zhang T, Zheng N, Wu Z. EVs containing host restriction factor IFITM3 inhibited ZIKV infection of fetuses in pregnant mice through Trans-placenta delivery. Mol Ther 2021; 29(1): 176-90.
[http://dx.doi.org/10.1016/j.ymthe.2020.09.026] [PMID: 33002418]

[79] Zhou L, Zhou J, Chen T, *et al.* Identification of Ascomycin against Zika virus infection through screening of natural product library. Antiviral Res 2021; 196: 105210.
[http://dx.doi.org/10.1016/j.antiviral.2021.105210] [PMID: 34801589]

[80] Yu W, Zhang B, Hong X, *et al.* Identification of desoxyrhapontigenin as a novel antiviral agent against congenital Zika virus infection. Antiviral Res 2023; 211: 105542.
[http://dx.doi.org/10.1016/j.antiviral.2023.105542] [PMID: 36646387]

[81] Yan Y, Yang J, Xiao D, *et al.* Nafamostat mesylate as a broad-spectrum candidate for the treatment of flavivirus infections by targeting envelope proteins. Antiviral Res 2022; 202: 105325.
[http://dx.doi.org/10.1016/j.antiviral.2022.105325] [PMID: 35460703]

[82] Zou M, Liu H, Li J, *et al.* Structure-activity relationship of flavonoid bifunctional inhibitors against Zika virus infection. Biochem Pharmacol 2020; 177: 113962.
[http://dx.doi.org/10.1016/j.bcp.2020.113962] [PMID: 32272109]

[83]   Quan Y, Zhou R, Yang B, *et al.* Identification of an N-phenylsulfonyl-2-(piperazin-1-yl)m-thyl-benzonitrile derivative as Zika virus entry inhibitor. Bioorg Chem 2023; 130: 106265.
[http://dx.doi.org/10.1016/j.bioorg.2022.106265] [PMID: 36417826]

[84]   Majee P, Pattnaik A, Sahoo BR, *et al.* Inhibition of Zika virus replication by G-quadruplex-binding ligands. Mol Ther Nucleic Acids 2021; 23: 691-701.
[http://dx.doi.org/10.1016/j.omtn.2020.12.030] [PMID: 33575115]

[85]   Ferraris P, Wichit S, Cordel N, Missé D. Human host genetics and susceptibility to ZIKV infection. Infect Genet Evol 2021; 95: 105066.
[http://dx.doi.org/10.1016/j.meegid.2021.105066] [PMID: 34487865]

[86]   Bhardwaj U, Pandey N, Rastogi M, Singh SK. Gist of Zika Virus pathogenesis. Virology 2021; 560: 86-95.
[http://dx.doi.org/10.1016/j.virol.2021.04.008] [PMID: 34051478]

[87]   Tharappel AM, Cheng Y, Holmes EH, Ostrander GK, Tang H. Castanospermine reduces Zika virus infection-associated seizure by inhibiting both the viral load and inflammation in mouse models. Antiviral Res 2020; 183: 104935.
[http://dx.doi.org/10.1016/j.antiviral.2020.104935] [PMID: 32949636]

[88]   Xu MM, Wu B, Huang GG, *et al.* Hemin protects against Zika virus infection by disrupting virus-endosome fusion. Antiviral Res 2022; 203: 105347.
[http://dx.doi.org/10.1016/j.antiviral.2022.105347] [PMID: 35643150]

[89]   Espinoza JA, González PA, Kalergis AM. Modulation of antiviral immunity by heme oxygenase-1. Am J Pathol 2017; 187(3): 487-93.
[http://dx.doi.org/10.1016/j.ajpath.2016.11.011] [PMID: 28082120]

[90]   Valdes I, Gil L, Lazo L, *et al.* Recombinant protein based on domain III and capsid regions of zika virus induces humoral and cellular immune response in immunocompetent BALB/c mice. Vaccine 2023; 41(40): 5892-900.
[http://dx.doi.org/10.1016/j.vaccine.2023.08.035] [PMID: 37599141]

[91]   Shang Z, Song H, Shi Y, Qi J, Gao GF. Crystal structure of the capsid protein from zika virus. J Mol Biol 2018; 430(7): 948-62.
[http://dx.doi.org/10.1016/j.jmb.2018.02.006] [PMID: 29454707]

[92]   Ambroggio EE, Costa Navarro GS, Pérez Socas LB, Bagatolli LA, Gamarnik AV. Dengue and Zika virus capsid proteins bind to membranes and self-assemble into liquid droplets with nucleic acids. J Biol Chem 2021; 297(3): 101059.
[http://dx.doi.org/10.1016/j.jbc.2021.101059] [PMID: 34375636]

[93]   Saumya KU, Kumar D, Kumar P, Giri R. Unlike dengue virus, the conserved 14–23 residues in N-terminal region of Zika virus capsid is not involved in lipid interactions. Biochim Biophys Acta Biomembr 2020; 1862(11): 183440.
[http://dx.doi.org/10.1016/j.bbamem.2020.183440] [PMID: 32783888]

[94]   He Y, Wang M, Chen S, Cheng A. The role of capsid in the flaviviral life cycle and perspectives for vaccine development. Vaccine 2020; 38(44): 6872-81.
[http://dx.doi.org/10.1016/j.vaccine.2020.08.053] [PMID: 32950301]

[95]   Saumya KU, Gadhave K, Kumar A, Giri R. Zika virus capsid anchor forms cytotoxic amyloid-like fibrils. Virology 2021; 560: 8-16.
[http://dx.doi.org/10.1016/j.virol.2021.04.010] [PMID: 34020329]

[96]   Tan TY, Fibriansah G, Kostyuchenko VA, *et al.* Capsid protein structure in Zika virus reveals the flavivirus assembly process. Nat Commun 2020; 11(1): 895.
[http://dx.doi.org/10.1038/s41467-020-14647-9] [PMID: 32060358]

[97]   Lai M, La Rocca V, Iacono E, *et al.* Inhibiting immunoregulatory amidase NAAA blocks ZIKV maturation in Human Neural Stem Cells. Antiviral Res 2023; 216: 105664.

[http://dx.doi.org/10.1016/j.antiviral.2023.105664] [PMID: 37414288]

[98] Piomelli D, Scalvini L, Fotio Y, *et al.* *N* -Acylethanolamine Acid Amidase (NAAA): Structure, Function, and Inhibition. J Med Chem 2020; 63(14): 7475-90.
[http://dx.doi.org/10.1021/acs.jmedchem.0c00191] [PMID: 32191459]

[99] Xia Z, Wang L, Li S, *et al.* ML-SA1, a selective TRPML agonist, inhibits DENV2 and ZIKV by promoting lysosomal acidification and protease activity. Antiviral Res 2020; 182: 104922.
[http://dx.doi.org/10.1016/j.antiviral.2020.104922] [PMID: 32858116]

[100] Wang X, Wang H, Yi P, *et al.* Metformin restrains ZIKV replication and alleviates virus-induced inflammatory responses in microglia. Int Immunopharmacol 2023; 121: 110512.
[http://dx.doi.org/10.1016/j.intimp.2023.110512] [PMID: 37343373]

CHAPTER 9

Mycobacterium tuberculosis: Recent Advances in Drug Discovery and Targets – A SAR-Based Approach

Krupanshi Bharadava[2], Aviral Kaushik[2], Nigam Vyas[1,2], Tarun Kumar Upadhyay[3], C. Ratna Prabha[4] and Radhey Shyam Kaushal[2,*]

[1] *Department of Microbiology, Parul Institute of Applied Sciences, Parul University, Vadodara, Gujarat, India*

[2] *Department of Life Sciences, Parul Institute of Applied Sciences and Biophysics & Structural Biology Laboratory, Research & Development Cell, Parul University, Vadodara, Gujarat, India*

[3] *Department of Life Sciences, Parul Institute of Applied Sciences and Immuno-biochemistry Laboratory, Research & Development Cell, Parul University, Vadodara, Gujarat, India*

[4] *Department of Biochemistry, Maharaja Sayajirao University of Baroda, Vadodara, Gujarat, India*

Abstract: Tuberculosis (TB) is a highly contagious and potentially life-threatening infectious disease caused by the bacterium *Mycobacterium tuberculosis* (MTB). Despite significant progress in medical science, TB remains a global health concern, affecting millions of people worldwide. Efforts to combat this disease have led to the development of various treatment regimens, and research in TB drug discovery continues to be a crucial area of study. Identifying the new drug targets is essential in the fight against MDR TB, TDR TB, and XDR TB. Owing to the current situation, the key aspect of modern drug discovery is based on the concept of structural information along with functional activity relationships to combat tuberculosis disease. The structure-activity relationship (SAR) involves understanding the relationship between a compound's chemical structure and its biological activity. The line of treatment of MTB addresses multiple targets, such as various ribosomal targets, including the exit tunnel of the 50S subunit of ribosome, DNA gyrase (GyrB), Inosine-5'-monophosphate dehydrogenase (IMPD), Adenosine kinases (AK), Chorismate mutase (CM), and many other targets as well. This chapter provides a complete insight into the existing medications versus newly developed drug molecules based on SAR, their protein targets, modes of action, and mechanisms of resistance. By comprehending the intricate relationship between the chemical structure of drugs and their biological activity, it is possible to develop more effective therapies to combat this deadly disease.

* **Correspondence author Radhey Shyam Kaushal:** Department of Life Sciences, Parul Institute of Applied Sciences and Biophysics & Structural Biology Laboratory, Research & Development Cell, Parul University, Vadodara, Gujarat, India; E-mail: radhey.kaushal82033@paruluniversity.ac.in

Keywords: Drugs, *Mycobacterium tuberculosis*, Protein targets, Resistance mechanism, Structural activity relationship.

INTRODUCTION

Mycobacterium tuberculosis (MTB) is a pathogen that causes tuberculosis (TB), a major health problem of the world. According to the reports of WHO, 10.6 million humans had been diagnosed with TB in 2021 globally, up by 4.5% from 2020, while 1.6 million patients died because of the illness. Out of these cases, approximately 450000 cases were those of multidrug-resistant TB, which was 3.1% more in comparison to 2020 (437,000 cases). India, along with seven other countries, constituted over two-thirds of the total tuberculosis (TB) patient count (Fig. **1**).

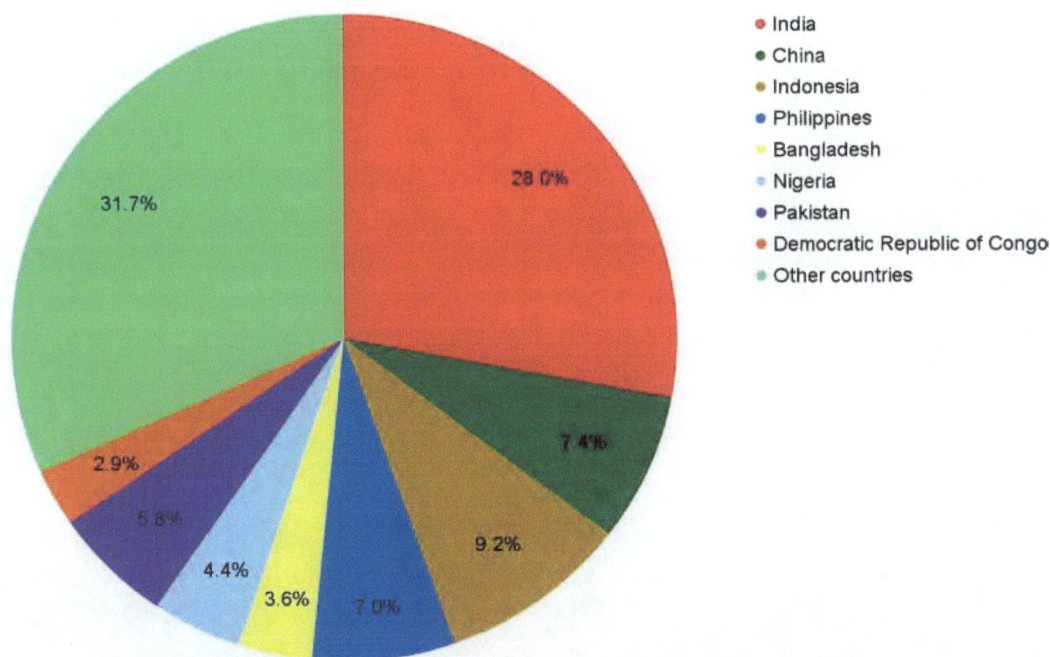

Fig. (1). Percentage distribution of Tuberculosis in India, China, Indonesia, Philippines, Bangladesh, Nigeria, Pakistan and Democratic Republic of Congo.

WHO aims to reduce cases by 80% and deaths by 90% by 2030. World TB Day 2023 theme is "Yes! We can end TB!" [1]. Discussing major characteristics of MTB, they are a human-specific, non-motile, rod-shaped, acid-fast bacterium with a slow growth rate [2]. The cell wall of MTB is a pivotal element in its pathogenesis and is involved in interactions with the host immune system and antimicrobial agents. Understanding the composition, architecture, and function of the MTB cell wall has been the subject of intense research due to its direct relevance to tuberculosis pathogenesis and drug resistance. A distinctive hallmark of the MTB cell wall is its high lipid content, notably mycolic acids, which comprise long-chain α-alkyl and β-hydroxy fatty acids, that form a unique, lipid-rich layer. This layer contributes significantly to the impermeability of the cell wall and its resilience against environmental stresses. Recent research has highlighted the involvement of mycolic acids in modulating the host cell responses and evading immune detection, thus playing a critical role in the establishment and persistence of MTB infection. Additionally, the MTB cell wall contains other essential components such as, teichoic acid arabinogalactan, LAM-lipoarabinomannan, lipopolysaccharide membrane-associated protein, lipoteichoic acid, outer membrane; peptidoglycan, plasma membrane, lipoprotein, and GL-glycolipid (Fig. **2**) [3 - 5].

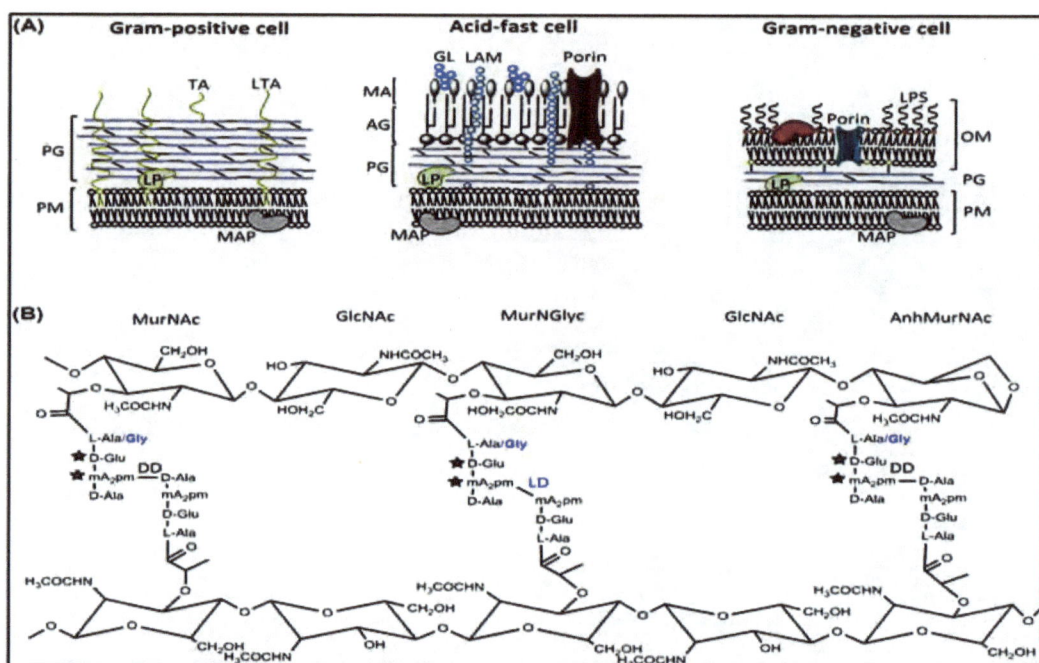

Fig. (2). (A) Comparison between various types of cell walls, here, TA-teichoic acid, AG - arabinogalactan, LAM-lipoarabinomannan, LPS-lipopolysaccharide, MAP-membrane-associated protein, LTA-lipoteichoic acid, MA-mycolic acid, OM, outer membrane; PG- peptidoglycan, PM, plasma membrane, LP-lipoprotein, GL-glycolipid (B) The distinctive characteristics of mycobacterial cells, indicated in blue, are revealed by the PG structure. The stars show remnants that go through amidation [5].

Indeed, emerging research has uncovered the significance of proteins embedded within the cell wall of MTB. These proteins, often referred to as "molecular machines," are essential for various critical processes, including nutrient uptake, transport, and secretion. Targeting these proteins holds promise for developing novel therapeutic strategies that selectively target MTB while minimizing damage to the host [6].

TB spreads through the air when an infected person talks, sneezes, coughs, or, releases infectious droplets into the atmosphere. Individuals nearby can inhale these droplets and become infected. Crowded and poorly ventilated spaces increase the risk of transmission, making TB a significant public health concern in densely populated areas [7, 8]. When MTB infects the host, the immune system initiates the formation of granulomas as a defensive response against the invading bacteria. These granulomas serve as organized immune structures, attempting to contain and control the mycobacterial infection [9]. The bacteria can persist in a dormant state within these granulomas, establishing latent tuberculosis infection (LTBI). In the latent phase, the bacteria remain viable but do not cause active disease. Various factors can contribute to the reactivation of latent TB, leading to the progression from latent infection to active tuberculosis disease [10]. One significant factor is a compromised or weakened immune system, which can occur due to immunosuppressive conditions, such as HIV infection, certain medications like corticosteroids, or immune disorders [11]. Several antibiotics can kill this pathogen, like rifampin, pyrazinamide, isoniazid, and ethambutol. The current major problem is its resistance to these antibiotics [12]. Nowadays, the major challenge is MTB's distinctive ability to become drug-resistant against antibiotics [13]. Drug resistance in MTB primarily arises due to several factors, including inadequate treatment regimens, inappropriate use of antibiotics, poor patient adherence to treatment, and the transmission of drug-resistant strains from person to person [12]. There are also some molecular factors that contribute to drug resistance, like some proteins known as heat-shock proteins and several other mechanisms like efflux pumps [14, 15].

In recent years, researchers have made significant progress in identifying novel drug targets within MTB, employing structure-activity relationship studies, high-throughput screening methods and repurposing existing drugs to tackle the disease. Combination therapy, short-course of treatment, exploring new drug classes, and investigating drug delivery systems have emerged as promising approaches to enhance treatment efficacy and patient compliance [16].

DRUG DISCOVERY AND ITS IMPORTANCE

Drug discovery is a multidisciplinary process aimed at identifying novel compounds for the treatment of diseases (Fig. **3**). It begins with target identification and validation, focusing on essential molecular pathways [17]. For example, in the context of TB, InhA, responsible for cell wall mycolic acid synthesis, is a potential target [18]. Next step is lead discovery, involving computational techniques and high-throughput screening to find substances that can interact with the target. Promising leads undergo rigorous testing for efficacy, safety, and selectivity. Lead optimization follows, with medicinal chemists fine-tuning compounds for enhanced potency and reduced toxicity. The preclinical phase involves safety and efficacy evaluations in lab and animal settings. Successful candidates move on to pivotal clinical trials, with Phase I assessing safety, Phase II optimizing dosages, and Phase III confirming therapeutic efficacy in larger patient populations. Only after successfully navigating through these phases and gaining regulatory approval can a compound be marketed and prescribed as a drug. It is important to note that from a pool of thousands of compounds, only a few may advance to be an actual drug [19].

Machine and deep learning algorithms are successfully applied in many aspects of discovery of drugs, including the process of synthesis of peptides, ligand-based virtual screening, drug repositioning, structure-based virtual screening, and toxicity prediction with drug monitoring and release, polypharmacology pharmacophore modeling, QSAR, and physiochemical activity assessment. These advancements in technology associated with the creativity and diligence of inventors have made these advances possible. The past achievements highlight deep learning and artificial intelligence's potential in this area. Furthermore, cutting-edge methods for data mining, curation, and management have substantially supported the advancement of modeling algorithms. Numerous AI-based algorithms and the development of web-based tools have been instrumental in drug repositioning. Examples include DrugNet, DRIMC, DPDR-CPI, PHARMGKB, PROMISCUOUS 2.0, and DRRS. These tools have enabled the identification of promising repurposed drugs for various medical conditions. Additionally, innovative approaches like multi-view graph attention models and multiciliary fusion algorithms have contributed to the success of drug repurposing [20].

IMPORTANCE OF DRUG TARGETS

Another major key point to winning this battle is to identify accurate and appropriate targets for MTB. Drug targets are essentially specific molecules or proteins within a microorganism that can be manipulated or inhibited to disrupt its normal function and growth. In case of tuberculosis, identifying and understanding these drug targets are crucial for developing a selected treatment that can effectually eliminate the bacteria while reducing damage to the host. Identifying viable drug targets is a meticulous process that combines cutting-edge technology, in-depth research, and a thorough understanding of the bacterium's biology. The selection of drug targets is a very complicated and tactful process.

Drug targets in MTB encompass certain biological molecules or functions that pharmaceuticals can target to inhibit bacterial development and eventually treat the infection. There are 6 well-known ways or 6 areas by which we can inhibit the growth of this bacterium (Fig. **4**). Researchers are harnessing the power of genomics, proteomics, and computational modeling to accelerate the identification of potential drug targets. The tendency of tuberculosis to gradually acquire resistance to certain medications is widely known. Combination drug treatment has been an effective way to overcome this problem. Simultaneously attacking several drug sites at once makes it much harder for the bacteria to acquire resistance.

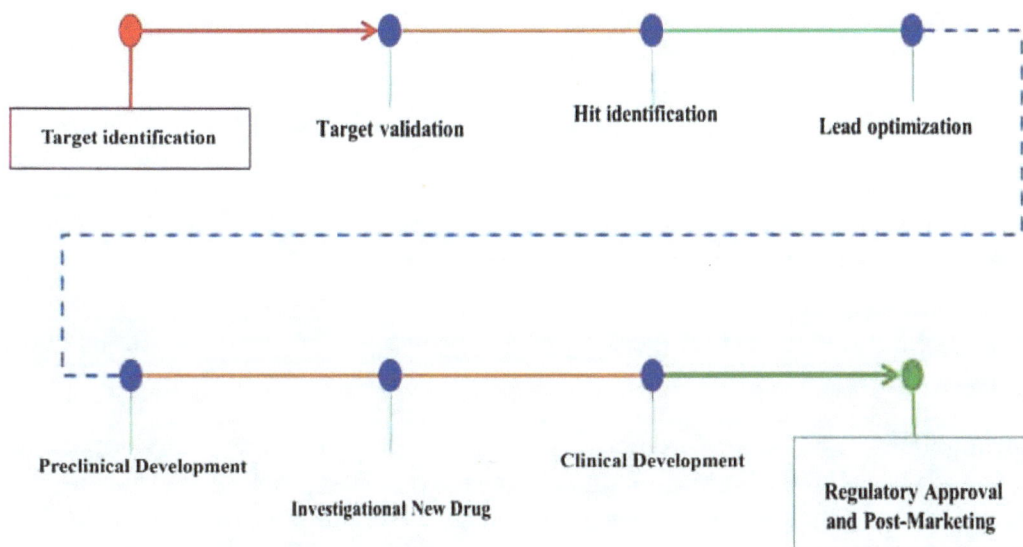

Fig. (3). Road Map of the Drug Discovery Process.

In the context of tuberculosis, there are several well-known targets like DNA gyrase. DNA gyrase is an essential bacterial enzyme in various bacterial species including *Mycobacterium.* The ATP-dependent enzyme plays a vital role by catalyzing negative supercoiling in DNA. Gyrase a heterodimer, possesses the subunits, GyrA and GyrB. The GyrA subunit functions to bind, break, and reseal the DNA while the function of the GyrB subunit provides the required energy by hydrolyzing ATP. Various studies concluded that the GyrB subunit serves as the conserved binding site for inhibiting the DNA repair mechanism of MTB. Since the resistance causing fluoroquinolones is beyond the range of the terminal domain of mutation in GyrB, therefore, the already existing resistant fluoroquinolones will not interfere with the inhibition of the DNA gyrase activity [21]. The fluoroquinolone-resistant *Mycobacterium tuberculosis*isolates so far reported have mutations in the residues 90, 91, and 94 in GgyrA and in the residues 495, 516, and 533 in GyrB [22].

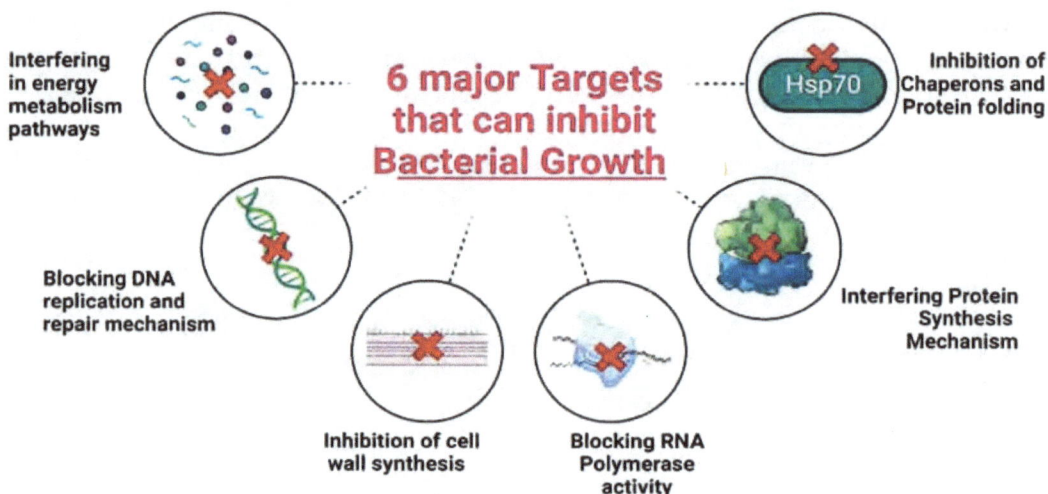

Fig. (4). Six major targets that can inhibit bacterial growth.

An anabolic pathway called the shikimate pathway, is utilized by plants, fungi, and bacteria for synthesizing phenylalanine, tyrosine, aromatic amino acids, and tryptophan. Chorismate mutase (CM), an enzyme, catalyzes a Claisen rearrangement, which proceeds with a chair-like geometry in the shikimate pathway. Due to the absence of the shikimate pathway, humans do not possess CM activity and thus it can be a principal target to develop the antibacterials. Four distinct synthetic compounds have been outlined as MTB CM inhibitors so far. However, none of them have gone through testing for anti-TB activity so far [7].

Adenosine kinases, a part of the purine salvage enzyme family, are responsible for catalyzing the reaction of adenosine-to-adenosine monophosphate conversion. The adenosine kinase of MTB is different from other adenosine kinases based on structural and biochemical properties. Besides, the MTB enzyme also functions to convert the adenosine analog into methyladenosine (methyl-ado), which initializes the metabolism of tuberculosis pathogens. The formation of methyl-ado provided us with a target against the salvage pathway to develop MTB inhibitors [23].

Inosine-5'-monophosphate (IMP) is a precursor generated through the *de novo* purine biosynthesis pathway, essential for adenine and guanine nucleotide synthesis. Inosine-5'-monophosphate dehydrogenase (IMPDH) catalyzes IMP's conversion into xanthosine 5'-monophosphate (XMP), a crucial initial step in producing guanine nucleotides. These guanine nucleotides play multifaceted roles in DNA and RNA synthesis, protein production, cell wall formation, and various cellular processes. Besides the *de novo* route, cells can resort to purine salvage to form guanosine 5'-monophosphate (GMP), bypassing biosynthetic steps. IMPDH is a major target for drug development against autoimmune diseases, cancers, and viral infections due to its central role in guanine nucleotide supply. Additionally, it is gaining attention as an antimicrobial drug target [24].

Ribosomes have a vital role in the protein synthesis in all living cells. Protein synthesis in bacteria involves 50S subunits, on the other hand, 40S and 60S subunits are required by humans. Since humans and bacteria require different subunits of ribosomes to carry out protein synthesis, the inhibitory action on the 50S subunit of the bacterial ribosome will not affect the protein synthesis of humans *i.e.*, 40S and 60S. Hence, the 50S ribosome subunit is taken as a target site in various studies to find a potent inhibitor against tuberculosis. There is a full family of erythromycin and its derivatives, which are found to block the 23S RNA of the 50S ribosomal subunit, which results in the inhibition of the protein synthesis in the pathogen [25].

Apart from these targets, MTB also has various other targets like MmpL3, Mmpl7, and Mmpl8 that serve as key examples of drug targets. Mycobacterial membrane protein large 3 is essential for the survival and virulence of MTB. MmpL3 is a transmembrane transporter protein in MTB, responsible for transporting unique long-chain fatty acids called mycolic acids from the inner cell membrane to the outer cell membrane. Mycolic acids are critical for the structural integrity of the mycobacterial cell wall, contributing to its impermeability and resistance to environmental stresses, including antibiotics and the host's immune system. MmpL3's role in maintaining the impermeable cell wall makes it a key contributor to drug resistance in MTB [26, 27]. Another target is SOD, which is an enzyme present in MTB, and it plays a role in the bacterium's defense against the host's immune system. It helps neutralize harmful reactive oxygen species (ROS) generated by the host's immune response, protecting the bacterium from oxidative stress. Targeting SOD has been explored as a potential avenue for developing new tuberculosis medications [27]. MPT64 is a protein unique to MTB. It has been studied as a potential antigen for the diagnosis of tuberculosis, particularly in serological tests. The detection of MPT64-specific antibodies in patient samples can indicate active tuberculosis infection [28]. Heat shock proteins (ex: Hsp60, Hsp70, Hsp90, HspX) are a family of molecular chaperones that play a critical role in maintaining protein homeostasis within cells, particularly during stressful conditions, including exposure to elevated temperatures. As chaperone proteins, Hsp60 (GroEL) and Hsp70 (DnaK) aid in the correct folding of other proteins, hampering their aggregation, and upholding protein quality control. Multiple client proteins involved in essential cellular functions are stabilized by Hsp90. By shielding MTB from oxidative and other stresses, HspX (Acr), a tiny Hsp, helps the bacterium survive inside host macrophages. In MTB, Hsps are promising drug targets in tuberculosis treatment. Inhibiting Hsps can lead to the misfolding and degradation of critical proteins required for MTB survival. The imbalance in protein quality control can disrupt bacterial replication and virulence, rendering the bacterium more susceptible to the host's immune system and other therapeutic interventions [29]. ESAT-6 (Early Secretory Antigenic Target 6) and CFP-10 (Culture Filtrate Protein 10) are the secretory proteins produced by MTB. They form a complex and play a role in the virulence of the bacterium and its ability to escape from infected host cells. ESAT-6 and CFP-10 are involved in the disruption of the phagosomal membrane within infected cells, allowing MTB to access the cytoplasm. ESAT-6 and CFP-10 themselves are not directly targeted by drugs, their secretion system, known as the ESX-1 (type VII) secretion system, has been considered as a potential target. Inhibiting the ESX-1 system could disrupt the pathogenicity of MTB and its ability to escape host immune cells. Next is a serine/threonine protein kinase known as protein kinase G (PknG), which is mostly found in the cytoplasm of the bacteria. It is essential to the pathophysiology of M. tuberculosis and its interactions with host cells. To assist MTB in evading immune responses, PknG modifies host-pathogen interactions. It prevents phagosome maturation, which keeps MTB alive in host cells. Furthermore, PknG controls survival mechanisms such as nutrient uptake and remodeling of the cell envelope, which helps MTB evade host defenses and successfully infect the host [30, 31]. The Antigen 85 Complex, often referred to as Ag85, is a group of 3 closely related proteins Ag85A, Ag85B, and Ag85C found in MTB and other mycobacterial species. The most critical role of the Antigen 85 Complex is its involvement in the biosynthesis of mycolic acids. Ag85A, Ag85B, and Ag85C are recognized by the host immune system and stimulate the production of antibodies and T-cell responses. The Antigen 85 Complex has been considered a potential drug target in tuberculosis treatment. Several drugs, such as isoniazid (INH) and ethionamide, have been designed to interfere with the function of the Ag85 proteins, particularly Ag85C [32]. The enzyme known as methyl-keto-mycolic acid synthase (MKM) is essential to the formation of mycolic acids. By blocking the production of mycolic acids, MKM synthase can be inhibited. This can weaken the cell wall of mycobacteria and make them more vulnerable to the host's immune system and antimicrobial agents [33]. Another target will be WecA, which is responsible for the synthesis of the arabinogalactan precursor. Researchers working with WecA are finding it as a promising target [34].

Elongation factor Tu (EF-Tu) is a highly conserved protein in bacteria, including MTB. It plays a crucial role in protein synthesis by facilitating the binding of aminoacyl-tRNAs to the ribosome, essential for incorporating amino acids into growing polypeptide chains. Targeting EF-Tu as a drug target in MTB is of interest for tuberculosis treatment. But it may need extreme specification otherwise the drug also can affect the host cell protein EF-1α, which is like EF-Tu [35]. One protein that is essential for recycling ribosomes following the completion of protein synthesis is called ribosome recycling factor, or RRF. It is responsible for the disassembly of post-termination ribosomal complexes, separating the ribosome's two subunits and recycling them for subsequent rounds of translation [36].

STRUCTURAL ACTIVITY RELATIONSHIP AND ITD IMPORTANCE

The goal of the Structure-Activity Relationship (SAR) approach is to create associations between the chemical structure and the biological activity (or target attribute) of the substances under investigation [21, 37]. By carefully and systematically modifying specific parts of a compound's structure, scientists can gain valuable insights into which structural features are essential for its effectiveness against pathogens. Therefore, SAR analysis can be exploited by researchers to explore the chemical elements that contribute to the potency of an anti-TB compound. By making strategic modifications and optimizations, they can boost its effectiveness in fighting against MTB infections, since the ultimate aim is to develop a more potent and efficient drug [38]. Between 2009 and 2018, the clinical trials had a pretty high failure rate of 84.6%, the main reason for these failures in both Phase 2 and 3 trials was that the drugs could not meet the-expected levels of efficiency, resulting in a lot of capital and resources being wasted. To improve the chances of making medicines that work, it is really important to find the right targets for the drugs [39]. SAR research continues to evolve with advances in technology. The integration of big data analytics, AI, and machine learning holds tremendous potential in deciphering complex SAR patterns [40]. These developments could accelerate the search for innovative therapies and enrich our understanding of the complex interaction between structure and activity. SAR studies disclose the direction of functional groups, the size and flexibility of molecular chains, and the presence of certain patterns. The activity of a molecule may be increased or decreased by systematically adjusting these properties, which allows researchers to identify which changes do so. This information assists scientists in creating substances with increased efficacy and fewer adverse effects, which is a requirement for effective medication development. Here are some key features of SAR listed below (Fig. 5). Several web-based tools and algorithms, including the QSAR-Co, FL-QSAR, VEGA platform, Meta-QSAR, Chemception, PubChem Transformer-CNN, Cloud 3D-QSAR, and, MoDeSuS have been developed to facilitate QSAR modeling. These tools and methods have been used in various research endeavors, including the prediction of small molecule properties, multi-target chemometric models, screening for potential inhibitors, and the prediction of antioxidant activities. In short QSAR in drug discovery and design processes has led to advancements and innovations in this field, allowing for more accurate and reliable modeling techniques [41].

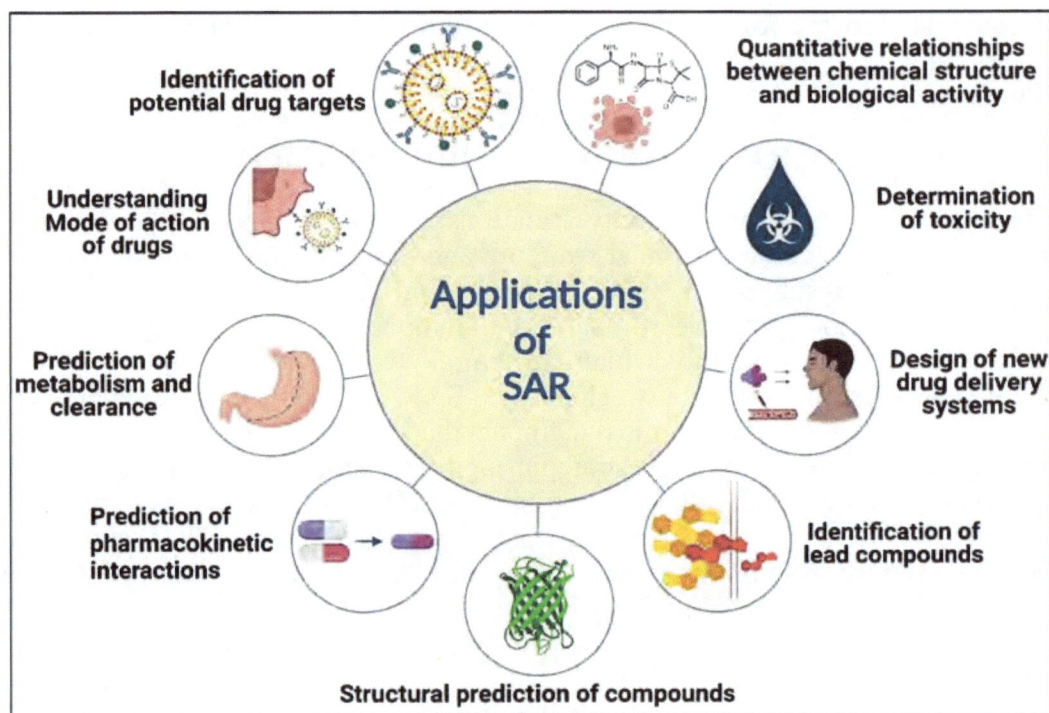

Fig. (5). Applications of Structural Activity Relationships.

Techniques Used in SAR Studies

For high-quality and accurate research, the techniques, and the accuracy of the scientific instruments play crucial roles. Researchers employ a range of experimental techniques that offer insights into the molecular world. All these techniques need accurate and expert handling to operate, and these efforts are responsible for positive results in the experiments performed. Here is a list of several important techniques that are essential for the study of SAR (Table **1**). High-throughput screening (HTS) expedites the exploration of vast compound libraries, enabling rapid identification of promising candidates. Complementing this, X-ray crystallography and Nuclear Magnetic Resonance (NMR) spectroscopy furnish atomic-level insights into molecular architectures [38]. Computational Modeling further validates and refines these structures while offering a virtual platform for predictive analyses. Mass spectrometry, high-performance liquid chromatography (HPLC), and isothermal titration calorimetry, adeptly quantify molecular interactions and binding affinities. Surface plasmon resonance (SPR) and microscale thermophoresis (MST) delve into real-time binding kinetics. Bioassays, including cell-based and electrophysiological assays, bridge the gap between molecular behavior and cellular response, lending physiological context. Thermal shift assay (TSA), circular dichroism (CD) spectroscopy, fluorescence resonance energy transfer (FRET), and surface-enhanced Raman spectroscopy (SERS) serve as versatile tools, probing structural changes, conformational dynamics, and vibrational fingerprints. Augmented by bioinformatics and data analysis, these techniques synergize, and empower comprehensive exploration of structure-activity relationships [42 - 61]. There are various techniques that are essential to understand the structure-activity relationship, some of them are represented in Table **1**.

STRUCTURE-ACTIVITY RELATIONSHIP OF DRUG TARGETS IN MTB

As discussed so far, there are various targets to inhibit bacterial growth. Our study focuses on three major targets: (i) blocking the DNA repair mechanism; (ii) interfering with the energy metabolism pathways and (iii) interfering with the protein synthesis mechanism. Some of the targets and drugs and their SAR are shown in Table **2**.

Table 1. Several techniques that are essential for the study of SAR.

S. No.	Technique	Application in Drug Discovery and Sar Studies	References
1	Protein engineering	To generate new target proteins with desired properties, such as increased expression, stability, or activity.	[42]
2	Enzyme kinetics studies (Mechanism of action assays for enzymes)	To understand the mechanism of action of target enzymes and to identify potential inhibitors or activators.	[43]
3	Thermal denaturation studies	To assess the stability of target proteins and to identify drugs that can stabilize or destabilize the protein.	[44]
4	Proteomics and genomics approaches	To identify potential drug targets and to characterize the molecular basis of disease.	[45]
5	Bioinformatics and data analysis	To mine large datasets for potential drug targets and to design new drugs.	[46]
6	High throughput screening (HTS)	To rapidly screen large libraries of compounds for activity against target proteins.	[47]
7	Bioassays and cell-based assays	To further evaluate the biological activity and efficacy of drug candidates in relevant cell models.	[48]

(Table 1) cont.....

S. No.	Technique	Application in Drug Discovery and Sar Studies	References
8	Electrophysiological assay	To study the effect of drug candidates on ion channels and membrane receptors.	[49]
9	Thermal shift assay (TSA)	To assess the stability of target proteins and the effect of drug candidates on protein stability.	[50]
10	Circular dichroism (CD) spectroscopy	for monitoring and evaluating chemical recognition phenomena in solution, as well as for figuring out the stereochemistry of chiral medicines and proteins.	[51]
11	Fluorescent nanoantennas	To study protein-protein interactions and conformational changes.	[52]
12	Surface-enhanced Raman spectroscopy (SERS)	To study the structure and interactions of drug candidates with proteins.	[53]
13	X-ray crystallography	To determine the 3-D structure of target proteins and their complexes with drug candidates.	[54]
14	Nuclear magnetic resonance (NMR) spectroscopy	To identify the 3-D structures of target proteins and how they interact with potential therapeutics.	[55]
15	Computational modeling	To predict the structure and properties of drug candidates and their interactions with target proteins.	[56]
16	Mass spectrometry	To characterize the mass and chemical composition of drug candidates.	[57]
17	High-performance liquid chromatography (HPLC)	To purify and analyze drug candidates.	[58]
18	Isothermal titration calorimetry	To study the thermodynamics of binding between drug candidates and target proteins.	[59]
19	Surface plasmon resonance (SPR)	To investigate how drug candidates and target proteins interact in real time.	[60]
20	Microscale thermophoresis (MST)	To study molecular interactions and binding affinities.	[61]

SAR of Mycobacterial Mycolic Acid Biosynthesis Proteins

Currently, established medications like isoniazid, prothionamide, ethionamide, thiacetazone, and perchlozone, which hinder mycolate biosynthesis and have historical or clinical usage in TB treatment, offer proof that investigations into targets related to mycolic acid synthesis are presently underway for their potential in chemotherapy [70]. Mycolic acid biosynthesis is a process that involves each Type I and Type II fatty acid synthase (FAS). FAS I oversees producing the α-chain of mycolates, whereas the FAS II system, which consists of several proteins (InhA, HadAB/HadBC, KasA, KasB, and MabA), oversees producing the extended chain of β-hydroxy fatty acid for mycolates. A variety of enzymes add methoxy, cyclopropane, or keto groups to the FAS II-generated meromycolate, and some of these specific enzymes have recently been identified as therapeutic targets due to their vital functions in modifying wall permeability, extending longevity, and influencing disease progression. Acyl-CoA carboxylase (ACC) and FadD32 then activate and load the FAS I and FAS II acyl chains onto polyketide synthase Pks13, resulting in the final condensation into an α-alkyl-β-ketoacyl derivative. Rv2509 then reduces this derivative to produce mycolic acid [71].

Table 2. SAR and targets of several drugs undergone repurposing.

S. No.	Target	Drug	Category	Mechanism Of Action	Key Sar	References
1	NADH dehydrogenase type 2 (NDH-2)	Clofazimine (Riminophenazine derivative)	Leprostatic, NSAID	Clofazimine (CFZ) is thought to function as a prodrug competing with menaquinone for reduction by NDH-2, which in turn releases the reactive oxygen species upon subsequent re-oxidation. CFZ may also have a specific impact on DNA and/or may interact with bacterial phospholipids A2 to work against mycobacteria.		[62]
		MTC420 (Quinoline/Quinolone derivative)	Anti-mycobacterial (diarylquinoline)	MTC 420 was gained as the lead compound after HTS of drugs and derivatives against MTB and its SAR revealed its functioning to inhibit the NDH2 target protein.		[63]
		Q203 (Telacebac) (Iodonium derivative)	Anti-infective (Investigational)	Telacebac functions by interrupting the electron transport chain of MTB by targeting the QcrB (CYP b subunit) and complex III (CYP bc1 complex). Later, because of HTS, Q203 was found to inhibit the NDH-2. It was found to be effective but rather toxic, so it requires further optimization.		[64]
2	Cytochrome bc1	Zolpidem	Sedative, Anti-TB (repurposed)	Zolpidem, a non-benzodiazepine compound, creates hypnosis by affecting the GABA neurotransmitter. As a result of drug repositioning, zolpidem also works as an anti TB agent by inhibiting the CYP bc1 complex at the QcrB level.		[65, 66]

(Table 2) cont.....

S. No.	Target	Drug	Category	Mechanism Of Action	Key Sar	References
3	Menaquinone Biosynthesis	DG70 (GSK1733953A)	Antituberculosis	A biphenyl amide, DG70, a chemotype compound possesses antiTB properties by inhibiting the catalytic methylation of demethylmenaquinone methyltransferase enzymes.		[67]
4	F₀F₁-ATP Synthase	Bedaquiline	Diarylquinoline	Bedaquiline is an anti-TB drug showing its biological function by binding to the c subunit of the ATP synthase, which is important for energy generation.		[68]
5	Cell wall synthesis	SQ109	Ethylenediamine Antibiotic	SQ109 possesses some different mechanisms of action to show antiTB effects. Inclusive of affecting multiple cellular pathways, the drug also inhibits cell wall synthesis.		[69]

SAR of InhA Protein by Tetrahydropyranyl Methylbenzamides

The pro-drug isoniazid targets the NADH-dependent enoyl acyl carrier protein (ACP) reductase produced by inhA. However, its clinical efficacy is compromised by frequent genetic variations in catalase-peroxidase (KatG) activation and diverse variations in human N-acetyltransferases, affecting drug metabolism [72]. The identification of InhA antagonists that do not need prodrug stimulation and do not have varied human metabolism would improve isoniazid's clinical value while addressing the issue of rising resistance frequencies [73].

GSK found tetrahydropyranyl methylbenzamides in the HTS campaign targeting InhA, with appropriate inhibition of enzymes and a low MIC (IC50 = 20 nM, MIC90 = 11.7 mM) (Fig. **6A**). It was found to have considerable cross-resistant properties towards isoniazid-resistant organisms that carry an inhA activator variant. Even though co-crystallization of tetrahydropyranyl methylbenzamides with InhA-NAD+ revealed identical affinity to thiadiazole inhibitor, this data was not useful in SAR research [75]. For SAR exploration (Fig. **6B**), eighteen analogues of tetrahydropyranyl methylbenzamides were synthesized and their pyrazole, phenyl, and thiazole cores were modified while the tetrahydropyranyl methyl benzamide core was left alone. Using various heteroaryl or heterocyclic rings in place of the pyrazole, as well as changing the linker between the phenyl and the pyrazole, did not increase activity, showing their protein connections observed in the crystal structure. When both aromatic rings were juxtaposed, the right-hand sides of B, as well as C, were more accessible for alterations. The most advanced analog (Fig. **6C**) was chosen as the most advanced compound with an adequate selectivity index (IC50 = 36 nM, MIC90 = 5 M). The efficacy of this scaffold over numerous other InhA inhibitors is still being determined [76].

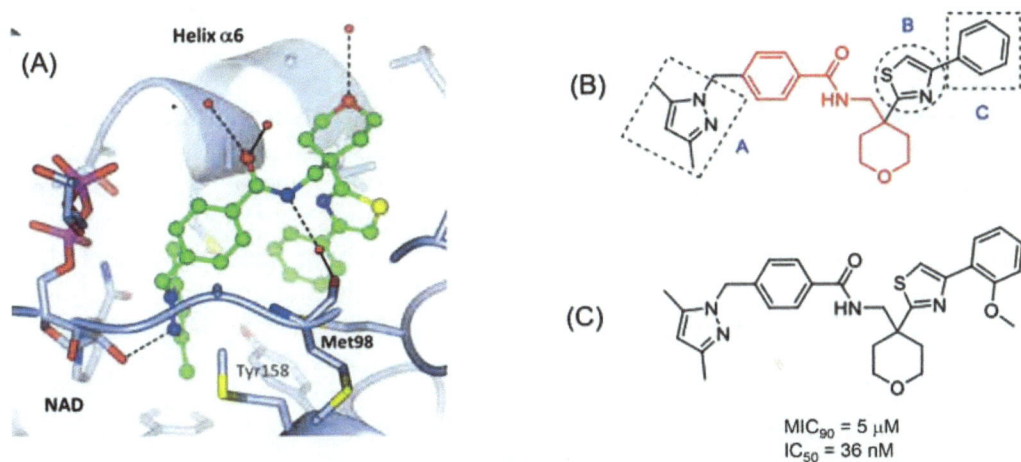

Fig. (6). (A) Tetrahydropyranyl methylbenzamides are attached to the active site of InhA. Represented by green ball-and-stick models, NAD is depicted with thick gray lines, and hydrogen bonds are illustrated with dashed lines. The structure reveals an organized helix α6, with emphasis on Met98 and Tyr158. Notably, Tyr158 assumes an apo orientation. (B) SAR plan from hit tetrahydropyranyl methylbenzamides (C) advanced analog of tetrahydropyranyl methylbenzamides [74].

SAR of InhA Protein by Thiadiazolyl Methylthiazoles

The tetracyclic InhA inhibitor, which is based on thiadiazole, was a significant lead in GSK's High-Throughput Screening (HTS) campaign aimed at discovering new InhA inhibitors. AstraZeneca subsequently confirmed its biological activity and revealed the binding mechanism at the active site by co-crystallizing it with InhA. Subsequent research efforts were focused on improving the physicochemical characteristics and drug-likeness of Thiadiazolyl methylthiazoles (with an IC50 of 4 nM and MIC90 of 0.2 M) [74].

The thiadiazole, which was situated in-between the thiadiazole and pyrazole rings, produced a hydrogen bond with the active site of InhA's, as did a thiazole on the right side, resulting in hydrogen bonding with the NAD+ cofactor's ribose (Fig. 7A). Because they had fewer interactions with InhA, the Structure-Activity Relationship (SAR) investigation focused primarily on altering the benzyl and pyrazole parts of the molecule. Although only the racemates were tested for SAR (Fig. 7B), the stereospecific (S)-hydroxyl group was found to be the drug's pharmacologically active enantiomer. Without altering the pyrazole, attempts to reduce lipophilicity in a library of tricyclic analogues by removing the A ring proved fruitless. The 2-pyridine demonstrated significant enzymatic and MTB inhibition when the pyrazole was swapped out for an aryl or heteroaryl ring, enabling the removal of the phenyl [74, 76]. The presence of hydrophobic and electron-withdrawing groups at the pyridine's α-position increased potency, and the racemic compound containing a 2-bromopyridine was chosen as the most promising. The most advanced chemical was validated by chiral separation. It was chosen despite the fact that 2-bromopyridines are typically avoided in medicinal chemistry due to their reactivity and potential toxicity. Surprisingly, the tricyclic compound analog was not more soluble than tetracyclic Thiadiazolyl methylthiazoles. Nonetheless, the compound analog had promising pharmacokinetics, good transparency, an acceptable CYP inhibition profile, and no hERG signal (Fig. **7C**). While the *in vivo* efficacy of analog in infected mice was constrained, this study is a fine illustration of reducing complicated structures using a co-crystal structure [74, 77].

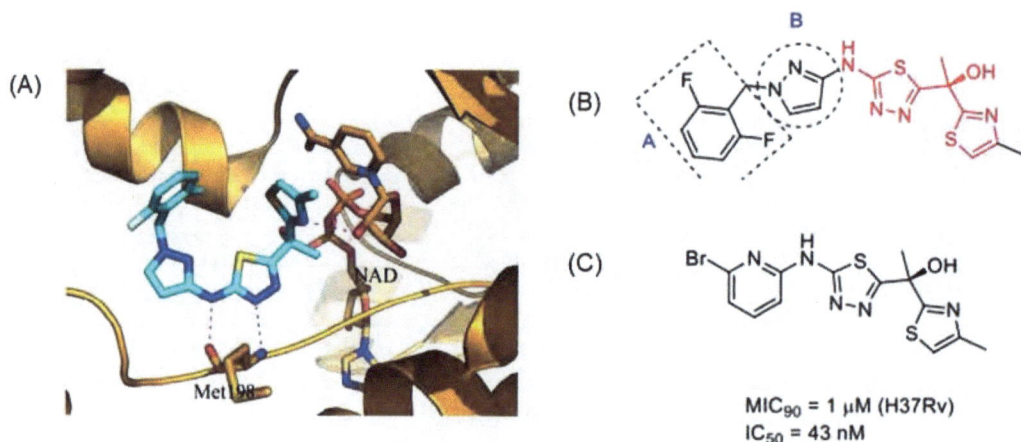

$MIC_{90} = 1 \ \mu M$ (H37Rv)
$IC_{50} = 43$ nM

Fig. (7). (**A**) Interaction between the thiadiazole within the active site of InhA (PDB ID: 4bqp). (**B**) SAR plan from hit of Thiadiazolyl methylthiazoles. (**C**) modified structure of Thiadiazolyl methylthiazoles [74].

SAR of Pks13 Protein by Benzofurans

The essential enzyme Pks13 in MTB plays a pivotal role by catalyzing the final Claisen-type condensation of fatty acid synthase I (FAS I), which generates a C26 α-alkyl branch, along with the production of C40-60 meromycolate precursors by fatty acid synthase II (FAS II). This enzymatic function involves a combination of two acyl carrier protein domains, a β-ketoacyl-synthase domain, an acyltransferase domain, and a thioesterase domain. Given that this polyketide synthase activity is unique to bacteria involved in mycolic acid synthesis, there was an anticipation of identifying selective inhibitors that would spare the host microbiome [78].

It has been demonstrated that a scaffold based on thiophene, incorporating a reactive pentafluorophenyl group that consistently targets Pks13, showed bactericidal effects in both *ex vivo* and *in vitro* experiments, emphasizing the potential of this target (Fig. **8A**). During a phenotypic screening of a commercial library against MTB (Fig. **8B**), the benzofuran scaffold was identified (Fig. **8C**), and resistance-conferring mutations were traced back to pks13. While the initial hit displayed satisfactory potency against MTB, it couldn't be utilized for *in vivo* drug efficacy studies due to the instability of its labile ethyl ester and poor metabolic stability, primarily attributed to phenyl group hydroxylation [79].

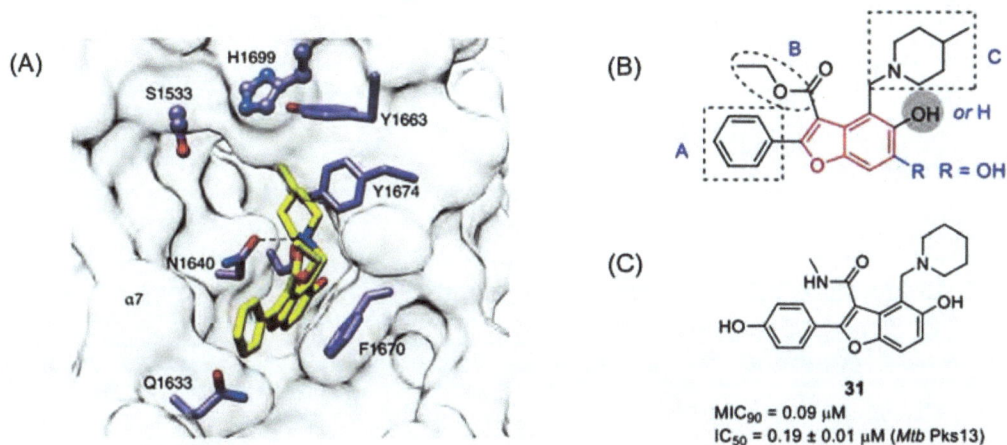

Fig. (8). (**A**) Inhibitor interactions reveal that the benzofuran core of TAM1 (depicted as yellow sticks) inserts itself between Phe1670 and. Asn1640, aligning its P3 group toward the catalytic site. Hydrogen bonds are indicated by dashed lines. (**B**) SAR plan from hit of benzofuran. (**C**) Benzofuran advanced analog [74].

It is shown that the benzofuran compound inhibited Pks13 catalytic activity (IC50 = 0.26 mM) and co-crystallized with the thioesterase domain, revealing that benzofuran binds to the acyl channel, which leads to the active site. This structural insight guided the development of benzofuran, focusing on maintaining or enhancing enzyme inhibition while addressing the labile · ethyl ester and modifying the phenyl group to reduce microsomal metabolism. The structural data showed that the p-phenol derivative (A) produced during microsomal metabolism could still interact with the thioesterase domain, as confirmed by the studies with the inhibition of the enzyme and MTB [80].

Replacing ester with methyl amide eliminated the methyl liability(B), which still inhibited the enzymes and exhibited whole-cell activity. Substituting other groups with the methyl piperidine was not a viable option, so the methyl group was removed. While these structural modifications did not enhance enzyme potency, they were crucial in exhibiting that the metabolic "liability" could be accepted by the generation of similarly active microsomal metabolite. MTB potency and enzyme activity showed a reasonable correlation. Through SAR studies of various analogs (MIC90 = 2.3 M, IC50 = 0.26 M), the most potent molecule, benzofuran-modified analog (MIC90 = 0.09 M, IC50 = 0.19 M), was identified. The derivative demonstrated promising ADMET (Absorption, Distribution, Metabolism, Excretion and Toxicity) characteristics, with plasma concentrations exceeding the MIC value [81]. It proved effective in both acute and chronic MTB infection models. While it showed no off-target effects against key human protein targets or primary CYP isoforms, it did inhibit the hERG assay—a marker for cardiovascular toxicity—and featured a Mannich base substructure. Addressing the hERG concern is crucial for future drug development endeavors using this platform. Drawing inspiration from natural product structures, transitioning to tetracyclic coumestans from the benzofuran derivative 30 resulted in the identification of compounds targeting Pks13 with favorable ADME-toxicity profiles [82].

SAR of KasA Protein by Indazole Sulfonamides

Natural compounds like cerulenin, platensimycin, and thiolactomycin (TLM) have been identified as inhibitors of mycobacterial β-ketoacyl ACP synthase I KasA, a vital component of the FAS II system in MTB [83]. However, these natural compounds have shown limited efficacy against MTB in whole-cell assays, and, in the case of cerulenin, exhibited toxicity to eukaryotic cells. As a result, there have been challenges in finding viable leads for therapeutic development [84]. The potential of KasA inhibitors lies in their clinical value, like isoniazid, and their ability to synergize with other FAS II inhibitors.

During chemical library screenings at GSK (Fig. **9A**), the indazole sulfonamide series surfaced as a promising prospect for drug discovery (Fig. **9B**). It displayed robust potential against MTB, selectivity, favorable physicochemical properties, and promising *in vitro* drug metabolism and pharmacokinetics (DMPK) profiles (Fig. **9C**). The pharmacokinetic assessment of indazole sulfonamide facilitated *in vivo* efficacy testing, demonstrating a decrease in bacterial burdens in a mouse model during both acute and chronic infection stages [85].

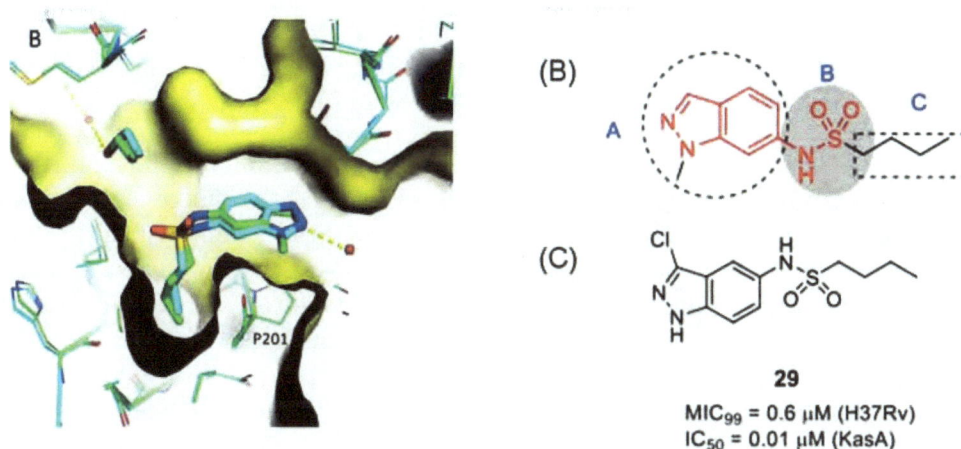

Fig. (9). (A) Superimposing KasA-1 with KasA bound to Indazole sulfonamides (shown in cyan) showcases a common binding pattern. In both compounds, the indazole ring occupies the same hydrophobic area above Pro20. (B) SAR strategy derived from Indazole sulfonamides hits. (C) Progressed analog of Indazole sulfonamides [74].

Employing diverse techniques, including mapping resistant mutants, target over-expression, evidence of suppressed mycolic acid production, and enzyme inhibition, KasA emerged as the target for indazole sulfonamide. The substance was discovered to attach within the channel that accommodates the meromycolate chain, immobilizing the enzyme in an exposed active site conformation [86]. Simultaneously, the same GSK hit was identified as a potent inducer of the iniBAC operon, suggesting its role in suppressing a facet of mycolyl-arabinogalactan biosynthesis. The research group identified resistance-inducing mutations in KasA, inhibited mycolate production, and conducted co-crystallization experiments to reveal the compound's binding mechanism with its target. The crystal structure demonstrated that the KasA homodimer bound four molecules of indazole sulfonamide in non-overlapping positions within the acyl channels, with the sulfonamides of two molecules forming hydrogen bonds with each other.

To address the compound's primary metabolic stability, a SAR investigation was carried out, especially considering relatively high microsome clearance rates. An elevated metabolic process turnover of indazole sulfonamide was attributed to indazole N-demethylation, which resulted in an inert molecule [87]. During SAR exploration, a range of N-substituted indazoles (A) was crafted. However, elongating this substitution notably diminished MTB effectiveness. Introducing additional functional groups in B, replacing the sulfonamide, diminished its potency, with only thiourea displaying modest efficacy. Extending the n-alkyl (C) chain past n-pentyl or adding bulkier groups led to diminished activity. Shifting the sulfonamide group from C-6 to C-5 produced a compound that bonded as a singular molecule per enzyme monomer, exhibiting marginally improved whole-cell activity [88].

Despite the SAR investigation, no advanced compounds with significantly improved metabolic stability were identified. Following the discovery of indazole sulfonamide, GSK initiated a lead optimization program, demonstrating that the demethylated derivative was equipotent to the initial hit. Despite these efforts, the integration of aniline in the indazole sulfonamide structure presented mutagenicity issues, and its *in vivo* production was detected in rat urine. Various attempts to substitute the nitrogen in the sulfonamide with linkers were ineffective [89]. To address the mutagenic potential, changes were made to the electrical environment of the sulfonamide linker through several substitutions of the indazole's 6-membered ring. These modifications resulted in compounds that were not rapidly converted into the amine derivative. However, all analogues proved to be inert. Modifying the indazole's 5-membered ring was tolerated, with repositioning the methyl group from N-1 to C-3 resulting in the most active analogues. These analogues, with methyl or halogen substitutions, exhibited equipotent whole-cell activity compared to the initial hit (MIC99 = 0.6 M). Notably, there was not always a direct correlation between whole-cell activity and *in vitro* enzyme inhibition, as certain modifications decreased MTB activity but preserved the potential for enzyme inhibition [87].

Despite attempts to reduce mutagenic risks, it was found that every active indazole and derivative core included a mutagenic amine, creating obstacles for continued development. The research concluded that optimizing structure-activity relationships (SAR) through phenotypic screening was the most successful strategy. This was driven by the recognition that unknown barriers in chemical absorption, efflux, or metabolism rendered certain compounds ineffective despite their enzyme-inhibitory properties [90, 91].

SAR of Mycobacterial GyrB ATPase inhibited by Pyrrolamides

Some studies showed that specific classes of antibiotics have the property of inhibiting GyrB activity, one of which includes quinolones. Moxifloxacin, a quinolone antibiotic, demonstrates effective activity against both drug-resistant and drug-sensitive TB, DNA gyrase, reinforced as a validated target against novel anti-TB agents. The crystal structures of GyrB from *E. coli* and *S. aureus* bound to pyrrolamide inhibitors were examined (Fig. **10**). Homology modeling was done for MTB H37Rv GyrB, which was based on the structure of *E. coli* GyrB. Docking studies within this model indicated close interactions of the pyrrole ring, piperidine linker, and thiazole acid on the left-hand side (LHS) like the pyrrolamide-bound *S. aureus* GyrB crystal structure (Fig. **11**). A water-mediated hydrogen bonding network was established between carbonyl groups and the pyrrole ring NH; and Ser208 and Asp118 of *M. tb* H37Rv GyrB. The thiazole ring formed π-cation bonds with Arg121, and its carboxylate group connected to Arg180 by a hydrogen bond [92].

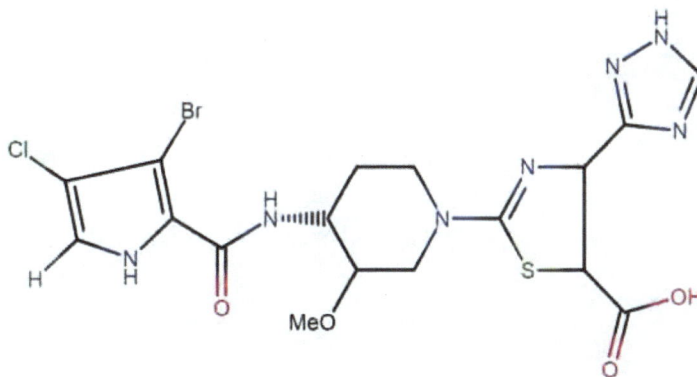

Fig. (10). Lead compound (pyrrolamide).

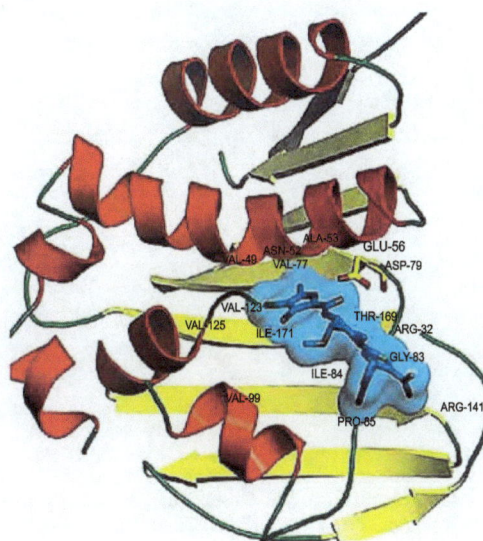

Fig. (11). Lead compound's (pyrrolamide) crystal structure (blue carbon atoms) binds to *M. smegmatis* GyrB in ribbon form [92].

For interactions with the active-site residues, the piperidine ring in the chair conformation allowed for the best possible placement of the LHS and RHS rings. These crucial interactions were then confirmed by comparing the cocrystal structure of the lead compound with a 22.7 kDa M. smegmatis GyrB fragment located at the N-terminus. The ligand occupied the ATP binding site, preserving contacts with a conserved water molecule and Asp79 in M. smegmatis GyrB (Asp118 in MTB H37Rv GyrB). Methoxy substitution at position 3 of the piperidine ring in the "cis" orientation resembled a notable increase in potency against MTB H37Rv MIC and M. smegmatis GyrB ATPase. The study examined the potential of lipophilic substituents possessing the electron-withdrawing characteristic, like bromine, to improve the pyrrole ring NH hydrogen bonding interaction with Asp118 [92].

SAR of MTB Chorismate Mutase Inhibited by Carvacrol Derivatives

Carvacrol was identified as a potential inhibitor by virtue of high-throughput screening of a small molecule database as shown in Fig. (**12**).

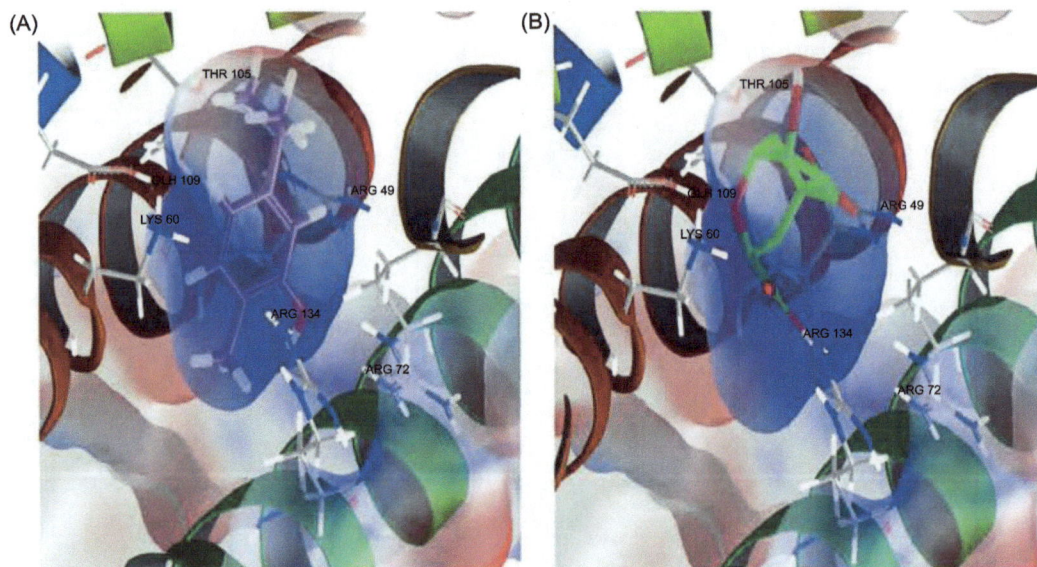

Fig. (12). MTB CM bound, (**A**) Carvacrol, and (**B**) transition site analog [93]. Carvacrol was found to interact with critical amino acids such as Arg134 and Arg72, believed to be essential for the enzyme's mechanism.

Carvacrol demonstrated excellent MTB CM inhibition in the enzyme inhibition studies, with an IC50 of 1.06-0.4 mM. Several carvacrol derivatives were tested *in vitro* to determine how well they could inhibit the MTB CM enzyme and entire MTB cells in order to investigate this possibility further. Since carvacrol is a natural phenolic compound, some other similar natural phenols were screened in the initial phase, and thymol, menthol, neo-isopulegol, eugenol, and vanillin were obtained. Thymol, eugenol, and vanillin were found to be less active; menthol had similar activity; and neo-isopulegol was two-fold more active when compared to carvacrol. In the second phase, an isomer of carvacrol, 3-isopropyl-5-methylphenol, was found to exhibit similar activity to that of carvacrol. It was also found that any further modification to the isomer structure resulted in the reduction of energy.

Carvacrol and thymol derivatives were further acetylated and methylated. Modifications of carvacrol resulted in the inactivity of the compounds, while enhanced potency was obtained in the case of thymol. However, thymol derivatives remained less potent than that of carvacrol [93].

SAR of Adenosine Kinase of MTB

The adenosine kinase, or Ado kinase, found in MTB is unique from other known Ado kinases in terms of structural and metabolic features. The purine salvage enzyme is essential for the first step in the transformation of 2-methyl-Ado (methyl-Ado), an adenosine analogue, into a metabolite with antitubercular characteristics. In order to fully use the potential of this enzyme, a thorough understanding of the structure of the active site is necessary in order to rationally design more powerful and selective substrates for Ado kinase. MTB Ado kinase demonstrated a considerable preference for conformations like carbocyclic-Ado or β-ṅ-ribofuranosyl (Fig. **13**).

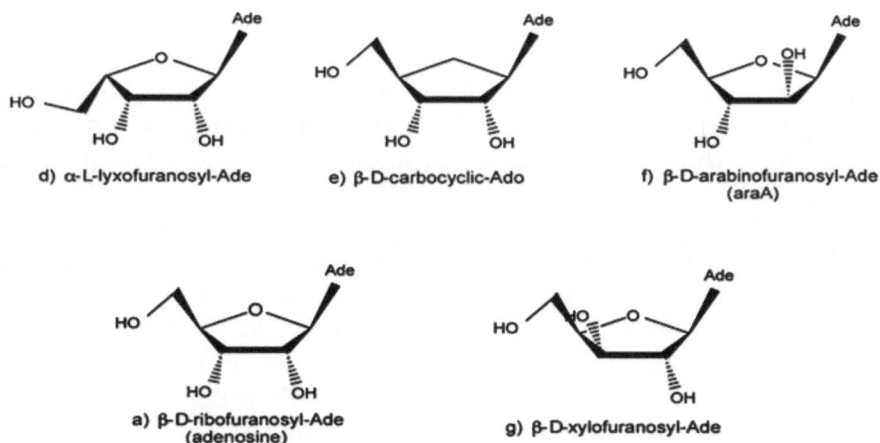

d) α-L-lyxofuranosyl-Ade   e) β-D-carbocyclic-Ado   f) β-D-arabinofuranosyl-Ade (araA)

a) β-D-ribofuranosyl-Ade (adenosine)   g) β-D-xylofuranosyl-Ade

Fig. (13). Sugar moiety structures utilized in SAR [94].

MTB Ado kinase has shown less activity with 2'-deoxy-Ado, in line with findings with human Ado kinase. The significant reduction in activity for 2'-deoxy-adenosine and 9-[β-D-arabinofuranosyl]-adenine (araA) indicates that the enzyme preferred the presence of the 20-hydroxyl moiety and its trans orientation to the adenine moiety. A few compounds with 2'-modifications were used as substrates; the most active ones were 2'-deoxy-2, 2'-difluoro-Ado, araA, and 2-fluoro-araA. The only 2'-substituted molecule that showed inhibition was 2-chloro-2'-deox--2'-fluoro-Ado, which is comparable to 2-chloro-adenosine.

MTB Ado kinase required a 3'-hydroxyl group in a trans orientation to the adenine moiety for substrate activity. Altering the 3'-hydroxyl group significantly affected substrate activity, while changes to the 2'-hydroxyl group had a lesser impact on this enzyme. Substituting the 3'-hydroxyl group with an amino or azido group eliminated activity, with 3'-deoxy-Ado exhibiting minimal activity. Conversely, a cis-conformation of the 3'-hydroxyl group, as seen in 9-[β-D-xylopyranosyl]-Ade, resulted in a specific activity. The necessity of a 3'-hydroxyl group in a trans orientation to the adenine moiety was crucial for both substrate recognition and inhibitor binding, indicating a potential role of steric hindrance at this site. The 4'-oxygen position exhibited high flexibility in substitutions within the ribose moiety, both in human and MTB Ado kinases. Carbocyclic-Ado (aristeromycin) (Fig. **13**) maintained similar activity in both human and MTB homologs. None of the carbocyclic compounds were effective inhibitors, with inhibitory effects not surpassing 81% at 100 mM. Reports indicated that 9-[α-L-lyxofuranosyl]-adenine was an inhibitor but not a substrate for human Ado kinase. 9-[β-D-5-methyl-(allo)-ribofuranosyl]-2-fluoro-adenine was approximately twice as active as 9-[--D-5-methyl-   (talo)-ribofuranosyl]-2-fluoro-adenine.   Among   all   sugar substitutions, the 5'-position yielded the most potent inhibitors, with 5'-amino- 5'-deoxy-Ado being the most competitive inhibitor, featuring a Ki of 0.8 ± 0.4 mM. This compound surpassed 5'-deoxy-Ado in inhibiting Ado phosphorylation. Moreover, compounds with an additional 5'-methyl group in the talo-conformation were roughly ten times less potent as inhibitors compared to their allo-conformers.

Ado kinase shed light on various observations (Fig. **14**), the crystal structure unveiled a pocket with a diameter of approximately 6.5 Å adjacent to Ado's 2-C, allowing substitutions at the 2-position. Regarding the mechanism of ATP's gamma-phosphate transfer to Ado, it remains to be fully elucidated. In other Ado kinases, such as the human variant, this transfer involves deprotonation of the 5'-hydroxyl group by an aspartic acid residue, followed by a water-mediated nucleophilic attack of the gamma-phosphate by the negatively charged O-5' atom. This leads to the formation of AMP and ADP *via* an SN2 reaction. There is no evidence suggesting a similar conformational change in MTB Ado kinase upon ATP binding [94].

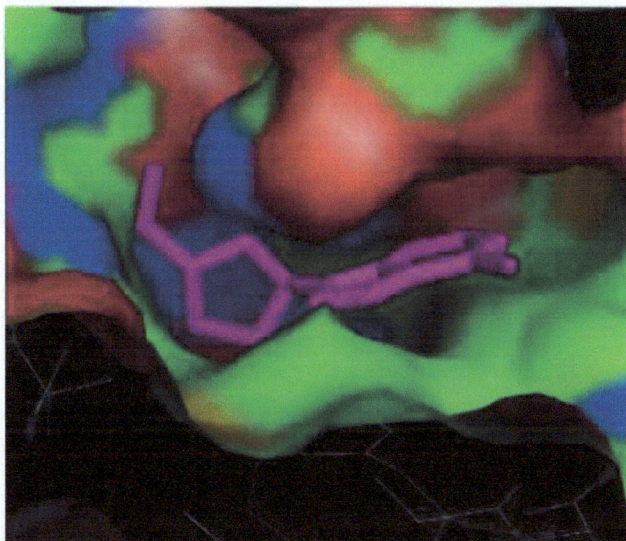

Fig. (14). Ligands docked in the active site of Ado kinase. One of the more favorable substrates, 9-[α-L-lyxofuranosyl]-adenine, offers a top-down perspective from the adenine base. A yellow highlight in the pocket near the 2-position of the adenine base indicates the space where a 2'-methyl or 2'-chloro group would reside [94].

SAR of MTB IMPDH Inhibited by 1-(5-isoquinoline Sulfonyl) Piperazine Analogues

The More Medicines for Tuberculosis (MM4TB) consortium monitored the discovery of cyclohexyl(4-(isoquinoline-5-sulfonyl) piperazine-1-yl) methanone (CISP), a novel antituberculosis drug with little toxicity to mammalian cells. CISP is a component of the well-known scaffold 1-(5-isoquinoline sulfonyl) homopiperazine (Fasudil), which inhibits Rho-associated protein kinase (ROCK). It was shown that this substance also prevents MTB from producing inosine-5--monophosphate dehydrogenase (IMPDH) [95].

The Fasudil analog, 5-(piperazin-1-yl sulfonyl) isoquinoline, displayed no Minimum Inhibitory Concentration (MIC) against MTB, underscoring the crucial role of the cyclohexyl group in CISP's activity. In the initial compound set, the cyclohexyl portion was retained, while the Fasudil-like section was altered to yield a compound (Fig. **15**). Substituting the isoquinoline with naphthalene, yielding the 1-naphthyl derivative or 2-naphthyl derivative, maintained modest enzyme activity but eliminated whole-cell activity, indicating the essential role of the nitrogen atom in the isoquinoline for compound uptake.

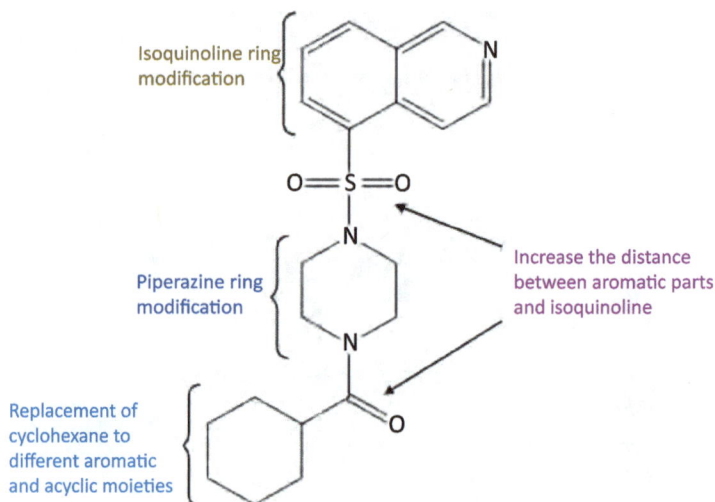

Fig. (15). Alteration of design of target compound series derived from piperazine analogues [95].

The introduction of a methyl group at the second position of the cyclohexyl ring modestly enhanced IMPDH inhibitory activity, while retaining some target-specific whole-cell effectiveness. A pharmacophore analysis highlighted interactions at critical hotspot regions (Fig. **16**).

Derivatives of phenylacetic acid were produced by inserting a methylene spacer between the cyclohexyl ring and the carbonyl group. Numerous compounds in this series demonstrated action against IMPDH, with the greatest potency being demonstrated by cyclohexylacetic acid 4-fluorophenylacetic acid (Fig. **17**). Substitution of the carboxamide group with the urea moiety resulted in the improvement of the inhibitory activities of the 3-substituted phenyl derivatives against the enzyme, although no improvement was seen in the whole cell activity.

Benzylurea derivatives were created to extend the distance between the carbonyl group and the cyclohexyl ring. As the most effective IMPDH inhibitor, a 3-methoxybenzylurea showed around three times the efficacy of the primary molecule. In MTB, 2-methyl benzylurea demonstrated remarkable anti-mycobacterial and biochemical efficacy while preserving target specificity. Despite the docking data indicating contact with the Y487' residue, it also demonstrated respectable activity against the resistant mutant, SRMV2.6. A benzoyl-urethane variation that was only one atom different from piperazine analogues maintained its activity against the enzyme but lost its whole-cell activity, highlighting the critical function that the nitrogen atom plays in binding the IMPDH target in MTB [95].

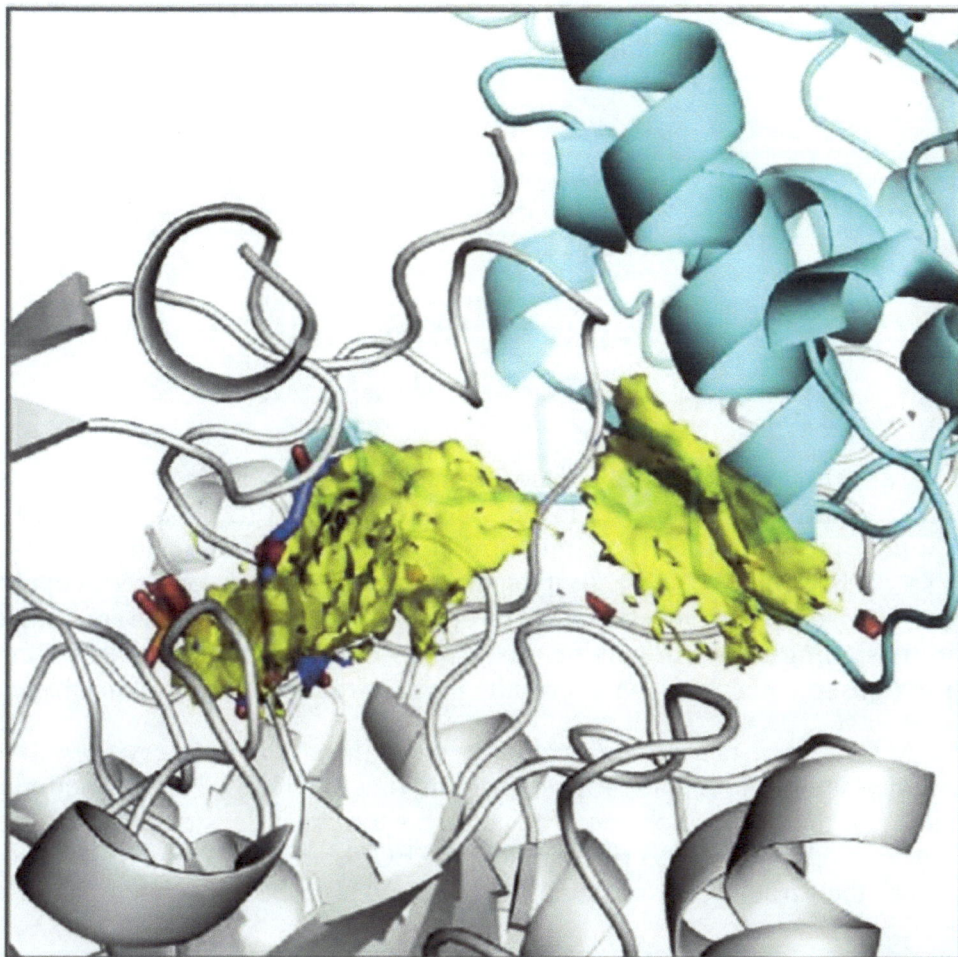

Fig. (16). Hotspot maps for IMP-bound IMPDH display hydrogen donor regions in blue, hydrogen acceptor regions in red, and non-polar regions in yellow [95]. The impact of two key modifications was examined: (i) extending the distance between the carbonyl group and the cyclohexyl ring or its analogs and (ii) replacing one of the nitrogen atoms in the piperazine ring with a carbon atom on the activity profile.

SAR of Protein Synthesis Inhibitor Sequanamycin Derivatives as Anti-TB Agents

Sequanamycin A, also known as SEQ-503, is a distinctive 14-membered ring macrolide related to the erythromycin family. It is synthesized by Allokutzneria albata, belonging to the Pseudonocardiaceae family in the Actinomycetales order. SEQ-503 possesses an impressively low minimum inhibitory concentration (MIC) of 1.4 mM against the tuberculosis-causing bacterium, MTB. Instead of cladinose, SEQ-503 boasts mycarose; it replaces desosamine with ketoallose and uniquely incorporates mycinose. SEQ-503's ability to bind within the ribosome's same pocket as erythromycin showcases its potential as an anti-tubercular agent. However, it presents some challenges.

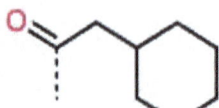

Cyclohexyl acetic acid   4-fluorophenylacetic acid

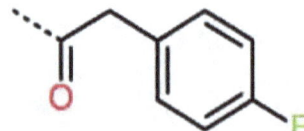

Fig. (17). Cyclohexylacetic acid and 4-fluorophenylacetic acid [95].

SEQ-9, a refined derivative, demonstrated favorable ADME properties. It exhibited improved stability, lower metabolic liabilities, and exceptional distribution into lung tissue. Additionally, it did not inhibit cytochrome 3A4 and had a safety margin. SEQ-9's activity against methylated ribosomes was explored, revealing its unique impact on MTB erm37 expression, which is linked to ribosome stalling or WhiB7 induction. Unlike other macrolides, SEQ-9 targets specific ribosome elements, which results in its distinct antibacterial mechanism.

As the MTB and *T. thermophilus* binding sites align (Fig. **18**), cryo-EM studies were undertaken to elucidate how sequanamycins overcome A2058 methylation resistance on the MTB ribosome. The goal was to reveal the structural features of the A2058-methylated MTB ribosome with SEQ-9 bound (PDB: 7KGB) and, for reference, the structure of the unmethylated MTB ribosome bound to SEQ-9 (PDB: 7SFR).

By growing MTB at subinhibitory erythromycin concentrations, ribosomal methylation was produced. The IC50 difference between methylated and unmethylated ribosomes was used to validate the methylation. Density corresponding to a methyl group at A2058's N6 position in the cryo-EM structure was observed (Fig. **18**), even though for A2057 or A2059, no comparable densities suggestive of methylation was seen.

Additionally, a displacement of SEQ-9 from A2058 was observed in the methylated ribosome compared to the unmethylated counterpart. The distance between A2058's N6 and SEQ-9's 3'-hydroxyl oxygen increased in the methylated ribosome to 3.7 Å, compared to 3.4 Å in the unmethylated ribosome. Similarly, in the methylated ribosome, the distance expanded from 3.4 Å to 4.5 Å between the N1 of A2059 and the oxygen linking the ketoallose group to the lactone ring at the C5 position.

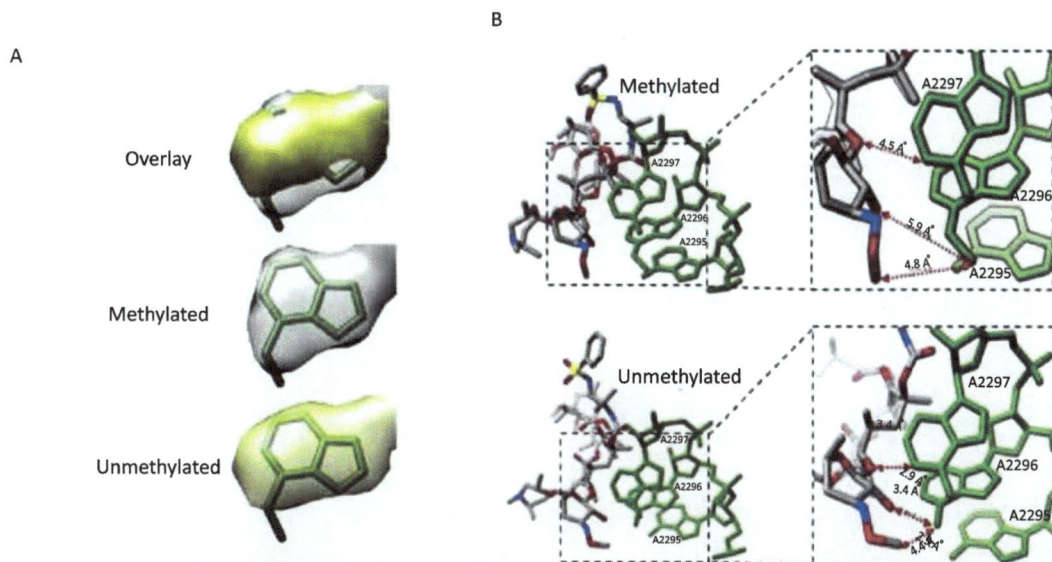

Fig. (18). Comparisons between the unmethylated and methylated MTB ribosome cyro-EM structures. (**A**) Cryo-EM density illustrates both unmethylated and methylated A2058, with SEQ-9 depicted in elemental coloring and nucleotides in green. In (**B**), the density at the methylated N-6 position of A2058 (labeled as A2296 in MTB numbering) is observed [96].

Comparing crystal structures, the macro-lactone and ketoallose groups occupy similar binding pockets in *T. thermophilus* and cryo-EM methylated MTB ribosomes. However, the methylated MTB ribosome exhibits varying conformations for the ketoallose's 3'-hydroxyl group and 4'-methyloxime. Examining interactions with mono-methylated A2058 in the MTB ribosome revealed a hydrogen bond between the hydroxyl group and the N1 of A2058, despite the observed shift in the 3'-hydroxyl group. As a result of this connection, A2058 was forced to relocate, changing its angle to SEQ-9 somewhat from when erythromycin was linked. Sequanamycins did not have a large dimethyl group next to the N6, hence there was no chance of a steric conflict. Chemical variations prevented sequanamycins from mimicking the shape of the water molecule which enables a tripartite interaction between erythromycin, A2058, and G2505. This resulted from the oxime group's unique sp^2 hybridization in sequanamycins as opposed to erythromycin's sp^3 dimethylamine. Moreover, the structural comparisons clearly show that the water molecule would be replaced by methylated A2058. A twofold bidentate contact between the methoxyl and hydroxyl groups of mycinose sugar and N6, NH$_2$ at C7 of G748 was also shown by the cryo-EM structure (Fig. **19**) [96].

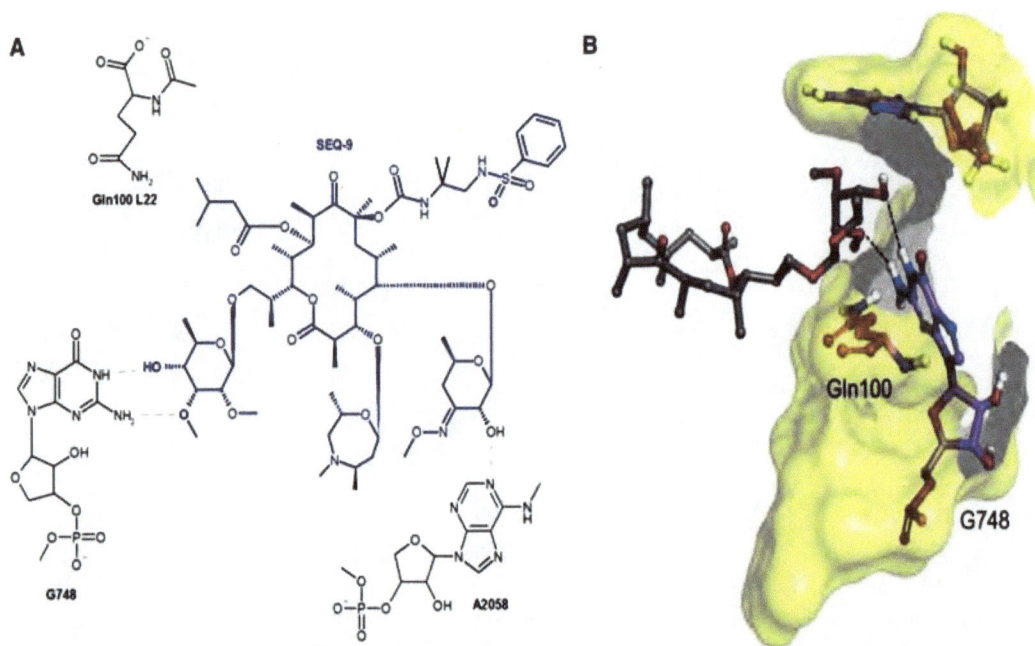

Fig. (19). Key interactions between MTB ribosome and SEQ-9 are shown in figure 19. H-bonds (dotted black lines). (**A**) The 2D interaction of SEQ-9. (**B**) the fringed interaction, formed by the MTB ribosome's mycinose C13 and G748. Furthermore, the equivalent of MTB L22 Arg90, Gln100, doesn't form a hydrogen bond with SEQ9 mycinose [96].

SEQ-9 exhibited strong antibacterial effectiveness against various strains of MTB. The SEQ-9 MIC values remained consistent across various MTB clinical isolates, including those resistant to specific first- or second-line TB drugs. Additionally, SEQ-9 demonstrated effectiveness against non-replicating MTB in hypoxic conditions, with a MIC of 0.6 mM [96].

CONCLUSION

In summary, the research on *Mycobacterium tuberculosis*, with an emphasis on recent breakthroughs in drug discovery and targeting using a structure-activity relationship (SAR) based method, underlines the crucial need for new solutions in the fight against tuberculosis. Tuberculosis continues as a global public health issue, with drug-resistant strains escaping the existing therapy unaffected. SAR-based approaches are a key aid in seeking new pharmaceutical candidates. Researchers can create more effective and tailored treatments by knowing the connection between the molecular makeup of chemicals and their biological action against Mycobacterium TB. Recent advancements in this sector have led to the identification of promising therapeutic options that target multiple stages of the *M. tuberculosis* life cycle, especially latent infections with drug-resistant strains. In addition, the study underlines the significance of discovering and targeting specific biochemical processes and proteins inside MTB, since this technique can facilitate the way for the creation of more accurate and precise medications. In this regard, the identification of new pharmacological routes and the creation of innovative therapies are important for the efficient eradication of tuberculosis. The SAR-based technique for discovering medicines offers a crucial step toward eliminating the molecular barriers imposed by MTB. In a recent breakthrough in tuberculosis research, the chemical Seqanamycin has emerged as a favorable candidate for the treatment of MTB. This development is established in comprehensive preclinical experiments, where Seqanamycin exhibited notable potency against MTB strains.

Seqanamycin, a naturally occurring macrolide belonging to the bacterial ribosome inhibitor class of antibiotics, shows a novel mode of action. Seqanamycin specifically binds to the MTB 50S ribosomal subunit, inhibiting protein synthesis by obstructing the polypeptide exit channel within the ribosome. Initial studies have emphasized its powerful antimycobacterial action while maintaining an acceptable safety profile in preclinical models. Observation of the drug's effectiveness in its early phases inspired the beginning of rigorous clinical trials, mainly aimed at analyzing its safety, pharmacokinetics, and therapeutic efficacy in human patients. Researchers are optimistic that Seqanamycin's unique molecular features offer a more tailored and efficacious drug for TB treatment, overcoming the obstacles of drug resistance. As Seqanamycin moves through clinical trials, the scientific community excitedly looks forward to its addition to the armory against TB, as a groundbreaking drug. The outcome of these trials holds promise for ushering in a new era of precision medicine in the treatment of TB, addressing a crucial global health challenge. While more work remains to be done, the advances discussed in this article hold promise for new therapeutics for the control and eradication of tuberculosis.

REFERENCES

[1]   Bagcchi S. WHO's Global Tuberculosis Report 2022. Lancet Microbe 2023; 4(1): e20.
[http://dx.doi.org/10.1016/S2666-5247(22)00359-7] [PMID: 36521512]

[2]   Gordon SV, Parish T. Microbe Profile: Mycobacterium tuberculosis: Humanity's deadly microbial foe. Microbiology (Reading) 2018; 164(4): 437-9.
[http://dx.doi.org/10.1099/mic.0.000601] [PMID: 29465344]

[3]   Vilchèze C. Mycobacterial cell wall: A source of successful targets for old and new drugs. Appl Sci (Basel) 2020; 10(7): 2278.
[http://dx.doi.org/10.3390/app10072278]

[4]   Jacobo-Delgado YM, Rodríguez-Carlos A, Serrano CJ, Rivas-Santiago B. *Mycobacterium tuberculosis* cell-wall and antimicrobial peptides: a mission impossible? Front Immunol 2023; 14: 1194923.
[http://dx.doi.org/10.3389/fimmu.2023.1194923] [PMID: 37266428]

[5]   Maitra A, Munshi T, Healy J, *et al.* Cell wall peptidoglycan in *Mycobacterium tuberculosis* : An Achilles' heel for the TB-causing pathogen. FEMS Microbiol Rev 2019; 43(5): 548-75.
[http://dx.doi.org/10.1093/femsre/fuz016] [PMID: 31183501]

[6]   Bendre AD, Peters PJ, Kumar J. Recent insights into the structure and function of mycobacterial membrane proteins facilitated by Cryo-EM. J Membr Biol 2021; 254(3): 321-41.
[http://dx.doi.org/10.1007/s00232-021-00179-w] [PMID: 33954837]

[7]   Forrellad MA, Klepp LI, Gioffré A, *et al.* Virulence factors of the *Mycobacterium tuberculosis* complex. Virulence 2013; 4(1): 3-66.
[http://dx.doi.org/10.4161/viru.22329] [PMID: 23076359]

[8]   Patterson B, Wood R. Is cough really necessary for TB transmission? Tuberculosis (Edinb) 2019; 117: 31-5.
[http://dx.doi.org/10.1016/j.tube.2019.05.003] [PMID: 31378265]

[9]   Churchyard G, Kim P, Shah NS, *et al.* What we know about tuberculosis transmission: An overview. J Infect Dis 2017; 216 (Suppl. 6): S629-35.
[http://dx.doi.org/10.1093/infdis/jix362] [PMID: 29112747]

[10]   Ehlers S, Schaible UE. The granuloma in tuberculosis: Dynamics of a host–pathogen collusion. Front Immun 2013. Available from: http://journal.frontiersin.org/article/10.3389/fimmu.2012.00411/abstract

[11]   Kiazyk S, Ball TB. Latent tuberculosis infection: An overview. Can Commun Dis Rep 2017; 43(3/4): 62-6.
[http://dx.doi.org/10.14745/ccdr.v43i34a01] [PMID: 29770066]

[12]   Pawlowski A, Jansson M, Sköld M, Rottenberg ME, Källenius G. Tuberculosis and HIV Co-Infection. PLoS Pathog 2012; 8(2): e1002464.
[http://dx.doi.org/10.1371/journal.ppat.1002464] [PMID: 22363214]

[13]   Kurz SG, Furin JJ, Bark CM. Drug-resistant tuberculosis. Infect Dis Clin North Am 2016; 30(2): 509-22.
[http://dx.doi.org/10.1016/j.idc.2016.02.010] [PMID: 27208770]

[14]   Jee B, Singh Y, Yadav R, Lang F. Small Heat Shock Protein16.3 of *Mycobacterium tuberculosis*: After Two Decades of Functional Characterization. Cell Physiol Biochem 2018; 49(1): 368-80.
[http://dx.doi.org/10.1159/000492887] [PMID: 30138912]

[15]   Laws M, Jin P, Rahman KM. Efflux pumps in *Mycobacterium tuberculosis* and their inhibition to tackle antimicrobial resistance. Trends Microbiol 2022; 30(1): 57-68.
[http://dx.doi.org/10.1016/j.tim.2021.05.001] [PMID: 34052094]

[16]   Seung KJ, Keshavjee S, Rich ML. Multidrug-resistant tuberculosis and extensively drug-resistant tuberculosis. Cold Spring Harb Perspect Med 2015; 5(9): a017863.
[http://dx.doi.org/10.1101/cshperspect.a017863] [PMID: 25918181]

[17]   Mi J, Gong W, Wu X. Advances in key drug target identification and new drug development for tuberculosis. BioMed Res Int 2022; 2022(1): 5099312.
[http://dx.doi.org/10.1155/2022/5099312] [PMID: 35252448]

[18]   Zhou SF, Zhong WZ. Drug design and discovery: Principles and applications. Molecules 2017; 22(2): 279.
[http://dx.doi.org/10.3390/molecules22020279] [PMID: 28208821]

[19]   Sabbah M, Mendes V, Vistal RG, *et al.* Fragment-based design of *Mycobacterium tuberculosis* InhA inhibitors. J Med Chem 2020; 63(9): 4749-61.

[http://dx.doi.org/10.1021/acs.jmedchem.0c00007] [PMID: 32240584]

[20] Hughes JP, Rees S, Kalindjian SB, Philpott KL. Principles of early drug discovery. Br J Pharmacol 2011; 162(6): 1239-49.
[http://dx.doi.org/10.1111/j.1476-5381.2010.01127.x] [PMID: 21091654]

[21] Gupta R, Srivastava D, Sahu M, Tiwari S, Ambasta RK, Kumar P. Artificial intelligence to deep learning: machine intelligence approach for drug discovery. Mol Divers 2021; 25(3): 1315-60.
[http://dx.doi.org/10.1007/s11030-021-10217-3] [PMID: 33844136]

[22] Pitaksajjakul P, Wongwit W, Punprasit W, Eampokalap B, Peacock S, Ramasoota P. Mutations in the gyrA and gyrB genes of fluoroquinolone-resistant *Mycobacterium tuberculosis* from TB patients in Thailand. Southeast Asian J Trop Med Public Health 2005; 36 (Suppl. 4): 228-37.
[PMID: 16438215]

[23] Melly G, Purdy GE, Mmp L. MmpL proteins in physiology and pathogenesis of *M. tuberculosis.* Microorganisms 2019; 7(3): 70.
[http://dx.doi.org/10.3390/microorganisms7030070] [PMID: 30841535]

[24] Cao XJ, Li YP, Wang JY, Zhou J, Guo XG. MPT64 assays for the rapid detection of *Mycobacterium tuberculosis.* BMC Infect Dis 2021; 21(1): 336.
[http://dx.doi.org/10.1186/s12879-021-06022-w] [PMID: 33838648]

[25] Kumar V, Roy S, Behera B, Das B. Heat shock proteins (Hsps) in cellular homeostasis: A promising tool for health management in crustacean aquaculture. Life (Basel) 2022; 12(11): 1777.
[http://dx.doi.org/10.3390/life12111777] [PMID: 36362932]

[26] Sreejit G, Ahmed A, Parveen N, *et al.* The ESAT-6 protein of *Mycobacterium tuberculosis* interacts with beta-2-microglobulin (β2M) affecting antigen presentation function of macrophage. PLoS Pathog 2014; 10(10): e1004446.
[http://dx.doi.org/10.1371/journal.ppat.1004446] [PMID: 25356553]

[27] Khan MZ, Bhaskar A, Upadhyay S, *et al.* Protein kinase G confers survival advantage to *Mycobacterium tuberculosis* during latency-like conditions. J Biol Chem 2017; 292(39): 16093-108.
[http://dx.doi.org/10.1074/jbc.M117.797563] [PMID: 28821621]

[28] Backus KM, Dolan MA, Barry CS, *et al.* The three *Mycobacterium tuberculosis* antigen 85 isoforms have unique substrates and activities determined by non-active site regions. J Biol Chem 2014; 289(36): 25041-53.
[http://dx.doi.org/10.1074/jbc.M114.581579] [PMID: 25028517]

[29] Holzheimer M, Buter J, Minnaard AJ. Chemical synthesis of cell wall constituents of *Mycobacterium tuberculosis.* Chem Rev 2021; 121(15): 9554-643.
[http://dx.doi.org/10.1021/acs.chemrev.1c00043] [PMID: 34190544]

[30] Mitachi K, Siricilla S, Yang D, *et al.* Fluorescence-based assay for polyprenyl phosphate-GlcNAc-1-phosphate transferase (WecA) and identification of novel antimycobacterial WecA inhibitors. Anal Biochem 2016; 512: 78-90.
[http://dx.doi.org/10.1016/j.ab.2016.08.008] [PMID: 27530653]

[31] Saikrishnan K, Kalapala SK, Varshney U, Vijayan M. X-ray structural studies of *Mycobacterium tuberculosis* RRF and a comparative study of RRFs of known structure. Molecular plasticity and biological implications. J Mol Biol 2005; 345(1): 29-38.
[http://dx.doi.org/10.1016/j.jmb.2004.10.034] [PMID: 15567408]

[32] Brown AC, Fraser TR. On the connection between chemical constitution and physiological action; with special reference to the physiological action of the salts of the ammonium bases derived from strychnia, brucia, thebaia, codeia, morphia, and nicotia. J Anat Physiol 1868; 2(2): 224-42.
[PMID: 17230757]

[33] Guha R. On exploring structure–activity relationships. In: Kortagere S, Ed. In Silico Models for Drug Discovery. Totowa, NJ: Humana Press 2013; pp. 81-94. Internet

[http://dx.doi.org/10.1007/978-1-62703-342-8_6]

[34]   Zhan B, Gao Y, Gao W, *et al.* Structural insights of the elongation factor EF-Tu complexes in protein translation of *Mycobacterium tuberculosis.* Commun Biol 2022; 5(1): 1052.
[http://dx.doi.org/10.1038/s42003-022-04019-y] [PMID: 36192483]

[35]   Ferreira L, Dos Santos R, Oliva G, Andricopulo A. Molecular docking and structure-based drug design strategies. Molecules 2015; 20(7): 13384-421.
[http://dx.doi.org/10.3390/molecules200713384] [PMID: 26205061]

[36]   Pun FW, Ozerov IV, Zhavoronkov A. AI-powered therapeutic target discovery. Trends Pharmacol Sci 2023; 44(9): 561-72.
[http://dx.doi.org/10.1016/j.tips.2023.06.010] [PMID: 37479540]

[37]   Bohr A, Memarzadeh K, Eds. Artificial intelligence in healthcare. London; San Diego, CA: Academic Press, imprint of Elsevier 2020.

[38]   Tobin P, Richards D, Callender R, Wilson C. Protein engineering: a new frontier for biological therapeutics. Curr Drug Metab 2015; 15(7): 743-56.
[http://dx.doi.org/10.2174/1389200216666141208151524] [PMID: 25495737]

[39]   Strelow J, Dewe W, Iversen PW, *et al.* Mechanism of action assays for enzymes. In: Markossian S, Grossman A, Brimacombe K, Arkin M, Auld D, Austin C, Eds. Assay Guidance Manual. Bethesda, MD: Eli Lilly & Company and the national center for advancing translational sciences 2004. Internet Available from: http://www.ncbi.nlm.nih.gov/books/NBK92001/

[40]   Llowarch P, Usselmann L, Ivanov D, Holdgate GA. Thermal unfolding methods in drug discovery. Biophys Rev (Melville) 2023; 4(2): 021305.
[http://dx.doi.org/10.1063/5.0144141] [PMID: 38510342]

[41]   Amiri-Dashatan N, Koushki M, Abbaszadeh HA, Rostami-Nejad M, Rezaei-Tavirani M. Proteomics applications in health: biomarker and drug discovery and food industry. Iran J Pharm Res 2018; 17(4): 1523-36.
[PMID: 30568709]

[42]   Xia X. Bioinformatics and drug discovery. Curr Top Med Chem. 2017;17(15):1709-1726.
[http://dx.doi.org/10.2174/1568026617666161116143440]   [PMID: 27848897]   [PMCID: PMC5421137]

[43]   Szymański P, Markowicz M, Mikiciuk-Olasik E. Adaptation of high-throughput screening in drug discovery-toxicological screening tests. Int J Mol Sci 2011; 13(1): 427-52.
[http://dx.doi.org/10.3390/ijms13010427] [PMID: 22312262]

[44]   Moore M, Ferguson J, Burns C. Applications of cell-based bioassays measuring the induced expression of endogenous genes. Bioanalysis 2014; 6(11): 1563-74.
[http://dx.doi.org/10.4155/bio.14.98] [PMID: 25046054]

[45]   Priest BT, Cerne R, Krambis MJ, *et al.* Automated electrophysiology assays. In: Markossian S, Grossman A, Brimacombe K, Arkin M, Auld D, Austin C, Eds. Assay Guidance Manual. Bethesda, MD: Eli Lilly & Company and the National Center for Advancing Translational Sciences 2004. Internet Available from: http://www.ncbi.nlm.nih.gov/books/NBK424997/

[46]   Hao J. Thermal shift assay for exploring interactions between fatty acid–binding protein and inhibitors. In: Posch A, Ed. Proteomic Profiling. New York, NY: Springer US 2021; pp. 395-409. Internet
[http://dx.doi.org/10.1007/978-1-0716-1186-9_24]

[47]   Bertucci C, Pistolozzi M, De Simone A. Circular dichroism in drug discovery and development: an abridged review. Anal Bioanal Chem 2010; 398(1): 155-66.
[http://dx.doi.org/10.1007/s00216-010-3959-2] [PMID: 20658284]

[48]   Harroun SG, Lauzon D, Ebert MCCJC, Desrosiers A, Wang X, Vallée-Bélisle A. Monitoring protein conformational changes using fluorescent nanoantennas. Nat Methods 2022; 19(1): 71-80.

[http://dx.doi.org/10.1038/s41592-021-01355-5] [PMID: 34969985]

[49]   Almehmadi LM, Valsangkar VA, Halvorsen K, Zhang Q, Sheng J, Lednev IK. Surface-enhanced Raman spectroscopy for drug discovery: peptide-RNA binding. Anal Bioanal Chem 2022; 414(20): 6009-16.
[http://dx.doi.org/10.1007/s00216-022-04190-5] [PMID: 35764806]

[50]   Carvalho AL, Trincão J, Romão MJ. X-ray crystallography in drug discovery. In: Roque ACA, Ed. Ligand-Macromolecular Interactions in Drug Discovery. Totowa, NJ: Humana Press 2010; pp. 31-56. Internet
[http://dx.doi.org/10.1007/978-1-60761-244-5_3]

[51]   Zloh M. NMR spectroscopy in drug discovery and development: Evaluation of physico-chemical properties. ADMET DMPK 2019; 7(4): 242-51.
[http://dx.doi.org/10.5599/admet.737] [PMID: 35359618]

[52]   Sliwoski G, Kothiwale S, Meiler J, Lowe EW Jr. Computational methods in drug discovery. Pharmacol Rev 2014; 66(1): 334-95.
[http://dx.doi.org/10.1124/pr.112.007336] [PMID: 24381236]

[53]   Dueñas ME, Peltier-Heap RE, Leveridge M, Annan RS, Büttner FH, Trost M. Advances in high-throughput mass spectrometry in drug discovery. EMBO Mol Med 2023; 15(1): e14850.
[http://dx.doi.org/10.15252/emmm.202114850] [PMID: 36515561]

[54]   Nikolin B, Imamović B, Medanhodžić-Vuk S, Sober M. High performance liquid chromatography in pharmaceutical analyses. Bosn J Basic Med Sci 2004; 4(2): 5-9.
[http://dx.doi.org/10.17305/bjbms.2004.3405] [PMID: 15629016]

[55]   Linkuvienė V, Krainer G, Chen WY, Matulis D. Isothermal titration calorimetry for drug design: Precision of the enthalpy and binding constant measurements and comparison of the instruments. Anal Biochem 2016; 515: 61-4.
[http://dx.doi.org/10.1016/j.ab.2016.10.005] [PMID: 27717855]

[56]   Olaru A, Bala C, Jaffrezic-Renault N, Aboul-Enein HY. Surface plasmon resonance (SPR) biosensors in pharmaceutical analysis. Crit Rev Anal Chem 2015; 45(2): 97-105.
[http://dx.doi.org/10.1080/10408347.2014.881250] [PMID: 25558771]

[57]   Magnez R, Bailly C, Thuru X. Microscale thermophoresis as a tool to study protein interactions and their implication in human diseases. Int J Mol Sci 2022; 23(14): 7672.
[http://dx.doi.org/10.3390/ijms23147672] [PMID: 35887019]

[58]   Watson JT, Sparkman OD. Introduction to mass spectrometry: instrumentation, applications and strategies for data interpretation. 4th ed., Chichester, England; Hoboken, NJ: John Wiley & Sons 2007.
[http://dx.doi.org/10.1002/9780470516898]

[59]   Srivastava M, Ed. High-performance thin-layer chromatography (HPTLC). Berlin, Heidelberg: Springer Berlin Heidelberg 2011. Internet
[http://dx.doi.org/10.1007/978-3-642-14025-9]

[60]   Thomson JA, Ladbury JE. Isothermal titration calorimetry: A tutorial. In: Ladbury JE, Doyle ML, Eds. Biocalorimetry 2. Wiley 2004; pp. 35-58. Internet
[http://dx.doi.org/10.1002/0470011122.ch2]

[61]   Schasfoort RBM. Front matter In: Handbook of Surface Plasmon Resonance. Cambridge: Royal Society of Chemistry 2017; pp. 1-4. Available from: http://ebook.rsc.org/?DOI=10.1039/9781788010283-FP001

[62]   Jerabek-Willemsen M, André T, Wanner R, et al. MicroScale Thermophoresis: Interaction analysis and beyond. J Mol Struct 2014; 1077: 101-13.
[http://dx.doi.org/10.1016/j.molstruc.2014.03.009]

[63]   Yano T, Kassovska-Bratinova S, Teh JS, et al. Reduction of clofazimine by mycobacterial type 2 NADH:quinone oxidoreductase: a pathway for the generation of bactericidal levels of reactive oxygen

species. J Biol Chem 2011; 286(12): 10276-87.
[http://dx.doi.org/10.1074/jbc.M110.200501] [PMID: 21193400]

[64]   Shirude PS, Paul B, Roy Choudhury N, Kedari C, Bandodkar B, Ugarkar BG. Quinolinyl pyrimidines: Potent inhibitors of NDH-2 as a novel class of anti-TB agents. ACS Med Chem Lett 2012; 3(9): 736-40.
[http://dx.doi.org/10.1021/ml300134b] [PMID: 24900541]

[65]   Pieroni M. Antituberculosis agents: Beyond medicinal chemistry rules. Annual Reports in Medicinal Chemistry. Elsevier 2019; pp. 27-69. Internet Available from: https://linkinghub.elsevier.com/retrieve/pii/S0065774319300089

[66]   Edinoff AN, Wu N, Ghaffar YT, *et al.* Zolpidem: Efficacy and Side Effects for Insomnia. Health Psychol Res 2021; 9(1): 24927.
[http://dx.doi.org/10.52965/001c.24927] [PMID: 34746488]

[67]   Moraski GC, Miller PA, Bailey MA, *et al.* Putting tuberculosis (TB) to rest: Transformation of the sleep aid, ambien, and "anagrams" generated potent antituberculosis agents. ACS Infect Dis 2015; 1(2): 85-90.
[http://dx.doi.org/10.1021/id500008t] [PMID: 25984566]

[68]   Adewumi AT, Soremekun OS, Ajadi MB, Soliman MES. Thompson loop: opportunities for antitubercular drug design by targeting the weak spot in demethylmenaquinone methyltransferase protein. RSC Advances 2020; 10(39): 23466-83.
[http://dx.doi.org/10.1039/D0RA03206A] [PMID: 35520325]

[69]   Lakshmanan M, Xavier AS. Bedaquiline – The first ATP synthase inhibitor against multi drug resistant tuberculosis. J Young Pharm 2013; 5(4): 112-5.
[http://dx.doi.org/10.1016/j.jyp.2013.12.002] [PMID: 24563587]

[70]   Sacksteder KA, Protopopova M, Barry CE III, Andries K, Nacy CA. Discovery and development of SQ109: a new antitubercular drug with a novel mechanism of action. Future Microbiol 2012; 7(7): 823-37.
[http://dx.doi.org/10.2217/fmb.12.56] [PMID: 22827305]

[71]   Abraham MJ, Murtola T, Schulz R, *et al.* GROMACS: High performance molecular simulations through multi-level parallelism from laptops to supercomputers. SoftwareX 2015; 1-2: 19-25.
[http://dx.doi.org/10.1016/j.softx.2015.06.001]

[72]   Marrakchi H, Bardou F, Lanéelle MA, Daffé M. A comprehensive overview of mycolic acid structure and biosynthesis. In: Daffé M, Reyrat JM, Eds. The Mycobacterial Cell Envelope. Washington, DC, USA: ASM Press 2014; pp. 41-62. Internet
[http://dx.doi.org/10.1128/9781555815783.ch4]

[73]   Kidder GW, Montgomery CW. Oxygenation of frog gastric mucosa *in vitro*. Am J Physiol 1975; 229(6): 1510-3.
[http://dx.doi.org/10.1152/ajplegacy.1975.229.6.1510] [PMID: 2018]

[74]   Oh S, Trifonov L, Yadav VD, Barry CE III, Boshoff HI. Tuberculosis drug discovery: A decade of hit assessment for defined targets. Front Cell Infect Microbiol 2021; 11: 611304.
[http://dx.doi.org/10.3389/fcimb.2021.611304] [PMID: 33791235]

[75]   Sim E, Abuhammad A, Ryan A. Arylamine N-acetyltransferases: from drug metabolism and pharmacogenetics to drug discovery. Br J Pharmacol 2014; 171(11): 2705-25.
[http://dx.doi.org/10.1111/bph.12598] [PMID: 24467436]

[76]   Pajk S, Živec M, Šink R, *et al.* New direct inhibitors of InhA with antimycobacterial activity based on a tetrahydropyran scaffold. Eur J Med Chem 2016; 112: 252-7.
[http://dx.doi.org/10.1016/j.ejmech.2016.02.008] [PMID: 26900657]

[77]   Shirude PS, Madhavapeddi P, Naik M, *et al.* Methyl-thiazoles: a novel mode of inhibition with the potential to develop novel inhibitors targeting InhA in Mycobacterium tuberculosis. J Med Chem

2013; 56(21): 8533-42.
[http://dx.doi.org/10.1021/jm4012033] [PMID: 24107081]

[78]   Šink R, Sosič I, Živec M, *et al.* Design, synthesis, and evaluation of new thiadiazole-based direct inhibitors of enoyl acyl carrier protein reductase (InhA) for the treatment of tuberculosis. J Med Chem 2015; 58(2): 613-24.
[http://dx.doi.org/10.1021/jm501029r] [PMID: 25517015]

[79]   Portevin D, de Sousa-D'Auria C, Houssin C, *et al.* A polyketide synthase catalyzes the last condensation step of mycolic acid biosynthesis in mycobacteria and related organisms. Proc Natl Acad Sci USA 2004; 101(1): 314-9.
[http://dx.doi.org/10.1073/pnas.0305439101] [PMID: 14695899]

[80]   Wilson R, Kumar P, Parashar V, *et al.* Antituberculosis thiophenes define a requirement for Pks13 in mycolic acid biosynthesis. Nat Chem Biol 2013; 9(8): 499-506.
[http://dx.doi.org/10.1038/nchembio.1277] [PMID: 23770708]

[81]   Ioerger TR, O'Malley T, Liao R, *et al.* Identification of new drug targets and resistance mechanisms in *Mycobacterium tuberculosis.* PLoS One 2013; 8(9): e75245.
[http://dx.doi.org/10.1371/journal.pone.0075245] [PMID: 24086479]

[82]   Aggarwal A, Parai MK, Shetty N, *et al.* Development of a novel lead that targets M. tuberculosis polyketide synthase 13. Cell 2017; 170(2): 249-259.e25.
[http://dx.doi.org/10.1016/j.cell.2017.06.025] [PMID: 28669536]

[83]   Zhang W, Lun S, Liu LL, *et al.* Identification of novel coumestan derivatives as polyketide synthase 13 inhibitors against *Mycobacterium tuberculosis.* part II. J Med Chem 2019; 62(7): 3575-89.
[http://dx.doi.org/10.1021/acs.jmedchem.9b00010] [PMID: 30875203]

[84]   Schiebel J, Kapilashrami K, Fekete A, *et al.* Structural basis for the recognition of mycolic acid precursors by KasA, a condensing enzyme and drug target from *Mycobacterium tuberculosis.* J Biol Chem 2013; 288(47): 34190-204.
[http://dx.doi.org/10.1074/jbc.M113.511436] [PMID: 24108128]

[85]   Parrish NM, Kuhajda FP, Heine HS, Bishai WR, Dick JD. Antimycobacterial activity of cerulenin and its effects on lipid biosynthesis. J Antimicrob Chemother 1999; 43(2): 219-26.
[http://dx.doi.org/10.1093/jac/43.2.219] [PMID: 11252327]

[86]   Ballell L, Bates RH, Young RJ, *et al.* Fueling open-source drug discovery: 177 small-molecule leads against tuberculosis. ChemMedChem 2013; 8(2): 313-21.
[http://dx.doi.org/10.1002/cmdc.201200428] [PMID: 23307663]

[87]   Kumar P, Capodagli GC, Awasthi D, *et al.* Synergistic Lethality of a Binary Inhibitor of Mycobacterium tuberculosis KasA. MBio 2018; 9(6): e02101-17.
[http://dx.doi.org/10.1128/mBio.02101-17] [PMID: 30563908]

[88]   Abrahams KA, Chung C, Ghidelli-Disse S, *et al.* Identification of KasA as the cellular target of an anti-tubercular scaffold. Nat Commun 2016; 7(1): 12581.
[http://dx.doi.org/10.1038/ncomms12581] [PMID: 27581223]

[89]   Cunningham F, Esquivias J, Fernández-Menéndez R, *et al.* Exploring the SAR of the β-Ketoacyl-ACP synthase inhibitor GSK3011724A and optimization around a genotoxic metabolite. ACS Infect Dis 2020; 6(5): 1098-109.
[http://dx.doi.org/10.1021/acsinfecdis.9b00493] [PMID: 32196311]

[90]   Lakhvich TT, Borava MI, Lakhvich AT. Structure activity relationship studies on KasA: aldonamides' affinity to receptor in context of TB drug design 2021; 87. Available from: https://elib.bsu.by/bitstream/123456789/269292/1/87.pdf

[91]   Machutta C, Tonge P. Slow onset inhibition of KasA by thiolactomycin: Mechanistic insights for lead optimization. FASEB J 2008; 22(S1) Available from: https://faseb.onlinelibrary.wiley.com/doi/10.1096/fasebj.22.1_supplement.792.6 [Internet].

[http://dx.doi.org/10.1096/fasebj.22.1_supplement.792.6]

[92]   P SH, Solapure S, Mukherjee K, *et al.* Optimization of pyrrolamides as mycobacterial GyrB ATPase inhibitors: structure-activity relationship and *in vivo* efficacy in a mouse model of tuberculosis. Antimicrob Agents Chemother 2014; 58(1): 61-70.
[http://dx.doi.org/10.1128/AAC.01751-13] [PMID: 24126580]

[93]   Alokam R, Jeankumar VU, Sridevi JP, *et al.* Identification and structure–activity relationship study of carvacrol derivatives as *Mycobacterium tuberculosis* chorismate mutase inhibitors. J Enzyme Inhib Med Chem 2014; 29(4): 547-54.
[http://dx.doi.org/10.3109/14756366.2013.823958] [PMID: 24090423]

[94]   Long MC, Shaddix SC, Moukha-Chafiq O, Maddry JA, Nagy L, Parker WB. Structure–activity relationship for adenosine kinase from Mycobacterium tuberculosis. Biochem Pharmacol 2008; 75(8): 1588-600.
[http://dx.doi.org/10.1016/j.bcp.2008.01.007] [PMID: 18329005]

[95]   Singh V, Pacitto A, Donini S, *et al.* Synthesis and Structure–Activity relationship of 1-(--isoquinolinesulfonyl)piperazine analogues as inhibitors of *Mycobacterium tuberculosis* IMPDH. Eur J Med Chem 2019; 174: 309-29.
[http://dx.doi.org/10.1016/j.ejmech.2019.04.027] [PMID: 31055147]

[96]   Zhang J, Lair C, Roubert C, *et al.* Discovery of natural-product-derived sequanamycins as potent oral anti-tuberculosis agents. Cell 2023; 186(5): 1013-1025.e24.
[http://dx.doi.org/10.1016/j.cell.2023.01.043] [PMID: 36827973]

Advances in the Medicinal Chemistry, 2025, 340-359

CHAPTER 10

Drug Discovery in *Fasciola hepatica*: Few Steps in the Last Ten Years

Ileana Corvo[1,*] and Mauricio Cabrera[1]

[1] *Laboratorio de I+D de Moléculas Bioactivas, Departamento de Ciencias Biológicas, Centro Universitario Regional Litoral Norte, Universidad de la República, Paysandú, Uruguay*

Abstract: Fascioliasis, caused by trematode parasites of the *Fasciola spp.* remains a significant global health concern, affecting both humans and livestock. This neglected tropical disease, along with other food-borne trematodes, impacts over 10% of the world's population, resulting in substantial economic losses exceeding $3 billion annually in the livestock industry. Since no vaccine has been developed so far, current disease control relies mainly on drugs, particularly triclabendazole, which although effective, faces challenges due to reported resistance in many regions. With *Fasciola hepatica* being the common fluke, its wide distribution and intricate life cycle, emphasize the importance of understanding parasite epidemiology and biology and addressing drug resistance. However, few efforts have been pursued in the last decade to develop new drugs against fascioliasis. There are different approaches to drug discovery. Screening methodologies may target essential parasite proteins through *in silico* or *in vitro* studies, employing protein docking and molecular dynamic simulations. This enables the rapid identification of potential drug candidates for subsequent *in vitro* or *in vivo* testing. Alternatively, phenotypic screenings with cultured parasites offer a broader understanding of drug efficacy but present challenges in terms of automation and the unknown mode of action of the drug candidates. Also, drug repurposing has emerged as a promising strategy in recent years. This approach accelerates the drug development process, addressing the lengthy timelines typically associated with bringing novel drugs to the market. This chapter provides a comprehensive overview of drug discovery efforts in the last ten years for fascioliasis treatment. In-depth discussions on drugs targeting specific *F. hepatica* molecular components are presented followed by phenotypic screenings with synthetic and natural compounds. The chapter concludes with a review of some scarce initiatives in drug repurposing, providing an overview of the various strategies employed to address drug discovery in fascioliasis.

Keywords: Anthelmintic, Cathepsin L, Drug development, Drug repurposing, *Fasciola gigantica*, *Fasciola hepatica*, Fascioliasis, Fasciolicide activity, Flukicidal activity, Foodborne trematode disease.

* **Corresponding author Ileana Corvo:** Laboratorio de I+D de Moléculas Bioactivas, Departamento de Ciencias Biológicas, Centro Universitario Regional Litoral Norte, Universidad de la República, Paysandú, Uruguay; E-mail: ilecorvo@gmail.com

Igor Jose dos Santos Nascimento & Ricardo Olimpio de Moura (Eds.)

INTRODUCTION

The discovery of new anthelmintics faces challenges that are unique to antiparasitic drug discovery. Less than five new classes of anthelmintics have been approved for animal use in the 21st century [1]. Fascioliasis, caused by trematodes parasites of the *Fasciola* genus, poses significant challenges for both human health and the livestock industry. The liver flukes, together with lung flukes and intestinal flukes, form a group known as the Food-Borne Trematodes, neglected tropical diseases affecting more than 10% of the world population [2]. Among these, *Fasciola hepatica* is known as the common fluke, it has a worldwide distribution, affecting a variety of hosts including ruminants, horses, wild animals like deer, rabbits, hares, and humans, resulting in substantial losses in production and clinical disease, with roughly estimated costs exceeding $3 billion annually for the global livestock industry [3]. It not only impacts animals but also represents a significant public health problem, especially in regions of South America, Asia, and Africa, where millions of people are estimated to be at risk of infection [2, 4]. Thus, the disease is not anymore considered merely as a secondary zoonosis but is also recognized as an important human parasitic disease.

The indirect life cycle of *F. hepatica*, involving lymnaeid snails as intermediate hosts, underscores the importance of understanding and addressing epidemiology and drug resistance. The parasite's ability to modulate the host's immune system and affect susceptibility and diagnosis of other diseases, such as bovine tuberculosis, adds complexity to the landscape [3]. Disease control relies primarily on the use of drugs, especially triclabendazole (TCBZ), which is effective against multiple stages of the parasite. However, resistance to this and other drugs reported in many countries has intensified the search for alternative control strategies [5]. Efforts to overcome TCBZ resistance led to the synthesis of TCBZ bioisosteres, among these, one of the most relevant is compound alpha (5-chloro-2-(methylthio)-6-(1-naphthyloxy)-1H-benzimidazole), whose fasciolicide activity has been demonstrated *in vivo* and is currently undergoing efficacy and safety studies, apparently being an alternative with reduced environmental contamination to control fascioliasis [6]. However, the urgency of developing new drugs and control measures is accentuated by growing concerns about flukicide resistance, as well as drug residues in meat and milk, leading to restrictions in use and longer withdrawal periods [3, 7].

DIFFERENT APPROACHES TO DRUG DISCOVERY IN *F. HEPATICA*

Drug screening approaches against the liver fluke may be directed to an isolated target, usually an enzyme or another essential parasite protein, or be performed on *in vitro* cultured flukes. The former studies have the advantage of being rapidly executed, they can be first done *in silico* through protein docking and molecular dynamic simulations, to narrow down the number of molecules to be then tested in an *in vitro* assay and allow the performance of high-throughput studies. This also, favors the optimization of the structure-activity relationship over the target. However, translation into *in vitro* flukicide activity is not always straightforward. In contrast, phenotypic screenings with cultured parasites have the advantage of overcoming this difficulty but are not easily automatized, and usually, the mode of action of the active compounds is unknown, which hinders drug structure optimization to eliminate unwanted effects without compromising its biological potency. Another strategy to overcome resistance is drug repurposing (testing of old drugs for new applications), which has become an attractive alternative in recent years since it shortens the long time required to bring novel drugs to the market.

This chapter will summarize the drug discovery efforts done over the last 10 years for fascioliasis treatment. First, the later findings about drugs that act over a specific *F. hepatica* molecular target and their structure-activity relationships are discussed in detail. Then, phenotypic screenings performed with different synthetic and natural compounds are presented. In the end, some efforts towards drug repurposing are depicted.

PROTEIN TARGETS FOR DRUG DEVELOPMENT

Cathepsin Ls

Cathepsin Ls are key protease enzymes secreted by the liver fluke *Fasciola hepatica,* which play a crucial role in the parasitic life cycle and pathogenesis. Cathepsins are integral to various physiological processes, including tissue invasion, immune evasion, and nutrient acquisition within the host organism [8, 9], which make them interesting molecular targets. *Fh*CL1 and *Fh*CL3 are the main enzymes secreted by the adult and newly excysted juvenile stages, respectively [10]. Cathepsin Ls are compact globular proteins consisting of an N-terminal prodomain and a catalytic domain connected by a flexible linker. The catalytic domain contains the active site, characterized by the triad Cys-His-Asn, which facilitates the enzyme's proteolytic activity. X-ray crystallography studies have provided high-resolution insights into the three-dimensional architecture of cathepsin L, highlighting its substrate-binding pockets and the structural basis for substrate specificity [11, 12]. Understanding the tridimensional structure of cathepsin L is pivotal for designing targeted inhibitors and developing therapeutic strategies. Both *in silico* and *in vitro* studies have been performed since enzyme activity can be easily measured by monitoring the cleavage of a fluorescent short peptide substrate over time [13]. Though peptide-based inhibitors were initially sought based on substrate preferences [14], small non-peptidic molecules have subsequently been explored to overcome the protease degradation of the formers. In a study by Hernández *et al.,* 2015 a virtual screening for potential *Fh*CL3 inhibitors was performed [15]. The generation of a 3D model for *Fh*CL3 involved a multiple sequence alignment of twelve papain-like proteases, using the crystal structure of pro*Fh*CL1 C25G as a template [12] (Stack *et al.* 2008). Molecular docking identified compounds HTS12701 (2-{[4-benzyl-5-(pyridin-4-yl)-4H-1,2,4-triazol-3-yl]sulfanyl}2-1-(1,2,3,4-tetrahydroquinolin-1-yl)ethan-1-one) and BTB03219 (1-N-[3,5-bis (trifluoromethyl) phenyl]-2-N-(1-ethynyl cyclohexyl) benzene-1,2-dicarboxamide) as the best potential inhibitors whose ΔGbind values suggest sub-micromolar and micromolar concentration bindings, respectively. These compounds exhibited a peptidomimetic scaffold, aromatic moieties, and heterocyclic rings, fostering hydrophobic and polar interactions within the binding site. HTS12701 and BTB03219 demonstrated selectivity for specific residues, potentially influencing inhibitor specificity. Structural insights highlighted the importance of *Fh*CL3 W69, a residue of the S3 binding pocket in ligand accommodation. This study provides valuable insights into *Fh*CL3-peptide interactions and identifies potential inhibitors, setting the stage for designing novel compounds targeting *Fh*CL3.

Other studies have employed both *Fh*CL1 and *Fh*CL3 to search for small-molecule inhibitors of both enzymes. Ferraro *et al.,* 2016 identified through *in vitro* enzyme inhibition screening, novel chalcones that inhibit *Fasciola hepatica* major cathepsins Ls [16]. Chalcones with heterocycles as B-ring and chalcones containing phenyl and naphtyl moieties were the most potent inhibitors. A hit was identified, **C34** (Fig. **1**), which resulted in a tight binding inhibitor of *Fh*CL3, not toxic to bovine sperm, with *in vitro* fasciolicide activity over cultured NEJ and *in vivo* activity in a murine model of *F. hepatica* infection [17]. In the same work, a related naphtylchalcone (**C31**, Fig. **1**) was also identified as a hit and its *in vitro* and *in vivo* biological activity was demonstrated [17], which encourages the further study of chalcones for fascioliasis drug development.

Another class of compounds that have shown *in vitro* F. hepatica cathepsin inhibition are quinoxaline 1,4-di-*N*-oxide (QNO) derivatives. It was found that those bearing a phenyl substituent in R2 were the best cathepsin inhibitors [18], which added to the fact that the best chalcone inhibitors were substituted by a naphthyl group on both rings, suggesting that the presence of bulky substituents and cyclic structures favors the inhibition of these enzymes, possibly by mimicking the peptide substrates. A recent study that describes a blind molecular docking strategy to pinpoint potential QNO derivatives targeting the *Fh*CL1 substrate binding site [19], supports this idea. Compounds with high affinity towards *Fh*CL1 share characteristics such as bulky groups, aliphatic, aromatic, and heterocyclic structures, halogenated substituents, and protonable amines in both open-chain and cyclic secondary amines. While predominantly hydrophobic, there are polar substituents like protonable amine, nitro, and hydroxyl groups, suggesting potential interaction with both hydrophobic and hydrophilic moieties. Analysis of *Fh*CL1 interactions with top-scored QNO derivatives reveals consistent engagement with specific residues and predominantly hydrophobic interactions are observed, with residues Asp232 and Gln244. Three of the five key interactions are shared with other reported *Fh*CL1 inhibitors, **C17** (a QNO) [18] and **C34** (a chalcone) [16], indicating a preference for the site determined by blind docking.

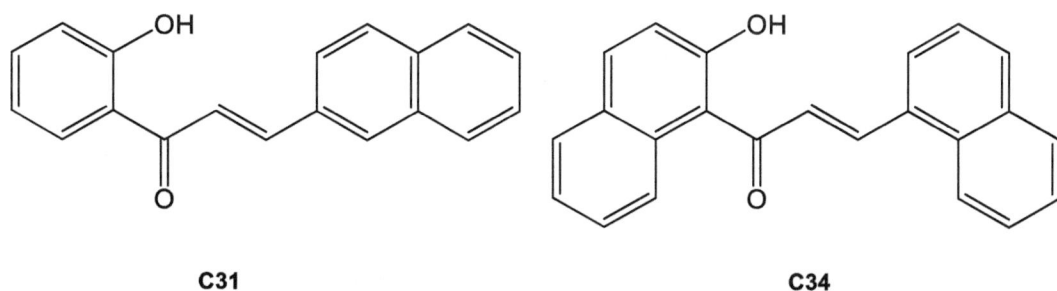

Fig. (1). Structure of the naphtylchalcones **C31** and **C34**.

Triosephosphate Isomerase

The glycolytic pathway is the main source of energy in the metabolism of trematode parasites, and a source of enzymes that are interesting drug targets. Among these, the triosephosphate isomerase (TPI) catalyzes the isomerization of glyceraldehyde-3-phosphate and dihydroxyacetone phosphate in the fifth step of the glycolytic pathway [20]. Like TPIs from most species, *Fh*TPI is a homodimer, each monomer consisting of eight parallel β-strands surrounded by eight α-helices that form the typical "TPI barrel" fold [13]. As the enzyme is active in its dimeric form, small molecules that interfere with the dimerization process or destabilize the dimeric interface will impair enzyme function. Lack of TPI leads to the build-up of dihydroxyacetone phosphate and redox toxicity, which results in reduced cell viability [21], suggesting the selective inhibition of TPI as a strategy for the design of novel drugs to target *F. hepatica*. Also, human TPI inhibition is a potential target in cancer therapy due to common post-translational modifications described in tumoral cells that can be selectively targeted [22].

TPI inhibitors against protozoan parasites and ticks have been described, whereas benzothiazole, benzoxazole, benzimidazole, and sulfhydryl derivatives are reported as the best inhibitors [23, 24]. They share structural characteristics as aromatic systems and symmetrical structures, which allows them to bind mainly at the TPI dimer interface and catalytic region, impairing enzyme function [24]. There are scarce studies of worm TPIs as potential anthelmintic drug targets [20, 25 - 27] and only one work has looked for *F. hepatica* and *S. mansoni* TPI inhibitors [28]. Here, a massive screening was conducted to identify molecules that destabilize the dimeric interface of *Fh*TPI. Several chemotypes, such as thiadiazines, thiosemicarbazides, and sulfone derivatives were found to be active against the parasite enzyme (Table **1**) [28].

Table 1. Thiadiazines, thiosemicarbazides, and sulfone derivatives inhibit *Fh*TPI with an IC$_{50}$<50 μM, including the best inhibitor compound 187 (adapted from [28]).

Compound ID	Structure	IC$_{50}$*Fh*TPI (μM)
110		7 ± 1
114		25 ± 8
115		8 ± 2
116		5 ± 1

(Table 1) cont.....

Compound ID	Structure	IC$_{50}$*Fh*TPI (μM)
128		5 ± 1
187		4 ± 0.2

Interestingly, most inhibitors possess aromatic systems and symmetrical structures as described before for molecules that interact at the TPI dimeric interface [24]. Among these, compound **187** was the best inhibitor with a high affinity for *Fh*TPI. This derivative showed selectivity for the parasitic enzyme compared to mammalian TPIs, no acute oral toxicity, and *in vivo* efficacy in mice infected with *F. hepatica,* comparable to the reference drug TCBZ [28].

Thioredoxin Glutathione Reductase

Flatworm parasites have a particular thioredoxin glutathione reductase (TGR) enzyme, which acts both in thioredoxin and glutathione-dependent pathways. These systems are key aspects of redox homeostasis and defense against oxidative damage, regulating DNA replication, cell growth, and apoptosis [29]. TGR is a selenoenzyme that has been validated as a drug target in *S. mansoni*. Though several inhibitors have been identified, most are reactive electrophiles targeting the selenocysteine-containing C-terminus and often show *in vivo* off-target effects because of the abundance of free thiols [30 - 32]. To our knowledge, in *F. hepatica* there is only one report of a high throughput screening of *Fh*TGR inhibitors, which led to the identification of oxadiazole *N*-oxides (furoxans), a quinoxaline and a thiadiazole, as potent inhibitors. They also inhibit *E. granulosus* TGR and their *in vitro* activity over flukes and tapeworms was confirmed [33]. The phenylsulfonyl moiety was present in many of the identified compounds, suggesting that this group is a potential pharmacophore to target flatworm TGRs. More recent work in *S. mansoni* identified noncovalent TGR inhibitors with efficacy against schistosome infections in mice [34]. A different inhibition mechanism of TGR was identified and non-covalent inhibitors that bind at the doorstop pocket of the enzyme and prevent the NADPH oxidation steps were designed, with activity in the nanomolar range [34]. These findings open new avenues for targeting parasite TGRs in other flatworms, and in particular, to continue exploring *Fh*TGR inhibitors as novel flukicide agents.

Promising Molecular Targets not Explored in *F. hepatica*

Other helminth proteins with pharmacological potential described for different parasites are known to have orthologs in *F. hepatica*. Some have just been identified at the gene level but many have been cloned and structurally characterized, for which there is still no report of the search for inhibitors or small molecules capable of interfering with their biological activity and hence disrupting the parasite life cycle. Among them, there is the glyceraldehyde 3-phosphate dehydrogenase (GAPDH), an enzyme that catalyzes one of the two steps in glycolysis, which generates the reduced coenzyme NADH, whose inhibition could be exploited to reduce parasitic energy generation [35 - 37]. Inhibitors of this enzyme have already been reported as antiprotozoal drug targets where epiandrosterone and dehydroepiandrosterone derivatives, 2-phenoxy-1-4-naphthoquinone and its analogs proved to be strong inhibitors of the protozoal enzyme [38, 39]. Though *Fh*GAPDH lacks the binding pocket that has been exploited in the design of novel antitrypanosomal compounds, oligomerization responses to ligand binding differ from the mammalian enzymes [35], which might be advantageous for the design of selective *F. hepatica* GAPDH inhibitors. Another metabolic enzyme that could be targeted for *F. hepatica* drug discovery is UDP-galactose 4'-epimerase (GALE), which catalyzes the conversion of UDP-galactose to UDP-glucose required for the Leloir pathway of galactose catabolism and is also implicated in the biosynthesis of UDP-N- acetylgalactosamine and UDP-N-acetylglucosamine, the precursors of the oligosaccharide units of glycoproteins and glycolipids [40]. GALE enzymes are typically homodimeric with two active sites and two tightly bound NAD+ cofactors. It is reported that a lack of GALE activity results in the accumulation of galactose 1-phosphate in cells at toxic concentrations, increased free radical production, and altered protein and lipid glycosylation. Though not yet validated as a drug target in *F. hepatica*, it leads to abnormal development in *Drosophila melanogaster* and defects in cell growth and division in trypanosomes (revised in [41]). Therefore, it seems reasonable to assume that selective inhibition of GALE would be detrimental to the liver flukes. There is only one report of six concentration-dependent inhibitors of *Fh*GALE obtained from the screening of the NCI DTP library, some with nanomolar IC_{50} values. Two of them (5-fluoroorotate and N-[(benzyloxy)carbonyl]leucyltryptophan) demonstrated selectivity for *Fh*GALE over the human enzyme. In spite of the conservation of GALE enzymes across different organisms, these results suggest it is possible to develop *Fh*GALE selective inhibitors [41].

On the other hand, G protein-coupled receptors (GPCRs) are well-studied druggable targets. They are one of the largest families of cell surface receptors spread along all organisms and play a major role in physiological responses and signal transduction [42]. Despite their potential for the development of new anthelmintics, there is still scarce functional and structural information on helminths GPCRs to aid drug design strategies. In a recent study, the first profile of GPCRs from the *F. hepatica* genome was described [43]. The liver fluke has a big cohort of 147 GPCRs, with 18 of them being highly diverged rhodopsins-type GPCRs which keep the core rhodopsin signatures but lack significant similarity with non-flatworm receptors, being an interesting group of potential flukicide targets. Despite one-third of human prescription medicines having a GPCR-based mode of action, so far, only one of the latest new anthelmintic approved for animal use against nematodes, the cyclic octa-depsipeptide emodepside [44], has GPCR-directed activity [45]. None of the *F. hepatica* GPCRs have been explored as drug targets, but flavonoids are reported to modulate GPCRs' activity by acting as allosteric ligands [46] and they are a class of compounds that have shown *in vitro* and *in vivo* activity against the liver fluke [16, 17]. Therefore, it could be investigated whether its mode of action might involve these receptors, and of course, massive screening of compound libraries against promising *F. hepatica* GPCRs is necessary to develop selective inhibitors of these receptors.

Finally, the cytochrome P450 (CYP) enzyme cannot be overlooked as a potential drug target against *F. hepatica*. CYP are essential enzymes for the biotransformation of xenobiotics and for the synthesis and degradation of signalling molecules in all living organisms. Free-living flatworms have several CYP coding genes, while flatworms have only one [47]. Antiparasitic activity of the FDA-approved CYP inhibitors miconazole, clotrimazole, and ketoconazole was tested in the liver fluke *Opisthorchis felineus* and in *Schistosoma mansoni*, finding a potency comparable to that of current drugs used for opisthorchiasis and schistosomiasis treatment [48]. This supports *F. hepatica* CYP enzyme as a promising drug target for the discovery of new anthelmintic agents or for the repurposing of known drugs.

PHENOTYPIC DRUG SCREENING

Several terpenoid derivatives have been evaluated against parasitic trematodes. In 2015, a diterpenoid isolated from *Lycium chinense*, 7-keto-sempervirol, was first described for its dual anthelmintic activity against the related trematodes *F. hepatica* and *S. mansoni* (Fig. **1**). As evaluated using microscopic phenotypic scoring matrices, 7-keto-sempervirol was effective against *in vitro* cultured *F. hepatica* newly excysted juveniles (NEJs, $EC_{50}=17.7\mu M$). Scanning electron microscopy assessment of adults treated with 7-keto-sempervirol also showed phenotypic abnormalities, including breaches in tegumental integrity and spines [49]. A subsequent study aimed to enhance the potency of 7-keto-sempervirol by synthesizing and screening 30 structural analogues against juvenile and adult lifecycle stages of both parasites. The most active analogue, **7d** (Fig. **2**), exhibited improved dual anthelmintic activity over 7-keto-sempervirol ($EC_{50} \approx 6$ µM for larval blood flukes; $EC_{50} \approx 3$ µM for juvenile liver flukes) and moderate selectivity (SI $\approx$ 4-5 for blood flukes, 8-13 for liver flukes compared to HepG2 and MDBK cells, respectively). Phenotypic studies using scanning electron microscopy revealed substantial tegumental alterations in both parasites when treated with **7d**. The compound activity was associated with a hydroxy group in position 12; however, when other substituents were added along with the hydroxy group, the activity was reduced [50]. Analogues of the diterpene abietic acid have been phenotypically evaluated against different stages of the liver fluke. From a screening of nineteen compounds, one, **MC010** (Fig. **2**), was identified as the most promising compound, showing flukicidal activity in all intra-mammalian stages: NEJ, 8-week immature adults, and 12-weeks adults (EC_{50} = 12.97 µM); however, the compound proved cytotoxic when evaluated on MDBK as a representative bovine cell (CC_{50} = 17.52 µM, SI = 1.35 for adult stage) [51]. Another study isolated a group of ten triterpenoids from *Abies procera* and assessed their anthelmintic activities against *F. hepatica* and *S.mansoni*. Among these, compound **700015** (Fig. **2**) was the most active against the three aforementioned stages of parasites (EC_{50} 0.7 µM–15.6 µM). Interestingly, this terpenoid derivative showed better selectivity indices for MDBK and HepG2 cell lines (SI = 13 for NEJ, 46 for immature, and 2 for mature flukes) [52]. More recently, five synthetic derivatives of hederagenin, isolated from *Hedera helix,* were selected from a screening of thirty-six compounds against *F. hepatica* NEJ and adult stages. Derivative **MC042** (Fig. **2**) was identified as the most active compound, with EC_{50} at 24h estimated as 1.07 µM and 13.02 µM for NEJ and adult flukes, respectively. Interestingly, **MC042** has good anthelmintic selectivity (44.37 for NEJ and 3.64 for adult flukes) relative to the *in vitro* cytotoxicity of the MDBK bovine cell line [53]. **MC042** has a morpholine-bound ureate, the non-basic oxygen of the morpholine fragment seems to correlate with better activity than the basic amino groups present in other less active derivatives. Similar ureates to those described in this study are well-known pharmacophores, suggesting that terpenoid derivatives possess suitable properties that merit further evaluation as potential flukicides.

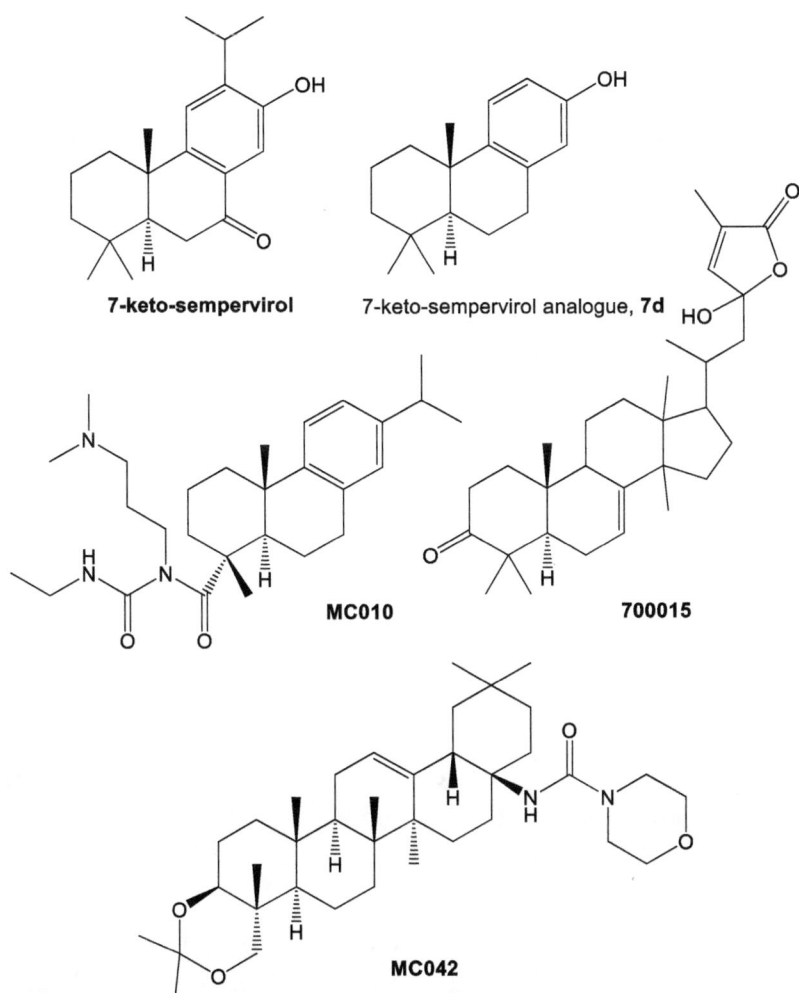

Fig. (2). Structures of the terpenes 7-keto-sempervirol and **7d** derivative, **MC010**, **700015**, and **MC042**.

On the other hand, an interesting naphthoquinone (5-hydroxy-2-methyl-1,4-naphthoquinone) derived from *Plumbago spp.* called plumbagin (Fig. **3**) is another candidate with flukicide activity. The efficacy of plumbagin and triclabendazole against NEJs and 4-weeks-old immature parasites of *Fasciola gigantica* through *in vitro* incubation for 1–24 hours has been compared. Results demonstrated that plumbagin-treated groups exhibited a more rapid decrease in motility, survival, and migration compared to triclabendazole-treated groups, causing greater tegumental damage, including swelling, blebbing, rupture of the tegument, loss of spines, erosion, lesion, and desquamation [54]. Also, plumbagin activity in other trematodes, such as *Schistosoma mansoni*, has been reported [55, 56]. These promising results open new avenues to explore plumbagin's potential as a novel anthelmintic against *Fasciola spp*. infection. However, a careful analysis is necessary, given the reported toxicity of this natural product. Plumbagin has a narrow therapeutic window, and literature reveals that the compound has genotoxic effects and other undesired activities [57, 58].

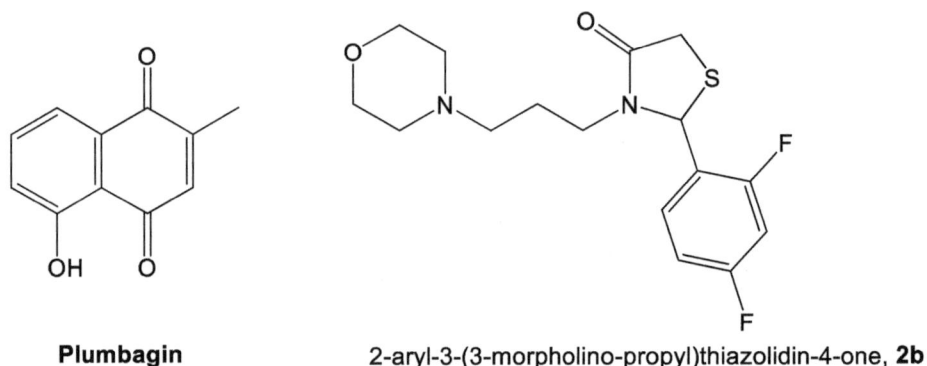

Plumbagin   2-aryl-3-(3-morpholino-propyl)thiazolidin-4-one, **2b**

Fig. (3). Structure of plumbagin and the thiazolidin-4-one **2b**.

In another phenotypic screening, two series of thiazolidin-4-ones were evaluated at different concentrations using the egg hatch assay (EHA) to test their ovicidal activity. Specifically, one compound, **2b** (Fig. **3**), showed 90% ovicidal activity and an excellent selectivity index when the viability of MDBK cells was assessed incubating at the same dose [59].

DRUG REPURPOSING FOR FASCIOLIASIS TREATMENT

Luckily for the drug development processes, evolution many times shapes proteins in a similar way between organisms, so it is often possible to find conserved features of binding and active sites among them. In this way, the pharmaceutical industry can take advantage of drugs that sometimes are able to bind targets that are structurally related to those they were originally designed to and test them for different pathologies, which is called drug repurposing. In *F. hepatica* drug development, a few examples of drug repurposing are found. One of them is the screening of the Pathogen Box for the discovery of new molecules with anti-*Fasciola hepatica* activity, an open-source collection of 400 drug-like compounds selected for their potential against several of the world's most important neglected tropical diseases [60, 61]. The screening was carried out by *in vitro* testing for fasciocidal activity on metacercariae and adult flukes, selecting three hit compounds (**MMV676380**, **MMV003270,** and **MMV690102**) on the basis of their micromolar range activity over both parasite stages and their nontoxic properties. These compounds have previously been reported as active against *Plasmodium falciparum, Ancylostoma ceylanicum, Trypanosoma cruzi,* and *Leishmania donovani.* For some of them, one or more targets have been proposed, and **MMV003270** (zoxazolamine) has 3 target proteins shared with TCBZ [60]. These compounds represent new lead candidates with a potential dual effect over NEJ and adult worms to be employed as anti-*F. hepatica* drugs.

There are other examples of drug repurposing in *F. hepatica.* Nitazoxanide is a thiazolide with a broad spectrum of activity against several intestinal protozoa and helminth parasites in humans, usually indicated for the treatment of diarrhea due to infection with *Giardia lamblia* or *Cryptosporidium parvum* [62]. Its efficacy in serving as an alternative to TCBZ in human fascioliasis treatment is questioned, since both successful reports [63 - 65], as well as partial success or lack of activity of nitazoxanide against TCBZ-resistant cases, are found in the literature [66, 67]. In this sense, more studies are needed in order to assess the efficacy of this drug for fascioliasis control. Another drug under repurposing studies is oxfendazole, a benzimidazole anthelmintic approved for treating nematode and cestode infections in ruminants and horses, as well as giardiasis in dogs. It has shown effectiveness against *F. hepatica* infections in sheep and pigs [68, 69] and the 'Oxfendazole Development Group' is carrying out clinical trials pursuing its registration for the treatment of *Fasciola hepatica, Taenia solium* cysticercosis, *Echinococcus granulosus* and STH, in particular *Trichuris* [70].

Another family of compounds with many old and few new advances in drug repurposing is the sesquiterpene endoperoxide, artemisinin (ART, Fig. **4**) isolated from *Artemisia annua* and its derivatives, first used for the treatment of malaria and human schistosomiasis [71]. Among other helminth parasites, ART-based drugs have proved to be effective against *Fasciola spp., Opisthorchis spp., and Clonorchis sinensis* (reviewed in [72]). Among these, artemether and artesunate were found to be effective against the liver flukes *Fasciola hepatica and C. sinensis,* progressing to exploratory phase-2 clinical trials in *Fasciola*-infected patients more than ten years ago, but unluckily failed to demonstrate acceptable efficacy. Since ART and its derivatives have short half-lives, compounds with improved half-lives and bioavailability, such as 1, 2, 4-trioxolane analogues (like OZ78) and 1, 2, 4, 5-tetraoxanes (like MT04) were developed attempting to gain better biological activity (Fig. **4**). Trials with infected sheep showed controversial results regarding MT04 efficacy, and an *in vivo* study on rats found around 50% worm burden reduction after OZ78 administration at a dose of 50 mg/kg (reviewed in [72]). In more recent work, *in vivo*,the fasciocidal activity of MT04 and OZ78 was confirmed over infected mice, which is increased by the presence of iron or hemin. Although they proved toxic to HepG2 cells, treated mice showed no signs of hepatotoxicity [73]. New trials could provide more information about the efficacy and safety of these derivatives to treat fascioliasis, either alone or in combination with other anthelmintics.

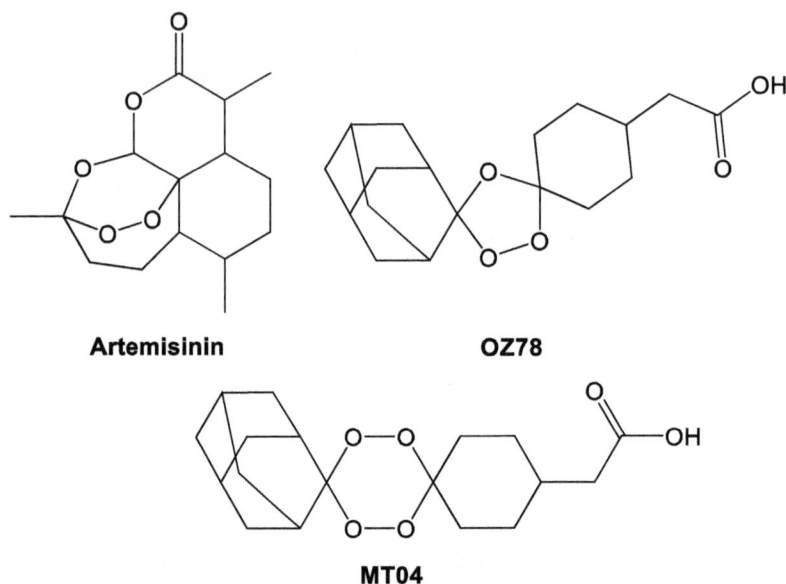

Fig. (4). Structure of artemisinin and its derivatives **OZ78** and **MT04**.

CONCLUDING REMARKS

Very few efforts have been made to advance towards new drugs for the control of fascioliasis. The increasing reports of resistance towards TCBZ, the only active drug against all stages of *F. hepatica,* make this an urgent necessity. However, in recent years, new druggable targets such as cathepsin L1, cathepsin L3, TPI, and thioredoxin glutathione reductase have been identified, and some inhibitors with flukicidal activity have been obtained. Many non-explored interesting molecular targets still remain to be exploited in the search for new fasciolicide drugs. Also, attempts have been made to obtain bioisosteric derivatives of TCBZ to improve its activity and avoid TCBZ-resistant strains. Studies aiming at drug repositioning have also been carried out, but none have passed phase II clinical trials. *in vitro* and *in vivo* phenotypic assays have been reported for several compounds, with different terpene derivatives standing out, but larger studies on nonspecific toxicity, mechanism of action, and preclinical development are needed. In light of these facts, the search for new drugs for the treatment of fasciolosis remains a priority.

REFERENCES

[1]   Nixon SA, Welz C, Woods DJ, Costa-Junior L, Zamanian M, Martin RJ. Where are all the anthelmintics? Challenges and opportunities on the path to new anthelmintics. Int J Parasitol Drugs

Drug Resist 2020; 14: 8-16.
[http://dx.doi.org/10.1016/j.ijpddr.2020.07.001] [PMID: 32814269]

[2]   Fairweather I, Brennan GP, Hanna REB, Robinson MW, Skuce PJ. Drug resistance in liver flukes. Int J Parasitol Drugs Drug Resist 2020; 12: 39-59.
[http://dx.doi.org/10.1016/j.ijpddr.2019.11.003] [PMID: 32179499]

[3]   Beesley NJ, Caminade C, Charlier J, *et al*. *Fasciola* and fasciolosis in ruminants in Europe: Identifying research needs. Transbound Emerg Dis 2018; 65(Suppl 1) (Suppl. 1): 199-216.
[http://dx.doi.org/10.1111/tbed.12682] [PMID: 28984428]

[4]   Mas-Coma S, Valero MA, Bargues MD. Fascioliasis. Adv Exp Med Biol 2019; 1154: 71-103.
[http://dx.doi.org/10.1007/978-3-030-18616-6_4] [PMID: 31297760]

[5]   Cwiklinski K, Dalton JP. Advances in *Fasciola hepatica* research using 'omics' technologies. Int J Parasitol 2018; 48(5): 321-31.
[http://dx.doi.org/10.1016/j.ijpara.2017.12.001] [PMID: 29476869]

[6]   Ibarra-Velarde F, Vera-Montenegro Y, Flores-Ramos M, *et al*. Assessment of the effective dose of an experimental intramuscular formulation against immature and adult *Fasciola hepatica* in sheep. Vet Parasitol 2018; 260: 38-44.
[http://dx.doi.org/10.1016/j.vetpar.2018.04.012] [PMID: 30197011]

[7]   Marcos L, Maco V, Terashima A. Triclabendazole for the treatment of human fascioliasis and the threat of treatment failures. Expert Rev Anti Infect Ther 2021; 19(7): 817-23.
[http://dx.doi.org/10.1080/14787210.2021.1858798] [PMID: 33267701]

[8]   Robinson M, Dalton J, Donnelly S. Helminth pathogen cathepsin proteases: it's a family affair. Trends Biochem Sci 2008; 33(12): 601-8.
[http://dx.doi.org/10.1016/j.tibs.2008.09.001] [PMID: 18848453]

[9]   Corvo I, Cancela M, Cappetta M, Pi-Denis N, Tort JF, Roche L. The major cathepsin L secreted by the invasive juvenile *Fasciola hepatica* prefers proline in the S2 subsite and can cleave collagen. Mol Biochem Parasitol 2009; 167(1): 41-7.
[http://dx.doi.org/10.1016/j.molbiopara.2009.04.005] [PMID: 19383516]

[10]   Cwiklinski K, Dalton JP, Dufresne PJ, *et al*. The *Fasciola hepatica* genome: gene duplication and polymorphism reveals adaptation to the host environment and the capacity for rapid evolution. Genome Biol 2015; 16(1): 71.
[http://dx.doi.org/10.1186/s13059-015-0632-2] [PMID: 25887684]

[11]   Fujishima A, Imai Y, Nomura T, Fujisawa Y, Yamamoto Y, Sugawara T. The crystal structure of human cathepsin L complexed with E-64. FEBS Lett 1997; 407(1): 47-50.
[http://dx.doi.org/10.1016/S0014-5793(97)00216-0] [PMID: 9141479]

[12]   Stack CM, Caffrey CR, Donnelly SM, *et al*. Structural and functional relationships in the virulence-associated cathepsin L proteases of the parasitic liver fluke, *Fasciola hepatica*. J Biol Chem 2008; 283(15): 9896-908.
[http://dx.doi.org/10.1074/jbc.M708521200] [PMID: 18160404]

[13]   Ferraro F, Cabrera MA, Álvarez GI, Corvo I. Drug targets: Screening for small molecules that inhibit *Fasciola hepatica* enzymes. Methods Mol Biol 2020; 2137: 221-31.
[http://dx.doi.org/10.1007/978-1-0716-0475-5_17] [PMID: 32399933]

[14]   Moran BW, Anderson FP, Ruth DM, Fágáin CÓ, Dalton JP, Kenny PTM. Fluorobenzoyl dipeptidyl derivatives as inhibitors of the *Fasciola hepatica* cysteine protease cathepsin L1. J Enzyme Inhib Med Chem 2010; 25(1): 1-12.
[http://dx.doi.org/10.3109/14756360902888184] [PMID: 20030504]

[15]   Hernández Alvarez L, Naranjo Feliciano D, Hernández González JE, de Oliveira Soares R, Barreto Gomes DE, Pascutti PG. Insights into the interactions of fasciola hepatica cathepsin L3 with a substrate and potential novel inhibitors through *in silico* approaches. PLoS Negl Trop Dis 2015; 9(5):

e0003759.
[http://dx.doi.org/10.1371/journal.pntd.0003759] [PMID: 25978322]

[16]   Ferraro F, Merlino A, dell'Oca N, *et al.* Identification of chalcones as *fasciola hepatica* cathepsin L inhibitors using a comprehensive experimental and computational approach. PLoS Negl Trop Dis 2016; 10(7): e0004834.
[http://dx.doi.org/10.1371/journal.pntd.0004834] [PMID: 27463369]

[17]   Artía Z, Ferraro F, Sánchez C, *et al. in vitro* and *in vivo* studies on a group of chalcones find promising results as potential drugs against fascioliasis. Exp Parasitol 2023; 255: 108628.
[http://dx.doi.org/10.1016/j.exppara.2023.108628] [PMID: 37776969]

[18]   Ferraro F, Merlino A, Gil J, *et al.* Cathepsin L inhibitors with activity against the liver fluke identified from a focus library of quinoxaline 1,4-di-*N*-oxide derivatives. Molecules 2019; 24(13): 2348.
[http://dx.doi.org/10.3390/molecules24132348] [PMID: 31247891]

[19]   González-González A, Méndez-Álvarez D, Vázquez-Jiménez LK, *et al.* Molecular docking and dynamic simulations of quinoxaline 1,4-di-*N*-oxide as inhibitors for targets from *Trypanosoma cruzi, Trichomonas vaginalis*, and *Fasciola hepatica. J* Mol Model 2023; 29(6): 180.
[http://dx.doi.org/10.1007/s00894-023-05579-4] [PMID: 37195391]

[20]   Zinsser VL, Hoey EM, Trudgett A, Timson DJ. Biochemical characterisation of triose phosphate isomerase from the liver fluke *Fasciola hepatica.* Biochimie 2013; 95(11): 2182-9.
[http://dx.doi.org/10.1016/j.biochi.2013.08.014] [PMID: 23973283]

[21]   Hrizo SL, Fisher IJ, Long DR, Hutton JA, Liu Z, Palladino MJ. Early mitochondrial dysfunction leads 289-96.
[http://dx.doi.org/10.1016/j.nbd.2012.12.020]

[22]   Enríquez-Flores S, De la Mora-De la Mora I, García-Torres I, Flores-López LA, Martínez-Pérez Y, López-Velázquez G. Human triosephosphate isomerase is a potential target in cancer due to commonly occurring post-translational modifications. Molecules 2023; 28(16): 6163.
[http://dx.doi.org/10.3390/molecules28166163] [PMID: 37630415]

[23]   Saporiti T, Cabrera M, Bentancur J, *et al.* Phenotypic and target-directed screening yields new acaricidal alternatives for the control of ticks. Molecules 2022; 27(24): 8863.
[http://dx.doi.org/10.3390/molecules27248863] [PMID: 36557996]

[24]   Vázquez-Jiménez LK, Moreno-Herrera A, Juárez-Saldivar A, *et al.* Recent advances in the development of triose phosphate isomerase inhibitors as antiprotozoal agents. Curr Med Chem 2022; 29(14): 2504-29.
[http://dx.doi.org/10.2174/0929867328666210913090928] [PMID: 34517794]

[25]   Zinsser VL, Farnell E, Dunne DW, Timson DJ. Triose phosphate isomerase from the blood fluke *Schistosoma mansoni* : Biochemical characterisation of a potential drug and vaccine target. FEBS Lett 2013; 587(21): 3422-7.
[http://dx.doi.org/10.1016/j.febslet.2013.09.022] [PMID: 24070897]

[26]   Son J, Kim S, Kim SE, Lee H, Lee MR, Hwang KY. Structural analysis of an epitope candidate of triosephosphate isomerase in *Opisthorchis viverrini.* Sci Rep 2018; 8(1): 15075.
[http://dx.doi.org/10.1038/s41598-018-33479-8] [PMID: 30305716]

[27]   Jimenez-Sandoval P, Castro-Torres E, González-González R, *et al.* Crystal structures of Triosephosphate Isomerases from *Taenia solium* and *Schistosoma mansoni* provide insights for vaccine rationale and drug design against helminth parasites. PLoS Negl Trop Dis 2020; 14(1): e0007815.
[http://dx.doi.org/10.1371/journal.pntd.0007815] [PMID: 31923219]

[28]   Ferraro F, Corvo I, Bergalli L, *et al.* Novel and selective inactivators of Triosephosphate isomerase with anti-trematode activity. Sci Rep 2020; 10(1): 2587.
[http://dx.doi.org/10.1038/s41598-020-59460-y] [PMID: 32054976]

[29]   Salinas G, Selkirk ME, Chalar C, Maizels RM, Fernández C. Linked thioredoxin-glutathione systems in platyhelminths. Trends Parasitol 2004; 20(7): 340-6.
[http://dx.doi.org/10.1016/j.pt.2004.05.002] [PMID: 15193566]

[30]   Kuntz AN, Davioud-Charvet E, Sayed AA, *et al.* Thioredoxin glutathione reductase from *Schistosoma mansoni*: an essential parasite enzyme and a key drug target. PLoS Med 2007; 4(6): e206.
[http://dx.doi.org/10.1371/journal.pmed.0040206] [PMID: 17579510]

[31]   Sayed AA, Simeonov A, Thomas CJ, Inglese J, Austin CP, Williams DL. Identification of oxadiazoles as new drug leads for the control of schistosomiasis. Nat Med 2008; 14(4): 407-12.
[http://dx.doi.org/10.1038/nm1737] [PMID: 18345010]

[32]   Fata F, Silvestri I, Ardini M, *et al.* Probing the surface of a parasite drug target thioredoxin glutathione reductase using small molecule fragments. ACS Infect Dis 2021; 7(7): 1932-44.
[http://dx.doi.org/10.1021/acsinfecdis.0c00909] [PMID: 33950676]

[33]   Ross F, Hernández P, Porcal W, *et al.* Identification of thioredoxin glutathione reductase inhibitors that kill cestode and trematode parasites. PLoS One 2012; 7(4): e35033.
[http://dx.doi.org/10.1371/journal.pone.0035033] [PMID: 22536349]

[34]   Petukhova VZ, Aboagye SY, Ardini M, *et al.* Non-covalent inhibitors of thioredoxin glutathione reductase with schistosomicidal activity *in vivo.* Nat Commun 2023; 14(1): 3737.
[http://dx.doi.org/10.1038/s41467-023-39444-y] [PMID: 37349300]

[35]   Zinsser VL, Hoey EM, Trudgett A, Timson DJ. Biochemical characterisation of glyceraldehyde 3-phosphate dehydrogenase (GAPDH) from the liver fluke, Fasciola hepatica. Biochim Biophys Acta Proteins Proteomics 2014; 1844(4): 744-9.
[http://dx.doi.org/10.1016/j.bbapap.2014.02.008] [PMID: 24566472]

[36]   Chetri PB, Shukla R, Tripathi T. Identification and characterization of glyceraldehyde 3-phosphate dehydrogenase from *Fasciola gigantica.* Parasitol Res 2019; 118(3): 861-72.
[http://dx.doi.org/10.1007/s00436-019-06225-w] [PMID: 30706165]

[37]   Boreiko S, Silva M, Iulek J. Structure determination and analyses of the GAPDH from the parasite *Schistosoma mansoni*, the first one from a platyhelminth. Biochimie 2021; 184: 18-25.
[http://dx.doi.org/10.1016/j.biochi.2021.01.014] [PMID: 33524435]

[38]   Bruno S, Uliassi E, Zaffagnini M, *et al.* Molecular basis for covalent inhibition of glyceraldehyde--phosphate dehydrogenase by a 2-phenoxy-1,4-naphthoquinone small molecule. Chem Biol Drug Des 2017; 90(2): 225-35.
[http://dx.doi.org/10.1111/cbdd.12941] [PMID: 28079302]

[39]   Ortíz C, Moraca F, Laverriere M, Jordan A, Hamilton N, Comini MA. Glucose 6-phosphate dehydrogenase from trypanosomes: Selectivity for steroids and chemical validation in b*Trypanosoma brucei.* Molecules 2021; 26(2): 358.
[http://dx.doi.org/10.3390/molecules26020358] [PMID: 33445584]

[40]   Daenzer JMI, Sanders RD, Hang D, Fridovich-Keil JL. UDP-galactose 4′-epimerase activities toward UDP-Gal and UDP-GalNAc play different roles in the development of *Drosophila melanogaster.* PLoS Genet 2012; 8(5): e1002721.
[http://dx.doi.org/10.1371/journal.pgen.1002721] [PMID: 22654673]

[41]   Zinsser VL, Lindert S, Banford S, Hoey EM, Trudgett A, Timson DJ. UDP-galactose 4′-epimerase from the liver fluke, *Fasciola hepatica* : biochemical characterization of the enzyme and identification of inhibitors. Parasitology 2015; 142(3): 463-72.
[http://dx.doi.org/10.1017/S003118201400136X] [PMID: 25124392]

[42]   Santos R, Ursu O, Gaulton A, *et al.* A comprehensive map of molecular drug targets. Nat Rev Drug Discov 2017; 16(1): 19-34.
[http://dx.doi.org/10.1038/nrd.2016.230] [PMID: 27910877]

[43]   McVeigh P, McCammick E, McCusker P, *et al.* Profiling G protein-coupled receptors of Fasciola

hepatica identifies orphan rhodopsins unique to phylum Platyhelminthes. Int J Parasitol Drugs Drug Resist 2018; 8(1): 87-103.
[http://dx.doi.org/10.1016/j.ijpddr.2018.01.001] [PMID: 29474932]

[44]   Harder A, Samson-Himmelstjerna G. Activity of the cyclic depsipeptide emodepside (BAY 44-4400) against larval and adult stages of nematodes in rodents and the influence on worm survival. Parasitol Res 2001; 87(11): 924-8.
[http://dx.doi.org/10.1007/s004360100479] [PMID: 11728017]

[45]   Welz C, Harder A, Schnieder T, Hoglund J, von Samson-Himmelstjerna G. Putative G protein–coupled receptors in parasitic nematodes—potential targets for the new anthelmintic class cyclooctadepsipeptides? Parasitol Res 2005; 97(S1) (Suppl. 1): S22-32.
[http://dx.doi.org/10.1007/s00436-005-1441-4] [PMID: 16228272]

[46]   Chda A, Bencheikh R. Flavonoids as G Protein-coupled Receptors Ligands: New Potential Therapeutic Natural Drugs. Curr Drug Targets 2023; 24(17): 1346-63.
[http://dx.doi.org/10.2174/0113894501268871231127105219] [PMID: 38037994]

[47]   Pakharukova MY, Vavilin VA, Sripa B, Laha T, Brindley PJ, Mordvinov VA. Functional analysis of the unique cytochrome P450 of the liver fluke *Opisthorchis felineus*. PLoS Negl Trop Dis 2015; 9(12): e0004258.
[http://dx.doi.org/10.1371/journal.pntd.0004258] [PMID: 26625139]

[48]   Mordvinov VA, Shilov AG, Pakharukova MY. Anthelmintic activity of cytochrome P450 inhibitors miconazole and clotrimazole: *In-vitro* effect on the liver fluke *Opisthorchis felineus*. Int J Antimicrob Agents 2017; 50(1): 97-100.
[http://dx.doi.org/10.1016/j.ijantimicag.2017.01.037] [PMID: 28527633]

[49]   Edwards J, Brown M, Peak E, Bartholomew B, Nash RJ, Hoffmann KF. The diterpenoid 7-ket--sempervirol, derived from *Lycium chinense*, displays anthelmintic activity against both *Schistosoma mansoni* and *Fasciola hepatica*. PLoS Negl Trop Dis 2015; 9(3): e0003604.
[http://dx.doi.org/10.1371/journal.pntd.0003604] [PMID: 25768432]

[50]   Crusco A, Bordoni C, Chakroborty A, *et al.* Design, synthesis and anthelmintic activity of 7-ket--sempervirol analogues. Eur J Med Chem 2018; 152: 87-100.
[http://dx.doi.org/10.1016/j.ejmech.2018.04.032] [PMID: 29698860]

[51]   Chakroborty A, Pritchard D, Bouillon ME, *et al.* Flukicidal effects of abietane diterpenoid derived analogues against the food borne pathogen *Fasciola hepatica*. Vet Parasitol 2022; 309: 109766.
[http://dx.doi.org/10.1016/j.vetpar.2022.109766] [PMID: 35926239]

[52]   Whiteland HL, Chakroborty A, Forde-Thomas JE, *et al.* An *Abies procera*-derived tetracyclic triterpene containing a steroid-like nucleus core and a lactone side chain attenuates *in vitro* survival of both *Fasciola hepatica* and *Schistosoma mansoni*. Int J Parasitol Drugs Drug Resist 2018; 8(3): 465-74.
[http://dx.doi.org/10.1016/j.ijpddr.2018.10.009] [PMID: 30399512]

[53]   Chakroborty A, Pritchard DR, Bouillon ME, *et al.* Modified hederagenin derivatives demonstrate *ex vivo* anthelmintic activity against *fasciola hepatica*. Pharmaceutics 2023; 15(7): 1869.
[http://dx.doi.org/10.3390/pharmaceutics15071869] [PMID: 37514055]

[54]   Lorsuwannarat N, Piedrafita D, Chantree P, *et al.* The *in vitro* anthelmintic effects of plumbagin on newly excysted and 4-weeks-old juvenile parasites of *Fasciola gigantica*. Exp Parasitol 2014; 136: 5-13.
[http://dx.doi.org/10.1016/j.exppara.2013.10.004] [PMID: 24157317]

[55]   Lorsuwannarat N, Saowakon N, Ramasoota P, Wanichanon C, Sobhon P. The anthelmintic effect of plumbagin on *Schistosoma mansoni*. Exp Parasitol 2013; 133(1): 18-27.
[http://dx.doi.org/10.1016/j.exppara.2012.10.003] [PMID: 23085370]

[56]   Bakery HH, Allam GA, Abuelsaad ASA, Abdel-Latif M, Elkenawy AE, Khalil RG. Anti-inflammatory, antioxidant, anti-fibrotic and schistosomicidal properties of plumbagin in murine

schistosomiasis. Parasite Immunol 2022; 44(11): e12945.
[http://dx.doi.org/10.1111/pim.12945] [PMID: 36066812]

[57]   Thakor N, Janathia B. Plumbagin: A potential candidate for future research and development. Curr Pharm Biotechnol 2022; 23(15): 1800-12.
[http://dx.doi.org/10.2174/1389201023666211230113146] [PMID: 34967293]

[58]   Singh AP, Sharma A. Structural insights and pharmaceutical relevance of plumbagin in parasitic disorders: A comprehensive review. Recent Advances in Anti-Infective Drug Discovery 2022; 17(3): 187-98.
[http://dx.doi.org/10.2174/2772434417666220905121531] [PMID: 36065920]

[59]   Zehetmeyr FK, da Silva MAMP, Pereira KM, *et al.* Ovicidal *in vitro* activity of 2-aryl-3-(2-morpholinoethyl)thiazolidin-4-ones and 2-aryl-3-(3-morpholinopropyl)thiazolidin-4-ones against Fasciola hepatica (Linnaeus, 1758). Exp Parasitol 2018; 192: 60-4.
[http://dx.doi.org/10.1016/j.exppara.2018.07.012] [PMID: 30040962]

[60]   Machicado C, Soto MP, Timoteo O, *et al.* Screening the pathogen box for identification of new chemical agents with anti- *fasciola hepatica* activity. Antimicrob Agents Chemother 2019; 63(3): e02373-18.
[http://dx.doi.org/10.1128/AAC.02373-18] [PMID: 30602522]

[61]   Veale CGL. Unpacking the pathogen box—an open source tool for fighting neglected tropical disease. ChemMedChem 2019; 14(4): 386-453.
[http://dx.doi.org/10.1002/cmdc.201800755] [PMID: 30614200]

[62]   Fox LM, Saravolatz LD. Nitazoxanide: a new thiazolide antiparasitic agent. Clin Infect Dis 2005; 40(8): 1173-80.
[http://dx.doi.org/10.1086/428839] [PMID: 15791519]

[63]   Favennec L, Jave Ortiz J, Gargala G, Lopez Chegne N, Ayoub A, Rossignol JF. Double-blind, randomized, placebo-controlled study of nitazoxanide in the treatment of fascioliasis in adults and children from northern Peru. Aliment Pharmacol Ther 2003; 17(2): 265-70.
[http://dx.doi.org/10.1046/j.1365-2036.2003.01419.x] [PMID: 12534412]

[64]   Zumaquero-Ríos JL, Sarracent-Pérez J, Rojas-García R, *et al.* Fascioliasis and intestinal parasitoses affecting schoolchildren in Atlixco, Puebla State, Mexico: epidemiology and treatment with nitazoxanide. PLoS Negl Trop Dis 2013; 7(11): e2553.
[http://dx.doi.org/10.1371/journal.pntd.0002553] [PMID: 24278492]

[65]   Sah R, Khadka S, Khadka M, *et al.* Human fascioliasis by *Fasciola hepatica*: the first case report in Nepal. BMC Res Notes 2017; 10(1): 439.
[http://dx.doi.org/10.1186/s13104-017-2761-z] [PMID: 28870243]

[66]   Winkelhagen AJS, Mank T, de Vries PJ, Soetekouw R. Apparent triclabendazole-resistant human *Fasciola hepatica* infection, the Netherlands. Emerg Infect Dis 2012; 18(6): 1028-9.
[http://dx.doi.org/10.3201/eid1806.120302] [PMID: 22607719]

[67]   Ramadan HKA, Hassan WA, Elossily NA, *et al.* Evaluation of nitazoxanide treatment following triclabendazole failure in an outbreak of human fascioliasis in Upper Egypt. PLoS Negl Trop Dis 2019; 13(9): e0007779.
[http://dx.doi.org/10.1371/journal.pntd.0007779] [PMID: 31553716]

[68]   Gomez-Puerta LA, Gavidia C, Lopez-Urbina MT, Garcia HH, Gonzalez AE. Efficacy of a single oral dose of oxfendazole against Fasciola hepatica in naturally infected sheep. Am J Trop Med Hyg 2012; 86(3): 486-8.
[http://dx.doi.org/10.4269/ajtmh.2012.11-0476] [PMID: 22403323]

[69]   Ortiz P, Terrones S, Cabrera M, *et al.* Oxfendazole flukicidal activity in pigs. Acta Trop 2014; 136: 10-3.
[http://dx.doi.org/10.1016/j.actatropica.2014.03.024] [PMID: 24713198]

[70] Pfarr KM, Krome AK, Al-Obaidi I, *et al.* The pipeline for drugs for control and elimination of neglected tropical diseases: 1. Anti-infective drugs for regulatory registration. Parasit Vectors 2023; 16(1): 82.
[http://dx.doi.org/10.1186/s13071-022-05581-4] [PMID: 36859332]

[71] Muangphrom P, Seki H, Fukushima EO, Muranaka T. Artemisinin-based antimalarial research: application of biotechnology to the production of artemisinin, its mode of action, and the mechanism of resistance of *Plasmodium* parasites. J Nat Med 2016; 70(3): 318-34.
[http://dx.doi.org/10.1007/s11418-016-1008-y] [PMID: 27250562]

[72] Lam NS, Long X, Su X, Lu F. Artemisinin and its derivatives in treating helminthic infections beyond schistosomiasis. Pharmacol Res 2018; 133: 77-100.
[http://dx.doi.org/10.1016/j.phrs.2018.04.025] [PMID: 29727708]

[73] Brecht K, Kirchhofer C, Bouitbir J, Trapani F, Keiser J, Krähenbühl S. Exogenous iron increases fasciocidal activity and hepatocellular toxicity of the synthetic endoperoxides OZ78 and MT04. Int J Mol Sci 2019; 20(19): 4880.
[http://dx.doi.org/10.3390/ijms20194880] [PMID: 31581457]

SUBJECT INDEX

Z

www.ingramcontent.com/pod-product-compliance
Lightning Source LLC
Chambersburg PA
CBHW050802220326
41598CB00006B/92